Difficult Decisions in Surgery: An Evidence-Based Approach

Series Editor

Mark K. Ferguson
Department of Surgery, MC5040
University of Chicago
Chicago, Illinois, USA

The complexity of decision making in any kind of surgery is growing exponentially. As new technology is introduced, physicians from nonsurgical specialties offer alternative and competing therapies for what was once the exclusive province of the surgeon. In addition, there is increasing knowledge regarding the efficacy of traditional surgical therapies. How to select among these varied and complex approaches is becoming increasingly difficult. These multi-authored books will contain brief chapters, each of which will be devoted to one or two specific questions or decisions that are difficult or controversial. They are intended as current and timely reference sources for practicing surgeons, surgeons in training, and educators that describe the recommended ideal approach, rather than customary care, in selected clinical situations.

More information about this series at http://www.springer.com/series/13361

Peter Angelos • Raymon H. Grogan
Editors

Difficult Decisions in Endocrine Surgery

An Evidence-Based Approach

Springer

Editors
Peter Angelos
Department of Surgery and MacLean
Center for Clinical Medical Ethics
The University of Chicago
Chicago, IL
USA

Raymon H. Grogan
Michael E. DeBakey Department of Surgery
Baylor College of Medicine
Houston, TX
USA

ISSN 2198-7750 ISSN 2198-7769 (electronic)
Difficult Decisions in Surgery: An Evidence-Based Approach
ISBN 978-3-030-06535-5 ISBN 978-3-319-92860-9 (eBook)
https://doi.org/10.1007/978-3-319-92860-9

This Springer imprint is published by Springer Nature, under the registered company Springer International Publishing AG
The registered company address is: Gewerbestrasse 11, 6330 Cham, Switzerland

Dr. Grogan:
I dedicate this book to my wife Yuemi and my two beautiful girls Ivy and Emery. Thank you Yuemi for supporting me day in and day out even though I spend so many hours away from home. And thank you Ivy and Emery for being my own personal "Fountain of Youth." You truly are a joy, an inspiration, and a daily source of pride and motivation.

Dr. Angelos:
I dedicate this book to my wife Grace without whose support none of my efforts would have been possible and to my children. Without Audrey, Christian, Meghan, and son-in-law Zach, life would not be nearly as exciting nor as much fun. Thank you all for your understanding and support.

Acknowledgements

There are several people who helped make this book possible. First and foremost, we would like to say thank you to our friend and colleague Dr. Edwin Kaplan. We both have benefited tremendously from the wisdom, knowledge, and camaraderie of working next to Dr. Kaplan on a daily basis. His inquisitive nature and seemingly bottomless wealth of knowledge on the subject of endocrine surgery has certainly changed the way we (and many people throughout the world) practice. Without his friendship over the years it is safe to say that we would not be the same surgeons we are today, and thus, this book would be a different book.

We would also like to thank the unseen heroes who work hard day in and day out taking care of our patients and practice, because without them we truly would not have the time or energy to pursue an academic endeavor such as this book. Ms. Pat Schaddelee our administrative assistant who basically does everything for us, Mrs. Sandra Frausto our RN and practice manager who is the face of our practice for our patients, and Mrs. Joly Raju our nurse practitioner who knows more about endocrine surgery than many endocrinologists we know.

Finally, we would also like to say thank you to all the endocrine surgery fellows and research fellows we have worked with over the years, because again it is their hard work and dedication that help to make academic pursuits like this possible. But more than that it is the fellows that help shape the way we perceive and think of the future of endocrine surgery as a specialty, and their influence has helped shape the content of this book.

Introduction

> The practice of evidence based medicine means integrating individual clinical expertise with the best available external clinical evidence from systematic research—From "Evidence based medicine, what it is and what it isn't" BMJ Jan 13 1996 Volume 312

What Is a Difficult Decision?

Life is a constant stream of decision making. From the time we wake up until the time we go to bed, we are continually making decisions. Every action taken, every movement, every thought has derived in some way from the decision-making process. Decision making is so essential to everyday function that it seems like much of it happens without our consciously thinking about it. But have you ever stopped to think about what a decision is and how it is derived? When you stop to consider this for a moment, you realize that what seems like something simple and mundane, the act of making a choice, is actually quite complex. So complex that there are entire psychology departments, societies, and scientific journals dedicated to studying and understanding human decision making. For the context of this book, however, let us consider a simple definition. In essence, decision making is the process of selecting a course of action from among multiple alternative possibilities. The final result of this process being a choice that will ultimately lead to future consequences. In medical decision making, it is these future consequences that we are consciously and subconsciously weighing every time we give our advice or opinion to our patients. Decision making becomes difficult when there is uncertainty regarding the type or magnitude of the consequences of each alternative being weighed. The more uncertainty, or the bigger the possible consequence, the more difficult the decision. Uncertainty is inherent in the medical decision-making process. We as physicians expect that our tests are not perfect, good outcomes are not always guaranteed, and the risks and benefits of our interventions vary based on circumstance. After all, it often seems as if the whole point of learning about sensitivity, specificity, and receiver operator curves in medical school is to remind us of the fact that there is still a certain amount of "art" in the science of medicine.

What Is This Book About Anyway?

It is from this idea that a lack of information leads to difficult decisions that this book *Difficult Decisions in Endocrine Surgery* was created. We started with a simple premise, to identify clinical scenarios that we see in our academic endocrine surgery practice that made us pause for a minute and think "what in the world *are* the evidence-based data on *that*?" Fortunately for us as editors of this book, there is no paucity of unusual, rare, and interesting cases that come through a busy academic endocrine surgery practice. That aspect of endocrine surgery is in part what makes it such an interesting clinical practice and what drives so many interesting research questions. Aside from the rare and unusual we also felt that to keep the book contemporary and useful on a broader level it was important to include chapters on things that might be more common, but are still controversial. Once the questions were identified, we looked through available literature as well as past meetings of the American Association of Endocrine Surgeons to find our expert chapter authors. We asked these authors to use a strict set of guidelines to write evidence-based medicine chapters on each topic. The goal being to provide the reader with the highest level of evidence possible to allow for clinical decision making. You can think of this book almost as a premade literature search combined with an expert mentor giving his or her own take on that literature. At the time of the writing of this book, there really is no additional scientific evidence available on most of these topics outside of what you will find synthesized here.

What Is Evidence-Based Medicine Really?

A common theme you will see throughout this book is a lack of good, objective level 1 evidence for many of the topics being discussed. Using the definition of a "Difficult Decision" that we outlined above, it was inevitable that we would come up with a set of clinical scenarios that did not have much evidence to support their treatment or care. So you might reasonably ask, is this book then an evidence-based book? We would argue that yes, in fact, this is an evidence-based book of a high quality. We believe this to be the case because the meaning and purpose behind the idea of "evidence-based medicine" is often misunderstood. Evidence-based medicine is not a mechanical following of practice guidelines. As explained in an editorial by Dr. David Sackett, one of the pioneers and founders of the evidence-based medicine movement, "The practice of evidence based medicine means integrating individual clinical expertise with the best available external clinical evidence from systematic research." In endocrine surgery, because there are many things that are unusual and rare we deal daily with cases and scenarios that do not have high levels of research-based evidence. In these cases, we can still practice evidence-based medicine, but we do this by integrating what little evidence is known with our own clinical experience along with the clinical expertise of those among us who have the most experience dealing with these situations. In this way, we learn and grow as individual practitioners and expand the broader field of endocrine surgery. We hope you find this book informative and useful, as well as helpful for your patients. We also hope that you take the lack of evidence presented in this book not as a negative but as a positive motivator to continue to expand your own personal research endeavors, as well as those of the entire endocrine surgery community. It is the basic inquisitive nature that is at the core of what drives so many of the most important clinical research studies. If this book leaves you with more questions than answers, then perhaps, counterintuitively, we have done our job.

Contents

Contributors

Shabirhusain Abadin, MD, MPH Department of Surgery, John H. Stroger, Jr. Hospital of Cook County, Chicago, IL, USA

Zahraa Al-Hilli, MD Department of General Surgery, Cleveland Clinic, Cleveland, OH, USA

Abbas Al-Kurd, MD Department of Surgery, Hadassah-Hebrew University Medical Center, Jerusalem, Israel

Peter Angelos, MD, PhD, FACS Department of Surgery and MacLean Center for Clinical Medical Ethics, The University of Chicago, Chicago, IL, USA

Wesley Barnes, MD Department of Surgery, Oakland University William Beaumont School of Medicine, Beaumont Hospitals, Royal Oak, MI, USA

Eren Berber, MD Department of Endocrine Surgery, Cleveland Clinic, Cleveland, OH, USA

Glenda G. Callender, MD Department of Surgery, Yale University School of Medicine, New Haven, CT, USA

Tobias Carling, MD, PhD, FACS Section of Endocrine Surgery, Department of Surgery, Yale University School of Medicine, New Haven, CT, USA

Anthony J. Chambers, MS, FRACS Department of Surgical Oncology, St Vincent's Hospital and University of New South Wales, Sydney, NSW, Australia

Kathleen K. Christians, MD, FACS Pancreatic Cancer Program, Medical College of Wisconsin; Department of Surgery (Division of Surgical Oncology), Milwaukee, WI, USA

Nicole A. Cipriani, MD The University of Chicago, Department of Pathology, Chicago, IL, USA

Mark S. Cohen, MD Department of Surgery, Division of Endocrine Surgery, Taubman Center, Ann Arbor, MI, USA

Carlos R. Cordón-Fernández, MD Department of Surgical Oncology, Instituto Guatemalteco de Seguridad Social, Guatemala City, Guatemala

Travis M. Cotton, MD Department of Endocrine Surgery, Warren Alpert Medical School of Brown University, Providence, RI, USA

Peter F. Czako, MD Department of Surgery, Oakland University William Beaumont School of Medicine, Beaumont Hospitals, Royal Oak, MI, USA

Alan Dackiw, MD Department of Surgery, University of Texas Southwestern Medical Center, Dallas, TX, USA

Karen Devon, MD, MSc, FRCSC Department of Surgery, University of Toronto, Endocrine Surgical Oncology, Women's College Hospital and University Health Network, Toronto, ON, Canada

Paxton V. Dickson, MD, FACS Division of Surgical Oncology, University of Tennessee Health Science Center, Memphis, TN, USA

Konstantinos P. Economopoulos, MD, PhD Department of Surgery, Duke University, Durham, NC, USA

Douglas B. Evans, MD Pancreatic Cancer Program, Medical College of Wisconsin; Department of Surgery (Division of Surgical Oncology), Milwaukee, WI, USA

Liane S. Feldman, MD Department of Surgery, McGill University Health Center, Montreal, QC, Canada

Steinberg-Bernstein Centre for Minimally Invasive Surgery and Innovation, McGill University, Montreal, QC, Canada

Mark K. Ferguson Department of Surgery, University of Chicago, Chicago, IL, USA

Ben George, MD Pancreatic Cancer Program, Medical College of Wisconsin; Department of Surgery (Division of Surgical Oncology), Milwaukee, WI, USA

Jason A. Glenn, MD Department of Surgery, Medical College of Wisconsin Affiliated Hospitals, Milwaukee, WI, USA

Neha Goel, MD Department of Surgery, New York Presbyterian-Columbia University Medical Center, New York, NY, USA

Raymon H. Grogan, MD, MS, FACS Baylor College of Medicine, Michael E. DeBakey Department of Surgery, Endocrine Surgery, Baylor St. Luke's Medical Center, Houston, TX, USA

Marlon A. Guerrero, MD, FACS Department of Surgery, Banner University Medical Center, University of Arizona, Tucson, AZ, USA

Joshua A. Hemmerich, PhD Department of Medicine, The University of Chicago, Chicago, IL, USA

Miguel F. Herrera, MD, PhD UNAM at the Instituto Nacional de Ciencias Médicas y Nutrición Salvador Zubirán, Mexico City, Mexico

Elizabeth Holt, MD, PhD Department of Internal Medicine, Yale University School of Medicine, New Haven, CT, USA

Jessica Hwang, MD John H. Stroger, Jr. Hospital of Cook County, Department of Endocrinology and Diabetes, Chicago, IL, USA

Benjamin James, MD, MS Section of Endocrine Surgery, Division of Surgical Oncology, Department of Surgery, Beth Israel Deaconess Medical Center, Boston, MA, USA

Edwin L. Kaplan, MD Department of Surgery, The University of Chicago, Chicago, IL, USA

Electron Kebebew, MD Department of Surgery, School of Medicine, Stanford University, Stanford, CA, USA

Jennifer H. Kuo, MD Division of GI/Endocrine Surgery, Columbia University, New York, NY, USA

Terry C. Lairmore, MD, FACS Division of Surgical Oncology, Department of Surgery, Baylor Scott and White Health, Texas A&M University Health Science Center, Temple, TX, USA

Shi Lam, MBBS, MRCS Department of Surgery, The University of Hong Kong, Hong Kong SAR, China

Brian H. H. Lang, MBBS, MS, FRACS Department of Surgery, The University of Hong Kong, Hong Kong SAR, China

Division of Endocrine Surgery, Department of Surgery, Queen Mary Hospital, Hong Kong SAR, China

Alexander Langerman, MD, SM, FACS Vanderbilt University Medical Center, Nashville, TN, USA

James A. Lee, MD Columbia University Medical Center, Department of Surgery, New York, NY, USA

James Y. Lim, MD General Surgery, The Mount Sinai Hospital, New York, NY, USA

Carrie C. Lubitz, MD, MPH (CCL) Department of Surgery, Massachusetts General Hospital, Boston, MA, USA

Institute for Technology Assessment, Boston, MA, USA

Melanie L. Lyden, MD, MHPE Department of Surgery, Mayo Clinic Hospital, Rochester, MN, USA

Colleen Majewski, MD Division of Endocrinology, Department of Medicine, Northwestern University, Chicago, IL, USA

Jennifer Malinowski, PhD Department of Surgery, Yale University School of Medicine, New Haven, CT, USA

Haggi Mazeh, MD Endocrine and General Surgery, Department of Surgery, Hadassah-Hebrew University Medical Center, Jerusalem, Israel

Frédéric Mercier, MD Department of Surgical Oncology, Centre Hospitalier de l'université de Montréal, Montreal, QC, Canada

Elliot J. Mitmaker, MD, MSc, FRCSC, FACS Department of Surgery, Royal Victoria Hospital – Glen Site, McGill University Health Center, Montreal, QC, Canada

Jacob Moalem, MD University of Rochester Medical Center, Department of Surgery, Rochester, NY, USA

Sapna Nagar, MD Department of Surgery, Oakland University William Beaumont School of Medicine, Beaumont Hospitals, Royal Oak, MI, USA

Cheryl C. Nocon, MD Department of Surgery, Division of Otolaryngology-Head and Neck Surgery, NorthShore University HealthSystem, Kellogg Cancer Center, Evanston, IL, USA

Fiemu E. Nwariaku, MD, FACS Department of Surgery, University of Texas Southwestern Medical Center, Dallas, TX, USA

Sarah C. Oltmann, MD Parkland Memorial Hospital, University of Texas Southwestern Medical Center, Dallas, TX, USA

Janice L. Pasieka, MD, FRCSC, FACS Faculty of Medicine, University of Calgary and Tom Baker Cancer Centre, Calgary, AB, Canada

Jesse Pasternak, MD, MPH Department of Surgery, University of Toronto, University Health Network-Toronto General Hospital, Toronto, ON, Canada

Dhaval Patel, MD Endocrine Oncology Branch, National Cancer Institute, National Institutes of Health, Bethesda, MD, USA

Subhash Patel, MB, BS, FACS John H. Stroger, Jr. Hospital of Cook County, Department of Surgery, Chicago, IL, USA

Amudhan Pugalenthi, MD Department of Endocrine Surgery, Cleveland Clinic, Cleveland, OH, USA

Courtney E. Quinn, MD Section of Endocrine Surgery, Department of Surgery, Yale University School of Medicine, New Haven, CT, USA

Reese W. Randle, MD Section of Endocrine Surgery, Department of Surgery, University of Kentucky, Lexington, KY, USA

Benjamin R. Roman, MD, MSHP Department of Surgery, Head and Neck Service, Memorial Sloan Kettering Cancer Center, New York, NY, USA

Selyne Samuel, MD Department of Surgery, Banner University Medical Center, University of Arizona, Tucson, AZ, USA

David F. Schneider, MD, MS Section of Endocrine Surgery, Department of Surgery, University of Wisconsin, Madison, WI, USA

Ashok R. Shaha, MD Department of Surgery, Head and Neck Service, Memorial Sloan Kettering Cancer Center, New York, NY, USA

Jyotirmay Sharma, MD Department of Surgery, Emory University Hospital, Atlanta, GA, USA

Wen T. Shen, MD, MA Department of Surgery, University of California, San Francisco/Mt. Zion Medical Center, San Francisco, CA, USA

Sadeesh K. Srinathan, MD, MSc Winnipeg Health Sciences Centre, Department of Surgery, University of Manitoba, Winnipeg, MB, Canada

Insoo Suh, MD Department of Surgery, Section of Endocrine Surgery, UCSF Medical Center – Mount Zion, San Francisco, CA, USA

Paritosh Suman, MD NorthShore University HealthSystem/John H. Stroger Hospital of Cook County, Department of Surgery, Evanston, IL, USA

Anu Thakrar, MD Department of Radiation Oncology, John H. Stroger, Jr. Hospital of Cook County, Chicago, IL, USA

Susan Tsai, MD, MHS Pancreatic Cancer Program, Medical College of Wisconsin; Department of Surgery (Division of Surgical Oncology), Milwaukee, WI, USA

Kellie Van Voorhis Department of Medicine, The University of Chicago, Chicago, IL, USA

Tracy S. Wang, MD, MPH Department of Surgery, Division of Surgical Oncology, Section of Endocrine Surgery, Medical College of Wisconsin, Milwaukee, WI, USA

Collin Weber, MD Department of Surgery, Emory University School of Medicine, Atlanta, GA, USA

Feng Xie, PhD Department of Health Research Methods, Evidence and Impact, Faculty of Health Sciences, McMaster University, St. Joseph's Hospital, Hamilton, ON, Canada

Linwah Yip, MD Division of Endocrine Surgery, Department of Surgery, University of Pittsburgh School of Medicine, Pittsburgh, PA, USA

George Younan, MD Pancreatic Cancer Program, Medical College of Wisconsin; Department of Surgery (Division of Surgical Oncology), Milwaukee, WI, USA

Abbreviations

Misc

3HPT	Tertiary hyperparathyroidism
4DCT	Four-dimensional computed tomography
5-FU	Fluorouracil

A

AACE	American Association of Clinical Endocrinologists
AAES	American Association of Endocrine Surgeons
ACC	Adrenocortical carcinoma
ACS-NSQIP	American College of Surgeons' National Surgical Quality Improvement Program
ACTH	Adrenocorticotropic hormone
AIMAH	ACTH-independent macronodular adrenal hyperplasia
APA	Aldosterone-producing adenoma
ARR	Aldosterone-to-renin ratio
ATA	American Thyroid Association
ATC	Anaplastic thyroid cancer
AUC	Area under the curve
AUS	Atypia of undetermined significance
AVS	Adrenal vein sampling or adrenal venous sampling

B

BAH	Bilateral adrenal hyperplasia
BMAH	Bilateral macronodular adrenal hyperplasia
BMD	Bone mineral density
BNE	Bilateral neck exploration

C

CaSR	Calcium-sensing receptor
CDA	Clinical decision analysis
CgA	Chromogranin A
CHPA	Cryopreserved heterotopic parathyroid autotransplantation
CT	Completion thyroidectomy
CT	Computed tomography

D

DFI	Disease-free interval
DFS	Disease-free survival
DXA	Dual-energy X-ray absorptiometry

E

EBM	Evidence-based medicine
EBRT	External beam radiotherapy
ECOG	Eastern Cooperative Oncology Group
EDTA	Ethylenediaminetetra-acetic acid
EGFR	Epidermal growth factor receptor (EGFR)
ENSAT	European Network for the Study of Adrenal Tumor
ESMO	European Society of Medical Oncology
EUS	Endoscopic ultrasound

F

FHH	Familial hypocalciuric hypercalcemia
FIHP	Familial isolated hyperparathyroidism
FIRM-ACT	First international randomized trial in locally advanced and metastatic adrenocortical carcinoma reatment
FLUS	Follicular lesion of undetermined significance
FN	False-negative
FNA	Fine-needle aspiration
FNMTC	Familial non-medullary thyroid cancer
FP	False-positive
FTC	Follicular thyroid carcinoma

G

GAN	Greater auricular nerve
GEC	Gene-expression classifier
GLP-1	Glucagon-like peptide 1 analog
GRADE	Grades of recommendation, assessment, development, and evaluation
GRBAS	Grade, roughness, breathiness, asthenia, and strain
GY	Gray

H

HNR	Harmonics-to-noise ratio
HPF	High-power field
HPT	Primary hyperparathyroidism
HPT-JT	Hyperparathyroidism jaw tumor
HTC	Oncocytic or Hurthle cell variant of FTC
HTN	Hypertension
HypoCa	Hypocalcemia

I

IA	Interarytenoid
ICU	Intensive care unit
IDLE	Indolent lesions of epithelial origin
IHA	Idiopathic aldosteronism
IMRT	Intensity-modulated radiotherapy
IOPTH/IoPTH	Intraoperative parathyroid hormone
IOUS	Intraoperative ultrasound
^{131}I-MIBG	Iodine meta-iodobenzylguanidine
iPTH	Intact PTH
IRI	Immunoreactive insulin
IVC	Inferior vena cava

L

LA	Laparoscopic adrenalectomy
LCA	Lateral cricoarytenoid
LN	Lymph node
LOS	Length of stay
LSP	Less than subtotal parathyroidectomy
LTA	Laparoscopic transperitoneal adrenalectomy

M

MDCT	Multidetector CT
MEN 1	Multiple endocrine neoplasia type 1
MeSH	Medical subject headings
MGD	Multiple gland disease
MIBI	99mTc-sestamibi
MIP	Minimally invasive parathyroidectomy
MR	Mineralocorticoid receptor
MRI	Magnetic resonance imaging
MTC	Medullary thyroid carcinoma
mTOR	Mammalian target of rapamycin
MTNS	McGill thyroid nodule score
MWA	Microwave ablation

N

NANETS	North American Neuroendocrine Tumor Society
NCCN	National Comprehensive Cancer Network
NCDB	National Cancer Database
NED	No evidence of disease
NGS	Next-generation sequencing
NIFT-P	Noninvasive follicular thyroid neoplasm with papillary-like nuclear features
NIH	National Institutes of Health
NIS	Nationwide Inpatient Specimen
NPV	Negative predictive value
NR	Not reported
Ns	Not specified

P

PA	Primary aldosteronism
PAF1	Polymerase II–associated factor 1
PCA	Posterior cricoarytenoid
PCR	Polymerase chain reaction
PDC	Poorly differentiated thyroid carcinoma
PDGF	Platelet-derived growth factor
PDNET	Pancreaticoduodenal neuroendocrine tumors
PEI	Phonation efficiency index
PET-CT	Positron emission tomography–computed tomography
PFS	Progression-free survival
PHP	Primary (chief cell) hyperplasia

pHPT Persistent hyperparathyroidism
PICO Population, intervention, comparator, and outcome
PNET Pancreatic neuroendocrine tumor
PPAR Peroxisome proliferator-activated receptor
PPNAD Primary pigmented nodular adrenocortical disease
PPV Positive predictive value
PRA Posterior retroperitoneal adrenalectomy
PRO Patient-reported outcomes
PTC Papillary thyroid cancer
PTC-FV Follicular variant of PTC
PTH Parathyroid hormone
PTHrP Parathyroid hormone-related peptide
PTMC Papillary thyroid microcarcinomas
PTX Parathyroidectomy
PV/SMV Portal vein/superior mesenteric vein

Q

QALY Quality-adjusted life years
QOL Quality of life

R

R Retrospective
RCT Randomized controlled trials
RFA Radiofrequency ablation
RH Resistant hypertension
rHPT Recurrent hyperparathyroidism
RLN Recurrent laryngeal nerve
RPMI Roswell Park Memorial Institute
RPT Randomized, prospective trial
RTOG Radiation Therapy Oncology Group

S

SABR Stereotactic ablative body radiotherapy
SCIP Surgical Care Improvement Project
SEER Surveillance, epidemiology, and end results
SeS Sestamibi
SF-36 Short form 36
SP Subtotal parathyroidectomy
SPECT Single-photon emission computed tomography

SRI	Surgically remediable aldosteronism
SSA	Somatostatin analogue
SSI	Surgical site infections
SSTR	Somatostatin receptors
SUS	Surgeon-performed ultrasound
SV	Splenic vein
SVS	Selective venous sampling

T

TA	Thyroarytenoid
TP/AT	Total parathyroidectomy and autotransplantation
TSH	Thyroid-stimulating hormone
TT	Total thyroidectomies

U

UFC	Urinary free cortisol
UICC	Union for International Cancer Control
US	Ultrasonographic
US FDA	United States Food and Drug Administration
USG	Ultrasonography
USG-FNAC	USG-guided fine-needle aspiration cytology
UTC	Undifferentiated or anaplastic thyroid carcinoma
UTI	Urinary tract infection

V

VEGF	Vascular endothelial growth factor
VFA	Vertebral fracture assessment
VHI	Voice handicap index
VHL	von Hippel-Lindau type 1

W

WHO	World Health Organization

Evidence-Based Medicine and the GRADE Approach

1

Sadeesh K. Srinathan

Abstract

Evidence-based medicine (EBM) is a term which entered the lexicon of medical practice in 1992. It can be defined as "the conscientious, explicit, and judicious use of current best evidence in making decisions about the care of individual patients". In this chapter we illustrate how to practice EBM using a sequence of straight forward steps moving from phrasing a clinical question to making a judgment of the risk of bias in the evidence we encounter. We will then introduce and use the GRADE system of determining the quality of evidence to allow the surgeon a means of determining their confidence in the evidence that they use to guide their clinical practice.

Keywords

EBM · Evidence based medicine · GRADE · Bias · Study design · Systematic reviews · Trials

Introduction

Surgeons routinely make difficult decisions. In many cases, the difficulty lies in the need to make these decisions in the face of incomplete or unreliable information. An example of this in an individual patient is deciding to perform an exploratory laparotomy for an acute abdomen where the evidence from diagnostic studies may be

S. K. Srinathan
Winnipeg Health Sciences Centre, Department of Surgery, University of Manitoba, Winnipeg, MB, Canada
e-mail: ssrinathan@exchange.hsc.mb.ca

P. Angelos, R. H. Grogan (eds.), *Difficult Decisions in Endocrine Surgery*, Difficult Decisions in Surgery: An Evidence-Based Approach,
https://doi.org/10.1007/978-3-319-92860-9_1

incomplete or contradictory. Another example, in terms of policy, would be to decide on the appropriateness of screening for occult malignancies where the evidence for early detection may be closely matched by evidence for undesirable events such as overtreatment.

In this book, difficult scenarios commonly encountered by the endocrine surgeon are presented. The authors of each chapter lay out the available evidence and make a recommendation as to the appropriate responses in these scenarios. They have followed the principles of evidence-based medicine to come to their recommendations and the purpose of this chapter is to present an overview of the process which led to their recommendations.

The phrase Evidence Based Medicine (EBM) came into widespread use after 1992 following a publication by Guyatt et al. [1], and is now commonly agreed to mean: '…the conscientious, explicit, and judicious use of current best evidence in making decisions about the care of individual patients. The practice of evidence based medicine means integrating individual clinical expertise with the best available external clinical evidence from systematic research" it also means that "… thoughtful identification and compassionate use of individual patients' predicaments, rights, and preferences in making clinical decision…" [2].

The practice of EBM can be carried out by using the following principles: (1) ask a clinical question, (2) locate the evidence, (3) appraise and synthesize the evidence, and (4) apply the evidence [3].

Asking the Clinical Question

On the face of it, asking the clinical question is straightforward. A patient problem is presented, and a question arises. For example, Mrs. Smith is presenting with a multinodular goiter. Should this patient undergo a total thyroidectomy or a subtotal thyroidectomy?

Going directly to Google with the key words "thyroidectomy for goitre", we obtain 250,000 hits, while Wikipedia results in 17 hits. Clearly, neither of these extremes is satisfactory in helping us to determine a surgical approach. A useful step is to convert this specific clinical question about Mrs. Smith to a form that will allow us to search for the relevant evidence. The *PICO* format, which is used throughout this book, is a useful tool for this purpose.

The *P* stands for Patient or Population and specifies the patient group to which the question refers, in this case it may be: (a) all patients with a multinodular goitre, (b) adult patients with a multinodular goiter, (c) adult patients with a non-toxic multinodular goiter (d) adult patients with a non-toxic multinodular goiter who have had a previous operation in the neck. It is apparent that each iteration of the definition of the population is more and more specific. These details are important, but we may limit the information available to us if we define our population of interest too narrowly.

The *I* is for the Intervention or exposure of interest and specifies what has happened to a group of patients such as an operation, or a diagnostic test. In our example the intervention we are considering is a total thyroidectomy. However, there could also be specific issues that are considered important such as the use of drains.

The *C* refers to the comparator that we are interested in. In this case it is a subtotal total thyroidectomy, but again we should be mindful of specific details of the standard procedure that may be important for our specific question.

O stands for the Outcome of interest. It is very important to be specific about the outcome of interest as it is likely that various studies may have used different outcomes in the study design than the one you are interested. One study may have been focused on goiter recurrence, whereas another may have been focused on incidence of major complications. It is worthwhile to identify each outcome of interest in the specific clinical scenario and to order them in order of importance to the patient and surgeon so that an overall assessment of the utility of an intervention can be made.

Taking these features of the clinical question into account, we can frame the scenario for Mrs. Smith in the following PICO question:

> In an adult patient with a non-toxic goiter, does a total thyroidectomy result in 1) decreased mortality 2) lower or same goiter recurrence 3) fewer complications than a subtotal thyroidectomy?

P: Adults with a non-toxic multinodular goiter
I: total thyroidectomy
C: subtotal thyroidectomy
O: (1) operative mortality, (2) goiter recurrence, and (3) complications

It is worth considering when reviewing the chapters in this book, whether the PICO questions chosen by the authors are *sufficiently* similar to your own formulation of the question for their findings and recommendations to apply to your specific case.

Finding the Evidence

Often the first step in a literature search is to go to PubMed, the interface to access the Medline database of citations in the National Library of Medicine in the United States. However, a search of "total subtotal thyroidectomy" produces 776 citations. This is more than we can reasonably go through for the purposes of answering a specific question for a patient. But, if we use the Clinical Queries page in PubMed which uses an algorithm to deliver focused studies relevant to clinical practice [4], we obtain citations for 26 systematic reviews and 313 clinical studies, much better. Alternative search engines include TRIP database (http://www.tripdatabase.com/) and SUMsearch (http://sumsearch.org/), which use multiple databases including Medline, EMBASE, and databases of guidelines and technology may also be used. Last, but certainly not least is the expertise available through your local medical librarian who will be well versed in the methods of constructing a PICO question and finding the relevant information from the medical literature.

Appraising the Studies

Once we have found the studies of interest, the next step is to identify the "best evidence". The concept of "best evidence" assumes a hierarchy of evidence. But to apply a hierarchy, it is important to understand the types of study designs and their use in answering specific types of clinical questions. Grimes and Schulz [5] provide a useful taxonomy of study designs (Fig. 1.1). In general, questions related to the superiority of one intervention over another (or no intervention) are best answered by experimental studies where one group of patients are assigned to the intervention by a bias free method, while another receive a comparison intervention. The gold standard for the experimental study is a well-designed randomized trial. Other types of clinical questions such as that of prognosis are appropriately answered using cohort studies, while questions of diagnosis rely on comparing the performance of a diagnostic test to a gold standard.

All study types have the potential for any number of biases which may lead to a finding which deviates from the "truth" [6]. The tools of critical appraisal are used determine the type and extent of these biases in the design and conduct of the study and make a judgment of how it may have affected the findings of the study and the extent to which it undermines our confidence in the validity of the findings.

There are many excellent resources and tools to guide us in the specifics of appraising the medical literature and practicing EBM and these are listed in the recommended readings.

What happens when despite the best formulation of a question and literature search we are unable to find the high quality systematic review or randomized trial to guide us? Do we abandon the principles of EBM? Again from Sackett: "Evidence based medicine is not restricted to randomized trials and meta-analyses. It involves tracking down the best external evidence with which to answer our clinical questions.... However, some questions about therapy do not require randomized trials (successful interventions for otherwise fatal conditions) or cannot wait for the trials to be conducted. And if no randomized trial has been carried out for our patient's predicament, we must follow the trail to the next best external evidence and work from there." [3].

Although we can approach each problem we face by formulating a question and finding the best available evidence, individual clinicians are unlikely to have the time or resources to do this for all possible scenarios. To illustrate: our example PICO question generated 85 results using PubMed. To identify and read through the abstracts or articles for this one question can take a considerable amount of time. To then appraise each study for its quality and relevance will add more.

The alternative to searching for each question has been standard textbooks, which seek to distill the evidence and guide clinical practice. The authors of these textbooks have always made decisions about which studies to consider and judgments about their confidence in making recommendation based on this evidence. However, these judgments and decisions have not been transparent. And although there are many schemes in use which grade the level of evidence and have been increasingly used in textbooks, it is not clear on what basis these decisions of grade

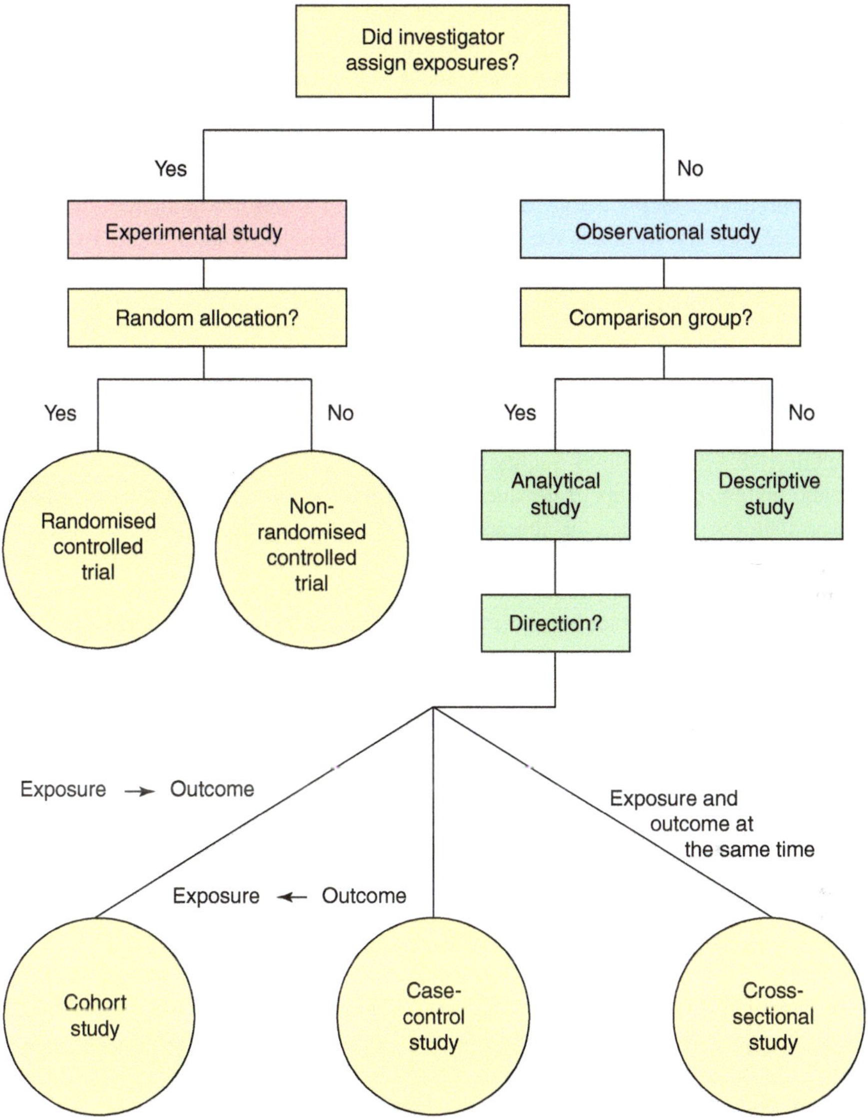

Fig. 1.1 Algorithm for classification of types of clinical research. From Grimes DA, Schulz KF. An overview of clinical research: the lay of the land. Lancet. 2002; 359(9300):57–61; with permission

were specifically arrived at [7]. A good systematic review makes transparent the question, the search strategy, and the rules for inclusion of studies and on what basis the quality of the study is determined. However, the final assessment of the overall quality of evidence and the subsequent recommendation arising from this evidence is often obscure.

To address this deficiency this book has adopted the GRADE system to make transparent the decision-making about the quality of evidence and the factors considered in making a recommendation and a statement about the strength of this recommendation. The reader may disagree with certain judgments made by the authors, but the reason for disagreement will hopefully be clear with the GRADE system and the reader can make up their own minds whether the conclusions drawn by the authors are on the whole reasonable or valid. The key component of GRADE is that it explicitly separates the process of evaluating the quality of the evidence for an intervention from the process of making a recommendation for its adoption (or not).

The Grade System

The GRADE system defines quality in the following way: "In the context of a systematic review, the ratings of the quality of evidence reflect the extent of our confidence that the estimates of the effect are correct. In the context of making recommendations, the quality ratings reflect the extent of our confidence that the estimates of an effect are adequate to support a particular decision or recommendation" [8]. It is the latter definition that applies in this book, and the authors have included a discussion of their clinical experience that brings into play the necessity of balancing conflicting factors in making a recommendation. A good discussion is provided by Andrews et al. and Brozek et al. [9, 10].

The GRADE table used in this book lays out the justification of why these decisions are made and it is instructive to describe in detail the components of the table. This example of a GRADE table (Table 1.1) is from Cirocchi et al. [11] who report on a systematic review comparing results between a total and subtotal thyroidectomy for multinodular goiter:

The Header The general title of the clinical question being considered.

Sub Heading A question broken up into the PICO format of patient or population, the setting the intervention and the comparison to which the intervention is being made. The question is that which is of interest to the author of the table and may or may not reflect the evidence which addresses this question.

Outcomes The key component of the GRADE process is to focus on the outcomes to which the evidence applies. Individual studies may focus on differing outcomes that are of interest. It is often the case that many studies address common outcomes reflecting benefit, but do not reliably report on other outcomes, especially on harm. It is possible that with the same questions and same group of studies, the quality of evidence supporting an intervention is high for one outcome but not others. This latter point is one of the reasons that when formulating the question it is useful to list in order of importance the outcomes of interest.

Table 1.1 Total or near-total thyroidectomy compared with subtotal thyroidectomy for multinodular nontoxic goitre in adults

Total or near-total thyroidectomy compared with subtotal thyroidectomy for multinodular non-toxic goitre in adults

Patient: Adults with multinodular non-toxic goitre
Settings: Tertiary referral centre
Intervention: (Near) total thyroidectomy
Comparison: Subtotal thyroidectomy

Outcomes	Illustrative comparative risks[a] (95% CI)		Relative effect (95% CI)	No of participants (studies)	Quality of the evidence (GRADE)	Comments
	Assumed risk	Corresponding risk				
	Subtotal thyroidectomy	(Near) total thyroidectomy				
All-cause mortality Follow-up: 1–10 years	See comment	See comment	See comment	1284 (4)	(a) ⊕⊕⊕◯ **moderate**[b]	No postoperative hospital deaths or deaths within the first 30 days occurred after total or subtotal thyroidectomy
(a) **Goitre recurrence** (b) **Re-intervention due to goitre recurrence** Follow-up: (a) 3–10 years, (b) 5 years	(a) **84 per 1000** (b) **8 per 1000**	(a) **5 per 1000** (1–19) (b) **5 per 1000** (1–48)	(a) **OR 0.05** (0.01 to 0.21) (b) **OR 0.66** (0.07 to 6.38)	(a) 1057 (3) (b) 570 (1)	(a) ⊕⊕⊕◯ **moderate**[c] (b) ⊕⊕◯◯ **low**[d]	–
Adverse events: (a) **Permanent recurrent laryngeal nerve palsy** (b) **Permanent hypoparathyroidism** Follow-up: (a) 1–10 years, (b) 1–10 years	(a) **8 per 1000** (b) **1 per 1000**	(a) **10 per 1000** (3–34) (b) **4 per 1000** (1–28)	(a) **OR 1.28** (0.38 to 4.36) (b) **OR 3.09** (0.45 to 21. 36)	(a)1275 (4) (b)1275 (4)	(a) ⊕⊕◯◯ **low**[e] (b) ⊕⊕◯◯ **low**[e]	–

(continued)

Table 1.1 (continued)

Total or near-total thyroidectomy compared with subtotal thyroidectomy for multinodular non-toxic goitre in adults						
Thyroid cancer incidence Follow-up: 1–5 years	**61 per 1000**	**79 per 1000** (50–123)	**OR** 1.32 (0.81 to 2.15)	1134 (3)	⊕⊕◯◯ **low**[e]	–
Health-related quality of life	See comment	See comment	See comment	See comment	See comment	Outcome not investigated
Socioeconomic effects	See comment	See comment	See comment	See comment	See comment	Outcome not investigated

GRADE Working Group grades of evidence
High quality: Further research is very unlikely to change our confidence in the estimate of effect
Moderate quality: Further research is likely to have an important impact on our confidence in the estimate of effect and may change the estimate
Low quality: Further research is very likely to have an important impact on our confidence in the estimate of effect and is likely to change the estimate
Very low quality: We are very uncertain about the estimate

From Cirocchi R, Trastulli S, Randolph J, Guarino S, Di Rocco G, Arezzo A, et al. Total or near-total thyroidectomy versus subtotal thyroidectomy for multinodular non-toxic goitre in adult. Cochrane Database Syst Rev. 2015 Aug 7;(8):CD010370

Assumed risk: mean control group risk across studies

CI confidence interval, ***OR*** odds ratio

[a]The basis for the **assumed risk** (e.g. the median control group risk across studies) is provided in footnotes. The **corresponding risk** (and its 95% confidence interval) is based on the assumed risk in the comparison group and the **relative effect** of the intervention (and its 95% CI)

[b]Downgraded by one level because of high risk of outcome reporting bias (no trial investigated all-cause mortality over longer periods of follow-up)

[c]Downgraded by one level because of small number of events and unknown risk of detection bias

[d]Downgraded by two levels because of high risk of outcome reporting bias (3 of 4 trials did not report re-interventions due to goitre recurrence), imprecision and one study only with small number of participants and low event rates

[e]Downgraded by two levels because of imprecision and low event rates

Justification for Quality Assessment In the GRADE system, a judgment is made whether the overall quality of evidence for each outcome is High, Moderate, Low, or Very Low. Initially evidence from RCTs is considered to be High quality evidence while observational studies start off as Low quality. Whether the overall body of evidence moves up or down the ranking is determined by the extent to which the studies have features which move them up or down and (Table 1.1) [7], specifies the features which move a study up or down the list.

Study Limitation The first judgment is related to the possible deficiency in the study designs themselves and these are determined during the critical appraisal process, features such as adequacy of randomization and blinding.

Inconsistency Different studies may come to different conclusions either qualitatively e.g. the intervention works vs. it doesn't or the degree to which a treatment works, i.e. the effect size differs. A measure of this in systematic reviews is the degree of heterogeneity often reported as the I^2. This heterogeneity can be due to differences in the patient population studied, the nature of the intervention, means of measuring outcomes or other study design features.

Directness This is the degree to which the studies address the question we are interested in. The results may be indirect because the study population is different from one we are interested in or the intervention differs substantially from what we are interested in.

Precision Studies may report effects with wide confidence intervals where the values at the upper and lower bounds would suggest the different clinical actions. In our example, the incidence of permanent recurrent nerve palsy is estimated to be between 3 and 34 cases per 1000 compared to an assumed risk of 8 per 1000 in subtotal thyroidectomy. In this case, total thyroidectomy may result in significantly fewer or significantly more recurrent nerve palsy than subtotal thyroidectomy. The wide confidence intervals are most often driven by event rate, related to small sample size in a study.

Publication Bias We may suspect publication bias when the preponderance of the available evidence comes from a number of small studies, most of which have been commercially funded. This may suggest that studies which not showing an effect have not been published which biases the evidence.

Features Increasing Quality of Observational Studies

Large magnitude of Effect In well-designed observation studies, if a large and plausible effect is observed (relative risk of greater than 5 or less than 0.2) there is reasonable confidence that the effect is not due to confounding. This is the reason why one doesn't really require a RCT to determine if parachutes are effective.

Dose Response Gradient A finding in observational studies that increases our confidence in a cause effect relationship is the demonstration of a dose response effect. For example, an increased risk of bleeding with increasing INR.

All Plausible Confounding Would Reduce the Demonstrated Effect or Increase It if No Effect Was Observed A confounder is a factor related to both a predictor and outcome but is not in the causal link between the predictor and outcome. If a likely confounder acts opposite to the way one would expect, then it is possible that the true effect is underestimated. For example, if high risk patients do at least as well with a surgical procedure as do those at low risk, it more strongly suggests that there is a true effect of the surgical intervention and would increase our confidence and thus the quality rating of the evidence.

The last column is a summary of findings where the estimate of relative effect, the baseline risk of the standard therapy and the absolute effects of the intervention are reported. A measure of the absolute effect is crucial for making a recommendation since one intervention may be more effective in comparison to another, the overall effect in terms of overall numbers may be small, in our example the absolute risk in recurrent nerve injury rises from 8 to 10 per 1000, or an absolute difference of 2 per 1000. Another example is if the baseline risk of pneumonia is 1% and with the addition of preoperative antibiotics drops down to 0.7%. A change in absolute risk of 0.3% is unlikely to be of clinical significance despite there being a 30% relative risk reduction, which in many cases would be considered of considerable "clinical significance".

From determining the quality of evidence, a recommendation is made. This is a separate process from determining quality of evidence. A recommendation is either strong or weak where "The strength of a recommendation is defined as the extent to which one can be confident that the desirable consequences of an intervention outweigh its undesirable consequences." [9]. In assessing the quality of the evidence necessary to make the recommendation, those making the recommendation should specify which of the various outcomes are crucial to making a recommendation, in our example there is a much higher risk of goiter recurrence with subtotal thyroidectomy (84 per 1000) than with total thyroidectomy (5 per 1000), at the same time there is a small increased risk of recurrent nerve injury.

A strong recommendation is one where from the clinicians' point of view; most patients should receive the intervention as the expected benefits comfortably outweigh the undesirable effects. In these situations, there is usually little need for extensive discussions about the merits of the intervention. Weak recommendations on the other hand, may be appropriate in some patients, but requires more thorough discussions about the benefits and adverse effects of the treatment (Table 1.2). In the following chapter on clinical decision analysis, we illustrate how this issue is dealt with quantitatively.

Ultimately, decisions about the care of individual patient falls to the surgeon and the patient which takes into account not just the external evidence for a particular course of action but crucially the patient's own preferences and values and the practical ability for the surgeon to deliver on this decision in their own specific environment.

Table 1.2 Implications of the two grades of strength of recommendations in the GRADE approach

Target group	Strong recommendations[a]	Conditional (weak) recommendations
Patients	Most people in your situation would want the recommended course of action and only a small proportion would not	The majority of people in your situation would want the recommended course of action, but many would not
Clinicians	Most patients should receive the recommended course of action	Recognize that different choices will be appropriate for different patients and that you must make greater effort to help each patient to arrive at a management decision consistent with his or her values and preferences; decision aids and shared decision making are particularly useful
Policy makers	The recommendation can be adopted as a policy in most situations	Policy making will require substantial debate and involvement of many stakeholders

GRADE grades of recommendation, assessment, development and evaluation

[a]Strong recommendations based on high-quality evidence will apply to most patients for whom these recommendations are made, but they may not apply to all patients in all conditions; no recommendation can take into account all of the unique features of individual patients and clinical circumstances

References

1. Guyatt G. Evidence-Based Medicine Working Group. Evidence-based medicine. A new approach to teaching the practice of medicine. JAMA. 1992;268(17):2420–5. https://doi.org/10.1001/jama.1992.03490170092032.
2. Sackett DL. Evidence-based medicine. Semin Perinatol. 1997;21(1):3–5.
3. Sackett DL, Rosenberg WMC, Gray JAM, Haynes RB, Richardson WS. Evidence based medicine: what it is and what it isn't. BMJ. 1996;312(7023):71–2. https://doi.org/10.1136/bmj.312.7023.71.
4. Haynes RB. Optimal search strategies for retrieving scientifically strong studies of treatment from Medline: analytical survey. BMJ. 2005;330(7501):1179–80. https://doi.org/10.1136/bmj.38446.498542.8F.
5. Grimes DA, Schulz KF. An overview of clinical research: the lay of the land. Lancet. 2002;359(9300):57–61. https://doi.org/10.1016/S0140-6736(02)07283-5.
6. Grimes DA, Schulz KF. Bias and causal associations in observational research. Lancet. 2002;359(9302):248–52. https://doi.org/10.1016/S0140-6736(02)07451-2.
7. Atkins D, Best D, Briss PA, Eccles M, Falck-Ytter Y, Flottorp S, et al. Grading quality of evidence and strength of recommendations. BMJ. 2004;328(7454):1490. https://doi.org/10.1136/bmj.328.7454.1490.
8. Balshem H, Helfand M, Schünemann HJ, Oxman AD, Kunz R, Brozek J, et al. GRADE guidelines: 3. Rating the quality of evidence. J Clin Epidemiol. 2011;64(4):401–6. https://doi.org/10.1016/j.jclinepi.2010.07.015.
9. Andrews J, Guyatt G, Oxman AD, Alderson P, Dahm P, Falck-Ytter Y, et al. GRADE guidelines: 14. Going from evidence to recommendations: the significance and presentation of recommendations. J Clin Epidemiol. 2013;66:719–25.
10. Brożek JL, Akl EA, Compalati E, Kreis J, Terracciano L, Fiocchi A, et al. Grading quality of evidence and strength of recommendations in clinical practice guidelines part 3 of 3. The

GRADE approach to developing recommendations. Allergy. 2011;66(5):588–95. https://doi.org/10.1111/j.1398-9995.2010.02530.x.

11. Cirocchi R, Trastulli S, Randolph J, Guarino S, Di Rocco G, Arezzo A, et al. Total or near-total thyroidectomy versus subtotal thyroidectomy for multinodular non-toxic goitre in adults. Cochrane Database Syst Rev. 2015;8:CD010370. https://doi.org/10.1002/14651858.CD010370.pub2.

Recommended Reading

CEBM website: http://www.cebm.net/.

EPIQ: https://www.fmhs.auckland.ac.nz/en/soph/about/our-departments/epidemiology-and-biostatistics/research/epiq.html.

GRADE website: http://www.gradeworkinggroup.org/index.htm.

Guyatt G, Rennie D, Meade M. JAMA users' guides the medical literature: essentials of evidence-based clinical practice. New York: McGraw-Hill; 2008.

Clinical Decision Analysis

2

Sadeesh K. Srinathan and Feng Xie

Abstract

Clinical decisions are often difficult as we try to balance the benefits or harms of one decision pathway compared to another possible pathway. Further, this has to be done in the face of incomplete information. In this chapter we describe a useful tool termed Clinical Decision Analysis to allow for a transparent and explicit description of the decision making process to guide us in identifying areas of uncertainty around the existing evidence.

Keywords

EBM · Evidence based medicine · GRADE · Bias · Study design · Systematic reviews · Trials

Introduction

This book is about difficult decisions; implicit in the title is that a clinician and the patient have to take action, even it that action is to wait for further information. The source of the difficulties lies in the uncertainties in the information upon which the decision is made. Heuristic methods of decision making do not explicitly and

S. K. Srinathan (✉)
Winnipeg Health Sciences Centre, Department of Surgery, University of Manitoba, Winnipeg, MB, Canada
e-mail: ssrinathan@exchange.hsc.mb.ca

F. Xie
Department of Health Research Methods, Evidence and Impact, Faculty of Health Sciences, McMaster University, St. Joseph's Hospital, Hamilton, ON, Canada
e-mail: fengxie@mcmaster.ca

P. Angelos, R. H. Grogan (eds.), *Difficult Decisions in Endocrine Surgery*, Difficult Decisions in Surgery: An Evidence-Based Approach,
https://doi.org/10.1007/978-3-319-92860-9_2

systematically identify the nature or extent of these uncertainties. These heuristic means of decision which often misinterprets statistical information, can lead to errors [1]. In this chapter we will present a useful tool, Clinical Decision Analysis (CDA), which allows a more transparent and explicit description of the decision-making process, a means of explicitly identifying available evidence and the uncertainty around existing evidence.

What Is Decision Analysis?

Decision analysis is a formal system that details all the possible outcomes and the clinical pathway leading to each outcome for a decision and its alternate and provides means of choosing the best course among the alternatives under uncertainty. Or to quote Weinstein "Decision analysis is a systematic approach to decision making under conditions of uncertainty" [2]. It is (1) explicit, (2) quantitative and (3) prescriptive.

The potential benefits of CDA are that (a) it is an explicit process where the logic and assumptions made in the analysis are made clear, (b) it highlights points of uncertainty and deficits of information by explicitly incorporating into the analysis, (c) it allows an exploration of the impact of the uncertainties on the final decision.

It must be kept in mind that although CDA models a problem, it does so only to aid in the decision-making process. By necessity, these models simplify the problem, and a number of simplifying assumptions are made, but the model assumptions are made explicit. A decision analysis is also not an explanatory model of a clinical scenario, and it does not explain the pathophysiology of a clinical situation.

A CDA is not an algorithm. Although they may appear similar, the branching structure of a decision tree are to allow for the calculation of the best possible decision at a specific point. In contrast, an algorithm provides a path to follow given certain information with multiple decision-making points.

A challenge with CDA is that it demands specification of the probabilities of outcomes and the values of the outcome. However, this is not limited to decision analysis and is inherent in all decision making. In fact, a major strength of the value of CDA is that this aspect of decision making is made explicit and a value is assigned to this uncertainty.

Many of these issues are common for any type of decision making, and the formality of the process ought not to lead to unreasonable expectations of the process.

Why Know About This?

As discussed in the previous chapter, EBM is about actually *using the best available* evidence in delivering patient care. Systematic reviews and guidelines go some way in guiding decisions, but they do not in themselves allow you to come to a specific decision in a given scenario. For example, a systematic review can state that a particular intervention may yield a 15% improvement in survival over a 5-year period but at the cost of a 5% increase in the risk of a major stroke. This information does not in itself tell you if the intervention should be carried out since the decision hinges on the positive value the patient places on the outcome of survival and on the negative value on the outcome of a stroke.

Clinical guidelines go further in providing recommendations, but they are predicated on "average" patients with "average risks" and assume that patients will make consistent value judgments. In the major grading systems such as GRADE, there is acknowledgment that different decisions can be made depending on the individual patient values and preferences and the strength of recommendation reflect this, but recommendations do not give a measure of the sensitivity of a clinical decision to these changes. Certainly, at a policy level and even in routine patient level care, it is valuable to have an understanding of the robustness of a decision to variations in factors considered important and relevant for the decision.

It may be challenging in carry out a formal analysis in making individual clinical decisions. However, we believe that familiarity with this process will at least make it easier to consider existing evidence and identify areas of uncertainty so that further effort can be made to reduce this uncertainty or to at least to raise a warning as to the degree of confidence that one can place on the decision one makes. Awareness of this process may also make it easier to "hang" medical evidence in a framework so that it can be integrated into clinical practice. Furthermore, this is a basic technique used by decision makers in health care and as such impact on every practicing surgeon.

Anatomy of Clinical Decision Analysis

The best decision is one that maximizes the preferred outcome. For instance, in business decision making, the best decision is one that maximizes profit. In general terms, a clinical decision maximizes health for a patient or population. The clinical decision is contingent on the probability of preferred outcomes occurring and the desirability assigned to the outcomes that may occur.

A Clinical Decision Analysis is composed of three main steps: (1) construct the decision analytic framework (Figs. 2.1 and 2.2), (2) carry out the calculations to

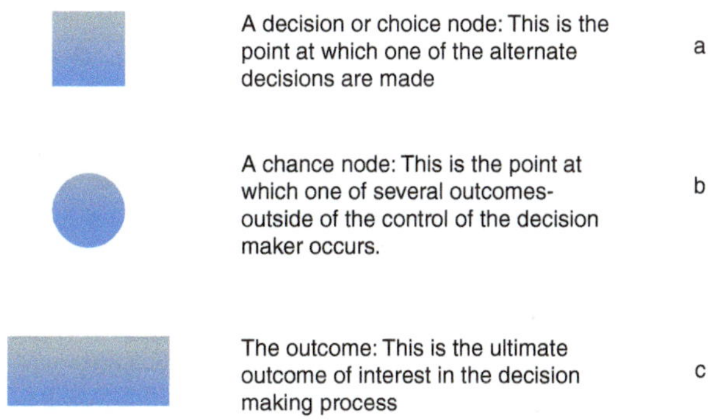

Fig. 2.1 Explanation of symbols used in clinical decision analysis. (**a**) A decision or choice node: This is the point at which one of the alternate decisions are made. (**b**) A chance node: This is the point at which one of several outcomes—outside of the control of the decision maker occurs. (**c**) The outcome: This is the ultimate outcome of interest in the decision making process

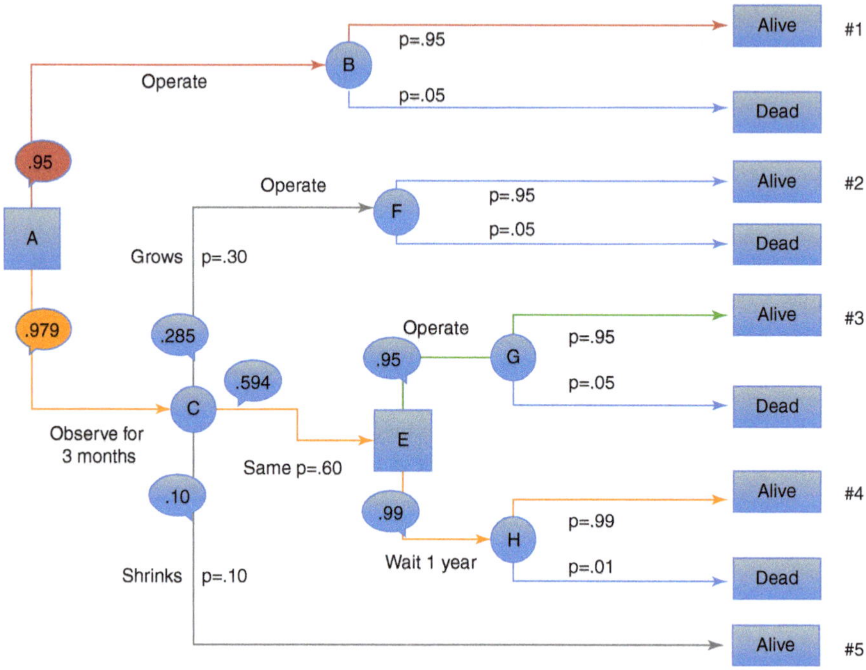

Fig. 2.2 Hypothetical CDA—should we operate on a tumour identified incidentally on imaging?

choose the best pathway or decision and (3) carry out a sensitivity analysis to determine the robustness of the decision, i.e. to what extent does the decision change across plausible values of probabilities of the outcome and the values assigned to the outcome.

Constructing the Decision Analytical Framework

The first step is to construct the decision analytical framework. This starts with framing the question of interest in terms of alternate possible decisions which are available to us at the outset, i.e. when the outcomes are unknowable. Nearly all scenarios in clinical practice present alternative scenarios and if these can be explicitly stated, then CDA can be applied. This initial point is the first decision node (Fig. 2.1a) and a key feature of the decision node is that it sets out what the alternative decisions are, and these alternatives at the decision node are mutually exclusive. The decision node is usually noted by a square box on a diagram.

To make a decision is to choose a specific path in the framework emanating from the decision node. The goal of CDA is to determine which of the paths taken at the first decision node is most likely to be the best one, i.e. will maximize the outcome, although there may be other decisions to be made subsequently throughout the framework.

Any decision results in, often multiple possible, consequences. This is reflected by the paths emanated from the nodes diagrammed as a circle (called "chance node) following each decision (Fig. 2.1b). A probability is attached to each of these consequences to show how likely one consequence occurs following a decision. The sum of the probabilities at each chance node is always 1. The framework ultimately terminates at the outcomes of interest, (Fig. 2.1c) which occurs as some defined point. This is usually diagrammed as a rectangle or triangle. The outcomes can be measured using relevant clinical measures or utility value to indicates its relative desirability. For instance, an ideal outcome such as being alive and well will have a value of 1, and death has a value of 0. An intermediate outcome such as alive but having suffered a major disability may have a value of 0.7, a value somewhere between well and dead.

Figure 2.2 provides a very simple, hypothetical CDA where the initial question is whether or not to operate on a tumour identified by an imaging test and where the outcome is to be determined over a 15-month time horizon. At the first decision node (A), the options are either to operate immediately (B) or alternatively, to reassess the tumour after 3 months (C). The possible outcomes associated with immediate surgery include alive after the operation with a utility value of 1, and postoperative death with utility value of 0. The probability of being alive is 0.95 and 0.05 for dying. If the decision is made to follow the tumour for 3 months at the outset, then possible outcomes include that the tumor either shrinks in which case nothing is done and the patient is always alive (outcome #5), remains unchanged in which case a further decision to be made (E), or the tumour grows, in which case an operation is always performed with the attendant risk of death. Each of these outcomes occurs with a probability of 0.30 for tumour growth, 0.60 for tumour size unchanged, and 0.10 for the tumour shrinkage. If the tumour size remains unchanged after the 3-month observation, then at the second decision node (E) the decision could be either to proceed to operation or to watch for a further 12 months. Again, the outcome of operation is either alive or dead with the same probabilities already stated. If the decision is to continue the observation, then the outcome is either stability which result in being alive with a probability of 0.99, or the tumor spreads leading to death with a probability of 0.01.

Determining Probabilities and Utility Values

From studying Fig. 2.2, the obvious question is where the values of the probabilities and utility come from? Probabilities and outcome measures are the critical inputs to the CDA and determining the probabilities of these outcomes occurring can be difficult. Ideally the information can be derived from clinical studies that report on outcomes after an intervention, such as from clinical trials that report the cure rate of an operation and also the risk of complication and mortality. Else but less ideal, the probability may have to be derived from a consensus among experts. The probability in a CDA, is ultimately a statement of belief about an outcome, and if there is objective means of establishing (e.g. clinical trials), then that is ideal. However, in the absence of this objective evidence, a statement of belief of the likelihood of an outcome occurring in itself can be used (e.g. expert opinions). Clearly, the confidence in the validity of the estimate of this probability will vary according to the source of this estimate of probability.

The patient and clinician are aware of the outcomes that are of interest, e.g. being alive, well and cured of a disease, or being cured of a disease but having suffered a complication, dying from the disease or dying from the treatment. The probability of the outcome may be discussed with patients, e.g. a 95% chance of being cured but a 4% chance of major complication and a 1% mortality, but the value that is placed on each of these outcomes by the patient are usually not discussed. Much like the probability of an outcome, the utility values used to measure the relative desirability of an outcome can be gleaned from the literature where patients were asked to rate their desirability of the outcome. Alternatively, one may ask the patient directly what their values are. This is not quite straightforward but is possible.

Calculating the Utility of Each Decision

The second step of CDA is coming to a decision by calculating the overall utilities associated with each of the decision. This overall utility of a decision is the sum of the product of the probabilities and the utility values assigned to the corresponding outcomes for all paths under each decision. Calculating the overall utility for each decision starts from the rightmost and then moves to the leftmost part of the framework (called "foldback"). We need to determine the probability and the utility value of the outcome at the end of each path. The utility is then multiplied by the probability of that outcome occurring. The probability of being alive after immediate surgery is 0.95. So in our framework, we have assigned utility values of 1 for alive and 0 for dead. So starting at outcome #1, at the chance node, the utility value is $0.95 \times 1 + 0.05 \times 0 = 0.95$. Since these leads directly to the first decision node, the utility expected from immediate operation is 0.95.

If we start at path #2 (i.e. the top branch following the chance node C). The probability of being alive after a surgery due to the tumour growth after the 3-month observation 0.285 (i.e. 0.95×0.3) and the probability of death 0.015 (i.e. 0.05×0.3). The expected utility for this path is then $0.285 \times 1 + 0.015 \times 0 = 0.285$.

It is important to note that there is another decision node (E) embedded in the framework, when we calculate the expected utility value for the middle path from chance node C. Following the above-mentioned method, the expected utility of choosing surgery (path #3) is 0.95 and 0.99 for continuing the observation for another 12 months at the decision note E (path #4). Since one path results in a higher expected utility value 0.99 than the other 0.95, we can ignore path #3 from further consideration and carry back only the utility value of 0.99 further towards the left. When the utility of the orange path is multiplied by the probability of ending up on this path, 0.60, then back at the chance node, the overall utility of this path is 0.594. The expected utility value for path #5 is 0.10. At the decision node, the overall value is now the sum of the total utility of each path emanating from the chance node C, 0.979 (i.e. 0.285 + 0.594 + 0.10).

When this is folded back towards the first decision node, we see that going straight to surgery, we obtain an expected utility value of 0.95, whereas if we waited for 3 months, then the expected utility of this path is 0.979. Since the waiting, gives a higher utility value, we determine that the best decision in this scenario is to wait for 3 months.

Our conclusions in this example are dependent on the values we selected for the probabilities of an event e.g. rate of post-operative deaths and also the desirability of the outcomes e.g. value of 1 for alive and 0 for dead. It is quite apparent that if post-operative mortality was lower than 0.05, then the decision to observe is likely to change. A formal exploration of how the decision will change according to the values of the inputs (the probability of the outcome and utility values associated with the outcome), is call sensitivity analysis and is a fundamental part of CDA. There are a number of ways in which this can be carried out, and an example from the literature demonstrates this.

Management of an Incidentaloma

Brunaud et al., carried out a clinical decision analysis which illustrates the features of a CDA [3]. The questions posed in their study is "What is the optimal management approach to a patient with a non-functioning adrenal "incidentaloma" with no suspicious image characteristics for a malignant adrenal neoplasm, and a tumor size between 4 and 6 cm?" They made clear that this question is one in which there is genuine uncertainty. In cases of tumours greater than 6 cm or those with suspicious features on imaging, there is little difference of opinion, so that the value of investing the effort on a CDA to those scenarios is limited. They provide two alternate decisions (Fig. 2.3), to observe the tumour or proceed to a unilateral laparoscopic adrenalectomy. A fundamental feature of CDA is that the decision to be made is explicitly stated and just as important, the alternative is explicitly stated. A not uncommon scenario in a guideline statement is that some course of action ought to be followed, but without explicitly stating what the alternatives are [4]. There is also an explicit statement of when the decision is to be made; in this case at the time the tumour is initially found. This allows the two alternative of proceeding to resection or waiting.

Next the authors describe how they calculate the expected utilities for each path. They then provide a table (Table 2.1) that lists the probabilities associated with each of the chance nodes which are derived from published studies and their own institutional experience. They include both a baseline value upon which they base the primary analysis and the range of values to be used for sensitivity analysis. They also state the utility values for the three possible outcomes, (1) a new indication for resection during the period of observation, (2) complications after adrenalectomy and (3) being alive during the observation without surgery, which assumed some degree of psychological morbidity associated with the uncertainty of the nature of

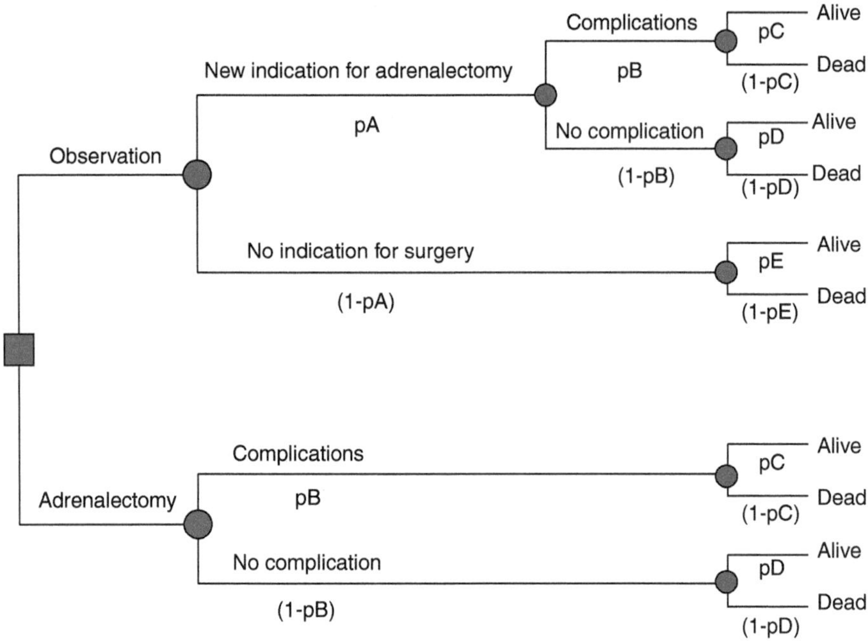

pA: P of developing new indication for adrenalectomy during observation
pB: P of complications from unilateral laparoscopic adrenalectomy
pC: P of being alive after a complicated adrenalectomy
pD: P of being alive after uncomplicated laparoscopic adrenalectomy
pE: P of being alive during observation without surgery

Fig. 2.3 Decision analysis framework for management of non-functional adrenal tumor. From Brunaud et al. [3] with permission

the mass. Since there were no published utility values for the outcomes, they undertook a survey of surgeons to estimate this. From this analysis they came to the conclusion that with the baseline values of the probabilities and utilities, the observation strategy had the highest expected utility. Although it may be reasonable to stop and come to a conclusion, at this point, it is quite clear that their conclusions will be expected to change if the values of the probabilities of the outcomes or the utility values ascribed to the outcomes change. In fact they found that if the complication rate for laparoscopic adrenalectomy was lower, as observed at their own institution, then the resection strategy was the preferred decision. To what extent does the decision change, and is there some value of one of the variables or of a number of variables at which the decision switches from one to another? To answer this question, a threshold analysis may be carried out which is a type of sensitivity analysis. Essentially, one calculates utility values for each value of the probability or utility both individually and as a combination and determines at what value or combination of values the decision changes.

Table 2.1 Values used for calculating probabilities and assigning utilities in the CDA for the management of a non-functioning adrenal tumor

Variables	Baseline (%)	Reported range (%)	Median (year)	Authors
Laparoscopic adrenalectomy				
Morbidity (pB)[a]	7.84	0–11	–	[5,20–27]
Mortality	0.36	0–2	–	
1 – mortality (pC)	99.64	98–100	–	[5,20–24]
Observation				
Indication for adrenalectomy during observation (pA)				
Malignancy	2.95	0–13	4.3	[4,28–34]
Size increase	6.91	0–25	3.6	[2,4,28–30,32,33,35–37]
Hypersecretion	1.19	0–20	2.8	[2,4,28,30,32,33,36–41]
Overall (pA)	3.13	0–25	3.6	
Surgeons questionnaire	68.00	30–90	–	

From Brunaud et al. [3] with permission

[a]Bleeding, wound (early and late), pulmonary, organ injury, gastrointestinal, urinary, thromboembolic, cardiac

An interesting and important finding from this analysis is the sensitivity of the conclusion to the utility value associated with observing the tumour. It was in fact the patient's perspective that had the most impact on which decision was best, but this was the one piece of the analysis which had large uncertainty (i.e. based on subjective, expert opinions). This illustrates very clearly the nature of the statement made in guidelines about the patient's perspectives and illustrates graphically the importance of this in clinical decision making.

Cost Effectiveness

In both individual patient care and in making policy, the role of the costs of different strategies is very important. Cost effectiveness analysis is helpful in addressing this issue. The analytical framework used in cost effectiveness analyses share a lot of similarities as in CDA but where resource utilization and costs are important extra information incorporated in the model. Cost effectiveness is a key piece of evidence to support health policymaking and its importance in clinical decision-making is being recognized. A description of cost effectiveness analysis through modeling is beyond the scope of this chapter.

Conclusion

This chapter was a brief overview of Clinical Decision Analysis. Much like a surgical procedure, the concepts of the procedure may be straightforward, but it is often in the carrying out of the procedures and the details that pose the challenge. However, it is still important to understand the main concepts, as this type of analysis is of great value in practicing evidence-based medicine and in doing the best for our patients.

References

1. Tversky A, Kahneman D. Judgment under uncertainty: heuristics and biases. Science. 1974;185(4157):1124–31. https://doi.org/10.1126/science.185.4157.1124.
2. Weinstein MC, Fineberg HV, Elstein AS, Frazier HS, Neuhauser D, Netura R, McNeil BJ. Clinical decision analysis. Philadelphia: W.B. Saunders; 1980.
3. Brunaud L, Kebebew E, Sebag F, Zarnegar R, Clark OH, Duh Q-Y. Observation or laparoscopic adrenalectomy for adrenal incidentaloma? A surgical decision analysis. Med Sci Monit. 2006;12(9):CR355–62.
4. Neumann I, Akl EA, Vandvik PO, Agoritsas T, Alonso-Coello P, Rind DM, et al. In: Guyatt G, Meade MO, Rennie D, Cook DJ, editors. Users' guides to the medical literature. New York, NY: McGraw-Hill Education; 2014.

Decision-Making from the Surgeon's Perspective

3

Karen Devon

Abstract

Advances in the treatment of endocrine diseases have brought about an array of choices for surgeons and patients. Surgical decision-making involves a clinical recommendation as well as the process of "shared decision-making" in order to reach the best outcome for a particular patient. This first part of this chapter will discuss factors related to surgical recommendations, the use of evidence and the quality of recommendations. The second part will focus on key elements of shared decision and informed consent such as disclosure and understanding, and highlight patient and surgeon factors which affect this process. A model for ethical decision-making that takes into account medical indications, patient preferences, quality of life and contextual features is described. Special issues in surgical decision-making discussed such as genetics, pediatrics, and end-of-life decision-making are also considered.

Keywords

Decision-making · Ethics · Informed consent · Surgery

Introduction

In 1848, Samuel Gross wrote about thyroid surgery: "no honest or sensible surgeon would ever engage in it". Since then the field of endocrine surgery has advanced substantially in terms of knowledge, safety and outcomes. The success of modern

K. Devon
Department of Surgery, University of Toronto, Endocrine Surgical Oncology, Women's College Hospital and University Health Network, Toronto, ON, Canada
e-mail: karen.devon@wchospital.ca

P. Angelos, R. H. Grogan (eds.), *Difficult Decisions in Endocrine Surgery*, Difficult Decisions in Surgery: An Evidence-Based Approach,
https://doi.org/10.1007/978-3-319-92860-9_3

medicine has increased treatment options so greatly that endocrine surgeons are faced with many clinical dilemmas on a daily basis. Resolving these dilemmas is a complex process with several distinct elements, that require attention to the personal and ethical dimensions of care, in addition to biomedical expertise. Good decisions are those where the result is a desired outcome for a particular patient [1] therefore surgical decision-making even when seen from the surgeon's perspective, cannot be discussed without including the patient. There are many definitions of decision-making as applied to surgeons. Likewise, decisions occurs both intra-operatively and peri-operatively, the latter being the focus of this chapter.

While most studies in the literature discuss "surgical decision-making" in reference to specific medical algorithms and indications, we will discuss two aspects of the decision-making process: the clinical recommendation and the practice of 'shared decision-making'. We will also provide a model for ethical decision-making and address special situations that may arise.

The Clinical Recommendation

The principle components of the surgical learning curve, and the focus of training programs, are the ability to operate and the ability to make sounds decisions [1] -also known as 'surgical judgment'. Surgeons reach decisions by collecting biomedical information including signs, symptoms, risk factors, test results, family history and non-biomedical information such as the patient's values. These are then interpreted with the multidimensional knowledge base and experience of the surgeon [2], and dependent on multiple factors.

Factors Influencing Surgeon Recommendations

Francis describes factors influencing clinical decisions (Table 3.1) [2]. These may be surgeon related or outside the control of the surgeon, as well as factors inherent to the decision itself. All of these factors should be acknowledged and optimized in order to achieve the best clinical recommendations. These factors also influence crucial and time-sensitive intra-operative decision-making.

Surgeon 'wisdom' or expertise is acquired and continues well past structured training programs and includes the development of excellent communication skills. Reflective practice may be an important component of developing such expertise [2]. Surgeons should take all opportunities to engage in continuing education through formal programs, colleagues and hands-on experiences. Experience-based knowledge combined with 'surgical-evidence' are the foundations of good clinical recommendations [2]. Surgeon factors also play a crucial role in the "shared decision-making" process and will be elaborated on further in the chapter.

Table 3.1 Factors influencing clinical decision making

Factors outside the control of the surgeon
The physical environment
Noise
Light
Temperature and humidity
Interruptions
The surgical team
Abilities and expertise
Personal interactions
Ability to work as a team
Organizational structures
Resources and facilities
Organizational culture, support and expectations
Need for prioritization
Ethical practices
Surgeon-related factors
Stress
Time pressure
Fatigue
Long working hours
Absence of adequate breaks between periods of work
Sleep deprivation
Illness
Mood and emotional state
Reasoning strategy
Gender
Age
Surgical wisdom
Factors inherent in the decision
Importance of the decision
Time pressure
Irreversibility
Range of options
Limited information on which to base the decision

From Francis DMA. Surgical decision making. ANZ J Surg. 2009;79:886–91; with permission

Application of Evidence

A good recommendation from a surgeon is based on sound knowledge or evidence. Surgeons have a professional obligation to seek the best available evidence related to a clinical problem [3]. The chapters that follow summarize the best evidence available to inform clinical recommendations in endocrine surgery. The application of evidence to medicine is an important skill for the practice of endocrine surgery given the many clinical pathways that are available. However, there are limitations inherent in using such evidence. In surgery there is a paucity of well-designed double-blind, randomized controlled trials, thought to be the gold standard of evidence [2, 4]. For example, in order to obtain evidence on a controversial practice, Carling et al. examined the feasibility of a prospective randomized controlled trial of prophylactic central lymph node dissection in cNO papillary thyroid cancer. They found that prohibitively large sample sizes would be required to for sufficient statistical power to demonstrate significant differences in outcomes [5].

One essential element of evidence-based medicine is assessing the validity of evidence [6, 7] and then applying this to a particular scenario. Aside from gaps described above the quality of trials and meta-analyses are variable. Furthermore, the variability of anatomy and pathology in surgical patients make interpretation and application of evidence particularly difficult [2]. Some evidence does attempt to take into account patient values systems, such as decision analyses and quality of life research, however patients values and desires may be equally as heterogeneous as their biologies. Thus, the concept of 'evidence-based medicine' now includes integration of individual clinical expertise with the best external evidence.

Quality of Recommendations

Poor clinical decisions may have significant impacts to patient and their families, as well as to institutions and the health care system at-large. Consequences may be physical, psychological, financial or medico-legal [2]. Individual surgeons, programs and institutions ought to have systems in place to audit decisions. While this may occur retrospectively, such as during a typical surgical morbidity or mortality conference, utilization of teams to assess and aid with decisions in a prospective manner, such as via a multidisciplinary tumor board, is encouraged.

Shared Decision-Making

The physician of free men "treats their disease by going into things thoroughly from the beginning in a scientific way and takes the patient into confidence. The physician does not give prescriptions until he has won the patient's support and when he has done so, he steadily aims at producing complete restoration to health…" [8, 9].

Now formally recognized as "patient-centered care", good decision-making has always been formed by a strong doctor-patient alliance that is respectful of and responsive to individual patient preferences, needs and values [10]. Some decisions may have clearly superior paths, however most medical options entail multiple combinations of treatments and sequelae and must be made by the patient and physician working as partners towards a common goal [11]. Shared decision-making is the model whereby clinicians, patients and often, other members of the health care team, friends or family, exchange information to reach an optimal decision [11].

Surgeons must respect a patients' autonomy while maintaining ethics principles of beneficence, non-maleficence and justice [9]. Shared decision-making has been increasingly endorsed as an ideal model [12] as it reconciles the demands of patient autonomy with the benefits of paternalism leading to greater trust, compliance, satisfaction and outcomes [9].

Informed Consent

A critical element of shared decision-making is informed consent [12]. This establishes a reciprocal relationship between participants formed by mutual respect and good communication [13, pp. 51–53]. Such a therapeutic alliance is beneficial to the patient as they have realistic expectations about treatment and become more willing to participate in their own care [13, pp. 51–53]. Informed consent ought to be regarded as an ongoing process that occurs between physician (or multidisciplinary team) and patient, rather than signatures on a document [14]. And while in the practice of surgery, the informed consent process often occurs during a distinct episode of care, this need not be the case when decision-making requires and allows for additional time.

Informed consent involves three aspects: disclosure, understanding, and the patient process of deciding [15].

Disclosure

Disclosure involves clear and honest information about a patient's diagnosis and available treatment alternatives, along with the risks and benefits of such interventions including the natural history of the disease without intervention [14]. Several standards for disclosure exist. The first is known as the 'professional community standard' [16; 17, p. 122]. Under this physician-oriented standard a patient should be told what an experienced physician would tell the patient. This standard has been gradually replaced by the 'reasonable person standard' [17, p. 123]. This standard requires that the information given to a patient should be based on what a reasonable patient would need to know about risks, benefits and alternatives in order to make a meaningful decision. However, definitions and agreement on exactly what a "reasonable" patient is has been controversial. A third, more subjective standard, requires tailoring information to a specific patient and is most consistent with the shared decision-making model of care [13, pp. 53–54; 17, p. 123]. Thus, discussions should be tailored to the capacity and preferences of individual patients. Patients should be asked what information they wish to receive as they may wish to limit information such information. Nonetheless, patients might not be able to specific information they need to know based on limited knowledge and thus this standard also has limitations [17, p. 124]. It is not necessary for a surgeon to "force" a patient to hear information that the surgeon deems to be important. Out of respect for autonomy it is vital to avoid altering the frame of reference, known as 'framing', to influence a patient's decision excessively [14; 17, p. 130]. For instance, in discussing the risk of bilateral recurrent laryngeal nerve injury during thyroid surgery, the surgeon might say: "it's possible but I've never seen it happen". This could imply that such a complication will not happen to this patient. A more appropriate description would be that "the risk is extremely low but present". Moreover, surgeons should avoid a particular type of framing refered to as "hanging of the crepe" whereby the gravity of a situation is emphasized in an effort to increase the perception of a successful outcome as attributable to the surgeon while decreasing responsibility for unsuccessful ones [18]. An example of this would be telling a patient that: "parathyroid glands are extremely difficult to find", thus setting the patient up for potential failure, when successful surgery is far more likely.

Understanding

It is the surgeon's responsibility to ensure the patient understands all important aspects of the nature of the decision that is being made including goals, recovery, complications, sequelae [14]. He or she should use appropriate vocabulary and allow and encourage patients to ask questions without fear of repercussions or judgment. It is also critical for surgeons to evaluate and ensure patients' decisional capacities, as well as recognize clinical diseases which may temporarily affect decisional capacity. For example, a patient with hypercalcemia from primary hyperparathyroidism may have cognitive disturbances which affect their understanding and capacity to make informed choices. On occasion, where there are concerns about decision capacity endocrine surgeons may need to involve psychiatry services [5]. When patients are known to have surrogate decision makers, the surrogate should be involved in the shared decision-making and abide by standards discussed further below.

Process of Deciding

Although the patient's preferences are paramount, the surgeon should assist the patient to develop an understanding of the value of different alternatives. Decision aids can be an adjunct that helps patients absorb clinical information and develop and communicate preferences [19]. Surgeons should tailor their recommendations based on better understanding of applicable factors.

Some patients may want more or less role in the decision-making process and this should also be respected [14] including the option of designating an alternate individual to participate in the process. Patients should be given the time and emotional support needed while undergoing the decision process [11] particularly when they are frightened or have just received difficult news about their medical condition.

When a patient chooses a treatment alternative that is less congruent with the surgeon's recommendation the surgeon should not be offended and cannot abandon the patient. They can however express concern and arrange subsequent visits or recommend a second opinion from another surgeon or other professional. Refusal of a recommendation is not in itself evidence of reduced decision-making capacity, and thoughtful questions from the surgeon can clarify the issues and factors relevant to the decision [14].

Patient Factors Affecting Shared Decision-Making

Many factors can affect decisions from the patient's standpoint, including culture, religion, information processing, and financial constraints.

Although cultural and religious issues may come into play and ought to be respected, surgeons should not make any assumptions about an individual patient's preferences based on cultural identity or stated religious group. On occasion, obtaining the patient's permission to invite a leader or respected member of the patient's community into the discussion can be beneficial.

Similarly, patients may seek out alternative or non-traditional forms of therapy. They should be encouraged to share this information with their surgeon so that both obtain a better understanding of the patients' beliefs and goals as well as ensure the safe conduct of medical care. Given that a key component of informed consent and shared decision-making is patient understanding, surgeons should be aware of and account for factors associated with the patients understanding. This may be as simple as information overload, or pre-conceptions from external sources or previous experiences. Furthermore, patients must be free of coercion or manipulation.

Unfortunately, financial constraints are a reality for many patients and play a role in decision-making. Such problems may be even more emphasized in the developing world. Poverty and social determinants of health account for a large variation in health care use [20–22]. Surgeons should make every attempt to mitigate financial factors while bearing them in mind as a significant feature of a patient's decision [13, pp. 161–223].

Surgeon Factors Affecting Shared Decision-Making

Wilson et al. surveyed of general surgeons including endocrine surgeons and measured the 'tendency to operate' in multiple clinical scenarios. Variation was found based on age, gender, race, specialty, and method of financial compensation [23]. Furthermore, a surgeon's training may cause additional bias regarding medical options and surgeons may vary in comfort level performing certain procedures [3]. For instance, a surgeon trained in retroperitoneal adrenalectomy from the posterior approach might consider this the "best" and most highly recommended approach, particularly if they do not feel comfortable with other approaches. When a surgeon knows of alternative options but is not able to provide them he or she is obligated to inform or refer the patient if that is appropriate.

Surgeons may be subject to other potential conflicts of interest. These include financial pressures and industry relationships, the obligation to train students, involvement in research and conflicts with other professionals. While surgeons do earn an income, they must ensure ethical conduct with respect to choice of treatment when there is clinical equipoise, irrespective of their own interests [3, 24]. American Thyroid Association Clinical and Professional Ethics Guidelines suggests disclosure of all potential or perceived industry relationships in order to maintain public trust [24].

Some surgeons are engaged in the teaching of students, residents or fellows. Shared decision-making necessitates that the surgeon disclose trainee involvement to the patient and that the patient understands the trainee's role in his or her care. Such involvement should not be presumed simply by way of practicing in part of a teaching institution [14].

Surgeons may be also lead or be involved in research studies. Research must be clearly distinguished from clinical treatment [13, pp. 203–211]. Explicit consent for research and innovation is critical in order to avoid therapeutic misconception-a misconception that participation in a trial is therapeutic in nature [17, p. 129]. All clinical research ought to abide by established research ethics standards. When possible, enrollment should be driven by a trained research assistant who is not directly involved in a patient's clinical care. When innovative treatments are recommend they require appropriate oversight and patients should understand that the treatment is not standard. Finally, clinical judgments between professionals in the same or different specialties can vary and lead to conflict. The surgeon's goal should not be to convince a patient of a particular point of view, but rather to strengthen the patient's autonomy in decision making by providing accurate clear information in an honest fashion [14]. In some cases, it may be helpful for all parties involved to meet in order to clarify issues and ensure patient understanding.

Model for Ethical Decision-Making

Jonsen et al. describe a practical approach to ethical decisions using a four-box model. This model encompasses the issues described above and takes into account Medical Indications, Patient Preferences, Quality of Life and Contextual Features (Table 3.2). It may be useful to use these topics to obtain a comprehensive picture of: diagnostic and therapeutic interventions being used to evaluate the medical problem, the choices of the patient or of those authorized to speak for the patient, features of a patient's life insofar as they are pertinent to medical decisions, and family, social, institutional, financial and legal setting within which the decision takes place [13].

Special Situations in Decision-Making

Genomic Issues

The use of genetic information to make medical decisions and tailor treatments to individual patients is becoming an increasingly important part of endocrine surgery. Specifically, genetic screening for hereditary syndromes and decisions about prophylactic surgery bring about additional challenges to decision making. Psychosocial barriers to genetic screening must be recognized and patients should be advised by certified genetic counselors [24]. Informed consent will be time consuming and must include the handling of incidental findings and false-positive or false-negative results as well as potential implications for family members [24, 25]. Once tested,

Table 3.2 A practical approach to ethical decisions using a four-box model

Medical indications	*Patient references*
The principles of beneficence and nonmaleficence 1. What is the patient's medical problem? Is the problem acute? chronic? critical? reversible? emergent? terminal? 2. What are the goals of treatment? 3. In what circumstances are medical treatments not indicated? 4. What are the probabilities of success of various treatment options? 5. In sum, how can this patient be benefited by medical and nursing care, and how can harm be avoided?	The principle of respect for autonomy 1. Has the patient been informed of benefits and risks, understood this information, and given consent? 2. Is the patient mentally capable and legally competent, and is there evidence of incapacity? 3. If mentally capable, what preferences about treatment is the patient stating? 4. If incapacitated, has the patient expressed prior preferences? 5. Who is the appropriate surrogate to make decisions for the incapacitated patient? 6. Is the patient unwilling or unable to cooperate with medical treatment? If so, why?
Quality of life	*Contextual features*
The principles of beneficence and nonmaleficence and respect for autonomy 1. What are the prospects, with or without treatment, for a return to normal life, and what physical, mental and social deficits might the patient experience even if treatment succeeds? 2. On what grounds can anyone judge that some quality of life would be undesirable for a patient who cannot make or express such a judgment? 3. Are there biases that might prejudice the provider's evaluation of the patient's quality of life? 4. What ethical issues arise concerning improving or enhancing a patient's quality of life? 5. Do quality-of-life assessments raise any questions regarding changes in treatment plans, such as forgoing life-sustaining treatment? 6. What are plans and rationale to forgo life-sustaining treatment? 7. What is the legal and ethical status of suicide?	The principles of justice and fairness 1. Are there professional, interprofessional, or business interests that might create conflicts of interest in the clinical treatment of patients? 2. Are there parties other than clinicians and patient, such as family members, who have an interest in ethical decisions? 3. What are the limits imposed on patient confidentiality by the legitimate interests of third parties? 4. Are there financial factors that create conflicts of interest in clinical decisions? 5. Are there problems of allocation of scarce health resources that might affect clinical decisions? 6. Are there religious issues that might influence clinical decisions? 7. What are the legal issues that might affect clinical decisions? 8. Are there considerations of clinical research and education that might affect clinical decisions? 9. Are there issues of public health and safety that affect clinical decisions? 10. Are there conflicts of interest within institutions and organizations (e.g., hospitals) that may affect clinical decisions and patient welfare?

Jonsen AR, Siegler M, Winslade WJ. Clinical ethics: a practical approach to ethical discussions in clinical medicine. 7th ed. New York: McGraw-Hill Medical; 2010; with permission

the threshold for recommending prophylactic surgery is variable and should be individualized based on several factors including: risk of disease (gene penetrance), age of onset, risks of surgery, alternative screening, and treatment options [25]. Guidelines for syndromes such as multiple endocrine neoplasia, should be used whenever available [26]. Testing in children brings about unique ethical challenges including timing and reporting of adult onset diseases in patients who are not able to provide informed consent [25]. The American College of Medical Genetics and American Academy of Pediatrics states that "diagnostic genetic testing should be driven by the best interest of the child and that carrier screening and pre-symptomatic testing of children at risk for adult-onset diseases should be deferred until the child reaches maturity [27, 28].

Pediatric Patients

Notwithstanding issues regarding genetic testing, pediatric patients may require endocrine surgery. Parents generally act as surrogates for pediatric patients however depending on age and maturity, children may begin to express their preferences. It is important to assess how reasonable and relevant these preferences are [13, pp. 51–65]. Parents are expected to act upon best interests of the child however in some instances this is unclear or disputed. In such cases a review by an ethics committee and on occasion recourse to the legal system may be required [13, pp. 80–87].

Surrogate Decision-Making

Important decisions may need to be made for patients who are unable to communicate desires about care, necessitating surrogates to speak on their behalf. Decisional capacity should be assessed during the informed consent and shared decision-making processes. Some patients may have a priori designated surrogates or durable powers of attorney for care, however in many jurisdictions there are legal statues that dictate who should be the surrogate decision-maker based on the relationship with the patient.

Several standards guide surrogate decision-makers. The first is called 'substituted judgment'. Substituted judgment dictates that when patient's preferences are known, the surrogate must use knowledge of these preferences to guide decisions [13, pp. 88–90]. The second is called the 'best interest standard'. When a patient's preferences are unknown, the surrogate must promote the best interest of the patient [13, pp. 88–90]. Best interests may not always be clear such as in the case of advanced anaplastic cancer, whereby there may be the ability to prolong life in the short term, however a patient's quality of life may decline substantially. A newer proposed model, the 'substituted interest' standard integrates both a patient's prior values into a decision about what might be in their best interests even when exact preferences are not known [29].

Unexpected Intraoperative Findings

Situations may arise when an unexpected intra-operative finding may require the surgeon make a value-based decision. For instance, a surgeon may, based on new pathology information confirming malignancy might consider performing a total thyroidectomy rather than a thyroid lobectomy for a particular patient. Ideally, scenarios that might arise in the course of an operation are addressed during the informed consent process however this is not always the case in practice. Decisions should take into all above factors however if time allows, the surgeon should not hesitate to consult with a colleague about the dilemma. Furthermore, the surgeon might consult with the patients' surrogate decision-maker, who should be determined and recorded in advance for all patients undergoing surgery.

End-of-Life Issues

Endocrine surgeons may be faced with guiding patients through difficult decision making at the end of life in the context of patients suffering from aggressive thyroid or adrenal cancers. Good decision-making includes advanced care planning where the following issues are discussed: prognosis, treatment options, code status and preferences regarding nutrition hydration and intubation, palliative care, and hospice care [24]. Again, it is often very worthwhile to involve other specialists and team members early on such as those who provide palliative care.

Allocation of Resources

Although surgeons ought to base clinical care decision on the individual patient with whom they have a direct fiduciary relationship, it is acknowledged that a large share of health care costs are controlled by physicians through medical decision making. Patients have a right to be informed of costs of treatments and management alternatives given that they now bear an increasing portion of these [13, pp. 186–187]. These costs may have negative financial and societal consequences if decisions are not made well [23].

Conclusion

In 1927 Peabody wrote: "The practice of medicine in its broadest sense includes the whole relationship of the physician with his patient. It is art, based to an increasing extent on the medical sciences.... The physician who attempts to take care of a patient while he neglects [emotional life] is as unscientific as the investigator who neglects to control...his experiment. The good physician knows his patients through and through... One of the essential qualities of the clinician is interest in humanity" [30]. With the expanding array of biomedical choices in patient care this may be even more relevant today. The Institute of Medicine calls patient-centered care a fundamental approach to improving the quality of health care [10]. Thus, decision-making from the surgeon's perspective must be one that emphasized not only biomedical expertise but is based on a model of shared decision-making in partnership with our patients. "For the secret of the care of the patient is in caring for the patient" [30].

References

1. Hall JC, Ellis C, Hamdorf J. Surgeons and cognitive processes. Br J Surg. 2003;90:10–6.
2. Francis DMA. Surgical decision making. ANZ J Surg. 2009;79:886–91.
3. Bernstein M, Jain VK. Ethical decision-making. In: Ammar A, Bernstein M, editors. Neurosurgical ethics in practice: value-based medicine. Berlin: Springer; 2014.
4. Horng S, Miller F. Is placebo surgery unethical? N Engl J Med. 2002;347:137–9.
5. Carling T, Carty SE, Ciarleglio MM, Cooper DS, Doherty GM, Kim LT, et al. American Thyroid Association design and feasibility of a prospective randomized controlled trial of prophylactic central lymph node dissection for papillary thyroid carcinoma. Thyroid. 2012;22:237–44.
6. Guyatt G, Haynes B, Jaeschke R, Cook DJ, Green L, Naylor CD, et al. Users' guides to the medical literature XXV. Evidence-based medicine: principles for applying the users' guides to patient care. J Am Med Assoc. 2000;284:1290–6.
7. Lacaine F. Evidence-based medicine in surgical decision making. World J Surg. 2005;29:588–91.
8. Plato. The laws. Taylor AE, translator. London: Dent; 1934. p. 104–5.
9. Siegler M. Searching for moral certainty in medicine: a proposal for a new model of the doctor-patient encounter. Bull N Y Acad Med. 1981;57:56–69.
10. National Research Council. Crossing the quality chasm: a new health system for the 21st century. Washington, DC: National Academies Press; 2001.
11. Barry MJ, Edgman-Levitan S. Shared decision making – the pinnacle of patient-centred care. N Engl J Med. 2012;366:780–1.
12. President's Commission for the Study of Ethical Problems in Medicine and Biomedical and Behavioral Research. Making health care decisions. A report on the ethical and legal implications of informed consent in the patient-practitioner relationship, vol. 1; 1982. p. 31–9.
13. Jonsen AR, Siegler M, Winslade WJ. Clinical ethics: a practical approach to ethical discussions in clinical medicine. 7th ed. New York: McGraw-Hill Medical; 2010.
14. McCullough LB, Jones JW, Brody BA. Informed consent: autonomous decision making of the surgical patient. In: McCullough LB, Jones JW, Brody BA, editors. Surgical ethics. New York: Oxford; 1998. p. 15–37.
15. Faden RR, Beauchamp TL. A history and theory of informed consent. New York: Oxford; 1986.
16. Rosovsky R. Consent to treatment: a practical guide. Boston: Little, Brown; 1984.
17. Beauchamp TL, Childress JF. Principles of biomedical ethics. 6th ed. New York: Oxford; 2009.
18. Siegler M. Pascal's wager and the hanging of crepe. N Engl J Med. 1975;23:853–7.
19. Stacey D, Bennett CL, Barry MJ, Col NF, Eden KB, Holmes-Rovner M, et al. Decision aids for people facing health treatment or screening decisions. Cochrane Database Syst Rev. 2011;10:CD001431.
20. Billings J, Zeitel L, Lukomnik J, Blank L, Newman AE, Carey TS. Impact of socioeconomic status on hospital use in New York City. Health Aff (Millwood). 1993;12:162–73.
21. Hofer TP, Wolfe RA, Tedeschi PJ, McMahon PJ. Use of community versus individual socioeconomic data in predicting variation in hospital use. Health Serv Res. 1998;33:243–59.

22. Cooper RA, Cooper MA, McGinley EL, Fan X, Rosenthal JT. Poverty, wealth and health care utilization: a geographic assessment. J Urban Health. 2012;89:828–47.
23. Wilson NP, Wilson FP, Neuman M, Epstein A, Bell R, Armstrong K, et al. Determinants of surgical decision making: a national survey. Am J Surg. 2013;206:970–8.
24. Rosenthal SM, Angelos P, Cooper DS, Fassler C, Finder SG, Hays MT, et al. Clinical and professional ethics guidelines for the practice of thyroidology. Thyroid. 2013;23:1203–10.
25. Devon KM, Lerner-Ellis JP, Ganai S, Angelos P. Ethics and genomic medicine, how to navigate decisions in surgical oncology. J Surg Oncol. 2015;111:1–6.
26. Rosenthal MS, Diekema DS. Pediatric ethics guidelines for hereditary medullary thyroid cancer. Int J Pediatr Endocrinol. 2011;2011:847603.
27. Green RC, Berg JS, Grody WW, et al. ACMG recommendations for reporting of incidental findings in clinical exome and genome sequencing. Genet Med. 2013;15:565–74.
28. American College of Medical Genetics and Genomics. Incidental findings in clinical genomics: a clarification. Genet Med. 2013;15:664–6.
29. Sulmasy DP, Snyder JD. Substituted interests and best judgments. An integrated model of surrogate decision making. J Am Med Assoc. 2010;304:1946–7.
30. Peabody FW. The care of the patient. J Am Med Assoc. 1927;88:877–82.

Involving Patients in Difficult Decisions About Having Surgery

4

Joshua A. Hemmerich†, Kellie Van Voorhis, and Mark K. Ferguson

Abstract

There is increasing involvement of patients participating in difficult decisions related to their health interventions, like whether or not to have surgery. Such patients must be informed about their treatment options and the risks and benefits that go along with each so that they can apply their preferences in making the decision. This process can be problematic in surgical clinics where time with patients is limited. Helping surgeons educate patients and incorporate the patient's preferences into the treatment choice is a major challenge that requires research and guidance.

Keywords

Shared decision making · Surgery · Patient education

Traditional healthcare was characterized by physician paternalism in guiding patients towards what treatment the physician determined was best to address the patient's condition [1]. Healthcare and decision making about treatments is evolving towards a practice referred to as Shared Decision Making (SDM), especially for problems for which there is no single standard of care. SDM requires the

† (Deceased)

J. A. Hemmerich · K. Van Voorhis
Department of Medicine, The University of Chicago, Chicago, IL, USA

M. K. Ferguson (✉)
Department of Surgery, The University of Chicago, Chicago, IL, USA
e-mail: mferguso@bsd.uchicago.edu

P. Angelos, R. H. Grogan (eds.), *Difficult Decisions in Endocrine Surgery*, Difficult Decisions in Surgery: An Evidence-Based Approach,
https://doi.org/10.1007/978-3-319-92860-9_4

participation of both the physician and the informed patient. This paradigm shift is expanding rapidly owing to the availability of patient-oriented information on the internet and through social media.

The change extends beyond the primary care setting, where patients and physicians often have a well-established relationship, to include surgical clinics, where the surgeon is charged with relatively limited, short-term care of the patient [2]. With more patients seeking an active role in SDM for difficult decisions, failing to ensure patients are sufficiently informed when taking part in SDM is likely to have negative, dramatic, and irreversible consequences in surgical care.

In decisions where relevant evidence is limited and patient values and goals can be diverse, informed patient preferences should be incorporated into making the choice. Consequently, this requires the sharing of information with the patient so that they are equipped with a good understanding of their situations and options. If the growing demand for SDM is to be met and executed appropriately, surgeons must be prepared to inform patients and foster healthy SDM.

What Is Shared Decision Making?

SDM is a clinical approach in which informed patients actively share in making choices about their own care with their physicians. SDM is specifically required when, due to limitations of medical evidence, none of the options is considered a true standard of care. For some health problems requiring SDM, there are trade-offs between options. Options are linked to various probabilistic outcomes that make the right decision reliant on patients' preferences [3]. The SDM process is a compound and ordered one that typically takes place in a face-to-face consultation between the patient and physician. The goal is to first deliver the important information and ensure its comprehension, then deliberate over the options to settle on the preferred course of action.

Driving this transition from traditional paternalism towards SDM is the evolution of the physician-patient relationship towards a more collaborative model. It likely reflects changes in population demography as more paternalistic pre-baby boomers pass away and are replaced by later generation autonomous healthcare consumers, but it also receives pro-active international advocacy from many medical care providers, researchers, and ethicists as a moral imperative.

Call for Shared Decision Making

The practice of SDM has gained proponents, critics and researchers from all around the world over the decades. An international panel of medical experts convening in Salzburg in 2010 came to a consensus and released the Salzburg Statement on Shared Decision Making declaring that the implementation of effective SDM would make the single most profound improvement to healthcare quality [4]. The statement included instructions for health policy makers as well as physicians and patients. It asserted that physicians have an ethical imperative to practice SDM with patients, engage in two way communication, field and answer patients' questions, and solicit patients' values and personal preferences. Physicians should also provide accurate and individually tailored information about options and the uncertainties, benefits, and harms of treatment options. They must allow patients sufficient time to consider their options and recognize that most decisions need not be made immediately. The Salzburg Statement implored patients to recognize their right to participate, to voice their concerns, questions, and values, and seek out and utilize the highest quality information available [4].

Survey data indicate that patients express a desire for SDM, but that significant variance still exists in patient preferences for decisional control, as some patients still desire the physician to take a guiding role [5]. A qualitative interview study indicated that older frail patients expressed a desire for information but not necessarily to have input into the treatment choice [6]. Cancer patients often desire to have important information even when they indicated that they don't prefer a very active role in settling on the treatment choice. Although there will continue to be an overall increasing desire for information and continuing evolution towards more patients wanting to be active participants in SDM, multiple decision making styles will persist.

Meeting the Requirement of Informed Patients in SDM

SDM is said to be performed effectively when patients accurately comprehend all of the necessary information regarding their options, identify their values and preferences, and determine which treatment choice gives them the best odds of realizing their goal [7]. Having a more equal informational footing, the patient and physician can often come to an agreement about what treatment best fits an individual patient's health state preferences and tolerance for risks, but if an agreement is not struck, the patient's preferences should ultimately prevail [4].

In much of the SDM literature, the "important information" is only vaguely if ever defined, but it is to some degree specific to the diagnosis and available treatment options. When considering surgery, it is important that the patient know the essential information at the critical time because this treatment cannot be discontinued and is irreversible. This is a serious concern with older patients who are observed to take different strategies in decision making and bias their attention in ways that younger patients do not [8].

Unfortunately, nationally representative survey data suggest that patients do not know the relevant information about a disease, prognosis and available options at multiple important points in care [9]. As a result, an entire decision support aid movement has started with the mission of developing and verifying the quality of tools intended to improve patient knowledge, including tools relevant to surgery [10, 11]. Many of these tools are intended to avoid ineffective SDM participation by uninformed or confused patients that could lead to treatment choices that do not match the patient's preferences and goals.

Several barriers to patient participation in SDM, which all could jeopardize patient education, have been identified and include dealing with multiple professionals unfamiliar with their preferences, diverse treatment strategies among physicians, fast patient turnover in hospitals, stressed medical personnel, and communication barriers [6]. All of these factors are risks that hinder the communication between patients and surgeons and contribute to leaving patients in a state of poor comprehension.

Impact of SDM on Clinical Outcomes

Currently, the downstream consequences for succeeding or failing to practice good SDM are not well-documented or understood. The rationale is that if a patient is to express their values, goals, and preferences and work with the physician to choose the treatment option that best fits, they must have an accurate model of the problem in their mind. There is some evidence that the quality of SDM is predictive of patient-centered, clinical and care-cost outcomes. Decision conflict is a construct that largely reflects how satisfied a patient is about their treatment decision shortly after making it and usually prior to fully realizing the outcome. There is debate about the tenability and value of lowering patients' decision conflict [12], but helping patients feel secure and confident in their treatment choice will benefit overall satisfaction with care.

Although, the ethics of SDM should make it immune to cost considerations, the potential to lower or raise costs is of growing interest. Good SDM could improve satisfaction and functional outcomes, but poorly executed SDM could disproportionately increase costs and worsen clinical outcomes, satisfaction with care, and quality of life. Patients are unlikely to be as influenced by financial incentives as much as physicians often are, but it is not a certainty how SDM will influence the cost of care until more appropriate and longitudinal data are available. Some theories have been proposed as to how SDM might lower costs, and one in particular, costs of litigation, is highly relevant to surgery. Some data indicate that it is health care professionals' style and not the content of their communication that predicts litigation. There is evidence that failures of SDM such as devaluing patient or family views, delivering information poorly, and failing to understand the patient's perspective of the problem were predictive of litigation [13–15]. Improving patient comprehension and participation in SDM could lower the high rate of litigation in surgery, and therefore potentially decrease health care costs.

The Need for SDM in Surgical Care

The global population is growing older because there are more people who are living to an older age. The U.S. population over age 65 is estimated to increase from 40 million in 2010 to 88 million in 2050 [16]. Surgeons deliberate over details, including patient age and frailty. They take into account the characteristics of the patient, their diagnosis, and the risks associated with surgery, and then formulate a recommendation about whether or not having surgery is the best course of action. Although there are professional and financial biases pushing surgeons to recommend surgery, they recognize when a patient is not an ideal surgical candidate and that it might be advisable to consider other options.

When presenting to a surgery clinic for a condition that can be treated surgically, patients are regularly evaluated on their surgical candidacy. Although surgery is quite common for some conditions, the decision about having surgery is not obvious when the patient is at higher risk for complications or less likely to benefit from resection. Without additional concerns, surgery is often preferred because it is definitive and is associated with improved quality of life and decreased mental anguish. However, the immediate and long-term risks associated with surgery provide reason for pause, and more thorough pre-surgical assessment reveals that not all patients prove to be good surgical candidates.

Surgical evaluation often involves assessment of physiologic performance thresholds that predict good immediate surgical outcomes, but lower scores are not prohibitive, and the clinical complexity and diversity of patients has made it intractable to identify criterion values below which the surgical risk level should be considered excessive for all patients. In addition, some operations result in important long-term functional impairment that is permanent, and communicating how such impairments affect quality of life is often challenging.

There are often alternatives to surgery, including medical therapy or radiation therapy, depending on the condition. Some patients may simply be observed if their condition doesn't require immediate intervention, and when intervention ultimately is warranted the treatment options may be more clear to both the patient and the surgeon.

Many of the data upon which treatment decisions are based are from studies that did not include random assignment and that under-represented specific populations such as older patients and women. Consequently, there are insufficient data to provide guidelines for a diverse patient population that presents a complex array of variables and co-morbid conditions.

Problems with SDM and Surgery

The claim that patients are to be informed participants in SDM brings new challenges for both patients and their physicians because appropriate training and infrastructure for good SDM has largely not been put into place. As well, patients are usually not prepared to get the most out of their face-to-face time with the surgeon. Many patients are already predisposed for or against surgery prior to their initial consultation with a surgeon. This may be a result of their conversations with non-surgical specialists, family influences, personal biases, or misinformation. Many patients with a diagnosis of cancer are predisposed to surgery even if evidence demonstrates that surgery is not their best treatment option [17].

Older patients are likely to have greater difficulty participating in SDM for multiple reasons. Older people represent a more diverse population than their younger counterparts because of the prevalence of a wide variety of medical conditions and physical functioning. Some older patients have a combination of medical conditions to be managed and an array of medications carrying various risks and side-effects. As the large influx of older patients floods into surgical clinics, these surgeons will be faced with tremendous challenges of delivering appropriate treatment to a diverse patient population, for which there are few data to guide treatment choices.

Patient Clinical Complexity

Many factors can increase surgical risk and render the decision about whether or not to have surgery more difficult. When the patient is not otherwise healthy, but instead has significant co-morbid health conditions or significantly diminished cardio-pulmonary function, they are less likely to benefit and are at higher risk for adverse outcomes. Outcomes can be expected to be worse in patients with more co-morbid burden [18], and scoring systems have been developed that demonstrate the relationship of cumulative deficits to adverse outcomes [19]. Advanced age itself has become a difficult issue in surgical decisions as people are living longer and the population of advanced age adults is one of diverse health. Some patients of advanced age are robust and highly functional, while others have difficulty with day to day endeavors and are vulnerable to further degradations of function and looming mortality.

There is a potentially important impact on surgical outcomes of the widely-recognized but poorly understood geriatric syndrome of physiological frailty [20–22]. Surgical clinics are becoming increasingly adept at assessing patient frailty through assessment of physical and cognitive factors. Surgeons also put the patient to the "eyeball test" regarding their fitness for surgery, assessing the patient's surgical candidacy more intuitively and beyond what is captured in traditional pre-surgical evaluations, but much remains to be learned about the impact of frailty on surgical outcomes and how to predict it [23].

There is no clear criterion cutoff for any pre-surgical or physical evaluation that expressly prohibits sending a patient to surgery and the available published data are not of sufficient quality to set sound practice guidelines for a clinically diverse patient population. The process of assessing risk and probable outcomes for imperfect surgical candidates is rather fuzzy and speculative and, even with information on frailty, there remains a high amount of uncertainty regarding an individual patient's fate. Consequently, without strict guidelines, SDM is called for so that patients know that their options lead to uncertain outcomes, but that there is information about their own surgical fitness worth knowing when deciding on treatment.

Difficulties in Patient Comprehension

Patients are never standing on the same ground as surgeons regarding foundational knowledge about disease and surgery. A substantial barrier to implementing effective SDM is helping patients understand the important facts about their disease and treatment options so that they are accurately informed at the time that they are participating in the decision making process. The devil is in the details because patients must know how their own clinical characteristics might impact the perioperative risks and probabilities of different outcomes. A verbatim detailed comprehension of risk statistics appears to be neither necessary nor sufficient to guide decisions of physicians or patients if they do not derive the proper meaning [24, 25]. Educational barriers are important obstacles to patient comprehension [26]. What is important is that patients understand what can be expected to happen if the disease goes untreated, what options are available to them to combat the disease, the goals of each treatment, the advantages and disadvantages of those options, and the uncertainty inherent in all. This is not always feasible for surgeons to convey or patients to comprehend [27].

Non-demented older patients process information differently and sometimes implement strategies that are unlike those used by their younger counterparts. As cognitive abilities change over the life span, there is sometimes a shift towards emotion-based information that can impact risk perception and decision making [8, 28]. Older adults often use religious coping for health related stressors, and that coping can come in positive or negative forms, such that they can either alleviate or bring on psychological morbidity [29]. However, it is not clear what impact religious thinking has on the treatment decisions of patients considering risky, but potentially curable, surgical treatment options with varying risk and promise.

Cancer patients deciding about surgery sometimes hold beliefs that contradict evidence-based medicine and can potentially misguide their decisions. In surgical oncology, some patients believe that cancer will spread during the surgery if the cancer, "hits the air" [30]. This belief is found to be retrospectively predictive of the decision to forego surgery [31] and it was found to be widespread among a national sample of healthy survey respondents [32]. It is clear that patients' abilities to process information and the mental representations that they ultimately construct can make a big difference in which choice they make about treatment.

Surgical Practice

The traditional practice of surgery might also provide barriers to effectively satisfying the requirement of an informed patient in SDM. Ultimately, the goal of all surgeons is to do the best that they can for their patients. However, this requires separating out the often influential institutional and financially-driven goals to more clearly determine what is preferred by the patient. It is likely that the professional culture of surgery has worked against the adoption of SDM as common practice. Surgeons focus on creating a feeling of confidence and optimism in their patients, which is somewhat at odds with delivering the "cold hard facts" and sometimes troubling risk information [2].

Surgeons strive to maintain an optimistic stance regarding the treatment that they provide and they often refer to an operation that removes all of the known cancer cells as a "cure" [1, 33]. This is thought to be integral part to the surgeon-patient relationship because putting patients into a positive state of mind is important to maximize hopes of a good outcome. The surgeon addresses the pre-surgical goal of comforting and convincing the patient that she or he is in good hands in the operating room and works to cultivate an optimistic attitude about surgery. The operation is typically performed only in cases in which the surgeon believes that it is justifiable, given the patients level of surgical risk, and the patient agrees to do what the surgeon believes is best. However, eliciting optimism in patients is difficult to balance with delivering important information about risk, uncertainty, or trade-offs that might be viewed as unfavorable by the patient in order to allow them to be fully informed participants.

Additionally, surgeons have other incentives to make specific choices [33]. There is little gain accrued when a patient is referred to radiation oncology, but surgeons receive financial incentives for patients going to the operating room [1]. Many factors cast doubt that popular current practices in surgical clinics effectively help patients to be informed and to share in difficult decisions about whether or not to undergo. Many of these motivations make assisting the patient in SDM a secondary concern, and even at odds with some of the surgeon's goals.

The Way Forward

It will become increasingly important for surgical clinic staff to be able to effectively educate patients on the important information and engage in SDM with patients, as it becomes the prevailing practice of healthcare. With a growing number of older, more clinically complex patients presenting to surgery clinics, some changes to surgical care practices will be necessary. These changes include a premium put on identification of patients' informational needs and desire for participation, well-designed external patient education resources, and decision support that is integrated into the individual patient's surgical consultation.

Surgeons should ascertain what level of involvement each of their patients want in the decision making process. Even when an older, sicker or frailer patient desires a passive role in SDM, the surgeon should take account of the patient's preferences and risk tolerances for different outcomes. For patients wishing to provide input into the choice, participation in SDM involves first education, confirming that they comprehend the essential information about their cancer diagnosis and treatment options, and inviting them to express their desires. Participation by an uninformed patient can be counterproductive and lead to choices that are a poor fit for patients' goals or leave them poorly prepared and in the dark about what lies ahead.

As difficult as it is to share such information, a patient should know the prognosis of their disease and the approximate time-frame in which it can be expected to advance and take their life. They should be told that there are options other than surgery, and that these might be worth exploring before making a choice, especially when they are not ideal surgical candidates. They should also know what treatment side-effects and health states are possible results from different treatments. A patient who wishes to eradicate their cancer in hopes of living as long as possible must be knowingly willing to accept a comparatively higher risk of treatment-related mortality and lasting morbidity. Such patients might choose to have surgery even if they are at a somewhat higher risk for complications or adverse outcomes because they desire what gives them the best hope of long-term survival. Conversely, a patient who believes that their remaining life-expectancy is too short to benefit from a high risk treatment offering a potential cure (5-year survival), should understand that they need not accept the risk of surgically-associated mortality and morbidities to do something to combat the malignancy, and instead could pursue radiation therapy which could slow the cancer's advancement and better preserve healthy lung tissue.

Further research is needed to understand SDM in surgery and how to improve and support it. The current theories of SDM and the instrumentation used to measure this process have been developed and used largely in primary care and, to a lesser degree, shown to be appropriate in oncology [34]. These instruments might not be well-tuned to measure and assess SDM or patient comprehension in surgical contexts and thus might have limited value in understanding the challenge that surgical professionals face when educating and sharing with their patients.

More research is needed to fully understand how to more reliably and consistently meet the unique decision support needs of older, clinically complex patients faced with a decision about curative surgery as they are likely to differ from those of patients in a primary care or medical oncology setting. The relatively short-term doctor patient relationship in surgical clinics, the trust required for effectively delivering surgical consultation, the high-risk/high-reward prospects of surgery, and the relative urgency with which surgical patients must be made informed, all make SDM a more difficult endeavor for surgical specialists than primary care physicians or even oncologists,

The specifics of each kind of surgery are important to SDM. There is limited support available for higher surgical risk early-stage cancer patients. The majority of the decision research that has examined SDM in surgical oncology has focused on breast cancer patients. A formal review of 25 empirical articles published between 1986 and 2006 on breast cancer patients making surgical decisions report that patients' information needs were consistent and ranked (in order) were: chances for a cure, stage of disease, and treatment options [35, 36]. Patient age and education predicted information needs and source use [37]. However, some research has examined patient-centered factors that predict a choice regarding surgery and shows that negative perceptions of the patient-physician interaction on a communication scale importantly influences patients' decisions [31]. More research and development of sound SDM support aids and patient education are required to meet the needs for the growing population of older and clinically diverse patients deciding about surgery.

For the time being, surgeons should strive to inform the patients presenting to their clinic that there is no standard of care and that multiple courses of action are justifiable. They should also ascertain the degree to which each patient wishes to actively weigh options and participate in making the choice. As in all areas of health care, physicians should express an eager willingness to answer any questions the patient has, allow them time to think over surgery and other options, and permit them to explore information in greater detail before making a decision.

Summary

Patients' desired role in difficult decisions, such as whether or not to undergo curative cancer resection when deemed to be less than ideal surgical candidates, continues to shift towards active and informed participation in SDM with the physician. This change brings profound challenges to a specialty already overtaxed on time and resources because good SDM requires that patients are accurately informed at the time of sharing in the decision. They must understand options, uncertainties, risks and potential tradeoffs. Currently, there appear to be significant risks that patients presenting to a surgical clinic are not accurately informed and have misconceptions that might steer them away from a treatment that might suit their goals and preferences. Further research can help to illuminate the problems in SDM for surgery and how to solve them. It is likely that the burden of preparing patients for effective SDM in surgical clinics will have to be shared with professionals other than the surgeons because the surgical clinics are too limited. For now, surgeons should be aware of the importance of striving to maximize patients' understanding about their disease and treatment options so that the patients' values and preferences guide a treatment choice that is right for them.

References

1. Katz P. The scalpel's edge: the culture of surgeons. Needham Heights, MA: Allyn and Bacon; 1999.
2. Hollingham R. Blood and guts: a history of surgery. 1st U.S. ed. New York: Thomas Dunne/St. Martin's; 2009. p. 319.
3. No Authorship. Taking shared decision making more seriously. Lancet. 2011;377(9768):784.
4. Salzburg Global Seminar. Salzburg statement on shared decision making. BMJ. 2011;342:d1745.
5. Singh JA, Sloan JA, Atherton PJ, Smith T, Hack TF, Huschka MM, et al. Preferred roles in treatment decision making among patients with cancer: a pooled analysis of studies using the Control Preferences Scale. Am J Manag Care. 2010;16(9):688–96.
6. Ekdahl AW, Andersson L, Friedrichsen M. "They do what they think is the best for me." Frail elderly patients' preferences for participation in their care during hospitalization. Patient Educ Couns. 2010;80(2):233–40.
7. Elwyn G, Miron-Shatz T. Deliberation before determination: the definition and evaluation of good decision making. Health Expect. 2010;13(2):139–47.
8. Peters E, Hess TM, Västfjäll D, Auman C. Adult age differences in dual information processes: implications for the role of affective and deliberative processes in older adults' decision making. Perspect Psychol Sci. 2007;2(1):1–23.
9. Fagerlin A, Sepucha KR, Couper MP, Levin CA, Singer E, Zikmund-Fisher BJ. Patients' knowledge about 9 common health conditions: the DECISIONS survey. Med Decis Making. 2010;30(5 Suppl):35S–52S.
10. Fagerlin A, Lakhani I, Lantz PM, Janz NK, Morrow M, Schwartz K, et al. An informed decision? Breast cancer patients and their knowledge about treatment. Patient Educ Couns. 2006;64(1–3):303–12.
11. Whelan T, Levine M, Willan A, Gafni A, Sanders K, Mirsky D, et al. Effect of a decision aid on knowledge and treatment decision making for breast cancer surgery: a randomized trial. JAMA. 2004;292(4):435–41.

12. Nelson WL, Han PKJ, Fagerlin A, Stefanek M, Ubel PA. Rethinking the objectives of decision aids: a call for conceptual clarity. Med Decis Making. 2007;27(5):609–18.
13. Ambady N, LaPlante D, Nguyen T, Rosenthal R, Chaumeton N, Levinson W. Surgeons' tone of voice: a clue to malpractice history. Surgery. 2002;132(1):5–9.
14. Levinson W, Roter DL, Mullooly JP, Dull VT, Frankel RM. Physician-patient communication: the relationship with malpractice claims among primary care physicians and surgeons. JAMA. 1997;277(7):553–9.
15. Beckman HB, Markakis KM, Suchman AL, Frankel RM. The doctor-patient relationship and malpractice. Lessons from plaintiff depositions. Arch Intern Med. 1994;154(12):1365–70.
16. Projections of the population by age and sex for the United States: 2010 to 2050 (NP2008-T12). In: Division P, editor. U.S. Census Bureau; August 14, 2008.
17. Fagerlin A, Zikmund-Fisher BJ, Ubel PA. Cure me even if it kills me: preferences for invasive cancer treatment. Med Decis Making. 2005;25(6):614–9.
18. Battafarano RJ, Piccirillo JF, Meyers BF, Hsu H-S, Guthrie TJ, Cooper JD, et al. Impact of comorbidity on survival after surgical resection in patients with stage I non-small cell lung cancer. J Thorac Cardiovasc Surg. 2002;123(2):280–7.
19. Velanovich V, Antoine H, Swartz A, Peters D, Rubinfeld I. Accumulating deficits model of frailty and postoperative mortality and morbidity: its application to a national database. J Surg Res. 2013;183(1):104–10.
20. Fried LP, Tangen CM, Walston J, Newman AB, Hirsch C, Gottdiener J, et al. Frailty in older adults: evidence for a phenotype. J Gerontol A Biol Sci Med Sci. 2001;56(3):M146–57.
21. Cicerchia M, Ceci M, Locatelli C, Gianni W, Repetto L. Geriatric syndromes in peri-operative elderly cancer patients. Surg Oncol. 2010;19(3):131–9.
22. Makary MA, Segev DL, Pronovost PJ, Syin D, Bandeen-Roche K, Patel P, et al. Frailty as a predictor of surgical outcomes in older patients. J Am Coll Surg. 2010;210(6):901–8.
23. Ferguson MK, Farnan J, Hemmerich JA, Slawinski K, Acevedo J, Small S. The impact of perceived frailty on surgeons' estimates of surgical risk. Ann Thorac Surg. 2014;98(1):210–6.
24. Reyna VF, Lloyd FJ. Physician decision making and cardiac risk: effects of knowledge, risk perception, risk tolerance, and fuzzy processing. J Exp Psychol Appl. 2006;12(3):179–95.
25. Reyna VF. A theory of medical decision making and health: fuzzy trace theory. Med Decis Making. 2008;28(6):850–65.
26. Gainer RA, Curran J, Buth KJ, David JG, Légaré JF, Hirsch GM. Toward optimal decision making among vulnerable patients referred for cardiac surgery: a qualitative analysis of patient and provider perspectives. Med Decis Making. 2017;37(5):600–10.
27. Mokhles S, Maat APWM, Aerts JGJV, Nuyttens JJME, Bogers AJJC, Takkenberg JJM. Opinions of lung cancer clinicians on shared decision making in early-stage non-small-cell lung cancer. Interact Cardiovasc Thorac Surg. 2017;25(2):278–84.
28. Finucane ML. Emotion, affect, and risk communication with older adults: challenges and opportunities. J Risk Res. 2008;11(8):983–97.
29. Pargament KI, Smith BW, Koenig HG, Perez L. Patterns of positive and negative religious coping with major life stressors. J Sci Study Relig. 1998;37(4):710–24.
30. DeLisser HM, Keirns CC, Clinton EA, Margolis ML. "The air got to it:" exploring a belief about surgery for lung cancer. J Natl Med Assoc. 2009;101(8):765–71.
31. Cykert S, Dilworth-Anderson P, Monroe MH, Walker P, McGuire FR, Corbie-Smith G, et al. Factors associated with decisions to undergo surgery among patients with newly diagnosed early-stage lung cancer. JAMA. 2010;303(23):2368–76.
32. Margolis M, Kaiser L, Christie J. Patient decisions to undergo surgery for early-stage lung cancer. JAMA. 2010;304(11):1165.
33. Axelrod DA, Goold S. Maintaining trust in the surgeon-patient relationship: challenges for the new millennium. Arch Surg. 2000;135(1):55–61.
34. Butow P, Juraskova I, Chang S, Lopez A-L, Brown R, Bernhard J. Shared decision making coding systems: how do they compare in the oncology context? Patient Educ Couns. 2010;78(2):261–8.

35. Goel V, Sawka CA, Thiel EC, Gort EH, O'Connor AM. Randomized trial of a patient decision aid for choice of surgical treatment for breast cancer. Med Decis Making. 2001;21(1):1–6.
36. Lantz PM, Janz NK, Fagerlin A, Schwartz K, Liu L, Lakhani I, et al. Satisfaction with surgery outcomes and the decision process in a population-based sample of women with breast cancer. Health Serv Res. 2005;40(3):745–68.
37. O'Leary KA, Estabrooks CA, Olson K, Cumming C. Information acquisition for women facing surgical treatment for breast cancer: influencing factors and selected outcomes. Patient Educ Couns. 2007;69(1–3):5–19.

Surgery vs Active Surveillance for Low-Risk Papillary Thyroid Carcinoma

5

Benjamin R. Roman and Ashok R. Shaha

Abstract

Low-risk papillary thyroid carcinomas (LR-PTC, tumors ≤1.5 cm) cause virtually no deaths, and are rapidly increasing in incidence due to overdiagnosis of subclinical disease. Herein we review the evidence base and the rationale behind a strategy of active surveillance of LR-PTC. We review natural history studies by Ito et al. and Tuttle et al., which to date form the backbone of literate on the subject. These studies provide good evidence supporting the hypothesis that LR-PTC is not a deadly disease even when observed. There is little additional evidence on patient reported outcomes (PROs, e.g. quality of life) and cost issues as they relate to an active surveillance strategy. We compare this body of literature to evidence regarding surgery for LR-PTC.

We conclude by highlighting the 2015 American Thyroid Association (ATA) Guideline recommendation *against* fine needle aspiration biopsy of thyroid nodules ≤1 cm without other concerning factors, and guideline recommendations regarding active surveillance. We recommend that patients who are diagnosed with LR-PTC be offered a choice of surgery or active surveillance, if there are no unfavorable or inappropriate features.

Keywords

Low risk papillary thyroid carcinoma · Papillary thyroid microcarcinoma · Overdiagnosis · Thyroidectomy · Active surveillance · Observation · Quality of life · Cost

B. R. Roman (✉) · A. R. Shaha
Head and Neck Service, Memorial Sloan Kettering Cancer Center, New York, NY, USA
e-mail: romanb@mskcc.org

P. Angelos, R. H. Grogan (eds.), *Difficult Decisions in Endocrine Surgery*,
Difficult Decisions in Surgery: An Evidence-Based Approach,
https://doi.org/10.1007/978-3-319-92860-9_5

Background

Papillary thyroid carcinoma is one of the least deadly human cancers. 97–99% of people with tumors confined to the thyroid are alive at 20 years [1]. Survival may be even higher for smaller papillary thyroid carcinomas confined to the thyroid (herein defined as low-risk papillary thyroid carcinoma, LR-PTC, tumor size ≤1.5 cm). Meanwhile, the incidence of LR-PTC has nearly tripled over the past 40 years, largely due to increased diagnostic scrutiny and overdiagnosis [2–5].

Overdiagnosis of cancer can occur when there is both a large reservoir of occult disease and increased diagnostic activity to find it. Both of these conditions are met in thyroid cancer. Autopsy studies demonstrate occult disease present in at least 5–10% of people at the time of death from other causes [6]. There is also evidence of increased use of ultrasonography, fine needle aspiration biopsy, and increased detection of "incidentalomas" both by imaging studies and by physical exam. Overdiagnosis in the fields of thyroid, breast, lung, and prostate among others has led to recommendations by some experts to change the definition of cancer to exclude what appear to be "IDLE" conditions (indolent lesions of epithelial origin) [7].

Another approach to seemingly occult lesions is active surveillance—a treatment strategy that avoids or delays invasive procedures and their attendant risks, harms, and costs. While already commonly accepted in prostate cancer, thyroid cancer active surveillance is not yet widely presented as an option for newly diagnosed patients.

Herein, we review the literature regarding active surveillance of LR-PTC, make recommendations for current practice, and discuss the potential future of this treatment strategy. Any new treatment strategies such as active surveillance for LR-PTC should be compared to standard treatment (i.e. thyroidectomy) based on the value of the new strategy: the benefit or outcomes provided to patients, divided by the associated harms and costs [8]. Concerning the treatment strategies of active surveillance versus surgery for LR-PTC, we review relevant literature regarding outcomes of survival and recurrence, patient reported outcomes such as quality of life issues, and financial costs, as per Table 5.1. We conclude with a discussion of the 2015 American Thyroid Association (ATA) guidelines, which for the first time recommend against biopsy of thyroid nodules <1 cm, and also for the first time endorse an active surveillance approach in selected patients with LR-PTC [9].

Table 5.1 PICO evidence-based clinical question

*P*opulation	Patients with PTC <1.5 cm (low-risk papillary thyroid cancer; LR-PTC)
*I*ntervention	Active surveillance (e.g. observation)
*C*omparator	Surgery
*O*utcomes	1. Survival, recurrence, progression of disease 2. PROs (patient reported outcomes e.g. quality of life) 3. Cost and harm

The Evidence Base: Survival, Recurrence, and Progression of Disease

To date, Yasuhiro Ito and colleagues in Japan, as well as R. Michael Tuttle at Memorial Sloan Kettering Cancer Center in New York are the only groups to publish data on the outcomes of patients choosing active surveillance for LR-PTC. Ito's first report was in 2003 [10]. This group offers active surveillance only to patients with tumors <1 cm. After diagnosis of LR-PTC via fine-needle aspiration biopsy in 732 patients between 1993 and 2001, active surveillance was chosen by 162 (28%) as a treatment strategy. It is important to note that active surveillance was not offered to patients with unfavorable features such as tumors located adjacent to the trachea or the recurrent laryngeal nerve, tumors showing high-grade malignancy on fine needle aspiration biopsy, and patients with clinically evident nodal metastases. Among patients in the active surveillance group, the tumor stayed the same size or shrank by ultrasonography in 72.3%. The tumor enlarged to greater than 1 cm in 18 patients (11.1%). Nine patients (5.6%) developed new lymph nodes suspicious for metastasis during active surveillance. Throughout the study period, 56 (34.6%) of patients in the active surveillance group underwent surgery, either for patient or physician preference. Among the 626 patients with microcarcinomas who chose immediate surgery, 594 underwent lymph node dissection, and metastasis was confirmed in 50.5%. The authors concluded that papillary microcarcinomas only rarely become clinically apparent, even if the disease is likely to have already spread to lymph nodes.

In 2010 Ito and colleagues published a follow-up study on the natural history of patients choosing active surveillance with an average of more than 6 years of observation [11]. Active surveillance was offered and chosen by 340 out of 1055 patients (32%) with LR-PTC without unfavorable features between 1993 and 2004. At 5 and 10-year follow up, 6.4% and 15.9% of patients, respectively, had enlargement of their tumor by more than 3 mm. 1.4% and 3.4% of patients at 5 and 10-years respectively developed new lymph nodes suspicious for metastases. 109 (32.1%) of patients in the active surveillance group eventually underwent thyroidectomy. None of these patients developed recurrences during the study period.

In 2013 Ito and colleagues published a study examining the impact of age on the progression of LR-PTC [12]. For this study, they defined "progression" as (1) any size enlargement; (2) novel appearance of lymph node metastasis; (3) progression to ≥12 mm; or clinically apparent lymph nodes. Between 2003 and 2011, 1235 patients were offered and chose observation, and were followed for an average of greater than 6 years. They stratified patients as young (<40 years, n = 169), middle-aged (40–59, n = 570), and old (≥60, n = 496). At 10 year follow up, any size enlargement was seen in 12.1% young/9.1% middle-aged/4.0% older patients. New lymph node metastases were seen in 16.1% young/2.3% middle-aged/0.5% older patients. Progression ≥12 mm or clinically apparent disease was seen in 22.5% young/4.9% middle-aged/2.5% older patients. Younger age therefore seemed to be related to various measures of faster progression, a relationship which held in multivariable analysis. Of 1235 patients being observed, 191 (15.5%) underwent surgery. Only one patient had recurrence in the thyroid bed, and none died of papillary thyroid carcinoma, meaning that faster progression in younger patients nonetheless did not portend a worse outcome.

Several key facts stand out from Ito's studies: First, patients eligible for active surveillance were carefully chosen; the strategy was not offered to patients with unfavorable features such as tumors located adjacent to the trachea or the recurrent laryngeal nerve, tumors showing high-grade malignancy on fine needle aspiration biopsy, or patients with clinically evident nodal metastases. Second, among carefully selected patients, active surveillance appears to be a viable treatment option, with no deaths from carcinoma observed in the group being followed. Third, it appears that younger patients choosing active surveillance are more likely to show progression of their disease compared to older patients, although their outcomes were not ultimately worse. Fourth, although some patients in the active surveillance group eventually had surgery, the proportion of patients who remained in active surveillance in the three studies increased over time, from 65.4% to 84.5%. The interpretation is that during the decade over which these studies took place, Ito and colleagues have become more comfortable observing patients for longer. This suggests that there may be additional room for an active surveillance strategy for patients with somewhat larger tumors or even for patients whose tumors show growth or progression over time. Ultimately, the appropriate limits of this strategy have not been fully identified, and will likely change with additional future inquiry.

R. Michael Tuttle at Memorial Sloan Kettering Cancer Center in New York recently published on a cohort of 291 patients with LR-PTC, with tumors up to ≤1.5 cm in size [13]. These patients were followed for a median of 25 months (range: 6–166). Using Ito's criteria of 3 mm of tumor growth, 11/291 (3.8%) experienced growth, with a cumulative incidence of 12.1% extrapolated at 5 years. Interestingly, 3-dimensional tumor volume assessment yielded earlier identification of tumor growth. Younger age correlated with increased likelihood of tumor growth. No patients in this cohort experienced lymph node or distant metastases while on an active surveillance approach, and there were no thyroid-cancer related deaths.

One additional study of the natural history of thyroid cancer not undergoing immediate surgical treatment is available from analysis of SEER data by Davies et al. [1]. In that study of 440 patients not receiving immediate surgery, most tumors with documented size were between 1.0 and 3.0 cm. These 440 patients had a 20 year cancer-specific survival of 97%.

The outcomes from an active surveillance strategy can be compared to an up-front surgical strategy in terms of survival and the need for future treatment (for progression in the case of active surveillance, or recurrence in the case of up-front surgery). From this perspective, outcomes are comparable: The survival was 100% in Ito's studies and 97% in Davies' SEER study (although the tumors in SEER were predominantly larger than 1 cm). For patients undergoing up-front surgery, Ito has published data on long-term outcomes including rate of tumor spread and survival [14]. In patients with tumors up to 2 cm in size, the rate of tumor spread to lymph nodes at 10 years was 1.9%, while the rate of spread to distant sites was 0.4%. Thyroid-cancer-related death occurred in 0.04% of patients with tumors <2 cm.

Two additional studies have examined outcomes of surgery for LR-PTC, using the SEER database. These studies have demonstrated >99% 5 and 10-year disease specific survival among patients with LR-PTC, [15, 16] regardless of the extent of surgery (hemi vs. total thyroidectomy) [15]. Other studies have verified that the extent of surgery does not affect outcomes [17–19]. Very few patients undergoing surgery for LR-PTC have recurrent disease requiring additional treatment [20]. Some reports suggest a difference in recurrence rates between microcarcinomas discovered incidentally and nonincidentally, [21] and differences based on multifocality, [19] but others have reported that radioactive iodine treatment did not affect recurrence [19, 22].

The Evidence Base: PROs Including Quality of Life (QOL)

Ito and colleagues have not studied PROs or QOL issues in their patients who choose not to undergo thyroidectomy. There is robust literature on quality of life in prostate cancer, and evidence that patients choosing active surveillance do not have burdensome levels of anxiety or other negative psychological effects of not undergoing treatment [23]; those prone to worry would not choose active surveillance. However extrapolation from prostate literature is difficult because there are major differences between the risks and benefits of active surveillance versus treatment for prostate and thyroid cancer. In short, the relatively common sexual and urinary dysfunction faced by men who choose treatment for prostate cancer would likely affect quality of life more than the common risks of thyroidectomy. One testable hypothesis regarding LR-PTC active surveillance is that patients may have improved PROs compared to those undergoing surgery because they can avoid sequelae of surgery such as a scar on the neck, need for lifetime thyroid hormone replacement, and temporary or permanent complications of vocal cord dysfunction and hypocalcemia. How such PROs might balance with the psychological concerns of choosing active surveillance has not been studied.

For patients who undergo surgery for LR-PTC, complications of thyroidectomy include temporary or permanent vocal cord dysfunction, rare need for tracheotomy, temporary or permanent hypocalcemia, and hematoma, along with complications related to general anesthesia [24]. The effect of these specific complications on PROs and QOL has not generally been studied. Regarding overall quality of life in patients undergoing thyroidectomy, a systematic review of 26 studies demonstrated a similar or slightly worse health-related quality of life compared to the normative population [25]. Affected domains on the Short Form 36 (SF-36) questionnaire include vitality, physical functioning, bodily pain, general health perceptions, physical role functioning, emotional role functioning, and mental health [26]. A thyroidectomy scar was shown to worsen scores on the Dermatology Life Quality Index [27]. PROs are worse among patients who have had a thyroidectomy if they also undergo neck dissection, including worse chewing and shoulder scores on the

University of Washington Quality of Life Questionnaire [28]. Worse PROs are also seen in multiple head and neck specific quality of life instruments among patients undergoing radioactive iodine ablation [28, 29].

The Evidence Base: Cost and Harm

By 2019, it is estimated that papillary thyroid cancer will become the third most common cancer in women of all ages in the United States, and will cost $18 to $21 billion dollars to treat. Compared to most cancers, however, the cost of treating one patient with thyroid cancer is relatively small, at an estimated $35,000 [30]. The lifetime costs of thyroidectomy are likely higher, since many estimates of cost do not take into account such issues of lifetime hormone replacement and loss of productivity from missed work, nor do they account for the impact of harms of treatment on quality-adjusted life years. Regarding the active surveillance strategy for LR-PTC, neither the projected nor the actual costs have been studied. Our estimate is that in time, as the appropriate regimens of active surveillance become more clear, this strategy will likely be less expensive than thyroidectomy.

Discussion

In summary, the rationale for an active surveillance approach to LR-PTC is that it allows patients to avoid the risks and complications of thyroidectomy without any apparent adverse effect on survival. This approach is not for every patient. Psychologically, a diagnosis of cancer will likely be too burdensome for certain patients to choose this strategy. The rationale for surgery for LR-PTC is that it allows most patients a definitive cure, with relatively low morbidity. The cost considerations of surgery versus active surveillance will need detailed studies as active surveillance with routine ultrasounds is needed even after surgery.

It should be noted that whereas the 2009 ATA Guidelines [31] left open the possibility of fine needle aspiration biopsy for patients with a high risk history and tumors >5 mm, the 2015 ATA Guidelines explicitly recommend against biopsy of nodules <10 mm [9]. Therefore, patients who might have LR-PTC are now not even recommended to determine whether their thyroid nodule is cancerous or not. If these guidelines are followed, patients with tumors <1 cm and ultrasonographic features highly suspicious for papillary thyroid carcinoma can be offered active surveillance without making a definitive diagnosis. Patients with tumors >1 cm who have been biopsied can be offered active surveillance.

The ATA 2015 guidelines also for the first time endorsed the active surveillance approach. The recommendation reads: "A cytology diagnostic for a primary thyroid malignancy will almost always lead to thyroid surgery. However, an active surveillance management approach can be considered as an alternative to immediate surgery in: (A) patients with very low risk tumors (e.g. papillary microcarcinomas); (B) patients at high surgical risk because of co-morbid conditions; (C) patients expected to have a relatively short remaining life span; (D) patients with concurrent medical or surgical issues that need to be addressed prior to thyroid surgery" [9].

In conclusion, active surveillance of LR-PTC, as well as any thyroid nodule less than 1 cm, is a viable option for patients. Even with a diagnosis of cancer, patients are very unlikely to die of this disease. However, much work remains to determine the best candidates for this approach, to develop decision-aids that will assist patients in choosing the best option for them, and in determining the optimal protocol for active surveillance. In addition, the role of BRAF and other molecular studies remains unclear at this time.

Recommendations

1. The American Thyroid Association (ATA) 2015 Guidelines recommend *against* fine needle aspiration biopsy of thyroid nodules ≤1 cm without other concerning factors.
   GRADE strength of recommendation: A, high: Further research is very unlikely to change our confidence in this recommendation.
2. The American Thyroid Association (ATA) 2015 Guidelines endorse active surveillance for selected patients, including those with "very low risk tumors," a group which includes (but is not necessarily limited to) tumors <1 cm (papillary microcarcinomas).
   GRADE strength of recommendation: B, moderate: Further research is likely to have an important impact on the outcome estimates.
3. Patients who are diagnosed with LR-PTC should be offered a choice of surgery or active surveillance if there are no unfavorable features (tumor adjacent to trachea or recurrent laryngeal nerve, pathology showing high-grade malignancy, or clinically evident lymph node metastases).
   GRADE strength of recommendation: B, moderate: Further research is likely to have an important impact on the outcome estimates.
4. Optimal active surveillance protocols have not been developed. Should active surveillance be chosen, the patient should ideally be enrolled in prospective data collection in order to further study this treatment approach.
   GRADE strength of recommendation: A, high: Further research is very unlikely to change our confidence in this recommendation.

References

1. Davies L, Welch HG. Thyroid cancer survival in the United States: observational data from 1973 to 2005. Arch Otolaryngol Head Neck Surg. 2010;136(5):440–4.
2. Davies L, Welch HG. Current thyroid cancer trends in the United States. JAMA Otolaryngol Head Neck Surg. 2014;140(4):317–22.
3. Morris LG, et al. The increasing incidence of thyroid cancer: the influence of access to care. Thyroid. 2013;23(7):885–91.

4. Chen AY, Jemal A, Ward EM. Increasing incidence of differentiated thyroid cancer in the United States, 1988–2005. Cancer. 2009;115(16):3801–7.
5. Davies L, Welch HG. Increasing incidence of thyroid cancer in the United States, 1973–2002. JAMA. 2006;295(18):2164–7.
6. Furuya-Kanamori L, Bell KJ, Clark J, Glasziou P, Doi SA. Prevalence of differentiated thyroid cancer in autopsy studies over six decades: a meta-analysis. J Clin Oncol. 2016;34(30):3672–9.
7. Esserman LJ, Thompson IM Jr, Reid B. Overdiagnosis and overtreatment in cancer: an opportunity for improvement. JAMA. 2013;310(8):797–8.
8. Roman BR, Awad MI, Patel SG. Defining value-driven care in head and neck oncology. Curr Oncol Rep. 2015;17(1):424.
9. Haugen BR, Alexander EK, Bible KC, et al. 2015 American Thyroid Association management guidelines for adult patients with thyroid nodules and differentiated thyroid cancer: the American Thyroid Association Guidelines Task Force on Thyroid Nodules and Differentiated Thyroid Cancer. Thyroid. 2016;26(1):1–133.
10. Ito Y, et al. An observation trial without surgical treatment in patients with papillary microcarcinoma of the thyroid. Thyroid. 2003;13(4):381–7.
11. Ito Y, et al. An observational trial for papillary thyroid microcarcinoma in Japanese patients. World J Surg. 2010;34(1):28–35.
12. Ito Y, et al. Patient age is significantly related to the progression of papillary microcarcinoma of the thyroid under observation. Thyroid. 2013;24(1):27–34.
13. Tuttle RM, Fagin JA, Minkowitz G, et al. Natural history and tumor volume kinetics of papillary thyroid cancers during active surveillance. JAMA Otolaryngol Head Neck Surg. 2017;143(10):1015–20.
14. Ito Y, Kudo T, Kihara M, et al. Prognosis of low-risk papillary thyroid carcinoma patients: its relationship with the size of primary tumors. Endocr J. 2012;59(2):119–25.
15. Wang TS, et al. Papillary thyroid microcarcinoma: an over-treated malignancy? World J Surg. 2014;38(9):2297–303.
16. Yu XM, et al. Should all papillary thyroid microcarcinomas be aggressively treated? An analysis of 18,445 cases. Ann Surg. 2011;254(4):653–60.
17. Lee J, et al. Long-term outcomes of total thyroidectomy versus thyroid lobectomy for papillary thyroid microcarcinoma: comparative analysis after propensity score matching. Thyroid. 2013;23(11):1408–15.
18. Lee CR, et al. Lobectomy and prophylactic central neck dissection for papillary thyroid microcarcinoma: do involved lymph nodes mandate completion thyroidectomy? World J Surg. 2014;38(4):872–7.
19. Hay ID, et al. Papillary thyroid microcarcinoma: a study of 900 cases observed in a 60-year period. Surgery. 2008;144(6):980–7. discussion 987–8.
20. Londero SC, et al. Papillary thyroid microcarcinoma in Denmark 1996–2008: a national study of epidemiology and clinical significance. Thyroid. 2013;23(9):1159–64.
21. Mehanna H, et al. Differences in the recurrence and mortality outcomes rates of incidental and nonincidental papillary thyroid microcarcinoma: a systematic review and meta-analysis of 21,329 person-years of follow-up. J Clin Endocrinol Metab. 2014;99(8):2834–43.
22. Kim HJ, et al. Radioactive iodine ablation does not prevent recurrences in patients with papillary thyroid microcarcinoma. Clin Endocrinol (Oxf). 2013;78(4):614–20.
23. Venderbos LD, et al. A longitudinal study on the impact of active surveillance for prostate cancer on anxiety and distress levels. Psychooncology. 2015;24(3):348–54.
24. Gopalakrishna Iyer N, Shaha AR. Complications of thyroid surgery: prevention and management. Minerva Chir. 2010;65(1):71–82.
25. Husson O, et al. Health-related quality of life among thyroid cancer survivors: a systematic review. Clin Endocrinol (Oxf). 2011;75(4):544–54.
26. Tan LG, et al. Health-related quality of life in thyroid cancer survivors. Laryngoscope. 2007;117(3):507–10.
27. Choi Y, et al. Impact of postthyroidectomy scar on the quality of life of thyroid cancer patients. Ann Dermatol. 2014;26(6):693–9.

28. Almeida JP, Vartanian JG, Kowalski LP. Clinical predictors of quality of life in patients with initial differentiated thyroid cancers. Arch Otolaryngol Head Neck Surg. 2009;135(4):342–6.
29. Dingle IF, et al. Salivary morbidity and quality of life following radioactive iodine for well-differentiated thyroid cancer. Otolaryngol Head Neck Surg. 2013;148:746–52.
30. Aschebrook-Kilfoy B, et al. The clinical and economic burden of a sustained increase in thyroid cancer incidence. Cancer Epidemiol Biomarkers Prev. 2013;22(7):1252–9.
31. Cooper DS, et al. Revised American Thyroid Association management guidelines for patients with thyroid nodules and differentiated thyroid cancer. Thyroid. 2009;19(11):1167–214.

Prospective Screening Protocol for FNMTC Family Members: Ultrasound Versus Physical Examination

6

Insoo Suh and Jesse Pasternak

Abstract

Non-medullary thyroid cancer (NMTC) of follicular cell origin make up 95% of thyroid cancers, of which 85% are papillary thyroid cancer (PTC). Generally, these tumors have an excellent prognosis. Since the first description of identical twins with papillary thyroid cancer in 1955, epidemiological data have shown that up to 8% of these tumors are familial in etiology, despite not being related to other known cancer syndromes.

Keywords

Thyroid nodule · Well-differentiated thyroid cancer · Familial non-medullary thyroid cancer · Cancer genetics · Thyroid ultrasound

Overview of Familial Non-medullary Thyroid Cancer (FNMTC)

Non-medullary thyroid cancer (NMTC) of follicular cell origin make up 95% of thyroid cancers, of which 85% are papillary thyroid cancer (PTC). Generally, these tumors have an excellent prognosis [1]. This chapter deals with the question of

I. Suh
Department of Surgery, Section of Endocrine Surgery, UCSF Medical Center – Mount Zion, San Francisco, CA, USA
e-mail: insoo.suh@ucsf.edu

J. Pasternak (✉)
Department of Surgery, Endocrine Surgery, University Health Network - TGH, Toronto, ON, Canada
e-mail: Jesse.Pasternak@uhn.ca

P. Angelos, R. H. Grogan (eds.), *Difficult Decisions in Endocrine Surgery*, Difficult Decisions in Surgery: An Evidence-Based Approach,
https://doi.org/10.1007/978-3-319-92860-9_6

ultrasound versus physical examination as the best screening protocol for FNMTC family members (Table 6.1).

Since the first description of identical twins with papillary thyroid cancer in 1955, epidemiological data have shown that up to 8% of these tumors are familial in etiology, despite not being related to other known cancer syndromes [2] (Table 6.2). First degree family members of patients with thyroid cancer have up to ninefold increase in also developing the disease [3, 4]. The classic definition of FMNTC describes the presence of NMTC in a family in which two or more first degree relatives are affected [5, 6]; however, there is no consensus agreement on this number of affected relatives, with other authors using different cutoffs for the number of affected relatives [5, 7]. Most of these tumors are PTC (>90%); in addition, other benign thyroid conditions such as goiter and thyroiditis are found in over 50% of cases [3, 6]. Swedish epidemiological data have found an over threefold and sixfold increased risk of NMTC in a PTC patient's parent and sibling, respectively [8].

There is much still to be understood regarding the inheritance of FNMTC; however, autosomal dominance with incomplete penetrance and variable expressivity continues to be generally accepted as the most likely pattern [9–13]. Families with two first degree relatives have between a 33% and 50% probability of belonging to an FNMTC kindred, and those with three or more first degree relatives have a 95% chance [14]. The dramatic increase in probability of FNMTC between a cutoff of 2 versus ≥3 affected family members is simply due to the difference in statistical possibility of these relatives sharing a diagnosis of NMTC but actually having separate incidences of sporadic disease.

Genetics of FNMTC

In contrast to other hereditary syndromes well described in the literature, FNMTC has less understood genome differences. Of the four other named cancer syndromes of which NMTC is a component, three are autosomal dominant (Gardner's

Table 6.1 PICO table

Population	Relatives of FNMTC patients
Intervention	Ultrasound screening
Comparator	Physical exam
Outcomes	Survival, recurrence, age at operation, size of tumor

Table 6.2 Author recommendations in the screening of FNMTC

Number of family members with WDTC	Recommendation
None	No screening
One	Physical exam yearly
Two	Ultrasound yearly
Three or more	Ultrasound yearly

syndrome, Cowden disease and Carney Complex) and one is autosomal recessive (Werner Syndrome). Each of these syndromes has a specific gene mutation [15–19]. It is important to note, however, that the risk of thyroid cancer within these entities is highly variable and even within each syndrome the range of reported risk of well differentiated thyroid cancer is very broad. FNMTC which as of yet has not been associated with a single mutation has not been as well described; one reason may be that other epigenetic mechanisms play a more significant role in the heredity of FNMTC. Nevertheless, several implicated genes and loci have been described, although it remains unclear whether these genetic alterations specifically cause thyroid cancer to develop, or rather that they are associated with increased thyroid follicular cell growth/function in general, since families with FNMTC also have higher rates of benign adenomas, Hashimoto's thyroiditis and multinodular goiters.

An overview of the genetic regions implicated in FNMTC is shown in Table 6.3 [20]. MNG1 was one of the first genetic loci to be associated with FNMTC; however, follow-up analysis showed that it was more closely related with familial multinodular goiters. The TCO, fPTC/PRN, and FTEN regions have had mixed results showing an association with FNMTC, with limited confirmatory datasets. NMTC1 has had multiple large studies showing its association with FNMTC, but particularly with follicular variant of PTC. A SNP array-based linkage analysis of 38 FNMTC kindreds revealed 2 loci on chromosomes 1q21 and 6q22, but these results have not been broadly validated [21]. Recently, there has been increased evidence for FOXE1 on chromosome 9q22.33 in several large FNMTC kindreds in both Europe and the U.S. Further, there has also been recent evidence that telomere telomerase complex may play a larger role in the genetics of familial thyroid cancer. The evidence however, is still limited and far from conclusive. Overall, the genetic underpinnings of FNMTC has yet to be fully characterized.

Prognostic Differences in FNMTC Patients

It is generally accepted that NMTC found in two family members may be more aggressive and portend a worse prognosis than those without a positive family history [22]. Several studies have supported this assertion. A retrospective analysis of 1262 patients of whom 113 (9%) were diagnosed with FNMTC found that those

Table 6.3 Genetic regions associated with familial nonmedullary thyroid cancer

Gene	Location
MNG1	14q31
TCO	19q13.2
fPTC/PRN	1q21
NMTC1	2q21
FTEN	8p23.1-p22
	1q21, 6q22
FOXE1	9q22.33
Telomere telomerase complex	

associated with FNMTC were associated with worse outcomes, particularly with respect to disease free survival [23]. McDonald et al. [24] echoed these findings, showing that FNMTC patients had higher rates of reoperation, additional treatment with radioactive iodine, distant metastasis, and death [24]. In addition, a multicenter matched case control series showed 48 patients with FNMTC compared with non-familial disease had shorter disease free survival [10]. Furthermore, Uchino et al. reviewed 6458 Japanese patients with NMTC and found 258 patients implicated in familial disease. In this study, disease free survival was worse overall in FNMTC patients, although the mechanism was unclear as rates of invasive tumors and lymph node metastasis were similar [7].

Screening for FNMTC

Detection of the Abnormal Thyroid

Before the introduction of ultrasound into clinical practice, the physical exam of the thyroid remained the mainstay of detection of suspicious goiters requiring intervention. Multiple studies done to assess the utility of clinical exam have been extremely variable. Studies looking at sensitivity of detecting presence of goiter by physical exam have be estimated to be as low as 64% [25, 26], and sensitivity for nodules as low as 31% [27]. On the other hand, assessment of specificity in detecting abnormal thyroid goiter has approached 100% in many studies [25, 28, 29]. Nevertheless the variability in physical examination's sensitivity led to widespread adoption of the use of ultrasound in detecting thyroid abnormalities. Since one of the first descriptions of use of ultrasound to view the thyroid gland in 1967, [30] the ultrasound rapidly became a central clinical tool in detecting pathology. Currently, ultrasound technology has integrated into the clinicians practice so much so that it has become an extension of the physical exam. Surgeon performed ultrasound has become accepted as an integral part of the assessment of thyroid nodules within national guidelines [31].

Defining the Population Most Likely to Benefit from Screening

There has been a growing concern regarding the overdiagnosis of thyroid cancer in the general population. The initiation of whole-population screening with thyroid ultrasound in South Korea has led to a striking increase in the diagnosis of thyroid cancer since the beginning of this millennium, but no change in cancer-related mortality. Although not nearly as dramatic, this phenomenon has been demonstrated to a lesser degree in the United States. This discrepancy between the rate of diagnosis versus rate of mortality has raised the concern that this detection strategy is leading to the workup and treatment of many smaller thyroid cancers which may otherwise never become clinically significant [32]. The implications on treatment-related complications/morbidity as well as costs and resources are evident.

On the other hand, FNMTC tumors do exhibit more aggressive behavior and confer a worse prognosis, as described above. In addition, it appears that early diagnosis and appropriate treatment in FNMTC patients increases their disease free and overall survival [5], which certainly suggests a benefit to screening at-risk family members. Therefore, any proposal for a screening strategy for FNMTC kindreds would do best to implement an adequately sensitive screening strategy for those families most at risk, while minimizing the pitfalls related to overdiagnosis and cost.

Identifying the FNMTC population most likely to benefit from screening depends critically upon whether FNMTC is defined as a family with ≥2 or 3 affected first-degree relatives. This is because the probability of a true genetic component in any given family with differentiated thyroid cancer increases (and that of a random sporadic cancer inversely decreases) as the number of known affected relatives increase [14] and (Table 6.3). Table 6.4 summarizes screening recommendations by breaking down the probability estimates of detecting a true FNMTC-related differentiated thyroid cancer using ultrasound versus physical exam, depending on the family history of a hypothetical screening subject. The key dependent variables in this model that were derived from the literature are (1) the prevalence of a thyroid nodule, (2) probability of a differentiated thyroid cancer in that nodule, (3) sensitivity of ultrasound versus physical exam in detecting this nodule/cancer, and (4) the likelihood that this cancer has a true heritable component (as opposed to a sporadic cancer). One limitation of this model is that the increased prevalence of a thyroid nodule and cancer in a subject with a positive family history remains static (52% and 20%, respectively) regardless of the number of affected family members. One would assume that there would be a more proportional relationship, but in the absence of robust evidence, the static prevalence numbers were left in place, and thought to represent a more conservative strategy from a cost-effectiveness standpoint.

Based on this model, it appears clear that any screening strategy for thyroid cancer (either ultrasound or physical exam) in the absence of any related family history would be ineffective, with an overall detection rate of 0.01%–0.02%. Conversely, ultrasound appears justified as an effective screening strategy for families with ≥2 affected members, with its ability to detect a true FNMTC-related cancer in 10% of this population. In comparison, screening strategies for colorectal cancer in the US addresses an approximately 1% cancer prevalence in people over the age of 50, and for breast cancer addresses a 3% prevalence in women over the age of 40.

For the prospective screening subject with only one affected first-degree family member with NMTC, however, it remains unclear whether the more modest improvement in sensitivity of ultrasound compared to physical exam (3.6% vs 1%) justifies the extra cost and resources. One could argue that these percentages are still within the range of those for general-population screening for colon and breast cancer; however, the consequences of delayed diagnosis are admittedly more severe in these cancers compared to either sporadic NMTC or FNMTC. Based on the current evidence, a firm recommendation cannot be made about the preferred screening modality for people with only one first-degree family member with NMTC.

Table 6.4 Understanding risks with numbers—hypothetical scenario of patient without known thyroid disease

Family members with WDTC, *N*	Overall chance of detected thyroid nodule, %	Chance of the nodule being a cancer, %	Chance ultrasound would detect cancer, %	Chance physical exam would detect cancer, %	Likelihood that identified cancer is associated with FNMTC, % (%)	Overall FNMTC-related cancer detection with ultrasound, %	Overall FNMTC-related cancer detection with physical exam, %	Difference, %
None	10	5	100	31[b]	4[c]	***0.021***	***0.007***	***0.14***
One	52[a]	20[a]	100	31[b]	35[c]	***3.6***	***1.1***	***2.5***
Two	52[a]	20[a]	100	31[b]	94[c]	***9.8***	***3.0***	***6.8***
Three	52[a]	20[a]	100	31[b]	100[c]	***10.4***	***3.2***	*7.2*

[a]Charkes 1998 and 2006 Thyroid [14]
[b]Eden et al. 2001 Med Pediatr Oncol [27]
[c]Uchino 2004 World J Surg [7]

Lastly, a key question also remains as to the proper timing of screening, both with respect to initiation and frequency. Limited evidence currently exists to support any frequency longer than yearly screening, and more studies are needed in order to address this.

Understanding Risks with Numbers: Hypothetical Scenario of Patient Without Known Thyroid Disease

As can be seen from Table 6.4, the hypothetical calculation above shows that comparing physical exam to ultrasound screening of patients with only one first degree relative having thyroid cancer shows a 3.6% vs 1.1% detection rate of thyroid cancer. This illustrates a potential miss rate of 2.5%. What is not calculated in this model is the cost of regular ultrasounds for many family members of thyroid cancer patients, as well as the rate of detection, workup and follow-up of benign or inconsequential thyroid nodules. Depending on the practice setting, the absolute risk reduction may or may not justify the extra costs associated with ultrasound screening in this cohort. Our tentative recommendation would be to.

On the other hand, it would be prudent to use ultrasound in families with two or more affected members with NMTC, due to the higher risks associated with a true FNMTC tumor. These are the patients who would most benefit from treatment and are least likely to belong to the category of patients with overdiagnosed thyroid cancer. According to this model, ultrasound would be effective in capturing the significantly higher proportion (~10%) of family members with FNMTC.

Fine Needle Aspiration of Thyroid Nodules

The American Thyroid Association recommends considering fine needle aspiration biopsy (FNAB) for all thyroid nodules >5 mm in patients with a first degree family member with NMTC (recommendation I—neither for nor against). Micropapillary thyroid cancer in the general population is an extremely indolent disease; however, little is known about these tumors in the context of FNMTC, and it is reasonable to assume that the more aggressive characteristics associated with FNMTC apply even to tumors <1 cm in size (Ito). We therefore suggest using the ATA recommendations specifically performing fine needle aspirations in thyroid nodules >5 mm with suspicious features or < 1 cm without (ATA recommendation A- strongly recommend and B—recommend respectively).

Conclusion

Although its genetics have yet to be elucidated, FNMTC is a clinically distinct entity with a worse prognosis compared to sporadic NMTC. For this reason, we recommend screening family members of FNMTC patients who are at risk for this disease; however it is important to stratify the modality of screening based on the overall probability of having FNMTC. There is a high variability in the sensitivity and specificity of physical exam, and an overall superior detection of suspicious thyroid nodules with ultrasonography. With no cost considerations, it is therefore clear that ultrasound is superior to physical exam. Further, as many studies have shown (Rosario etc), it is important to recognize these malignancies earlier as familial cancers portend a worse prognosis than sporadic ones. Without formal cost effective studies taking into consideration the prevalence of FNMTC, current recommendations suggest screening all those with a single first degree family member with NMTC. Considering that the prevalence of true FNMTC is relatively low, as well as the high cost of regular ultrasounds, biopsies and health professional follow-up, the authors recommend yearly ultrasound screening for those with ≥2 family members with NMTC, and physical exam with aggressive management of any detected thyroid nodules in those families with only one affected member with NMTC.

References

1. Mazzaferri EL. Long-term outcome of patients with differentiated thyroid carcinoma: effect of therapy. Endocr Pract. 2000;6(6):469–76.
2. Moses W, Weng J, Kebebew E. Prevalence, clinicopathologic features, and somatic genetic mutation profile in familial versus sporadic nonmedullary thyroid cancer. Thyroid. 2011;21(4):367–71.
3. Pal T, Vogl FD, Chappuis PO, Tsang R, Brierley J, Renard H, Sanders K, Kantemiroff T, Bagha S, Goldgar DE, Narod SA, Foulkes WD. Increased risk of nonmedullary thyroid cancer in the first degree relatives of prevalent cases of nonmedullary thyroid cancer: a hospital-based study. J Clin Endocrinol Metab. 2001;86:5307–12.
4. Goldgar DE, Easton DF, Cannon-Albright LA, Skolnick MH. Systematic population-based assessment of cancer risk in first-degree relatives of cancer probands. J Natl Cancer Inst. 1994;86:1600–8.
5. Triponez F, Wong M, Sturgeon C, Caron N, Ginzinger DG, Segal MR, Kebebew E, Duh QY, Clark OH. Does familial non-medullary thyroid cancer adversely affect survival? World J Surg. 2006;30(5):787–93.
6. Grossman RF, Tu SH, Duh QY, Siperstein AE, Novosolov F, Clark OH. Familial nonmedulary thyroid cancer. An emerging entity that warrants aggressive treatment. Arch Surg. 1995;130:892–7. discussion 898–899.
7. Uchino S, Noguchi S, Yamashita H, Murakami T, Watanabe S, Ogawa T, et al. Detection of asymptomatic differentiated thyroid carcinoma by neck ultrasonographic screening for familial nonmedullary thyroid carcinoma. World J Surg. 2004;28:1099–102.
8. Hemminki K, Eng C, Chen B. Familial risks for nonmedullary thyroid cancer. J Clin Endocrinol Metab. 2005;90(March):5747–53.
9. Loh KC. Familial nonmedullary thyroid carcinoma: a meta-review of case series. Thyroid. 1997;7:107–13.
10. Alsanea O, Wada N, Ain K, et al. Is familial non-medullary thyroid carcinoma more aggressive than sporadic thyroid cancer? A multicenter series. Surgery. 2000;128:1043–50. discussion 1050–1051.
11. Burgess JR, Duffield A, Wilkinson SJ, Ware R, Greenaway TM, Percival J, Hoffman L. Two families with an autosomal dominant inheritance pattern for papillary carcinoma of the thyroid. J Clin Endocrinol Metab. 1997;82:345–8.

12. Lupoli G, Vitale G, Caraglia M, et al. Familial papillary thyroid microcarcinoma: a new clinical entity. Lancet. 1999;353:637–9.
13. Malchoff CD, Malchoff DM. Familial nonmedullary thyroid carcinoma. Cancer Control. 2006;13(2):106–10. https://doi.org/10.1089/thy.2013.0079.
14. Charkes ND. On the prevalence of familial non-medullary thyroid cancer in multiply affected kindreds. Thyroid. 2006;16:181–6.
15. Stratakis CA, Kirschner LS, Taymans SE, et al. Carney complex, Peutz-Jeghers syndrome, Cowden disease, and Bannayan-Zonana syndrome share cutaneous and endocrine manifestations, but not genetic loci. J Clin Endocrinol Metab. 1998;83:2972–6.
16. Bonora E, Tallini G, Romeo G. Genetic predisposition to familial nonmedullary thyroid cancer: an update of molecular findings and state-of-the-art studies. J Oncol. 2010;2010:385206.
17. Liaw D, Marsh DJ, Li J, Dahia PL, Wang SI, Zheng Z, Bose S, Call KM, Tsou HC, Peacocke M, Eng C, Parsons R. Germline mutations of the PTEN gene in Cowden disease, an inherited breast and thyroid cancer syndrome. Nat Genet. 1997;16:64–7.
18. Cetta F, Montalto G, Gori M, Curia MC, Cama A, Olschwang S. Germline mutations of the APC gene in patients with familial adenomatous polyposis-associated thyroid carcinoma: results from a European cooperative study. J Clin Endocrinol Metab. 2000;85:286–92.
19. Richards ML. Thyroid cancer genetics: multiple endocrine neoplasia type 2, non-medullary familial thyroid cancer, and familial syndromes associated with thyroid cancer. Surg Oncol Clin N Am. 2009;18:39–52. viii.
20. Mazeh H, Sippel R. Familial nonmedullary thyroid carcinoma. Thyroid. 2013;23(9):1049–58.
21. Suh I, Filetti S, Vriens MR, Guerrero MA, Tumino S, Wong M, Shen WT, Kebebew E, Duh QY, Clark OH. Distinct loci on chromosome 1q21 and 6q22 predispose to familial nonmedullary thyroid cancer: a SNP array-based linkage analysis of 38 families. Surgery. 2009;146:1073–80.
22. Wang X, Cheng W, Li J, Su A, Wei T, Liu F, Zhu J. Accepted Preprint first posted on 30 January 2015 as Manuscript EJE-14-0960 Familial nomeduallary thyroid carcinoma is a more aggressive disease: a systematic review and meta-analysis. 2015;(January):1–20.
23. Lee Y, Yoon JH, Yi O, Sung T, Chung K, Kim WB, Hong SJ. Familial history of non-medullary thyroid cancer is an independent prognostic factor for tumor recurrence in younger patients with conventional papillary thyroid carcinoma. J Surg Oncol. 2014;109:168–73.
24. McDonald TJ, Driedger AA, Garcia BM, Van Uum SH, Rachinsky I, Chevendra V, Breadner D, Feinn R, Walsh SJ, Malchoff CD. Familial papillary thyroid carcinoma: a retrospective analysis. J Oncol. 2011;2011(948786):17.
25. Perrild H, Hegedüs L, Baastrup PC, Kayser L, Kastberg S. Thyroid function and ultrasonically determined thyroid size in patients receiving long-term lithium treatment. Am J Psychiatry. 1990;147(11):1518–21.
26. Siminoski K. Does this patient have a goiter? JAMA. 1995;273:813–7.
27. Eden K, Mahon S, Helfand M. Screening high-risk populations for thyroid cancer. Med Pediatr Oncol. 2001;36(5):583–91. Review.
28. Hegedus L, Hansen JM, Luhdorf K, Perrild H, Feldt-Rasmussen U, Kampmann JP. Increased frequency of goitre in epileptic patients on long-term phenytoin or carbamazepine treatment. Clin Endocrinol. 1985;23(4):423–9.
29. Hegedus L, Karstrup S, Veiergang D, Jacobsen B, Skovsted L, Feldt-Rasmussen U. High frequency of goitre in cigarette smokers. Clin Endocrinol. 1985;22(3):287–92.
30. Fujimoto Y, Oka A, Omoto R, Hirose M. Ultrasound scanning of the thyroid gland as a new diagnostic approach. Ultrasonics. 1967;5:177–80.
31. Cooper DS, Doherty GM, Haugen BR, Kloos RT, Lee SL, Mandel SJ, Tuttle RM. Revised American Thyroid Association management guidelines for patients with thyroid nodules and differentiated thyroid cancer. Thyroid. 2009;19(11):1167–214.
32. Ahn HS, Kim HJ, Welch HG. Korea's thyroid-cancer "epidemic"--screening and overdiagnosis. N Engl J Med. 2014;371(19):1765–7.

Operative Management Versus Observation for Thyroid Nodules Larger than 4 cm with Benign Cytology

7

Nicole A. Cipriani

Abstract

Workup of thyroid nodules usually involves a multi-disciplinary approach, including fine needle aspiration (FNA) biopsy. The Bethesda System for Reporting Thyroid Cytopathology (TBSRTC) was devised to stratify patients into tiers with increasing risk for cancer, based on features identified on FNA. A number of studies have attempted to correlate thyroid nodule size with intrinsic risk of malignancy, as well as with false negative rates (nodules with a benign diagnosis on cytology but a malignant diagnosis on final surgical pathology following resection). The aims of this chapter are (1) to review studies that have evaluated the false negative rate of thyroid nodules based on size, (2) to summarize, analyze, and grade the published data, and (3) to make recommendations for treatment of large thyroid nodules.

Keywords

Fine-needle aspiration (FNA) · Ultrasonography · Thyroid nodules · False negative rates

Introduction

Workup of thyroid nodules usually involves a multi-disciplinary approach, and may involve serologic thyroid function testing, manual palpation, ultrasonographic (US) evaluation, and fine needle aspiration (FNA) biopsy. The Bethesda System for Reporting Thyroid Cytopathology (TBSRTC) was devised to stratify patients into

N. A. Cipriani
The University of Chicago, Department of Pathology, Chicago, IL, USA
e-mail: Nicole.Cipriani@uchospitals.edu

P. Angelos, R. H. Grogan (eds.), *Difficult Decisions in Endocrine Surgery*, Difficult Decisions in Surgery: An Evidence-Based Approach,
https://doi.org/10.1007/978-3-319-92860-9_7

Table 7.1 PICO table

Population	Patients with cytologically benign (Bethesda II) thyroid nodules >3 cm or >4 cm in size on ultrasound
Intervention	Observation
Comparator	Surgical resection
Outcomes	Cancer rate, quality of life, progression of disease

tiers with increasing risk for cancer, based on features identified on FNA [1] (Table 7.1). Nodules are placed into six diagnostic categories: nondiagnostic (Bethesda I), benign (Bethesda II), atypia of undetermined significance (AUS) or follicular lesion of undetermined significance (FLUS) (Bethesda III), follicular neoplasm or suspicious for follicular neoplasm (Bethesda IV), suspicious for malignancy (Bethesda V), or malignant (Bethesda VI). Estimated risks of malignancy in categories II through VI are up to 3%, 15%, 30%, 75%, and 99%, respectively [1, 2]. Actual percentages may vary based on practices of both cytopathologists and surgical pathologists, and have been shown to vary by institution [3, 4].

Surgical resection is recommended by the American Thyroid Association (ATA) for thyroid nodules with a definitive FNA) diagnosis of malignancy, with the exception of low risk microcarcinomas, patients with high surgical risk or short life expectancy, or patients whose other comorbid conditions need more urgent treatment [2]. Contrarily, for nodules with a benign FNA diagnosis in asymptomatic patients, additional immediate workup or treatment is not recommended. Follow-up may vary based on ultrasonographic features: for highly suspicious nodules, repeat US with FNA within 1 year is recommended; for minimally suspicious nodules, the utility of surveillance is limited, and repeat US should be performed no sooner than 2 years. Resection of cytologically benign nodules is not routinely recommended, but may be considered in the context of growth, patient symptoms, or other clinical concern [2]. A number of studies have attempted to correlate thyroid nodule size with intrinsic risk of malignancy, as well as with false negative rates (nodules with a benign diagnosis on cytology but a malignant diagnosis on final surgical pathology following resection). Some authors report higher rates of malignancy or false negative rates in larger nodules (>3 cm or >4 cm), whereas others report the opposite, or no difference based on size. The ATA guidelines find the current data unsatisfactory, and make no recommendation on treatment of cytologically benign nodules based on size: "Based on the evidence, it is still unclear if patients with thyroid nodules ≥4 cm and benign cytology carry a higher risk of malignancy and should be managed differently than those with smaller nodules" [2].

The aims of this chapter are (1) to review studies that have evaluated the false negative rate of thyroid nodules based on size, (2) to summarize, analyze, and grade the published data, and (3) to make recommendations for treatment of large thyroid nodules.

Methodology

A literature search in PubMed was performed using the words *false negative thyroid size*, resulting in 114 articles, of which 105 were written in English. Thirty-seven potentially-relevant articles were identified, and an additional 13 articles were identified within the references, for a total of 50 potentially-relevant articles. Potentially-relevant articles were reviewed and included if they contained: (1) Size stratification of thyroid nodules using 3 cm or 4 cm cutoffs. (2) Final diagnosis (benign or malignant) confirmed by histologic examination. Malignant diagnoses included papillary thyroid carcinoma (PTC), follicular variant of PTC (PTC-FV), follicular thyroid carcinoma (FTC), oncocytic or Hurthle cell variant of FTC (HTC), poorly differentiated thyroid carcinoma (PDC), undifferentiated or anaplastic thyroid carcinoma (UTC), medullary thyroid carcinoma (MTC), or other malignant neoplasms. (3) Nodules with Bethesda II (benign) diagnoses, or nodules with ALL Bethesda diagnoses. (4) Numeric documentation of total nodules with benign cytology including those with malignant histology, stratified by size (i.e. false negatives). Articles not meeting these criteria were excluded, resulting in 21 articles meeting criteria. Articles were relatively recent: all were published between 1995 and 2016, including 15 between 2010 and 2016. Based on authors, institutions, and time-frames, the data in two articles was identical [5, 6], however, one specifically compared females to males. When applicable, these two articles are reported together.

Results of Literature Review and Data Analysis

Patients with large thyroid nodules (>3 cm or >4 cm) may undergo lobectomy or thyroidectomy in the context of a malignant or suspicious FNA, compressive symptoms, patient preference, or other relevant indications. Should patients with large nodules, benign FNA, and no other indication undergo operative resection? Is there a higher risk of false negative results on FNA in larger nodules? In other words, is there a higher risk of finding malignancy on final pathologic examination in these larger nodules compared to smaller nodules? If so, how great is the risk and is it worth a surgical procedure? In our literature search, 12 articles directly compared false negative rates in small versus large nodules. Nine articles evaluated false negative rates in large nodules only.

Nodules Larger Than 4 cm

Fourteen articles evaluated cytologically benign nodules using a size cutoff of 4 cm. Seven articles directly compared false negative rates in nodules <4 cm versus >4 cm [6–12]. The total number of nodules with benign cytology that were evaluated ranged from 74 to 417 (39–319 in small, 35–113 in large nodules). False negative rates in small nodules ranged from 1.3 to 28.2%; false negative rates in large nodules ranged from 4.1 to 20%. Seven articles only evaluated false negative rates in nodules >4 cm [5, 13–18] (the data in Parikh et al. [5] is evaluated with Albuja-Cruz et al. [6]). The number of large nodules with benign cytology that were evaluated ranged from 71 to 123. False negative rates in these large nodules ranged from 0.8 to 12.7%. When considering all 14 articles, false negative diagnoses were reported in 9. Of the seven articles that documented false negative diagnoses in large nodules, the most frequently-reported diagnosis was PTC-FV (25 cases), followed by FTC (14 cases, including 3 HTC), PTC (11 cases), PTMC (3 within the index nodule), 1 MTC, and 3 other (including 1 lymphoma and 2 unspecified). Two articles reported false negative diagnoses without specifying size: 20 PTC, 2 PTMC (within the index nodule), 5 FTC, 1 MTC, and 1 UTC.

Authors of 9 articles (9/14, 64%) did not recommend surgical resection of nodules >4 cm with benign cytology [6–11, 13–15]. Koo et al. and Carrillo et al. additionally recommended repeat ultrasound-guided biopsy or consideration of surgery in the event of nodule growth [11]. Rosario et al. additionally recommended that each institution calculate its own false negative rate in large thyroid nodules and determine patient management in this context [15]. One author (1/14, 7%) suggested surgical resection in women (not men), due to apparent higher false negative rates in large nodules in women compared to men (17% (17/98) in women versus 0% in men (0/9)) [5]. However, this difference may be biased by the higher prevalence of thyroid nodules in women, rather than a true gender difference in false negative rates. Authors of 3 articles (3/14, 21%) advocated surgical resection of all cytologically benign thyroid nodules >4 cm [16–18] due to perceived high false negative rates. Khalife et al. made no recommendation regarding resection, as the main aim of their paper was to evaluate the McGill Thyroid Nodule Score (MTNS) [12].

Overall, false negative rates in nodules >4 cm were variable, ranging from 0.8 to 20%. Interestingly, the highest false negative rate in an article that did not recommend resection (20%, Carrillo et al.) was *higher* than that of the highest false negative rate in an article that did recommend resection (12.7%, McCoy et al.) [11, 18]. All articles that *compared* false negative rates in large and small nodules did not recommend resection, as the rates between small and large nodules were not significantly different. Half of articles that did not compare rates (i.e. only evaluated large nodules) recommended resection.

Nodules Larger Than 3 cm

Seven articles evaluated cytologically benign nodules using a size cutoff of 3 cm. Five articles directly compared false negative rates in nodules <3 cm versus >3 cm [19–23]. The total number of nodules with benign cytology that were evaluated ranged from 42 to 323 (12–83 in small, 30–240 in large nodules). False negative rates in small nodules ranged from 0 to 21.9%; false negative rates in large nodules ranged from 6.7 to 16.7%. One article reported unusually high false negative rates (43.7 and 77.3% in small and large nodules, respectively), however, they did include PTMC *outside* the index nodule as a "false negative," likely contributing to these high rates [20]. Two articles only evaluated false negative rates in nodules >3 cm [24, 25]. The number of large nodules with benign cytology that were evaluated were 112 and 145. False negative rates in these large nodules were 0.7 and 1.8%. When considering all seven articles, false negative diagnoses were reported in five. Of the four articles that documented false negative diagnoses in large nodules, the most frequently-reported diagnosis was PTC-FV (19 cases), followed by FTC (8 cases, including 1 HTC), PTC (4 cases, including 1 oxyphilic, 1 tall cell, and 1 with "mixed" histologic patterns), 2 PTMC (outside the index nodule), 2 UTC, and 1 PDC. One of these also reported 4 PTC-FV in nodules <3 cm [23]. One additional article reported false negative diagnoses without specifying size: 5 PTC-FV, 2 FTC, and 1 PTC.

Overall, false negative rates in nodules >3 cm were variable, ranging from 0.7 to 16.7%. Authors of 4 articles (4/7, 57%) did not recommend surgical resection of nodules >3 cm with benign cytology [19, 21, 24, 25]. Mehanna et al. additionally recommended repeat ultrasound-guided biopsy or consideration of surgery [21]. Authors of 3 articles (3/7, 43%) advocated surgical resection of all cytologically benign thyroid nodules >3 cm [20, 22, 23] due to higher false negative rates. Excluding the article that included PTMC outside nodule [20], the highest false negative rate in an article that did not recommend resection (10.9%, Mehanna) was slightly lower than that of the highest false negative rate in an article that did recommend resection (16.7%, Meko) [21, 22].

Summary and Limitations

Considering all 21 articles that evaluated false negative rates in cytologically benign thyroid nodules using size cutoffs of 3 or 4 cm, 13 (62%) did *not* recommend immediate surgical resection of large, cytologically benign nodules, as they found that false negative rates in large nodules were low, or were not significantly different from false negative rates in smaller nodules. In this group, three suggested repeat ultrasound-guided biopsy to identify any possible indeterminate or malignant nodules, and one recommended institution-dependent management (determining need for surgical resection based on false negative rates within one's own institution). One article considered preferential resection in women rather than men. Six of 21 (29%) advocated surgical resection of *all* large cytologically benign nodules due to false negative rate findings.

Most authors evaluated small to moderate numbers of large nodules (range 12–240, mean 87, median 84), likely due to low resection rates of cytologically benign nodules in standard practice. All but two studies were retrospective, leading to a significant selection bias in most studies. One study claimed to prospectively recruit patients, however, the management of patients did not appear different from the standard of care [7]. In other words, *not* all cytologically benign nodules were resected, and "surgery was to remove or exclude malignant goiter." Therefore, the patient population in this study is similar to that in retrospective studies [7]. Only one study appeared to be truly prospective, such that *all patients* with thyroid nodules >4 cm on ultrasound and no contraindication to or refusal of surgery proceeded to surgical resection regardless of the FNA result [15]. In this prospective study, false negative rates in large nodules were low (3.6%), and 2 of 3 were PTC-FV. A number of retrospective studies reported that surgical resection was routinely *offered* to patients with large nodules [13, 17–19, 21, 23], however, they do not claim that all patients with large nodules actually underwent resection; therefore, some level of selection bias is likely still present in these studies.

Another limitation is that only 8 of 21 articles included a pathologist amongst the authors [10–12, 17–19, 21, 24]. This rate seems low, given that the focus was to compare diagnoses on cytology to surgical pathology. This type of comparison is not always straightforward, and difficulties may arise when confirming that the nodule sampled on FNA was correlated to the surgical specimen, i.e. that the aspirated nodule was able to be identified based on the gross and microscopic surgical pathology report. Inclusion of a pathologist to assist with pathologic correlation would be encouraged.

Two articles that strongly recommended resection of large nodules made their recommendations not only based on perceived high false negative rates (5.8% and 12.7%, similar to other studies), but also claimed that benign cytology may miss or incorrectly classify "follicular lesions," namely follicular adenomas (including oncocytic or Hurthle cell adenomas) [16, 18]. McCoy et al. found 19 adenomas in their group of 71 cytologically benign nodules >4 cm [18]; Pinchot et al. found 22 adenomas in their group of 52 cytologically benign nodules >4 cm [16]. Pinchot also reported that none of the patients with a missed follicular lesion had a *malignant* follicular neoplasm. All missed cancers were PTC. Since follicular neoplasms require resection for determination of follicular adenoma versus carcinoma, they claim that follicular adenomas with benign cytology may be inappropriately treated non-surgically. There are a few issues with this statement: (1) We cannot assume that follow-up of patients with cytologically benign nodules is not needed. If a follicular neoplasm with benign cytology is not immediately resected, repeat FNA or subsequent resection may be prompted by growth, worrisome ultrasonographic features, or other patient symptoms. One may argue that a benign follicular adenoma that remains in the patient and does not grow, does not cause symptoms, and has no worrisome imaging features is likely not a significant threat. (2) We cannot assume that all follicular adenomas are highly cellular or composed of microfollicles, such that they would be called FLUS or follicular neoplasm on FNA). In fact, The Bethesda System specifically comments that "FNA is unable to distinguish NG [nodular goiter] from a colloid-rich, macrofollicular adenoma, so the latter will often be diagnosed cytologically as a BFN [benign follicular nodule]" [26]. In other words, a follicular adenoma composed of large follicles with abundant colloid will likely be classified as colloid nodule on FNA. (3) We cannot assume that all pathologists diagnose follicular adenoma in the same way. According to the World Health Organization Classification of Tumours of Endocrine Organs, follicular adenoma is "typically enclosed in a fibrous capsule of variable thickness…[and] may have been referred to as 'normofollicular', 'macrofollicular' and 'microfollicular', reflecting the size of the of the follicles comprising the tumor" [27]. Furthermore, the "distinction between follicular adenoma and adenomatoid nodule (cellular colloid nodule) is sometimes rather arbitrary." In light of the vague criteria and wide histologic spectrum (from follicular adenoma to adenomatoid nodule to hyperplastic nodule to colloid nodule), we cannot assume that identical diagnostic criteria are used by all pathologists, and what one may call a follicular adenoma, another may call a hyperplastic nodule. The only way to determine if a nodule is a true clonal neoplasm (i.e. adenoma) is via genetic analysis, which is not routinely performed on benign thyroid. In a clonality analysis using X-inactivation, Apel et al. found that 18 of 27 histologically hyperplastic thyroid nodules were monoclonal, and morphologically identical to the polyclonal cases [28]. Additionally, it is well-known that benign adenomatoid or histologically hyperplastic nodules harbor clonal *RAS* point mutations [29]. Due to the interobserver variability amongst both surgical pathologists and cytopathologists, caution must be exercised when evaluating so-called "missed follicular lesions," as the significance is unclear and negative impact on patient care may be minimal [3, 30].

Lastly, the prevalence of follicular variant of papillary thyroid carcinoma (PTC-FV) requires discussion. Considering all 14 articles that reported false negative diagnoses within the index nodule, PTC-FV was the most frequent (53/132, 40%). The proposed nomenclature revision for PTC-FV will affect these rates. Namely, neoplasms formerly classified as encapsulated, noninvasive PTC-FV, should, according to the proposal, now be classified as noninvasive follicular thyroid neoplasm with papillary-like nuclear features (NIFTP) as long as strict diagnostic criteria are met [31]. Infiltrative PTC-FV or encapsulated, invasive PTC-FV should not be classified as NIFTP and will still be considered cancers. True NIFTPs will no longer be classified or treated as cancers, but will be followed akin to follicular adenomas. Arguably, surgical resection is required for definitive diagnosis (similar to follicular neoplasms), however, the same concepts discussed above for follicular adenomas pertain to NIFTP: (1) not all are microfollicular or highly cellular; some are macrofollicular or colloid-rich; (2) a clinically aggressive but cytologically benign NIFTP could also be brought to attention (repeat FNA or resection) by worrisome clinical or radiographic features. Some studies have evaluated NIFTP in the context of the Bethesda system, and upon histologic re-review, decreases in the malignancy rates of cytologically benign (Bethesda II) nodules have been reported by various institutions (ranging from 3% to 60% relative percent decrease with removal of NIFTPs) [32, 33]. Not all historic PTC-FV would fall into the NIFTP category, however, some certainly will. False negative rates in this context are, therefore, expected to decrease.

Recommendations

Patients with cytologically benign (Bethesda II) thyroid nodules >3 cm or >4 cm in size on ultrasound need not undergo immediate surgical resection, in light of three main factors: (1) False negative rates in larger nodules are widely variable and, in most studies, are not significantly different from false negative rates in smaller nodules; (2) False negative rates are highly institution- and pathologist-dependent; (3) False negative rates are expected to decrease in light of new recommendations on the nomenclature of NIFTP versus PTC-FV. Although number needed to treat or cost-benefit analysis was not performed, surgical resection may lead to increased morbidity (physical, psychological, and possibly financial) compared to close clinical follow-up of cytologically benign nodules (including repeat ultrasound and/or FNA).

Quality of recommendation: (low quality evidence; weak recommendation).

Personal View

Rates of malignancy in cytologically benign nodules are highly variable, and depend upon individual and institutional practices of surgeons, endocrinologists, radiologists, and pathologists. First, false negative rates may be affected by variability in sampling practices: FNA under ultrasound guidance by an interventional radiologist with adequacy assessment by a cytopathologist is favored at our institution, in order to more accurately qualify the imaging characteristics of the nodule and target the nodule or region of interest. Palpation-guided aspiration is not recommended and is hypothesized to result in an increased number of inadequate or inappropriately-sampled specimens [34, 35]. At our institution, false negative rates in nodules <4 cm versus >4 cm are 2.5% and 5.4%, respectively, which is not a statistically significant difference (years 2011–2013) [36]. Second, interobserver variability amongst cytopathologists and surgical pathologists may affect false negative rates: A large study by Cibas et al. evaluated differences between an academic cytopathology panel and local community cytopathologists and found that overall concordance in the standard six-category Bethesda system was 64%. Furthermore, they found that local pathologists made fewer benign cytologic diagnoses, but their risk for malignancy was slightly higher; in other words, academic pathologists made more benign diagnoses with no increase in final false negative rate. Additionally, overall concordance in a 2-tier histopathology system (benign versus malignant) was 90.7%, with the most common disagreements being in PTC and PTC-FV [3].

It is my personal view that patients with cytologically benign but large thyroid nodules need not undergo immediate surgical resection, based on the reasons listed above: (1) False negative rates in larger nodules are widely variable and, in most studies, are not significantly different from false negative rates in smaller nodules; (2) False negative rates are highly institution- and pathologist-dependent; (3) False negative rates are expected to decrease in light of new recommendations on the nomenclature of NIFTP versus PTC-FV. Close clinical follow-up can identify patients who ultimately require resection, and those with indolent disease may avoid surgery for benign but large thyroid nodules.

Abstracted Recommendation for Box

Patients with cytologically benign (Bethesda II) thyroid nodules >3 cm or >4 cm in size on ultrasound need NOT undergo immediate surgical resection. Close clinical follow-up is advised. (low quality evidence; weak recommendation).

References

1. Cibas ES, Ali SZ. The Bethesda system for reporting thyroid cytopathology. Am J Clin Pathol. 2009;132(5):658–65.
2. Haugen BR, Alexander EK, Bible KC, Doherty GM, Mandel SJ, Nikiforov YE, Pacini F, Randolph GW, Sawka AM, Schlumberger M, Schuff KG, Sherman SI, Sosa JA, Steward DL, Tuttle RM, Wartofsky L. 2015 American Thyroid Association management guidelines for adult patients with thyroid nodules and differentiated thyroid cancer: the American Thyroid Association guidelines task force on thyroid nodules and differentiated thyroid cancer. Thyroid. 2016;26(1):1–133.
3. Cibas ES, Baloch ZW, Fellegara G, LiVolsi VA, Raab SS, Rosai J, Diggans J, Friedman L, Kennedy GC, Kloos RT, Lanman RB, Mandel SJ, Sindy N, Steward DL, Zeiger MA, Haugen BR, Alexander EK. A prospective assessment defining the limitations of thyroid nodule pathologic evaluation. Ann Intern Med. 2013;159(5):325–32.
4. Krauss EA, Mahon M, Fede JM, Zhang L. Application of the Bethesda classification for thyroid fine-needle aspiration: institutional experience and meta-analysis. Arch Pathol Lab Med. 2016;140(10):1121–31.
5. Parikh PP, Allan BJ, Lew JI. Sex variability of fine-needle aspiration reliability in the diagnosis of malignancy in thyroid nodules ≥4 cm. Am J Surg. 2013;206(5):778–82.
6. Albuja-Cruz MB, Goldfarb M, Gondek SS, Allan BJ, Lew JI. Reliability of fine-needle aspiration for thyroid nodules greater than or equal to 4 cm. J Surg Res. 2013;181(1):6–10.
7. Kuru B, Gulcelik NE, Gulcelik MA, Dincer H. The false-negative rate of fine-needle aspiration cytology for diagnosing thyroid carcinoma in thyroid nodules. Langenbeck's Arch Surg. 2010;395(2):127–32.
8. Bohacek L, Milas M, Mitchell J, Siperstein A, Berber E. Diagnostic accuracy of surgeon-performed ultrasound-guided fine-needle aspiration of thyroid nodules. Ann Surg Oncol. 2012;19(1):45–51.
9. Varshney R, Forest V-I, Zawawi F, Rochon L, Hier MP, Mlynarek A, Tamilia M, Payne RJ. Ultrasound-guided fine-needle aspiration of thyroid nodules: does size matter? Am J Otolaryngol. 2014;35(3):373–6.
10. Koo DH, Song K, Kwon H, Bae DS, Kim J-H, Min HS, Lee KE, Youn Y-K. Does tumor size influence the diagnostic accuracy of ultrasound-guided fine-needle aspiration cytology for thyroid nodules? Int J Endocrinol. 2016;2016(5):3803647–6.
11. Carrillo JF, Frias-Mendivil M, Ochoa-Carrillo FJ, Ibarra M. Accuracy of fine-needle aspiration biopsy of the thyroid combined with an evaluation of clinical and radiologic factors. Otolaryngol Head Neck Surg. 2000;122(6):917–21.
12. Khalife S, Bouhabel S, Forest V-I, Hier MP, Rochon L, Tamilia M, Payne RJ. The McGill thyroid nodule Score's (MTNS+) role in the investigation of thyroid nodules with benign ultrasound guided fine needle aspiration biopsies: a retrospective review. J Otolaryngol Head Neck Surg. 2016;45(1):29.
13. Raj MD, Grodski S, Woodruff S, Yeung M, Paul E, Serpell JW. Diagnostic lobectomy is not routinely required to exclude malignancy in thyroid nodules greater than four centimetres. ANZ J Surg. 2012;82(1–2):73–7.
14. Kulstad R. Do all thyroid nodules >4 cm need to be removed? An evaluation of thyroid fine-needle aspiration biopsy in large thyroid nodules. Endocr Pract. 2016;22(7):791–8.
15. Rosario PW, Salles DS, Bessa B. Low false-negative rate of cytology in thyroid nodules> 4 cm. Arq Bras Endocrinol Metabol. 2009;53(9):1143–5.
16. Pinchot SN, Al-Wagih H, Schaefer S, Sippel R, Chen H. Accuracy of fine-needle aspiration biopsy for predicting neoplasm or carcinoma in thyroid nodules 4 cm or larger. Arch Surg. 2009;144(7):649–55.
17. Wharry LI, McCoy KL, Stang MT, Armstrong MJ, LeBeau SO, Tublin ME, Sholosh B, Silbermann A, Ohori NP, Nikiforov YE, Hodak SP, Carty SE, Yip L. Thyroid nodules (≥4 cm): can ultrasound and cytology reliably exclude cancer? World J Surg. 2014;38(3):614–21.

18. McCoy KL, Jabbour N, Ogilvie JB, Ohori NP, Carty SE, Yim JH. The incidence of cancer and rate of false-negative cytology in thyroid nodules greater than or equal to 4 cm in size. Surgery. 2007;142(6):837–44. discussion 844.e1–3.
19. Ucler R, Usluogulları CA, Tam AA, Ozdemir D, Balkan F, Yalcın S, Kıyak G, Ersoy PE, Guler G, Ersoy R, Cakır B. The diagnostic accuracy of ultrasound-guided fine-needle aspiration biopsy for thyroid nodules three centimeters or larger in size. Diagn Cytopathol. 2015;43(8):622–8.
20. Ucar AE, Sarikaya SM, Parlak Ö, Yalcin A. Effect of nodule size on the reliability of fine-needle aspiration biopsy in thyroid nodules. Turk J Med Sci. 2014;44(6):1002–9.
21. Mehanna R, Murphy M, McCarthy J, O'Leary G, Tuthill A, Murphy MS, Sheahan P. False negatives in thyroid cytology: impact of large nodule size and follicular variant of papillary carcinoma. Laryngoscope. 2013;123(5):1305–9.
22. Meko JB, Norton JA. Large cystic/solid thyroid nodules: a potential false-negative fine-needle aspiration. Surgery. 1995;118(6):996–1003. discussion 1003–4.
23. Giles WH, Maclellan RA, Gawande AA, Ruan DT, Alexander EK, Moore FD, Cho NL. False negative cytology in large thyroid nodules. Ann Surg Oncol. 2015;22(1):152–7.
24. Porterfield JR, Grant CS, Dean DS, Thompson GB, Farley DR, Richards ML, Reading CC, Charboneau JW, Vollrath BK, Sebo TJ. Reliability of benign fine needle aspiration cytology of large thyroid nodules. Surgery. 2008;144(6):963–8. discussion 968–9.
25. Yoon JH, Kwak JY, Moon HJ, Kim MJ, Kim E-K. The diagnostic accuracy of ultrasound-guided fine-needle aspiration biopsy and the sonographic differences between benign and malignant thyroid nodules 3 cm or larger. Thyroid. 2011;21(9):993–1000.
26. Ali SZ, Cibas E. The Bethesda system for reporting thyroid cytopathology: definitions, criteria and explanatory notes. New York: Springer; 2010. p. 23.
27. Delellis RA, Lloyd RV, Heitz PU, Eng C, editors. World Health Organization classification of tumours. Lyon: IARC Press; 2004. p. 99.
28. Apel RL, Ezzat S, Bapat BV, Pan N, LiVolsi VA, Asa SL. Clonality of thyroid nodules in sporadic goiter. Diagn Mol Pathol. 1995;4(2):113–21.
29. Daniels GH. What if many follicular variant papillary thyroid carcinomas are not malignant? A review of follicular variant papillary thyroid carcinoma and a proposal for a new classification. Endocr Pract. 2011;17(5):768–87.
30. Cipriani NA, Nagar S, Kaplan SP, White MG, Antic T, Sadow PM, Aschebrook-Kilfoy B, Angelos P, Kaplan EL, Grogan RH. Follicular thyroid carcinoma: how have histologic diagnoses changed in the last half-century and what are the prognostic implications? Thyroid. 2015;25(11):1209–16.
31. Nikiforov YE, Seethala RR, Tallini G, Baloch ZW, Basolo F, Thompson LDR, Barletta JA, Wenig BM, Ghuzlan Al A, Kakudo K, Giordano TJ, Alves VA, Khanafshar E, Asa SL, El-Naggar AK, Gooding WE, Hodak SP, Lloyd RV, Maytal G, Mete O, Nikiforova MN, Nosé V, Papotti M, Poller DN, Sadow PM, Tischler AS, Tuttle RM, Wall KB, LiVolsi VA, Randolph GW, Ghossein RA. Nomenclature revision for encapsulated follicular variant of papillary thyroid carcinoma: a paradigm shift to reduce overtreatment of indolent tumors. JAMA Oncol. 2016;2(8):1023–9.
32. Strickland KC, Howitt BE, Marqusee E, Alexander EK, Cibas ES, Krane JF, Barletta JA. The impact of noninvasive follicular variant of papillary thyroid carcinoma on rates of malignancy for fine-needle aspiration diagnostic categories. Thyroid. 2015;25(9):987–92.
33. Faquin WC, Wong LQ, Afrogheh AH, Ali SZ, Bishop JA, Bongiovanni M, Pusztaszeri MP, VandenBussche CJ, Gourmaud J, Vaickus LJ, Baloch ZW. Impact of reclassifying noninvasive follicular variant of papillary thyroid carcinoma on the risk of malignancy in the Bethesda system for reporting thyroid cytopathology. Cancer Cytopathol. 2016;124(3):181–7.
34. Can AS, Peker K. Comparison of palpation-versus ultrasound-guided fine-needle aspiration biopsies in the evaluation of thyroid nodules. BMC Res Notes. 2008;1:12.
35. Wu M. A comparative study of 200 head and neck FNAs performed by a cytopathologist with versus without ultrasound guidance: evidence for improved diagnostic value with ultrasound guidance. Diagn Cytopathol. 2011;39(10):743–51.
36. Cavallo A, Johnson DN, White MG, Siddiqui S, Antic T, Mathew M, Grogan RH, Angelos P, Kaplan EL, Cipriani NA. Thyroid nodule size at ultrasound as a predictor of malignancy and final pathologic size. Thyroid. 2017;27(5):641–50.

Lobectomy Versus Total Thyroidectomy for Follicular Microcarcinomas

8

Linwah Yip

Abstract

The diagnosis of follicular thyroid cancer <1 cm is most likely to occur after initial thyroid lobectomy. High risk features include widely invasive, extensive angioinvasion (≥4 foci), or presence of distant metastasis and are the primary predictors of poor prognosis. In the absence of these features, thyroid lobectomy is likely adequate for treatment.

Keywords

Follicular thyroid carcinoma · Microcarcinoma · Extent of thyroidectomy · Thyroid surgery · Thyroid cancer

Follicular thyroid carcinoma (FTC) has historically represented 10–15% of diagnosed thyroid cancers [1]. FTC is more common in areas with endemic goiter and is associated with iodine deficiency. Therefore, the incidence is estimated to be lower (~5%) in iodine-replete geographic regions [2]. The incidence of FTC may be increasing nationally but at a rate that is slower than for papillary thyroid cancer (PTC) [3]. In contrast to the lymphatic spread characteristic of PTC, FTC spreads hematogenously to bone and lung. The relative 10-year survival for FTC is 85–90% and is lower than for PTC although patients with AJCC TNM stage I/II disease have an outstanding prognosis with mortality <1% [1]. Although there is a significant

L. Yip
Division of Endocrine Surgery, Department of Surgery, University of Pittsburgh School of Medicine, Pittsburgh, PA, USA
e-mail: yipl@upmc.edu

P. Angelos, R. H. Grogan (eds.), *Difficult Decisions in Endocrine Surgery*, Difficult Decisions in Surgery: An Evidence-Based Approach,
https://doi.org/10.1007/978-3-319-92860-9_8

increase in small (<1 cm) differentiated thyroid cancers, this is predominantly in PTC and overall, ~2% of <1 cm thyroid cancers are FTC [4, 5]. The aim of this review is to discuss the evidence available to guide treatment recommendations for FTC <1 cm (Table 8.1).

FTC incidence has been variable as a result of changes in histologic classification criteria. A cellular pattern of macro- or microfollicles without nuclear features of papillary thyroid cancer (PTC) is characteristic of both follicular adenoma (FA) and FTC [6]. The differentiating feature of carcinoma is the presence of capsular and/or vascular invasion. The criteria for diagnosing these invasive features are specific; for example, vascular invasion is defined by tumors cells in association with thrombus formation and tumor plugs within the vascular space is not in itself considered sufficient for vascular invasion [6]. Whether capsular invasion without vascular invasion has malignant potential is also debated although patients with capsular invasion alone have been reported to have distant metastatic disease.

Another histologic change that has caused variability in the incidence of FTC is the recognition of follicular-variant PTC (FV-PTC) as a clinically distinct entity. Microscopically, these lesions are predominantly follicular patterned but also have nuclear features of PTC [6]. The nuclear features associated with FV-PTC may be focal instead of diffuse, lack papillae, and may be entirely encapsulated. Thus, many of these lesions were likely misdiagnosed as FTC or FA. In a study by Cipriani et al. which histologically re-reviewed 66 FTC diagnosed over a 40 year time period, 70% were reclassified as PTC, FA, or poorly differentiated thyroid cancer (PDTC) [7]. In another study by Liu et al., ~30% of follicular neoplasms diagnosed from 1980 to 1995 were reclassified by a single pathologist to FV-PTC [8]. The changing histologic classification associated with follicular lesions has impacted FTC diagnosis in particular, and has implications for accurate interpretation of both population level data and historic retrospective studies that have not utilized histologic re-review [2, 9].

Because the diagnostic criteria rely on histologic features, FTC can only be diagnosed after thyroidectomy. For nodules >1 cm, often preoperative fine needle aspiration (FNA) biopsy is cytologically indeterminate (Bethesda III: atypia or follicular lesion of undetermined significance or IV: follicular neoplasm [10]) and at minimum, initial thyroid lobectomy has been performed [6]. Ultrasound features that have been described to associate with FTC include hypervascularity, hypoechogenicity, absence of a hypoechoic halo, calcifications, solid component, and larger nodule size, and these features may be most clinically helpful in directing need for FNA biopsy [11]. Available adjuncts such as FNA molecular marker testing or immunocytochemical analysis, lack sufficient accuracy to definitively differentiate FA from FTC. In the 2015 American Thyroid Association (ATA) Guidelines, FNA

Table 8.1 PICO table

Population	Patients with follicular thyroid cancer <1 cm
Intervention	Lobectomy
Comparator	Total thyroidectomy
Outcomes	Survival, quality of life, disease progression

biopsy is not recommended for nodules <1 cm [12] and small nodules are now less likely to undergo preoperative FNA biopsy. Recommendations for active observation versus thyroid lobectomy are proposed for differentiated thyroid cancer <1 cm however, it is unlikely, given the need for histologic evaluation, that FTC <1 cm will be diagnosed solely on radiographic, molecular, and/or cytologic criteria. Thus, the most likely current clinical scenarios for diagnosing FTC <1 cm is either incidentally or in the evaluation of distant metastatic disease.

Incidental Diagnosis of FTC

FTC is subclassified by the World Health Organization as either minimally or widely invasive [13]. Minimally invasive FTC without vascular invasion have indolent behavior with 97–98% disease-free survival at 10 years [14]. The presence of even minimal vascular invasion is a poorer prognostic factor and reduces the 10-year disease free survival to 80% [15–18]. In contrast, widely invasive FTC have <50% 10-year disease free survival [14, 19, 20] (Table 8.2). Thus, the degree of invasiveness and the presence as well as extent of vascular invasion are essential histologic variables.

Other disease-related factors that are associated with poorer outcomes include older age at diagnosis, larger size of the primary tumor, and completeness of resection [19]. Conventional staging systems such as AMES, AJCC TNM and even MACIS can provide accurate prognostic information for FTC patients [21–23]. Among patients with minimally-invasive FTC, variables that are associated with poor prognosis also include older age, larger tumor size (>4 cm), male gender, and extensive vascular invasion (≥4 foci) [16, 24, 25]. Lymph node metastasis are rare in FTC but have been reported in ~10% of patients at presentation [26]. Nodal disease does not appear to impact prognosis and does not correlate with distant metastasis. The presence of distant metastasis is the most important prognostic indicator; synchronous distant metastasis has been reported to occur in 3–20% and develop metachronously in 10–20% of patients [19, 27].

In a single institution series from Machens et al. which compared FTC to PTC outcomes after stratifying by tumor size, the cumulative risk of distant metastasis was equal for the two types of cancer and was directly proportional to tumor size. However, distant metastasis was not observed for PTC or FTC <2 cm in size [28]. Poorer outcomes were observed despite small tumor size in a population-level

Table 8.2 Classification of follicular thyroid carcinoma and prognosis

	10-year overall survival
All	85–90%
Minimally invasive	95–98%
Capsular only	98–100%
Angioinvasive	60–75%
Widely invasive	50–75%
Distant metastasis	20–40%

database study from Kuo et al. which evaluated histologic variables and for PTC, FTC, and Hurthle cell carcinomas (HCC) <1 cm [29]. This series specifically excluded minimally invasive FTC. The rate of distant metastasis for FTC <1 cm was 5.4% and overall 10-year disease specific survival was 95% which was lower than the 10-year disease specific survival for patients with PTC < 1 cm (99%). The study concluded that having HCC or FTC histology was an independent predictor of decreased survival even when tumor size was small [29]. Because the study utilized data from the SEER database (1988–2009) which does not mandate a centralized pathologic review, there is likely significant interobserver variability and potential overdiagnosis associated with FTC diagnosis that was not accounted for and which may be a confounder particularly for small tumors.

Synchronous Distant Metastasis

FTC can present with bone, lung, or more unusually, liver, brain, or soft tissue metastasis. The diagnosis can be challenging in the absence of a known history of thyroid cancer. Histologically, biopsy of the metastatic site will have follicular cells with a background of colloid, and immunohistochemical staining will be thyroid transcription factor-1 and thyroglobulin positive. When diagnosed, the initial treatment should include stabilization of bone disease associated with impending fracture or neurologic compromise, and total thyroidectomy which will allow for radioactive iodine (RAI) ablation therapy [12]. The prognosis of patients who present with metastatic FTC is dependent on degree of iodine avidity.

Surgical Treatment for FTC <1 cm

As mentioned, if synchronous metastasis is known, then total thyroidectomy should be the extent of initial thyroidectomy. Without a pre-existing diagnosis of synchronous metastasis, thyroid lobectomy has typically already been performed in order to reach the diagnosis of FTC. Completion thyroidectomy is considered for thyroid cancer if RAI ablation is needed and/or to facilitate surveillance [12]. FTC with concerning histologic features such as widely invasive or extensive vascular invasion (≥4 foci) are considered high risk for recurrence and metastatic disease, and should be treated with completion thyroidectomy followed by RAI ablation [12]. *TERT* promoter mutations have been found in up to 15% of FTC and are independent markers of aggressive disease including distant and persistent disease [30]. It is not yet known if *TERT* positive FTC without other histologic high-risk features should be treated more aggressively with total thyroidectomy and RAI ablation.

Minimally-invasive FTC have excellent long-term outcomes and current guidelines classify these as low risk tumors that could likely be treated with lobectomy alone [12, 31]. Sugino et al. evaluated a comparison cohort study of patients who had minimally-invasive FTC; 101 patients had total thyroidectomy and 223 patients had lobectomy alone [32]. The primary criteria for recommending completion thyroidectomy was patient age ≥45 years. The extent of surgery did not affect cause-specific survival regardless of patient age at diagnosis however, no patient age ≥45 years who had total thyroidectomy had disease-related mortality. The study concluded that completion thyroidectomy can be recommended for older patients with minimally-invasive FTC although the study was likely underpowered to show the true impact of extent of thyroidectomy on disease outcomes [32].

In a population-level analysis using the SEER database (2000–2009), 1200 patients with minimally-invasive FTC were evaluated and survival was not impacted by extent of thyroidectomy or use of RAI ablation [33]. The overall survival of patients with minimally-invasive FTC mirrored that of the U.S. general population regardless of type of treatment suggesting that thyroid lobectomy was likely adequate treatment. Megwalu et al. also queried the SEER database during a different time frame (1988–2009) to evaluate if extent of thyroidectomy was associated with outcomes in patients with FTC <1 cm (n = 203) [34]. Multifocal disease was rare (4%) and 5-year survival was the same in the lobectomy (98%) and total thyroidectomy (99%) cohorts. This study did not stratify tumors by degree of invasiveness but the findings suggested that small FTC are overall likely indolent [34].

Quality of life following thyroid cancer treatment has been reported to be decreased and is similar to survivors of other cancers with poorer prognosis such as colon, breast, and gynecologic cancers [35, 36]. However, there are no studies that have specifically compared quality of life in patients who had thyroid lobectomy versus total thyroidectomy. Quality of life is impacted by factors such as treatment related complications, need for testing, concern for recurrence and other physical and psychosocial components that contribute to well-being. Although operative risks are lower with lobectomy, it is unclear whether lobectomy instead of total thyroidectomy for low risk FTCs would impact quality of life.

In summary, FTC <1 cm are typically encountered after initial lobectomy has already been performed but can also rarely be diagnosed by the presence of synchronous distant metastasis. Extent and type of invasiveness has prognostic implications and guides subsequent treatment. Minimally invasive FTC has an outstanding long-term prognosis, and is likely adequately treated by lobectomy. Total thyroidectomy should be reserved for those patients with high risk widely-invasive FTC, or FTC with extensive vascular invasion which may still be associated with distant metastasis (up to 5%) even when size <1 cm.

References

1. Hundahl SA, Fleming ID, Fremgen AM, Menck HR. A National Cancer Data Base report on 53,856 cases of thyroid carcinoma treated in the U.S., 1985-1995 [see comments]. Cancer. 1998;83(12):2638–48. PMID: 9874472.
2. Franc B, de la Salmoniere P, Lange F, Hoang C, Louvel A, de Roquancourt A, et al. Interobserver and intraobserver reproducibility in the histopathology of follicular thyroid carcinoma. Hum Pathol. 2003;34(11):1092–100. PMID: 14652809.
3. Aschebrook-Kilfoy B, Grogan RH, Ward MH, Kaplan E, Devesa SS. Follicular thyroid cancer incidence patterns in the United States, 1980–2009. Thyroid. 2013;23(8):1015–21. PMID: 23360496. PMCID: 3752506.

4. Aschebrook-Kilfoy B, Ward MH, Sabra MM, Devesa SS. Thyroid cancer incidence patterns in the United States by histologic type, 1992–2006. Thyroid. 2011;21(2):125–34. PMID: 21186939. PMCID: 3025182.
5. Brito JP, Al Nofal A, Montori VM, Hay ID, Morris JC. The impact of subclinical disease and mechanism of detection on the rise in thyroid cancer incidence: a population-based study in Olmsted County, Minnesota during 1935 through 2012. Thyroid. 2015;25(9):999–1007. PMID: 26103159. PMCID: 4560845.
6. LiVolsi VA, Baloch ZW. Follicular-patterned tumors of the thyroid: the battle of benign vs. malignant vs. so-called uncertain. Endocr Pathol. 2011;22(4):184–9. PMID: 22072271.
7. Cipriani NA, Nagar S, Kaplan SP, White MG, Antic T, Sadow PM, et al. Follicular thyroid carcinoma: how have histologic diagnoses changed in the last half-century and what are the prognostic implications? Thyroid. 2015;25(11):1209–16. PMID: 26440366. PMCID: 4948203.
8. Liu J, Singh B, Tallini G, Carlson DL, Katabi N, Shaha A, et al. Follicular variant of papillary thyroid carcinoma: a clinicopathologic study of a problematic entity. Cancer. 2006;107(6):1255–64. PMID: 16900519.
9. Lloyd RV, Erickson LA, Casey MB, Lam KY, Lohse CM, Asa SL, et al. Observer variation in the diagnosis of follicular variant of papillary thyroid carcinoma. Am J Surg Pathol. 2004;28(10):1336–40. PMID: 15371949.
10. Cibas ES, Ali SZ. The Bethesda system for reporting thyroid cytopathology. Thyroid. 2009;19(11):1159–65. PMID: 19888858.
11. Sillery JC, Reading CC, Charboneau JW, Henrichsen TL, Hay ID, Mandrekar JN. Thyroid follicular carcinoma: sonographic features of 50 cases. AJR Am J Roentgenol. 2010;194(1):44–54. PMID: 20028904.
12. Haugen BRM, Alexander EK, Bible KC, Doherty G, Mandel SJ, Nikiforov YE, et al. American Thyroid Association Management Guidelines for Adult Patients with Thyroid Nodules and Differentiated Thyroid Cancer. Thyroid. 2015. PMID: 26462967.
13. DeLellis R, Lloyd RV, Heitz PU, Eng C. WHO/IARC classification of tumours. 3rd ed. Lyon: IARC Press; 2004.
14. D'Avanzo A, Treseler P, Ituarte PH, Wong M, Streja L, Greenspan FS, et al. Follicular thyroid carcinoma: histology and prognosis. Cancer. 2004;100(6):1123–9. PMID: 15022277.
15. O'Neill CJ, Vaughan L, Learoyd DL, Sidhu SB, Delbridge LW, Sywak MS. Management of follicular thyroid carcinoma should be individualised based on degree of capsular and vascular invasion. Eur J Surg Oncol. 2011;37(2):181–5. PMID: 21144693.
16. Lee YM, Lee YH, Song DE, Kim WB, Sung TY, Yoon JH, et al. Prognostic impact of further treatments on distant metastasis in patients with minimally invasive follicular thyroid carcinoma: verification using inverse probability of treatment weighting. World J Surg. 2017;41(4):1144. PMID: 28101608.
17. Kim HJ, Sung JY, Oh YL, Kim JH, Son YI, Min YK, et al. Association of vascular invasion with increased mortality in patients with minimally invasive follicular thyroid carcinoma but not widely invasive follicular thyroid carcinoma. Head Neck. 2014;36(12):1695–700. PMID: 24115217.
18. Ito Y, Hirokawa M, Masuoka H, Yabuta T, Kihara M, Higashiyama T, et al. Prognostic factors of minimally invasive follicular thyroid carcinoma: extensive vascular invasion significantly affects patient prognosis. Endocr J. 2013;60(5):637–42. PMID: 23327839.
19. Sugino K, Ito K, Nagahama M, Kitagawa W, Shibuya H, Ohkuwa K, et al. Prognosis and prognostic factors for distant metastases and tumor mortality in follicular thyroid carcinoma. Thyroid. 2011;21(7):751–7. PMID: 21615311.
20. Podda M, Saba A, Porru F, Reccia I, Pisanu A. Follicular thyroid carcinoma: differences in clinical relevance between minimally invasive and widely invasive tumors. World J Surg Oncol. 2015;13:193. PMID: 26041024. PMCID: 4458056.
21. Lo CY, Chan WF, Lam KY, Wan KY. Follicular thyroid carcinoma: the role of histology and staging systems in predicting survival. Ann Surg. 2005;242(5):708–15. PMID: 16244545. PMCID: 1409851.

22. D'Avanzo A, Ituarte P, Treseler P, Kebebew E, Wu J, Wong M, et al. Prognostic scoring systems in patients with follicular thyroid cancer: a comparison of different staging systems in predicting the patient outcome. Thyroid. 2004;14(6):453–8. PMID: 15242573.
23. Lang BH, Lo CY, Chan WF, Lam KY, Wan KY. Prognostic factors in papillary and follicular thyroid carcinoma: their implications for cancer staging. Ann Surg Oncol. 2007;14(2):730–8. PMID: 17103065.
24. Sugino K, Kameyama K, Ito K, Nagahama M, Kitagawa W, Shibuya H, et al. Outcomes and prognostic factors of 251 patients with minimally invasive follicular thyroid carcinoma. Thyroid. 2012;22(8):798–804. PMID: 22853727.
25. Lee YM, Song DE, Kim TY, Sung TY, Yoon JH, Chung KW, et al. Risk factors for distant metastasis in patients with minimally invasive follicular thyroid carcinoma. PLoS One. 2016;11(5):e0155489. PMID: 27171147. PMCID: 4865049.
26. Asari R, Koperek O, Scheuba C, Riss P, Kaserer K, Hoffmann M, et al. Follicular thyroid carcinoma in an iodine-replete endemic goiter region: a prospectively collected, retrospectively analyzed clinical trial. Ann Surg. 2009;249(6):1023–31. PMID: 19474675.
27. Ito Y, Hirokawa M, Higashiyama T, Takamura Y, Miya A, Kobayashi K, et al. Prognosis and prognostic factors of follicular carcinoma in Japan: importance of postoperative pathological examination. World J Surg. 2007;31(7):1417–24. PMID: 17534542.
28. Machens A, Holzhausen HJ, Dralle H. The prognostic value of primary tumor size in papillary and follicular thyroid carcinoma. Cancer. 2005;103(11):2269–73. PMID: 15856429.
29. Kuo EJ, Roman SA, Sosa JA. Patients with follicular and Hurthle cell microcarcinomas have compromised survival: a population level study of 22,738 patients. Surgery. 2013;154(6):1246–53. discussion 53-4. PMID: 23993409.
30. Melo M, da Rocha AG, Vinagre J, Batista R, Peixoto J, Tavares C, et al. TERT promoter mutations are a major indicator of poor outcome in differentiated thyroid carcinomas. J Clin Endocrinol Metab. 2014;99(5):E754–65. PMID: 24476079. PMCID: 4191548.
31. Dionigi G, Kraimps JL, Schmid KW, Hermann M, Sheu-Grabellus SY, De Wailly P, et al. Minimally invasive follicular thyroid cancer (MIFTC)--a consensus report of the European Society of Endocrine Surgeons (ESES). Langenbecks Arch Surg. 2014;399(2):165–84. PMID: 24233345.
32. Sugino K, Kameyama K, Nagahama M, Kitagawa W, Shibuya H, Ohkuwa K, et al. Does completion thyroidectomy improve the outcome of patients with minimally invasive follicular carcinoma of the thyroid? Ann Surg Oncol. 2014;21(9):2981–6. PMID: 24770681.
33. Goffredo P, Cheung K, Roman SA, Sosa JA. Can minimally invasive follicular thyroid cancer be approached as a benign lesion?: a population-level analysis of survival among 1,200 patients. Ann Surg Oncol. 2013;20(3):767–72. PMID: 23111705.
34. Megwalu UC, Green RW. Total thyroidectomy versus lobectomy for the treatment of follicular thyroid microcarcinoma. Anticancer Res. 2016;36(6):2899–902. PMID: 27272803.
35. Aschebrook-Kilfoy B, James B, Nagar S, Kaplan S, Seng V, Ahsan H, et al. Risk factors for decreased quality of life in thyroid cancer survivors: initial findings from the North American thyroid cancer survivorship study. Thyroid. 2015;25(12):1313–21. PMID: 26431811. PMCID: 4684649.
36. Applewhite MK, James BC, Kaplan SP, Angelos P, Kaplan EL, Grogan RH, et al. Quality of life in thyroid cancer is similar to that of other cancers with worse survival. World J Surg. 2016;40(3):551–61. PMID: 26546191.

9 Initial Total Thyroidectomy Versus Lobectomy with Intraoperative Frozen Section for Thyroid Nodules That Are "Suspicious for PTC"

Jason A. Glenn and Tracy S. Wang

Abstract

The optimal surgical management for a thyroid nodule that is 'suspicious for papillary thyroid carcinoma (PTC)' remains unclear. Surgical options include (1) lobectomy with intraoperative frozen section or (2) initial total thyroidectomy. To help address this clinical question we employ the GRADE approach. The current literature was reviewed, and outcomes were assessed for their impact on clinical decision-making as related to thyroid surgery. Based on our review of the literature, it is clear that there is currently a paucity of high-to-moderate quality evidence regarding the treatment of patients with thyroid nodules that are 'suspicious for PTC'. Important aspects to consider in the decision-making process are (1) accuracy of diagnosis and (2) relative risk of surgery. When considering the available evidence, assuming relatively low complication rates by experienced surgeons, initial total thyroidectomy may be recommended.

Keywords

Papillary thyroid carcinoma · Suspicious for malignancy · Total thyroidectomy · Thyroid lobectomy · Frozen section · Thyroidectomy cost

J. A. Glenn
Department of Surgery, Medical College of Wisconsin Affiliated Hospitals, Milwaukee, WI, USA

T. S. Wang (✉)
Department of Surgery, Division of Surgical Oncology, Section of Endocrine Surgery, Medical College of Wisconsin, Milwaukee, WI, USA
e-mail: tswang@mcw.edu

P. Angelos, R. H. Grogan (eds.), *Difficult Decisions in Endocrine Surgery*, Difficult Decisions in Surgery: An Evidence-Based Approach, https://doi.org/10.1007/978-3-319-92860-9_9

Introduction

The incidence of thyroid nodular disease is increasing, largely attributed to an aging population and the increased use of cross-sectional imaging of the neck and chest [1]. Thyroid nodules are detected in up to 10% of the United States population, of whom 5–30% are found to have a malignancy requiring thyroidectomy (up to 90% are papillary thyroid carcinoma, PTC) [2, 3]. As the societal cost for thyroid cancer treatment is projected to reach $3.1 billion by 2020, there continues to be controversy regarding the optimal surgical management of PTC [4, 5]. To help define the current clinical question, the Population, Intervention, Comparator, and Outcome (PICO) strategy was employed (Table 9.1).

Current Status of Thyroid Cancer Diagnosis

Fine-needle aspiration (FNA) is the gold standard for the preoperative assessment of thyroid nodules, as it is rapid and cost-effective [6]. However, due to sampling errors, histological variants (e.g. follicular variant PTC), and variable interpretations from non-expert cytopathologists (overall intra-observer accordance rate as low as 64%), the rate of agreement between FNA cytology and final surgical histopathology has been reported to be under 73% [7, 8]. In 2009, the Bethesda System for Reporting Thyroid Cytopathology was introduced to help increase the reproducibility of FNA diagnoses (Table 9.2) [9, 10].

Table 9.1 PICO table

Population	Node-negative patients with no family history of thyroid cancer or prior neck irradiation, who present with a unifocal, 1–4 cm thyroid nodule diagnosed as 'suspicious for PTC' on FNA
Intervention	Diagnostic lobectomy with intraoperative frozen section
Comparator	Initial total thyroidectomy
Outcomes	Diagnostic accuracy; patient quality-of-life; cost/time benefits

Table 9.2 Incidence of malignancy according to The Bethesda System for Reporting Thyroid Cytopathology [7, 9, 10]

Category	Intra-observer accordance (%)	Incidence of malignancy (%)	Management
I. Non-diagnostic	69	1–4	Repeat FNA
II. Benign	82	0–3	Clinical follow-up
III. Atypia or follicular lesion of undetermined significance	35	5–15	Repeat FNA
IV. Follicular neoplasm	66	15–30	Diagnostic lobectomy
V. Suspicious for malignancy (suspicious for PTC)	37	50–75	Total thyroidectomy or diagnostic lobectomy
VI. Malignant	94	97–99	Total thyroidectomy

FNA fine-needle aspiration, *PTC* papillary thyroid carcinoma

Previously grouped into an 'indeterminate' category, a new designation of 'suspicious for malignancy' (Bethesda Category V) was proposed by the Bethesda System. For a nodule to be confirmed as PTC (Bethesda Category VI) on FNA, cytology must demonstrate sheets of epithelial cells, enlarged nuclei, intra-nuclear inclusions, nuclear grooves, and papillary structures [9, 10]. If only a few of these characteristics are present, if the features are not widespread throughout the cell population, or if the specimen is sparsely cellular, a malignant diagnosis cannot be established and the specimen is considered 'suspicious for PTC' [9, 10]. Up to 7% of all nodules are diagnosed as 'suspicious for PTC', anywhere from 29 to 95% of which have been reported to harbor thyroid cancer on final surgical histopathology [10–16]. Despite the widespread implementation of the Bethesda System classification, the intra-observer accordance has been reported to be as low as 37% for a diagnosis of 'suspicious for PTC' [7]. Therefore, due to lack of diagnostic reproducibility and varying reports of malignancy incidence, the optimal surgical management for thyroid nodules that are 'suspicious for PTC' remains unclear.

Optimal Surgical Management of Thyroid Nodules That Are 'Suspicious for PTC'

According to the 2015 Revised American Thyroid Association (ATA) guidelines, thyroid lobectomy is indicated for patients with a solitary, cytologically indeterminate nodule (R19; Strong recommendation) [17]. However, due to an increased risk for disease recurrence and the potential need for radioactive iodine adjuvant therapy and/or use of serum thyroglobulin to identify recurrent PTC, initial total thyroidectomy is indicated for patients that have large (>4 cm) nodules, gross extrathyroidal extension, metastatic disease, a family history of thyroid cancer, or a personal history of neck irradiation (R20 and R35; Strong recommendations) [17]. For nodules that are 'suspicious for malignancy' on FNA, these guidelines suggest that total thyroidectomy *may* be preferred, as long as completion thyroidectomy would be indicated based on malignant histopathology (R20; Strong recommendation) [17].

Advocates of initial thyroid lobectomy cite advantages in outcomes such as overall cost, operative time, and quality-of-life, as a subset of patients may not require total thyroidectomy. Intraoperative frozen section is typically performed, with immediate completion thyroidectomy if a malignancy is identified [18–20]. Thyroid lobectomy may prevent patients with benign pathology from requiring life-long thyroid hormone replacement and spare them from the potential morbidity of total thyroidectomy, which can include hypoparathyroidism and bilateral recurrent laryngeal nerve (RLN) injury. Alternatively, those who advocate initial total thyroidectomy report relatively high variability in the diagnostic accuracy of frozen section, noting very little advantage over FNA diagnosis in some studies [21, 22]. A report by Akhtar et al. noted that while FNA and frozen section had 100% specificity for detecting malignancy at their institution, both diagnostic adjuncts had relatively low sensitivity (50% and 64%, respectively) and overall accuracy (68% and 77%, respectively) [23]. Due to the risk of multifocality with thyroid cancer, completion thyroidectomy is recommended for high risk tumors (e.g. extrathyroidal extension, locoregional metastases, BRAF mutation); false-negative frozen sections (benign on frozen section but malignant on final pathology) would require a second operation, often performed at least 8 weeks after initial surgery to minimize potential morbidity [17]. This not only increases potential morbidity but also requires a second recovery, increasing loss of productivity.

Evaluation of Surgical Management Options

The GRADE approach for literature review systematically defines a clinical question, ranks the importance of various outcomes, stratifies the quality of published evidence, and summarizes the authors' confidence in the estimate of treatment effect to support a particular clinical decision [24]. To help define the current clinical question, the Population, Intervention, Comparator, and Outcome (PICO) strategy was employed. The target population is defined as patients with no family history of thyroid cancer, prior neck irradiation, or clinical evidence of metastatic lymphadenopathy, who present with a unifocal, 1–4 cm thyroid nodule that is diagnosed as 'suspicious for PTC' on FNA cytology. The intervention being studied is lobectomy with intraoperative frozen section and the comparator is initial total thyroidectomy (Table 9.1). In the following sections, several outcomes that influence thyroid cancer clinical decision-making are considered. The primary outcome evaluated was 'diagnostic accuracy' (the probability that a thyroid nodule that is 'suspicious for PTC' on FNA cytology is in fact malignant on final surgical histopathology, or the probability that a nodule that is benign on frozen section is in fact benign on final surgical histopathology), as this is paramount in determining the extent of initial operation for nodules that are 'suspicious for PTC'. Outcomes such as patient quality-of-life and cost/time benefits were also assessed.

Search Strategy

A comprehensive review of the literature was performed. Searches were conducted in the PubMed Medline database using the key words: suspicious for papillary thyroid carcinoma, indeterminate thyroid nodules, total thyroidectomy, thyroid lobectomy, hemithyroidectomy, thyroid intraoperative frozen section, and thyroidectomy cost. Searches were limited to the English language, human subjects, and literature published within the last 10 years. Our search returned 953 studies. A total of 26 articles were critically reviewed; these studies included information related to the diagnostic accuracy of FNA and/or frozen section for nodules that are 'suspicious for PTC', information on patient quality-of-life when comparing total thyroidectomy to thyroid lobectomy with frozen section, or information analyzing cost/time outcomes for thyroid surgery. Clinical practice guidelines from the ATA were included for reference.

Diagnostic Accuracy

First introduced about 85 years ago, FNA has proven to be a simple, cost-effective tool in the evaluation of thyroid nodules [18, 23]. When a nodule is diagnosed as either 'benign' (Bethesda Category II) or 'malignant' (Bethesda Category VI) on FNA cytology, the rate of agreement with the final surgical histopathology is >97% [25]. However, when a nodule is diagnosed as 'suspicious for PTC', the rate of agreement varies widely between studies [10–16]. This discrepancy is largely due to a lack of diagnostic reproducibility for suspicious nodules (FNA cytology that experienced cytopathologists label as benign or malignant, are instead labeled as suspicious by less experienced cytopathologists) [7]. Thus, an institution's rate of agreement between FNA cytology and final surgical histopathology should help guide the optimal initial surgical management at that particular institution.

Accuracy of FNA in Thyroid Nodules That Are 'Suspicious for PTC'

The Bethesda System for Reporting Thyroid Cytopathology reports a 50–75% incidence of malignancy in nodules that are 'suspicious for PTC' [9, 10]. However, as noted in several recent studies, this incidence can range anywhere from 33% to 87%, and is largely contingent on the expertise of the respective cytopathologists in determining malignancy when all cytological criteria for PTC diagnosis are not met (Table 9.3) [14, 18–20, 25–33]. All of these recent studies were retrospective institutional reviews with relatively small sample sizes; therefore, the quality of available evidence for determining the accuracy of FNA in our target patient population is limited.

In a report by Kwak et al., five off-site pathologists, specializing in thyroid cytopathology, reviewed 10,487 FNAs performed over a 4-year period [33]. They diagnosed 394 (4%) of these nodules as 'suspicious for PTC', and 303 (77%) subsequently underwent thyroidectomy. The rate of agreement between FNA cytology and final surgical histopathology for these patients was 84% [33]. Moon et al. echoed these findings in another recent report, where over a one and a half-year period, nine expert cytopathologists reviewed 10,338 FNAs; 410 (4%) nodules were diagnosed as 'suspicious for PTC', and 217 (53%) subsequently underwent thyroidectomy [20]. The rate of agreement between FNA cytology and final surgical histopathology for these patients was 87% [20].

Several smaller studies have suggested that the accuracy of FNA for diagnosing nodules that are 'suspicious for PTC' may be significantly less than what has been reported above; however, these studies consist of much smaller sample sizes and rarely comment on the expertise of cytopathologists [14, 19, 26, 28, 30]. In a report by Huber et al., ten pathologists, without mention of thyroid cytopathology expertise, reviewed 201 FNAs obtained at a single institution over a two and a half-year period [28]. In a total of 15 thyroid nodules diagnosed as 'suspicious for malignancy', the agreement rate between FNA cytology and final surgical histopathology

Table 9.3 Diagnostic accuracy of FNA and frozen section for suspicious thyroid nodules

Study (year)	Population	Study type	Number of suspicious FNAs	Incidence of malignancy; n, %	Number of frozen sections	Frozen section false-negatives; n, % (NPV)	Quality of evidence[a]
Basolo et al. (2007) [18]	Suspicious for PTC	Retrospective	14	12, 86%	4	0, 0% (100)	Low
Baynes et al. (2014) [25]	Suspicious for malignancy	Retrospective	94	53, 56%	NR	NR	Low
Chao et al. (2007) [26]	Suspicious for malignancy	Retrospective	56	26, 46%	56[b]	4, 7%[b] (88)	Low
Chiu et al. (2012) [27]	Suspicious for PTC	Retrospective	44	28, 64%	NR	NR	Low
Haymart et al. (2008) [19]	Suspicious for PTC	Retrospective	30	17, 57%	26	2, 8% (85)	Low
Huber et al. (2007) [28]	Suspicious for malignancy	Retrospective	15	5, 33%	11	3, 27% (70)	Low
Kwak et al. (2008) [33]	Suspicious for PTC	Retrospective	303	255, 84%	NR	NR	Low
Makay et al. (2007) [29]	Suspicious for PTC	Retrospective	24	19, 79%	NR	NR	Low
Mittendorf et al. (2006) [14]	Suspicious for malignancy	Retrospective	45	18, 40%	14	0, 0% (100)	Low
Moon et al. (2009) [20]	Suspicious for PTC	Retrospective	217	189, 87%	217	14, 7% (50)	Mod
Raj et al. (2010) [30]	Suspicious for malignancy	Retrospective	51	24, 47%	NR	NR	Low
Sangalli et al. (2006) [32]	Suspicious for malignancy	Retrospective	65	50, 77%	NR	NR	Low
Yoder et al. (2006) [31]	Suspicious for malignancy	Retrospective	17	11, 65%	NR	NR	Low

NR not reported, *FNA* fine-needle aspiration, *NPV* negative-predictive value, *PTC* papillary thyroid carcinoma

[a] Rating of quality of evidence based on GRADE approach [24]

[b] Data abstracted from other findings in study, actual results may vary slightly

was only 33%. When considering the results of the larger and smaller studies together, these findings suggest that a high institutional volume of suspicious thyroid nodules, as well as physician expertise in thyroid cytopathology, improve the diagnostic accuracy of FNA for nodules that are 'suspicious for PTC'.

Accuracy of Frozen Section in Thyroid Nodules That Are 'Suspicious for PTC'

Frozen section has been in use since 1818; however, it was not until the introduction of cryostat in 1960 that it became widely used in the intraoperative evaluation of indeterminate thyroid nodules [18]. Despite its relative popularity, the 2015 Revised ATA guidelines does not recommend intraoperative frozen section in the management of nodules that are 'suspicious for malignancy' [17]. This omission leaves the utility of frozen section up for debate and ultimately at the discretion of the surgeon. The goal of intraoperative frozen section is to identify benign nodules and rule out the presence of malignancy. As a result, the negative predictive value (NPV) of intraoperative frozen section is of critical importance. With respect to thyroid frozen section, NPV denotes the proportion of lesions interpreted as benign on frozen section that are also benign on final surgical histopathology *(NPV = true negatives/(true negatives + false negatives))*. Therefore, a low NPV (more false-negatives) results in a higher proportion of patients that require completion thyroidectomy.

Several recent studies have examined the diagnostic accuracy of intraoperative frozen section for nodules that are 'suspicious for PTC' [14, 18–20, 26]. The NPV in these studies ranged from 50 to 100%; however, the quality of available evidence was limited, as only two studies reported >30 intraoperative frozen sections during their study period (Table 9.3) [14, 18–20, 26]. Chao et al. evaluated 569 intraoperative frozen sections performed over a two and a half-year period, which included 56 thyroid nodules that were 'suspicious for malignancy' [26]. They reported that the NPV of intraoperative frozen section at their institution was 88%, but also noted a rate of agreement between FNA cytology and final surgical histopathology of only 46% [26]. In the previously mentioned study by Moon et al., 217 intraoperative frozen sections were performed on nodules that were 'suspicious for PTC' [20]. They reported that the NPV at their institution was only 50% for suspicious nodules, whereas the rate of agreement between FNA cytology and final surgical histopathology was 87% [20]. Due to the relative inaccuracy of FNA cytology and a high NPV of frozen section in the Chao et al. study, initial thyroid lobectomy with frozen section may be recommended as the preferred management at that institution. Conversely, accurate FNA cytology and a relatively low NPV of frozen section reported in the Moon et al. study suggests that total thyroidectomy may be the preferred initial management at that institution.

In a recent cost-effectiveness study by Leiker et al., a Markov decision model was created to compare the incremental cost-utility of total thyroidectomy versus lobectomy with intraoperative frozen section as the initial surgical management for thyroid nodules that are 'suspicious for PTC' [34]. The authors found that

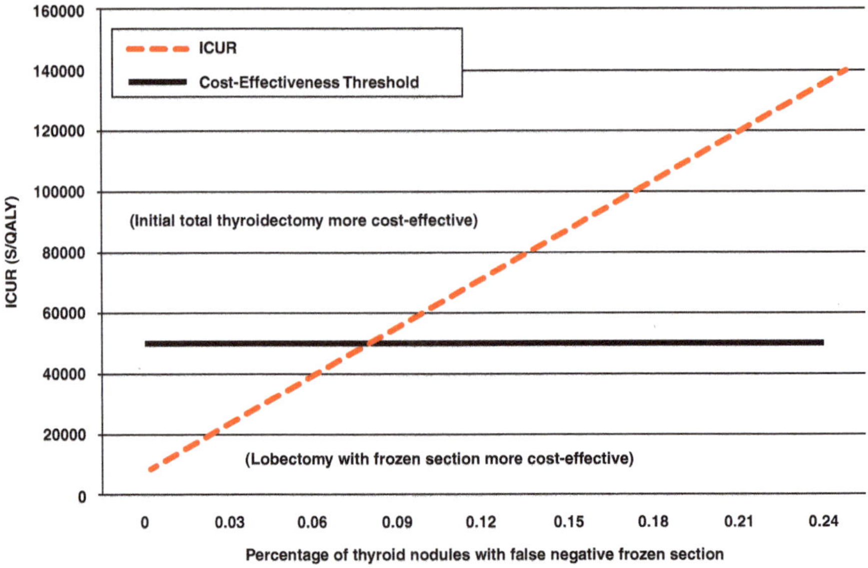

Fig. 9.1 Sensitivity analysis of the negative predictive values of frozen section in the diagnosis of nodules that are 'suspicious for PTC'. *ICUR* incremental cost-utility ratio, *QALY* quality-adjusted life-year; *Adapted with permission of Leiker et al. [34]

lobectomy with intraoperative frozen section becomes the favored initial surgical procedure only when the percentage of false-negative frozen sections is ≤8%; otherwise, initial total thyroidectomy dominates as the preferred surgical management (Fig. 9.1) [34]. As the included studies reported values above and below this threshold, each institution should evaluate their own frozen section NPV to determine if lobectomy with intraoperative frozen section is advantageous over FNA cytology alone for the treatment of nodules that are 'suspicious for PTC'.

Use of Molecular Markers in Thyroid Nodules That Are 'Suspicious for PTC'

In an effort to better characterize the malignant potential of 'indeterminate' thyroid nodules, there has been increased utilization of molecular markers as preoperative adjuncts in recent years [35]. Preliminary data suggests that the greatest influence of mutational analysis on surgical decision-making comes when the pre-test probability of malignancy is relatively low (i.e. atypical/follicular lesions of undetermined significance or follicular neoplasms) [17]. In these cases, a positive test result would likely favor initial total thyroidectomy, and a negative result may or may not facilitate decision-making, depending on the sensitivity of test being used and the clinical context (nodule size, ultrasound characteristics, etc.). The role for the molecular profiling of nodules that are 'suspicious for malignancy' remains less clear, as the sensitivity for many of these tests approximate the estimated risk of malignancy based on cytological analysis alone (up to 75%) [17, 35].

Several molecular profiling platforms have been developed over the past 10 years, a few of which are now commercially available. Gene-Expression Classifier (GEC) tests measure the expression of >160 thyroid gene transcripts, for which somatic mutations have been identified in >70% of PTCs [17, 36–38]. In a prospective, double blind, multicenter study, Alexander et al. found that GEC testing correctly identified 92% of malignant thyroid nodules, and they noted a NPV of 85% in 55 nodules that were 'suspicious for malignancy'. However, a positive predictive value (PPV) of 76%, which is similar to that of FNA cytology alone, suggests that GEC may not significantly change surgical decision-making for nodules that are 'suspicious for malignancy' [39–42].

Next-Generation Sequencing (NGS) panels offer simultaneous detection of >1000 known mutation hotspots and >40 gene fusion sites for multiple thyroid cancer-related genes [17, 43, 44]. In studies evaluating the diagnostic accuracy of NGS for 'indeterminate' thyroid nodules, Nikiforov et al. found that the residual risk of malignancy in thyroid nodules that are 'suspicious for malignancy' and have a negative NGS panel, is approximately 20% [43, 44]. Additionally, several retrospective single institution studies have reported a specificity up to 96% and PPV up to 95% when using NGS panels that include BRAF, RAS, RET/PTC, and PAX8/PPARγ [17, 45–47]. As such, the 2015 Revised ATA guidelines recommend that mutational testing for BRAF, or the use of an NGS panel, *may* be considered in nodules that are 'suspicious for malignancy' if the results are expected to alter surgical decision-making (R17; Weak recommendation) [17].

Recommendation

The diagnostic accuracy of FNA and intraoperative frozen section for nodules that are 'suspicious for PTC' ranges widely in the literature, and is likely to be institution and cytopathologist-dependent. If the data obtained by FNA is deemed to be sufficiently accurate for suspicious nodules and/or if the proportion of false-negative frozen sections is >8%, then total thyroidectomy may be recommended as the preferred initial surgical management. If the data obtained by FNA is deemed to be relatively inaccurate, then frozen section or molecular testing may offer a diagnostic benefit over FNA cytology alone. Due to the important impact that diagnostic accuracy has in determining the optimal surgical management of thyroid nodules, the authors rate this outcome as 'critical for decision-making'. However, when taken together, due to a small sample size and lack of prospective studies, the overall quality of available evidence for this outcome is low. For each study reviewed, a summary of the quality of evidence is included in Table 9.3.

Quality of Life

Patient quality-of-life is an important determinate for any clinical decision. When assessing the optimal extent of thyroid resection, factors such as perioperative morbidity and the need for life-long thyroid hormone replacement must be considered. The most common complications after thyroidectomy include recurrent laryngeal nerve (RLN) injury, hypoparathyroidism, and iatrogenic hypothyroidism [48, 49]. There is a relative paucity of data specifically reporting these complications in those treated for nodules that are 'suspicious for PTC'; therefore, the following sections will include a general overview of recent literature evaluating total thyroidectomy, lobectomy, and completion thyroidectomy associated complications.

Recurrent Laryngeal Nerve Injury

Although RLN injury is a relatively rare complication of thyroid surgery, it potentially has the greatest effects on overall patient quality-of-life [50]. The life-threatening complication of bilateral RLN injury, rarely seen following total thyroidectomy, has led many clinicians to favor lobectomy with intraoperative frozen section as the initial surgical management of suspicious nodules. Several recent studies have reported on the incidence of RLN injury following thyroid surgery, noting a permanent RLN injury rate of up to 1.9% for total thyroidectomy, up to 0.9% for lobectomy, and up to 3.1% for completion thyroidectomy (Table 9.3) [48, 49, 51–55]. In the two studies that directly compared total thyroidectomy with completion thyroidectomy, the latter was associated with increased RLN injury rates (0 vs 0.5% and 1.4 vs 2.5%, respectively) [52, 55]. This higher injury rate following completion thyroidectomy may suggest that total thyroidectomy represents the preferred initial surgical management of thyroid nodules that are 'suspicious for PTC'. Similarly, Leiker et al. noted that total thyroidectomy remained the more cost-effective approach, unless rates of unilateral and bilateral RLN injury exceeded 5% and 2%, respectively; these rates were not observed in any of the reviewed studies and are higher than what would be clinically acceptable [34].

Hypoparathyroidism

Hypoparathyroidism is the most commonly reported procedure-related complication following thyroid surgery [48, 49]. Although total thyroidectomy has previously been associated with higher rates of hypoparathyroidism when compared to lobectomy, concerns over an increased risk of hypoparathyroidism following completion thyroidectomy has led many clinicians to favor initial total resection [51]. Several recent studies have reported on the incidence of hypoparathyroidism following thyroid surgery, for which the rates of permanent hypoparathyroidism have ranged from 3.3 to 16.1% for total thyroidectomy, 1.4–7.1% for lobectomy, and 2.5–4.0% for completion thyroidectomy (Table 9.4) [48, 49, 51–55].

In a study by Vaiman et al., hypoparathyroidism was noted following 3.5% of 3834 total thyroidectomies, 1.4% of 1051 lobectomies, and 4.0% of 194 completion thyroidectomies [55]. Despite a relatively small sample size of completions, there were no significant differences in hypoparathyroidism rates between total and completion thyroidectomies in this study. In another recent study, Rafferty et al. reported a higher rate of postoperative hypoparathyroidism following total thyroidectomy

(3.3%) when compared to completion thyroidectomy (2.5%) [52]. While varying rates of parathyroid re-implantation may be a potential confounder of this data, improved surgical techniques and an increased overall volume of thyroid surgery have likely resulted in hypoparathyroidism rates that are comparable for total and completion thyroidectomies. In a prospective, randomized study by Cayo et al., no significant differences were found in rates of postoperative hypoparathyroidism based on the surgical procedure performed (total versus completion thyroidectomy), the frequency of parathyroid re-implantation, or the frequency of central compartment neck dissection [56].

Hypothyroidism

When determining the optimal surgical management for suspicious thyroid nodules, a reported advantage of lobectomy is that if the intraoperative frozen section is benign, half of the gland is preserved, allowing for an endogenous source of thyroid hormone. However, recent data suggests that many of these patients still require thyroid hormone replacement following lobectomy. A meta-analysis by Kandil et al. examined the need for thyroid hormone replacement following lobectomy; their review included 32 studies and a total of 15,412 lobectomies [57]. They reported an overall incidence of hypothyroidism ranging from 11 to 49% across studies (Table 9.4), noting an increased occurrence in patients with thyroiditis and in those with a high-normal preoperative TSH (relative risk of 3.2 for TSH >2.5 μIU/L).

Recommendation

Based on a slightly higher rate of RLN injury following completion thyroidectomy and the significant proportion of lobectomy patients that become hypothyroid, initial total thyroidectomy may be recommended, assuming relatively low complication rates with experienced surgeons. However, this data is generalized and does not specifically encompass those patients in our target population (thyroid nodules that are 'suspicious for PTC'). Due to relatively small differences in complication rates, the authors rate this outcome as 'important, but not critical for decision-making'. When taken together, the overall quality of available evidence for this outcome is low. For each study reviewed, a summary of the quality of evidence is included in Table 9.4.

Cost/Time Benefits

It is undeniable that we are in an era of increasing health care regulation and oversight by federal and private insurance agencies. With the ballooning costs of thyroid cancer diagnosis and treatment, hospitals are held self-accountable to provide efficient and

Table 9.4 Complication rates following thyroidectomy

Study (year)	Study type	Number of TT (Group A)	Number of lobectomies (Group B)	Number of CT (Group C)	RLN injuries (%)	Hypo-parathyroidism (%)	Hypo-thyroidism (%)	Quality of evidence[a]
Glockzin et al. (2012) [54]	Retrospective	NR	NR	128	C: 3.1	C: 3.1	NR	Low
Hauch et al. (2014) [48]	Observational(NIS)	36,316	26,406	NR	A: 1.3 B: 0.6	A: 16.1 B: 7.1	NR	Mod
Kandil et al. (2013) [57]	Meta-analysis (32 studies)	NR	15,412	NR	NR	NR	C: 10.9–48.8	Mod
Lefevre et al. (2007) [51]	Retrospective	NR	NR	685	C: 1.5	C: 2.5	NR	Low
Rafferty et al. (2007) [52]	Retrospective	149	NR	201	A: 0 C: 0.5	A: 3.3 C: 2.5	NR	Low
Vaiman et al. (2010) [55]	Retrospective	3834	1051	194	A: 1.4 B: 0.9 C: 2.5	A: 3.5 B: 1.4 C: 4.0	NR	Low
Vashishta et al. (2012) [49]	Observational (NIS)	31,862	19,725	NR	A: 1.1 B: 0.6	A: 8.6 B: 2.1	NR	Mod
Zerey et al. (2009) [53]	Observational (NIS)	9616	4238	NR	A: 1.9 B: 0.8	A: 10.6 B: 3.5	NR	Mod

NR not reported, *TT* total thyroidectomies, *CT* completion thyroidectomies, *RLN* recurrent laryngeal nerve, *NIS* Nationwide Inpatient Specimen
[a]Rating of quality of evidence based on GRADE approach [24]

cost-effective patient care [4]. To determine the optimal initial surgical management of thyroid nodules that are 'suspicious for PTC', clinicians must consider patient and institutional costs, as well as loss of time and productivity, from a societal perspective. Costs related to frozen section, operative time, length of hospital stay, workdays lost, thyroid hormone replacement, reoperation, and surveillance must be considered in order to make an informed clinical decision. However, most studies do not address these factors in the setting of thyroid nodules that are 'suspicious for PTC'.

Costs for the Treatment of Thyroid Nodules That Are 'Suspicious for PTC'

A report by Leiker et al. was the only study in our review that addressed the effects of cost and time on the surgical management of thyroid nodules that are 'suspicious for PTC' [34]. Using Medicare reimbursement schedules, they examined quality-adjusted life-years (QALY) and cost differentials between total thyroidectomy and lobectomy with intraoperative frozen section. They assigned base monetary values to perioperative variables based on QALY and used an incremental cost ratio with a threshold of $50,000/QALY to signify cost-effectiveness. Overall, they found that total thyroidectomy was the most cost-effective initial treatment of thyroid nodules that are 'suspicious for PTC'. However, if complication rates were unacceptably high or if the percentage of false-negative frozen sections was ≤8%, lobectomy with intraoperative frozen section could be the most cost-effective option (Fig. 9.1) [34].

Total Thyroidectomy Versus Lobectomy with Intraoperative Frozen Section

All other studies in our review did not specifically encompass patients with thyroid nodules that are 'suspicious for PTC'; however, several will be included in this discussion for completeness [53, 58–60]. When comparing procedural costs for total thyroidectomy versus lobectomy with intraoperative frozen section, total thyroidectomy was associated with an increased cost of 8–32% [53, 58–60]. Also, when evaluating hospital length-of-stay, Marino et al. reported that when compared to same-day surgery, an overnight 23-h admission was associated with an increased admission cost of 22% for total thyroidectomy and 18% for lobectomy [58]. As these studies include data from Canada and the United States, relative cost and reimbursement differentials between health care systems may account for inconsistencies in outcome reporting.

In a series examining the societal cost for the treatment of follicular thyroid nodules, Zanocco et al. used Medicare reimbursement schedules to construct a Markov decision model to evaluate the cost-effectiveness of lobectomy with intraoperative frozen section [60]. They assigned base monetary values to perioperative variables based on QALY and used an incremental cost ratio with a threshold of $100,000/QALY to signify cost-effectiveness. Overall, they found that total thyroidectomy was the most cost-effective initial treatment of follicular nodules. However, if the

FNA malignancy risk becomes >43%, the cost of lobectomy becomes <$8990, the cost of completion thyroidectomy becomes >$11,787, the hourly cost of missed patient work becomes >$410, the additional work lost to undergo completion thyroidectomy becomes >12 days, or life-expectancy becomes <2 years, then lobectomy with intraoperative frozen section could be the most cost-effective [60].

Recommendation

Based on the two cost-utility models reviewed (one for nodules that are 'suspicious for PTC' and one for follicular nodules), initial total thyroidectomy is cost-effective and may be recommended; however, this is contingent on low overall complication rates, especially for that of RLN injury. As the effect that this outcome has on clinical decision-making is highly conditional and is not universally applicable to all surgical practices, the authors rate this outcome as 'important, but not critical for decision-making'. Most previous studies have evaluated surgical decision-making in the setting of follicular or 'indeterminate' nodules, and not specifically for nodules that are 'suspicious for PTC'. Therefore, more moderate-to-high quality evidence is required to be able to make confident treatment recommendations based on cost/time benefits for the surgical management of nodules that are 'suspicious for PTC'. When taken together, due to theoretical nature of cost-utility models and the relative paucity of data related to cost/time outcomes for our targeted patient population, the overall quality of available evidence for this outcome is low.

Conclusions

To determine the optimal initial surgical management of thyroid nodules that are 'suspicious for PTC' on FNA cytology, one must consider the diagnostic accuracy of FNA and frozen section, patient quality of life, and cost/time benefits for total thyroidectomy versus lobectomy with intraoperative frozen section. Based on our review of the literature, it is clear that there is currently a paucity of high-to-moderate quality evidence regarding this patient population. However, when considering the available evidence, assuming relatively low complication rates by experienced surgeons, initial total thyroidectomy may be recommended, as long as completion thyroidectomy would be otherwise be indicated based on histopathology.

Summary of Recommendations

Diagnostic accuracy of FNA and intraoperative frozen section

- Outcome rating: Critical for decision-making
- Quality of available evidence: Low

- If the data obtained by FNA is deemed to be sufficiently accurate for suspicious nodules and/or if the proportion of false-negative frozen sections is >8%, then total thyroidectomy may be recommended as the preferred initial surgical management, as long as completion thyroidectomy would be indicated based on histopathology
- If the data obtained by FNA is deemed to be relatively inaccurate, then frozen section or molecular testing may offer a diagnostic benefit over FNA cytology alone.

Patient quality-of-life

- Outcome rating: Important, but not critical for decision-making
- Quality of available evidence: Low
- Based on a higher rate of RLN injury following completion thyroidectomy and the significant proportion of lobectomy patients that become hypothyroid, initial total thyroidectomy may be recommended, assuming relatively low complication rates with experienced surgeons.

Cost/time benefits

- Outcome rating: Important, but not critical for decision-making
- Quality of available evidence: Low
- Initial total thyroidectomy is cost-effective and may be recommended; however, this is contingent on low overall complication rates, especially for that of RLN injury.

References

1. Davies L, Welch HG. Increasing incidence of thyroid cancer in the United States, 1973–2002. JAMA. 2006;295(18):2164–7.
2. Bakhos R, Selvaggi SM, DeJong S, Gordon DL, Pitale SU, Herrmann M, et al. Fine-needle aspiration of the thyroid: rate and causes of cytohistopathologic discordance. Diagn Cytopathol. 2000;23(4):233–7.
3. Grant CS. Papillary thyroid cancer: strategies for optimal individualized surgical management. Clin Ther. 2014;36(7):1117–26.
4. Lubitz CC, Kong CY, McMahon PM, Daniels GH, Chen Y, Economopoulos KP, et al. Annual financial impact of well-differentiated thyroid cancer care in the United States. Cancer. 2014;120(9):1345–52.
5. Aschebrook-Kilfoy B, Schechter RB, Shih YC, Kaplan EL, Chiu BC, Angelos P, et al. The clinical and economic burden of a sustained increase in thyroid cancer incidence. Cancer Epidemiol Biomark Prev. 2013;22(7):1252–9.
6. Cooper DS, Doherty G, Haugen B, Kloos R, Lee S, Mandel S, et al. Revised American Thyroid Association management guidelines for patients with thyroid nodules and differentiated thyroid cancer. Thyroid. 2009;19(11):1167–214.
7. Cibas ES, Baloch ZW, Fellegara G, LiVolsi VA, Raab SS, Rosai J, et al. A prospective assessment defining the limitations of thyroid nodule pathologic evaluation. Ann Intern Med. 2013;159(5):325–32.

8. Jing X, Michael CW. Potential pitfalls for false suspicion of papillary thyroid carcinoma: a cytohistologic review of 22 cases. Diagn Cytopathol. 2012;40(Suppl 1):E74–9.
9. Baloch ZW, Cibas ES, Clark DP, Layfield LJ, Ljung BM, Pitman MB, et al. The National Cancer Institute thyroid fine needle aspiration state of the science conference: a summation. Cytojournal. 2008;5:6.
10. Cibas ES, Ali SZ. The Bethesda system for reporting thyroid cytopathology. Am J Clin Pathol. 2009;132(5):658–65.
11. Mahajan A, Lin X, Nayar R. Thyroid Bethesda reporting category, 'suspicious for papillary thyroid carcinoma', pitfalls and clues to optimize the use of this category. Cytopathology. 2013;24(2):85–91.
12. Yang J, Schnadig V, Logrono R, Wasserman PG. Fine-needle aspiration of thyroid nodules: a study of 4703 patients with histologic and clinical correlations. Cancer. 2007;111(5):306–15.
13. Goldstein RE, Netterville JL, Burkey B, Johnson JE. Implications of follicular neoplasms, atypia, and lesions suspicious for malignancy diagnosed by fine-needle aspiration of thyroid nodules. Ann Surg. 2002;235(5):656–62. discussion 62–4.
14. Mittendorf EA, Khiyami A, McHenry CR. When fine-needle aspiration biopsy cannot exclude papillary thyroid cancer: a therapeutic dilemma. Arch Surg. 2006;141(10):961–6. discussion 6.
15. Marchevsky AM, Walts AE, Bose S, Gupta R, Fan X, Frishberg D, et al. Evidence-based evaluation of the risks of malignancy predicted by thyroid fine-needle aspiration biopsies. Diagn Cytopathol. 2010;38(4):252–9.
16. Olson MT, Boonyaarunnate T, Altinboga AA, Ali SZ. 'Suspicious for papillary thyroid carcinoma' before and after the Bethesda system for reporting thyroid cytopathology: impact of standardized terminology. Acta Cytol. 2014;58(1):15–22.
17. Haugen BRM, Alexander EK, Bible KC, Doherty G, Mandel SJ, Nikiforov YE, et al. American Thyroid Association management guidelines for adult patients with thyroid nodules and differentiated thyroid cancer. Thyroid. 2015; 2015.
18. Basolo F, Ugolini C, Proietti A, Iacconi P, Berti P, Miccoli P. Role of frozen section associated with intraoperative cytology in comparison to FNA and FS alone in the management of thyroid nodules. Eur J Surg Oncol. 2007;33(6):769–75.
19. Haymart MR, Greenblatt DY, Elson DF, Chen H. The role of intraoperative frozen section if suspicious for papillary thyroid cancer. Thyroid. 2008;18(4):419–23.
20. Moon HJ, Kwak JY, Kim EK, Kim MJ, Park CS, Chung WY, et al. The combined role of ultrasound and frozen section in surgical management of thyroid nodules read as suspicious for papillary thyroid carcinoma on fine needle aspiration biopsy: a retrospective study. World J Surg. 2009;33(5):950–7.
21. Antic T, Taxy JB. Thyroid frozen section: supplementary or unnecessary? Am J Surg Pathol. 2013;37(2):282–6.
22. Boyd LA, Earnhardt RC, Dunn JT, Frierson HF, Hanks JB. Preoperative evaluation and predictive value of fine-needle aspiration and frozen section of thyroid nodules. J Am Coll Surg. 1998;187(5):494–502.
23. Akhtar S, Awan MS. Role of fine needle aspiration and frozen section in determining the extent of thyroidectomy. Eur Arch Otorhinolaryngol. 2007;264(9):1075–9.
24. Apoorva Krishna Chandar YF-Y. Difficult decisions in thoracic surgery. 1 DiSABle, editor. London: Springer; 2014.
25. Baynes AL, Del Rio A, McLean C, Grodski S, Yeung MJ, Johnson WR, et al. Fine-needle aspiration of the thyroid: correlating suspicious cytology results with histological outcomes. Ann Surg Oncol. 2014;21(5):1653–8.
26. Chao TC, Lin JD, Chao HH, Hsueh C, Chen MF. Surgical treatment of solitary thyroid nodules via fine-needle aspiration biopsy and frozen-section analysis. Ann Surg Oncol. 2007;14(2):712–8.
27. Chiu CG, Yao R, Chan SK, Strugnell SS, Bugis S, Irvine R, et al. Hemithyroidectomy is the preferred initial operative approach for an indeterminate fine needle aspiration biopsy diagnosis. Can J Surg. 2012;55(3):191–8.

28. Huber GF, Dziegielewski P, Matthews TW, Warshawski SJ, Kmet LM, Faris P, et al. Intraoperative frozen-section analysis for thyroid nodules: a step toward clarity or confusion? Arch Otolaryngol Head Neck Surg. 2007;133(9):874–81.
29. Makay O, Icoz G, Gurcu B, Ertan Y, Tuncyurek M, Akyildiz M, et al. The ongoing debate in thyroid surgery: should frozen section analysis be omitted? Endocr J. 2007;54(3):385–90.
30. Raj MD, Grodski S, Martin SA, Yeung M, Serpell JW. The role of fine-needle aspiration cytology in the surgical management of thyroid cancer. ANZ J Surg. 2010;80(11):827–30.
31. Yoder BJ, Redman R, Massoll NA. Validation of a five-tier cytodiagnostic system for thyroid fine needle aspiration biopsies using cytohistologic correlation. Thyroid. 2006;16(8):781–6.
32. Sangalli G, Serio G, Zampatti C, Bellotti M, Lomuscio G. Fine needle aspiration cytology of the thyroid: a comparison of 5469 cytological and final histological diagnoses. Cytopathology. 2006;17(5):245–50.
33. Kwak JY, Kim EK, Kim MJ, Hong SW, Choi SH, Son EJ, et al. The role of ultrasound in thyroid nodules with a cytology reading of "suspicious for papillary thyroid carcinoma". Thyroid. 2008;18(5):517–22.
34. Leiker AJ, Yen TW, Cheung K, Evans DB, Wang TS. Cost analysis of thyroid lobectomy and intraoperative frozen section versus total thyroidectomy in patients with a cytologic diagnosis of "suspicious for papillary thyroid cancer". Surgery. 2013;154(6):1307–13. discussion 13–4.
35. Noureldine SI, Olson MT, Agrawal N, Prescott JD, Zeiger MA, Tufano RP. Effect of gene expression classifier molecular testing on the surgical decision-making process for patients with thyroid nodules. JAMA Otolaryngol Head Neck Surg. 2015;141(12):1082–8.
36. Moon HJ, Kwak JY, Kim EK, Choi JR, Hong SW, Kim MJ, et al. The role of BRAFV600E mutation and ultrasonography for the surgical management of a thyroid nodule suspicious for papillary thyroid carcinoma on cytology. Ann Surg Oncol. 2009;16(11):3125–31.
37. Jara SM, Bhatnagar R, Guan H, Gocke CD, Ali SZ, Tufano RP. Utility of BRAF mutation detection in fine-needle aspiration biopsy samples read as "suspicious for papillary thyroid carcinoma". Head Neck. 2014;37(12):1788–93.
38. Ahmadieh H, Azar ST. Controversies in the management and followup of differentiated thyroid cancer: beyond the guidelines. J Thyroid Res. 2012;2012:512401.
39. Moses W, Weng J, Sansano I, Peng M, Khanafshar E, Ljung BM, et al. Molecular testing for somatic mutations improves the accuracy of thyroid fine-needle aspiration biopsy. World J Surg. 2010;34(11):2589–94.
40. Franco C, Martinez V, Allamand JP, Medina F, Glasinovic A, Osorio M, et al. Molecular markers in thyroid fine-needle aspiration biopsy: a prospective study. Appl Immunohistochem Mol Morphol. 2009;17(3):211–5.
41. Musholt TJ, Fottner C, Weber MM, Eichhorn W, Pohlenz J, Musholt PB, et al. Detection of papillary thyroid carcinoma by analysis of BRAF and RET/PTC1 mutations in fine-needle aspiration biopsies of thyroid nodules. World J Surg. 2010;34(11):2595–603.
42. Alexander EK, Kennedy GC, Baloch ZW, Cibas ES, Chudova D, Diggans J, et al. Preoperative diagnosis of benign thyroid nodules with indeterminate cytology. N Engl J Med. 2012;367(8):705–15.
43. Nikiforova MN, Wald AI, Roy S, Durso MB, Nikiforov YE. Targeted next-generation sequencing panel (ThyroSeq) for detection of mutations in thyroid cancer. J Clin Endocrinol Metab. 2013;98(11):E1852–60.
44. Nikiforov YE, Carty SE, Chiosea SI, Coyne C, Duvvuri U, Ferris RL, et al. Highly accurate diagnosis of cancer in thyroid nodules with follicular neoplasm/suspicious for a follicular neoplasm cytology by ThyroSeq v2 next-generation sequencing assay. Cancer. 2014;120(23):3627–34.
45. Nikiforov YE, Steward DL, Robinson-Smith TM, Haugen BR, Klopper JP, Zhu Z, et al. Molecular testing for mutations in improving the fine-needle aspiration diagnosis of thyroid nodules. J Clin Endocrinol Metab. 2009;94(6):2092–8.
46. Liu S, Gao A, Zhang B, Zhang Z, Zhao Y, Chen P, et al. Assessment of molecular testing in fine-needle aspiration biopsy samples: an experience in a Chinese population. Exp Mol Pathol. 2014;97(2):292–7.

47. Nikiforov YE, Ohori NP, Hodak SP, Carty SE, LeBeau SO, Ferris RL, et al. Impact of mutational testing on the diagnosis and management of patients with cytologically indeterminate thyroid nodules: a prospective analysis of 1056 FNA samples. J Clin Endocrinol Metab. 2011;96(11):3390–7.
48. Hauch A, Al-Qurayshi Z, Randolph G, Kandil E. Total thyroidectomy is associated with increased risk of complications for low- and high-volume surgeons. Ann Surg Oncol. 2014;21(12):3844–52.
49. Vashishta R, Mahalingam-Dhingra A, Lander L, Shin EJ, Shah RK. Thyroidectomy outcomes: a national perspective. Otolaryngol Head Neck Surg. 2012;147(6):1027–34.
50. Gardner GM, Smith MM, Yaremchuk KL, Peterson EL. The cost of vocal fold paralysis after thyroidectomy. Laryngoscope. 2013;123(6):1455–63.
51. Lefevre JH, Tresallet C, Leenhardt L, Jublanc C, Chigot JP, Menegaux F. Reoperative surgery for thyroid disease. Langenbeck's Arch Surg. 2007;392(6):685–91.
52. Rafferty MA, Goldstein DP, Rotstein L, Asa SL, Panzarella T, Gullane P, et al. Completion thyroidectomy versus total thyroidectomy: is there a difference in complication rates? An analysis of 350 patients. J Am Coll Surg. 2007;205(4):602–7.
53. Zerey M, Prabhu AS, Newcomb WL, Lincourt AE, Kercher KW, Heniford BT. Short-term outcomes after unilateral versus complete thyroidectomy for malignancy: a national perspective. Am Surg. 2009;75(1):20–4.
54. Glockzin G, Hornung M, Kienle K, Thelen K, Boin M, Schreyer AG, et al. Completion thyroidectomy: effect of timing on clinical complications and oncologic outcome in patients with differentiated thyroid cancer. World J Surg. 2012;36(5):1168–73.
55. Vaiman M, Nagibin A, Olevson J. Complications in primary and completed thyroidectomy. Surg Today. 2010;40(2):114–8.
56. Cayo AK, Yen TW, Misustin SM, Wall K, Wilson SD, Evans DB, et al. Predicting the need for calcium and calcitriol supplementation after total thyroidectomy: results of a prospective, randomized study. Surgery. 2012;152(6):1059–67.
57. Kandil E, Krishnan B, Noureldine SI, Yao L, Tufano RP. Hemithyroidectomy: a meta-analysis of postoperative need for hormone replacement and complications. ORL J Otorhinolaryngol Relat Spec. 2013;75(1):6–17.
58. Marino M, Spencer H, Hohmann S, Bodenner D, Stack BC Jr. Costs of outpatient thyroid surgery from the University HealthSystem Consortium (UHC) database. Otolaryngol Head Neck Surg. 2014;150(5):762–9.
59. Shrime MG, Goldstein DP, Seaberg RM, Sawka AM, Rotstein L, Freeman JL, et al. Cost-effective management of low-risk papillary thyroid carcinoma. Arch Otolaryngol Head Neck Surg. 2007;133(12):1245–53.
60. Zanocco K, Heller M, Elaraj D, Sturgeon C. Cost effectiveness of intraoperative pathology examination during diagnostic hemithyroidectomy for unilateral follicular thyroid neoplasms. J Am Coll Surg. 2013;217(4):702–10.

Primary Repair Versus No Repair for Transected Recurrent Laryngeal Nerve

10

Alexander Langerman and Cheryl C. Nocon

Abstract

This chapter will examine the data regarding this rare but serious complication of thyroid surgery. We evaluated the available literature for recommendations regarding immediate primary repair versus no repair in patients with an identified transected RLN during thyroid surgery.

Keywords

Recurrent laryngeal nerve transection · Vocal cord paralysis · Thyroidectomy complication

Introduction

Injury to the recurrent laryngeal nerve (RLN) is a known complication of thyroid surgery that can have a significant impact on a patient's quality of life. Even in an experienced surgeon's hands, a temporary palsy of the RLN can occur in 2.5–5% of patients [1]. This may be the result of inadvertent nerve traction, stretching, electrothermal injury, or transient ischemia; in all of these cases despite the injury the nerve is still intact. Full recovery is expected and may be supplemented by temporary measures.

A. Langerman (✉)
Department of Otolaryngology, Vanderbilt University Medical Center, Nashville, TN, USA
e-mail: alexander.langerman@vanderbilt.edu

C. C. Nocon
Department of Surgery, Division of Otolaryngology-Head and Neck Surgery, NorthShore University HealthSystem, Kellogg Cancer Center, Evanston, IL, USA
e-mail: cnocon@northshore.org

P. Angelos, R. H. Grogan (eds.), *Difficult Decisions in Endocrine Surgery*, Difficult Decisions in Surgery: An Evidence-Based Approach,
https://doi.org/10.1007/978-3-319-92860-9_10

The incidence of complete RLN transection (planned and unplanned) and permanent paralysis is much less common at 1–1.5% after total thyroidectomy [1]. Disease-specific risk factors for nerve transection include thyroid malignancy, concurrent neck dissection, substernal goiter and thyroiditis [2]. In planned transection, a patient either presents with obvious tumor invasion of the RLN or surgical exploration reveals adherence of a cancerous thyroid gland. In both cases sacrifice of the nerve is often made in favor of a complete oncologic resection. Inadvertent iatrogenic transection of the RLN also occurs, and is made more likely by recurrence and re-operation, and distorted anatomy caused by large nodules or goiters.

The Recurrent Laryngeal Nerve and Management Options for Nerve Transection

The RLN innervates all intrinsic laryngeal muscles except the cricothyroid muscle. This includes adductor muscles—thyroarytenoid (TA), lateral cricoarytenoid (LCA), interarytenoid (IA)—and abductor muscles—posterior cricoarytenoid (PCA). The sequelae of RLN injury and vocal fold denervation are well known, including vocal fold immobility, flaccidity and subsequent muscle atrophy [3]. A height disparity between the paralyzed and intact vocal fold may also result from destabilization of the cricoarytenoid joint. This produces glottis incompetence, which can clinically manifest as hoarseness, shortened phonation and aspiration [4].

The surgical management options following known RLN transection include medialization procedures as well as primary nerve repair with re-innervation procedures. Vocal cord medialization improves vocal quality by improving glottal competence. Such procedures include thyroplasty, arytenoid adduction and vocal cord injection [5–7]. Re-innervation procedures, on the other hand, aim to restore neural integrity. Even when the nerve is repaired, normal movement of the vocal cord is not restored [3]. Within the RLN there is no spatial segregation of the nerve fibers. Therefore, even with direct anastomosis of severed nerve endings, nerve fibers regenerate but it occurs in a misdirected fashion among adductor and abductor fibers. This process, called synkinesis, results in the cross-innervation of adductor muscle fibers into abductor axons, or vice versa [8]. The degree of synkinesis after reinnervation is hard to predict. But because there is a 3:1 axonal distribution of adductors and abductors, laryngeal adduction predominates over abduction and the re-innervated cords are normally fixed at the median [8].

Re-innervation, however, is the only procedure that prevents muscle atrophy and therefore is worthwhile to perform if nerve transection occurs. Voice improvement occurs by restoration of motor tone to the flaccid TA muscle [3]. It can also allow for some vocal cord adduction from the LCA and IA, though this is not the primary benefit of re-innervation. Tonic action of the PCA can also be preserved, which may have a stabilizing effect on the cricoarytenoid joint [3]. Although RLN re-innervation does not restore geometric symmetry to the glottis as a medialization procedure can, it can achieve viscoelastic symmetry of the vocal cord which improves phonatory function [9].

Types of Primary Repair

Direct re-innervation should be performed when the length of the defect in the transected RLN is small enough (typically <5 mm) to allow for a tension-free primary anastomosis. The nerve is carefully traced out distally and proximally to provide the mobility necessary to minimize tension. Using loupe magnification or an operating microscope, 2–4 fine monofilament sutures (8-0 to 10-0) are carefully placed in the epineurium. However, if tension-free re-approximation of transected nerve endings cannot be performed, then several graft options are available to achieve re-innervation.

A common neurorrhaphy alternative is the ansa cervicalis-to-RLN anastomosis. This technique can be employed when the proximal RLN is not available for nerve repair. Using the same thyroidectomy incision, the ipsilateral sternocleidomastoid muscle is mobilized laterally to identify the ansa cervicalis loop overlying the internal jugular vein. Branches to the strap muscles are transected and then the ansa cervicalis itself is divided and anastomosed to the distal RLN as described previously. When the ipsilateral ansa cervicalis is unavailable, the contralateral nerve can also be used. Similarly, if the ipsilateral vagus is sacrificed proximal to the RLN branch secondary to a neck or chest tumor excision, the proximal vagus stump can be reflected medially and anastomosed to the distal RLN.

When the proximal and distal ends of the RLN are intact, and re-innervation with the ansa cervicalis is not possible, a free cable graft can be used to repair the RLN. The most commonly and easily harvested donor is the greater auricular nerve (GAN). The same thyroidectomy incision can again be utilized and the GAN is identified overlying the ipsilateral sternocleidomastoid muscle. A segment of nerve can be harvested to fit the transected portion of the RLN. Anastomosis is performed at both the distal and proximal ends of the RLN. Postoperatively, patients should be alerted that they will have permanent periauricular numbness, especially the earlobe, and that they should be careful to protect against injury to the numb ear (common causes are burns from curling irons and frostbite).

This chapter will examine the data regarding this rare but serious complication of thyroid surgery. We evaluated the available literature for recommendations regarding immediate primary repair versus no repair in patients with an identified transected RLN during thyroid surgery (Table 10.1).

Methods

We conducted a comprehensive review of the literature related to the treatment of RLN transection during thyroid surgery. Literature searches were conducted in the PubMed database using the key words: recurrent laryngeal nerve injury, recurrent laryngeal nerve transection, recurrent laryngeal nerve management, immediate recurrent laryngeal nerve repair, neurorraphy, recurrent laryngeal nerve reconstruction, thyroidectomy complications, laryngeal re-innervation, vocal fold paralysis treatment. Searches were limited to the English language, human subjects over

Table 10.1 Studies comparing immediate RLN repair with no repair

Author (year)	Study type	Population	No. patients: primary repair	No. patients: no repair	Types of repair	Follow-up time	Outcome measures	Evidence strength
Hong et al. (2013) [17]	Retrospective	Thyroid surgery for malignancy	10	4	Direct (±injection laryngoplasty)	12 months	MPT, glottal gap, GRBAS, aspiration, VHI	Low
Miyauchi et al. (2009) [19]	Retrospective	Thyroid surgery for malignancy	88	27	Direct, ansa, vagus, free nerve graft	12 months	MPT, PEI	Low
Yumoto et al. (2006) [20]	Prospective	Thyroid surgery for malignancy	9	9	Direct, free nerve graft	9–29 months	HNR, jitter, shimmer, MPT, glottal gap	Low
Chou et al. (2003) [4]	Retrospective	Thyroid surgery for malignancy and benign disease; parathyroid surgery for benign disease	8	4	Direct	6–24 months	GRBAS, aspiration, MPT, glottal gap, vocal cord tone	Low
Miyauchi et al. (1998) [18]	Retrospective	Thyroid surgery for malignancy, other[a]	34	26	Direct, ansa, vagus, free nerve graft	1.1–10.7 years	MPT	Low

MPT maximum phonation time, *GRBAS* grade, roughness, breathiness, asthenia and strain, *VHI* vocal handicap index, *PEI* phonation efficiency index, *HNR* harmonics-to-noise ratio

[a]Eleven patients (Surgery for thymic cancer, parathyroid cancer, vagal tumor, lung cancer, aortic aneurysm)

18 years old, and literature published in the last 20 years. We excluded articles on RLN injury that occurred exclusively during non-thyroid surgeries (i.e.: cardiac, esophageal, trauma), and articles that focused solely on non-nerve repair treatments (i.e.: medialization procedures). Reference lists of identified articles were screened for additional relevant studies. There were no related articles found in the Cochrane Library using the same search key words.

Measurement of Clinical Outcomes

There are various methods to clinically measure nerve repair outcomes following injury. This includes the Voice Handicap Index (VHI), a validated self-administered questionnaire that measures the functional, emotional and physical impact of a voice disorder on patient quality of life [10]. Perceptual voice quality is measured by a speech language pathologist using the grade, roughness, breathiness, asthenia and strain (GRBAS) scale. Acoustic analysis and mean phonation time (MPT) are other common measures of phonatory function. Finally, laryngoscopic examination, including the use of videostroboscopy, is used to objectively evaluate vocal function.

Immediate Management of Transected RLN

There are no current national guidelines or consensus statements for the management of RLN transection identified intra-operatively during thyroid surgery. The majority of studies focusing on this specific clinical situation are observational cohort studies or case series. There are only a handful of review articles on the management of vocal fold paralysis following all types of surgery [11–13], and specifically thyroid surgery [14–16], but none that look at primary nerve repair in the immediate setting.

Several studies have examined the natural history of denervation and compared it to outcomes following primary nerve repair. In a small cohort study, Chou et al. [4] studied subjective and objective vocal outcomes in patients with complete RLN injury who had either immediate direct anastomosis or no repair following thyroid surgery. Immediate repair was prohibited by extensive cancer involvement of the distal RLN. Although all patients demonstrated an immobilized vocal cord on post-operative laryngoscopy, only the patients who underwent direct repair showed significantly improved voice quality, aspiration, GRBAS scales, and MPT at 6 months follow-up compared to 3 months; patients who did not undergo repair did not show improvement in any of these measures. Laryngoscopic findings, including glottic gap size and vocal cord muscle tone, also improved over time only in the repair group. All patients in the no repair group eventually underwent medialization laryngoplasty to achieve better vocal quality.

A similar study comparing direct anastomosis with no repair was replicated recently by Hong et al. [17], with the noted difference that all patients in both groups routinely underwent injection medialization 2–6 months post-operatively. Even so, the re-innervation group still had objective improvement in phonatory function, with significantly longer MPT and smaller glottal gap than the non-innervation group at 12 months. These indices also improved significantly over time from 3 to 12 months in the re-innervation group, suggesting progressive laryngeal re-innervation that provides persistent clinical benefit even after the temporary effects of injection laryngoplasty diminish. In addition, no patient showed laryngoscopic evidence of vocal cord atrophy. Subjective outcomes, including GBRAS scales, VHI and aspiration scores, were all significantly better in the re-innervation group overall, and showed significant improvement at 12 months compared to 3 months post-operatively.

In two larger cohort studies, Miyauchi et al. [18, 19] studied thyroid cancer patients who had unilateral RLN resection in order to achieve oncologic control. Functional outcomes were compared among patients who underwent various types of RLN re-innervation, patients who did not have any repair, and normal controls. Patients who underwent repair demonstrated MPT values that were longer than those without repair, and comparable to normal controls [18]. Serial measurements of MPT demonstrated a clear increase around 3–5 months after reconstruction. To account for differences in lung function when measuring MPT, the authors utilized another measurement called the phonation efficiency index (PEI), which takes into account pulmonary vital capacity. Similar to MPT, the PEI was greater in patients who underwent repair, and comparable to normal controls [19]. Among patients who had pre-operative vocal cord paralysis and ultimately underwent repair, the PEI was found to be greater at 1 year post-operatively than the PEI before surgery in 45 of 51 patients, demonstrating good recovery of phonatory function even when pre-operative paralysis exists [19].

The long-term effects of immediate RLN reconstruction on acoustic measurements of the voice were examined by Yumoto et al. [20]. Acoustic analysis is an objective measurement of vocal parameters that reflect the vibratory patterns of the vocal cords. Measurements such as jitter, shimmer and harmonics-to-noise ratio (HNR) are indices of vocal stability and clinically translate into the severity of dysphonia or hoarseness. Compared to a group of thyroidectomy patients who did not undergo any RLN repair, the group that underwent RLN reconstruction with either direct anastomosis or GAN free graft had significantly greater HNR, less jitter and trended toward less shimmer, all of which indicate improved vocal quality. The reconstructed group also demonstrated significantly greater MPT and smaller glottal gap on laryngoscopy. The mean follow-up period was 17 months.

Recommendations

Studies that compare primary nerve repair to no repair in the setting of a recognized intra-operative RLN transection are limited to small observational cohort studies. They demonstrate the improvement in various clinical measures of vocal function and quality in patients who undergo immediate repair. Because it is performed immediately, the patient is spared a second surgery and anesthetic, while adding only a small increase in operative time. It avoids a re-operative surgical bed, and the tissue fibrosis and adhesions associated with higher complications, and is the only procedure that prevents muscle atrophy and the loss of muscle tension and bulk, providing good long-term results. However, immediate primary repair requires an intact distal RLN and it does not produce vocal improvement for several months. If the microsurgical expertise is available, a transected RLN with favorable anatomy should be reconstructed.

Selection of Re-innervation Technique

There have been several studies that compare the different RLN re-innervation techniques following transection during thyroid surgery. Overall, no single technique has demonstrated significantly better outcomes. The main determinant of technique selection has been anatomic limitations. Two recent prospective studies by Lee et al. [21] and Dzodic et al. [22] showed no difference between direct and ansa cervicalis-to-RLN anastomosis in various clinical measures, including glottal gap, acoustic analyses, MPT, VHI and perceptual voice quality. Dzodic noted improved phonation at 1 month for patients who underwent direct anastomosis, and 2–6 months for ansa cervicalis-to-RLN patients. Lee noted sustained results up to 2 years following reconstruction, with an overall mean time to improvement of 4.3 months. The only systematic review of different laryngeal re-innervation techniques found the mean time to the first signs of re innervation to be 4.5 months [12].

Comparisons between ansa-to-RLN anastomosis and free nerve grafting have also demonstrated good vocal outcomes, with improved phonation by both subjective and objective measures [23–28]. In addition to the GAN, other donor nerve grafts included transverse cervical, supraclavicular and ansa cervicalis. There were no outcome differences between techniques and among donor nerves. These findings were confirmed in a systematic review of different laryngeal innervation techniques. Of note, these studies showed no difference in outcomes between those patients who demonstrated pre-operative vocal fold paralysis and those who did not, although the time to improvement was slightly longer in the former group. While this supports the effectiveness of re-innervation techniques even in the presence of ongoing nerve degeneration, what is less clear is the optimal time to re-innervation after the onset of vocal fold paralysis, with two large retrospective studies reporting success up to 2 years after injury [29, 30].

Studies on ansa cervicalis-to-RLN reconstruction comprise the majority of case series examining the outcomes of laryngeal re-innervation. Overall, all re-innervation techniques achieve good acoustic, perceptual and visual outcomes, whether it is performed immediately or delayed, and in the setting of both thyroid and non-thyroid surgery. However, it is important to note that there is great heterogeneity in the literature with regard to surgical timing, indications, technique, possible concomitant procedures, and follow-up, precluding the ability to make strong recommendations regarding one technique over another [11–14].

The only randomized controlled trial that studied re-innervation for the management of unilateral vocal fold paralysis was performed by Paniello et al. [31], which compared medialization laryngoplasty to delayed ansa cervicalis-to-RLN reconstruction in patients with a paralyzed vocal cord at least 6 months after initial surgery. Unfortunately the study was prematurely closed due to administrative and consent issues and only enrolled 24 patients. Nonetheless, it showed a greater improvement in perceptual, acoustic and quality of life scores in re-innervation patients under age 52 compared to those over age 52 and medialization patients of all ages, underscoring the role of age in outcomes. A retrospective study of 349 patients who underwent delayed ansa cervicalis-to-RLN repair following primary thyroid surgery corroborated this finding of age-dependent vocal outcomes, with decreased effectiveness in those over age 60 [29]. Finally, the complication rate of nerve reconstruction is low, even when compared to medialization procedures [11, 13, 32].

Recommendations

There are no completed randomized trials comparing immediate re-innervation techniques of a transected RLN during thyroid surgery. Existing data on the various techniques of repair are heterogeneous and limited to observational cohort studies. The few available systematic reviews comparing management strategies that include nerve reconstruction evaluate it as a delayed intervention. Anatomic limitations and surgeon expertise should dictate which technique is used to repair the RLN, as there are no significant differences in vocal outcomes or safety profiles among the different techniques.

Summary of Recommendations

Immediate Management of Transected RLN

Primary repair is recommended in the setting of a transected RLN identified during thyroid surgery (evidence quality low; weak recommendation). Primary repair is the only management strategy that prevents muscle atrophy and preserves muscle tension and bulk, resulting in long-term vocal improvement (evidence quality low; weak recommendation). Primary repair alone should not be performed if immediate vocal improvement is desired, given the recognized delay in vocal outcomes associated with primary repair (evidence quality low; weak recommendation).

Selection of Re-innervation Technique

There are no vocal outcome or safety differences among re-innervation techniques, and technique selection should be dependent on anatomic limitations and surgeon expertise (evidence quality low; weak recommendation). Limited data suggest that primary repair be recommended for younger patients, and used with caution in older patients (evidence quality low; weak recommendation).

Conclusion

We discuss the immediate management of RLN transection incurred during thyroid surgery. While high-quality data examining this particular situation is lacking, the available data suggest the benefit of immediate re-innervation compared to no repair, and the comparable outcomes from different re-innervation techniques. The current state of literature highlights the need for prospective studies.

References

1. Flint PW. Cummings otolaryngology head and neck surgery. 6th ed. Philadelphia: Elsevier; 2015.
2. Chiang FY, Wang LF, Huang YF, Lee KW, Kuo WR. Recurrent laryngeal nerve palsy after thyroidectomy with routine identification of the recurrent laryngeal nerve. Surgery. 2005;137:342–7.
3. Paniello RC. Laryngeal reinnervation. Otolaryngol Clin North Am. 2004;37:161–81.
4. Chou F, Su C, Jeng S, Hsu K, Lu K. Neurorrhaphy of the recurrent laryngeal nerve. J Am Coll Surg. 2003;197:52–7.
5. Isshiki N, Taira T, Kojima H, Shoji K. Recent modifications in thyroplasty type I. Ann Otol Rhinol Laryngol. 1989;98:777–9.
6. Isshiki N, Tanabe M, Sawada M. Arytenoid adduction for unilateral vocal cord paralysis. Arch Otolaryngol. 1978;104:555–8.
7. McCulloch TM, Andrews BT, Hoffman HT, Graham SM, Karell MP, Minnick C. Long-term follow-up of fat injection laryngoplasty for unilateral vocal cord paralysis. Laryngoscope. 2002;112:1235–8.
8. Gibbons N. The evolution of laryngeal reinnervation, the current state of science and thoughts for future treatments. J Voice. 2014;28:793–8.
9. Titze IR. Comments on the myoelastic-aerodynamic theory of phonation. J Speech Hear Res. 1979;23:495–510.
10. Solomon NP, Helou LB, Henry LR, et al. Utility of the voice handicap index as an indicator of postthyroidectomy voice dysfunction. J Voice. 2013;27:348–54.
11. Siu J, Tam S, Fung K. A comparison of outcomes in interventions for unilateral vocal fold paralysis: a systematic review. Laryngoscope. 2015;126:1616–24.
12. Aynehchi BB, McCoul ED, Sundaram K. Systematic review of laryngeal reinnervation techniques. Otolaryngol Head Neck Surg. 2010;14:749–59.
13. Misono S, Merati AL. Evidence-based practice: evaluation and management of unilateral vocal fold paralysis. Otolaryngol Clin N Am. 2012;45:1083–108.
14. Lynch J, Parameswaran R. Management of unilateral recurrent laryngeal nerve injury after thyroid surgery: a review. Head Neck. 2017;39:1470–8.
15. Chen X, Wan P, Yu Y, Li M, Xu Y, Huang P, Huang Z. Types and timing of therapy for vocal fold paresis/paralysis after thyroidectomy: a systematic review and meta-analysis. J Voice. 2014;28:799–808.
16. Hartl DM, Travagli J, Leboulleux S, Baudin E, Brasnu DF, Schlumberger M. Current concepts in the management of unilateral recurrent laryngeal nerve paralysis after thyroid surgery. J Clin Endocrinol Metab. 2005;90:3084–8.

17. Hong JW, Roh TS, Yoo H, et al. Outcome with immediate direct anastomosis of recurrent laryngeal nerves injured during thyroidectomy. Laryngoscope. 2013;124:1402–8.
18. Miyauchi A, Matsusaka K, Kihara M, et al. The role of ansa-to-recurrent-laryngeal nerve anastomosis in operations for thyroid cancer. Eur J Surg. 1998;164:927–33.
19. Miyauchi A, Inoue H, Tomoda C, et al. Improvement in phonation after reconstruction of the recurrent laryngeal nerve in patients with thyroid cancer invading the nerve. Surgery. 2009;146:1056–62.
20. Yumoto E, Sanuki T, Kumai Y. Immediate recurrent laryngeal nerve reconstruction and vocal outcome. Laryngoscope. 2006;116:1657–61.
21. Lee SW, Park KN, Oh SK, Jung C, Mok J, Kim C. Long-term efficacy of primary intraoperative recurrent laryngeal nerve reinnervation in the management of thyroidectomy-related unilateral vocal fold paralysis. Acta Otolaryngol. 2014;134:1179–84.
22. Dzodic R, Markovic I, Santrac N, Buta M, Djurisic I, Lukic S. Recurrent laryngeal nerve liberations and reconstructions: a single institution experience. World J Surg. 2016;40:644–51.
23. Sanuki T, Yumuto E, Minoda R, Kodama N. The role of immediate recurrent laryngeal nerve reconstruction for thyroid cancer surgery. J Oncol. 2010;2010:846235.
24. Kumai Y, Kodama N, Murakami D, Yumoto E. Comparison of vocal outcome following two different procedures for immediate RLN reconstruction. Eur Arch Otorhinolaryngol. 2016;273:967–72.
25. Miyauchi A, Yokozawa T, Kobayashi K, Hirai K, Matsuzuka F, Kuma K. Opposite ansa cervicalis to recurrent laryngeal nerve anastomosis to restore phonation in patients with advanced thyroid cancer. Eur J Surg. 2001;167:540–1.
26. Miyauchi A, Ito Y, Miya A, et al. Lateral mobilization of the recurrent laryngeal nerve to facilitate tracheal surgery in patients with thyroid cancer invading the trachea near Berry's ligament. World J Surg. 2007;31:2081–4.
27. Miyauchi A, Masuoka H, Tomoda C, et al. Laryngeal approach to the recurrent laryngeal nerve involved by thyroid cancer at the ligament of Berry. Surgery. 2012;152:57–60.
28. Rohde SL, Wright CT, Muckala JC, Wiggletone J, Rousseau B, Netterville JL. Voice quality after recurrent laryngeal nerve resection and immediate reconstruction. Otolaryngol Head Neck Surg. 2012;147:733–6.
29. Li M, Chen D, Song X, et al. The effect of patient age on the success of laryngeal reinnervation. Eur Arch Otorhinolaryngol. 2014;271:3241–7.
30. Wang W, Chen D, Chen S, et al. Laryngeal reinnervation using ansa cervicalis for thyroid surgery-related unilateral vocal fold paralysis: a long-term outcome analysis of 237 cases. PLoS One. 2011;6:e19128.
31. Paniello RC, Edgar JD, Kallogjeri D, Piccirillo JF. Medialization vs. reinnervation for unilateral vocal fold paralysis: a multicenter randomized clinical trial. Laryngoscope. 2011;121:2172–9.
32. Blumin JH, Merati AL. Laryngeal reinnervation with nerve-nerve anastomosis versus laryngeal framework surgery alone: a comparison of safety. Otolaryngol Head Neck Surg. 2008;138:217–20.

Surgery Versus Observation for Papillary Thyroid Microcarcinoma

11

Shi Lam and Brian H. H. Lang

Abstract

Papillary thyroid carcinoma (PTC) is the most common malignancy arising from the follicular cells and its age-adjusted incidence has doubled over the past two decades. As a result, it imposes a cost burden to the society in general. However, despite the rapid rise in incidence, the actual mortality (or the chance of dying) from PTC has remained relatively unchanged in the same period.

Keywords

Papillary thyroid carcinoma (PTC) · Papillary thyroid microcarcinoma (PTMC)

Introduction

Papillary thyroid carcinoma (PTC) is the most common malignancy arising from the follicular cells and its age-adjusted incidence has doubled over the past two decades [1]. As a result, it imposes a cost burden to the society in general [1]. However, despite the rapid rise in incidence, the actual mortality (or the chance of dying) from PTC has remained relatively unchanged in the same period [2]. One explanation for this seemingly-contradictory phenomenon is that this observed increase could have been a result of an increasing detection of small and harmless

S. Lam
Department of Surgery, The University of Hong Kong, Hong Kong SAR, China

B. H. H. Lang (✉)
Department of Surgery, The University of Hong Kong, Hong Kong SAR, China

Division of Endocrine Surgery, Department of Surgery, Queen Mary Hospital, Hong Kong SAR, China
e-mail: blang@hku.hk

P. Angelos, R. H. Grogan (eds.), *Difficult Decisions in Endocrine Surgery*, Difficult Decisions in Surgery: An Evidence-Based Approach,
https://doi.org/10.1007/978-3-319-92860-9_11

PTCs rather than clinically-significant PTCs (i.e. those larger than 1 cm with nodal or distant metastasis). Small and harmless PTCs are often referred to as incidental papillary thyroid microcarcinoma (PTMC) because they are incidental and usually not larger than 10 mm [3]. In fact, it is known that PTMC can be found frequently in the healthy general population. The estimated prevalence of PTMC at autopsy examination ranged widely between 2 and 35.6% [3] depending on how thorough the thyroid gland was sectioned. With improved ultrasonography (USG) technique and increased accuracy in USG-guided fine-needle aspiration cytology (USG-FNAC), it is possible to detect a PTMC as little as 2–3 mm in diameter in an otherwise normal thyroid lobe [4]. Therefore, one could postulate that over time, the prevalence of PTC would eventually approach that of the autopsy series. In fact, if a massive USG screening program of the thyroid gland were to be carried out in an otherwise healthy asymptomatic female population aged 30 years or older, the actual prevalence of PTMC (or the chance of finding a small PTC) would come close to 4% [5]. This is in contrast to the low prevalence observed for clinical PTC (1.9 to 11.7 per 100,000 females) [6]. Therefore, the prevalence of incidental PTMCs (or "incidentalomas") could be up to 500–1000 times higher than that of clinical PTC. Following this observation, some have questioned whether immediate surgery is necessary for these incidental PTMCs because most would probably not cause any symptoms or harm over one's lifetime. Some investigators have even gone further to propose that perhaps close observation might be a better alternative to surgery [7, 8]. However, given that PTMCs could behave unpredictably with some tumors having high rates of multicentricity and nodal metastases on presentation and even causing deaths [9, 10] several centers in Japan initiated observation trials in the 1990s to evaluate the natural behavior of these incidental PTMC over time. The purposes of this chapter are to critically review the results on these ongoing trials and make management recommendations if any based on the review (Table 11.1).

Background and Details of These Active Observation Trials

Akira Miyauchi was the pioneer of these trials. He first proposed nonsurgical treatment for low-risk PTMC at the Kuma Hospital in 1993. In the same year, the "active" observation trial was started at the Kuma hospital [11]. His idea of nonsurgical treatment for low-risk PTMC was adopted by another Japanese group (Sugitani et al. at Cancer Institute Hospital in Tokyo) in 1995 [11]. However, to be eligible for these observation trials, the incidental PTMC had to be considered "low-risk" which

Table 11.1 PICO table

*P*opulation	Patients with FNA proven papillary thyroid microcarcinoma
*I*ntervention	Active observation
*C*omparator	Immediate surgery
*O*utcomes	Disease progression, survival

by their definition, meant that the tumor was located away from the trachea and the recurrent laryngeal nerve and had no evidence of nodal or distant metastases on presentation. The reason for having these exclusions was that in case the tumor did progress over time under active observation, it would not have posed any added patient risk or morbidity. Therefore, tumors with any one of these features were immediately surgically resected. The other inclusion criterion was that the incidental tumor had to be PTC on FNAC and not other higher grade cancers like tall cell variant or poorly differentiated cancers. Therefore, all eligible tumors had to be biopsied before the start of the trial.

Figure 11.1 describes the overall design of these trials. As these trials were non-randomized, patients with proven PTC on FNAC were given the choice of either active observation or immediate surgery. For those who chose active observation, they underwent regular USG examination of the thyroid gland every 6–12 months and during each examination, the size of the primary tumor and the regional lymph node status were carefully assessed and recorded by a dedicated radiologist. If the primary tumor size increased by 3 mm or more (relative to the original dimension) or reached above 12 mm in diameter or a new metastatic lymph node was found, immediate surgery was offered. Based on their experience, the rationale for choosing a cut-off of 3 mm or above was because the inter-observer variation even among expert radiologists was 2 mm and so a ≥3 mm enlargement represented a "real" size enlargement [12].

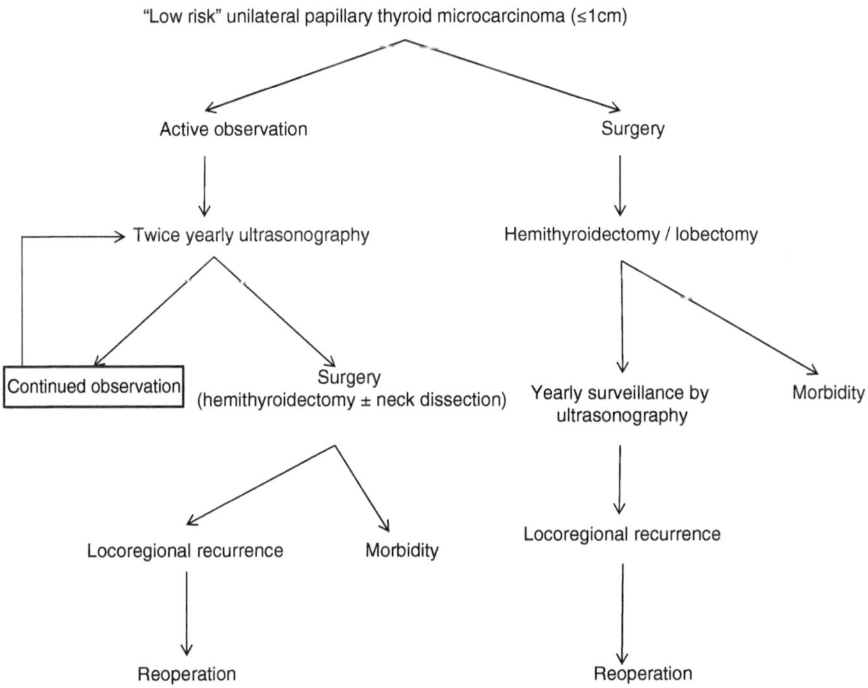

Fig. 11.1 Overall design of the trials reviewed

Results of These Observation Trials for Low-Risk PTMC

Table 11.2 summarizes the results of these trials. The first report was published in 2003 from the Kuma Hospital, Kobe [7]. In that particular report, of the 732 eligible patients, 162 (22.1%) patients chose to undergo active observation and after a mean period of 46.5 months, more than 70% did not experience any size change or reduction. However, there were around 10% whose tumors enlarged to >10 mm and 1.2% developing new lymph node metastasis in the lateral compartment. In the surgical arm, 570 (77.9%) patients chose surgical treatment at diagnosis while 56 (34.6%) patients in the observation group eventually chose surgery after a period of observation. Of these 626 patients, lymph node dissection was performed in 594 patients, and metastasis was confirmed histologically in 50.5%. Multiple tumor formation was seen in 42.8% of patients. In this surgical group, the recurrence rate was 2.7% at 5 years and 5.0% at 8 years after surgery. The authors concluded that PTMC did not frequently become clinically apparent, and that patients may choose observation while their tumors are not progressing. These data were later superseded by a more recent report published in 2014 [13]. In that later report, Miyauchi et al. recruited a total of 1235 patients with incidental PTMC at Kuma Hospital from 1993 to 2011. These patients were placed under observation for 18 months or longer. Their data showed that 58 (4.7%) showed size enlargement, 19 (1.5%) showed a novel appearance of lymph node metastasis (four in central and 15 in lateral compartments) and 43 (3.5%) showed progression to clinical disease. None of the patients developed distant metastasis or died of thyroid cancer, and one patient in the operated group developed recurrence with stable disease on follow-up. Interestingly, the proportion of patients with PTMC progression was lowest in the older patients while it was

Table 11.2 A comparison of progression and nodal metastasis in PTMCs undergoing active observation only

First author (year)	Number of patients or PTMCs observed	Surgical comparative group	Mean observation period (months)	% patients/ PTMCs with enlargement (≥3 mm)	% patients/ PTMCs with nodal metastasis
Ito (2003) [7]	162	626	46.5	10.2	1.2
Ito (2007) [11]	346	n/a	54	6.7	1.7
Sugitani (2010) [8]	300[a]	56	60	7.3[a]	1.0
Ito (2014) [13]	1235	n/a	75	4.7	1.5
Sugitani (2014) [14]	415[a]	n/a	78	6.0[a]	0.9

n/a not available, *PTMC* papillary thyroid microcarcinoma
[a]Expressed as number of PTMCs

highest in the young patients. Older (>60) patients had a 2.2% chance of size enlargement while younger (<40) and middle-aged (40–59) patients had 5.9% and 5.7% chances, respectively, of size enlargement. Similarly, for new nodal metastasis, the incidence in young, middle-aged and older aged patients were 5.3%, 1.4% and 0.4%, respectively. In fact, on multivariate analysis, young age was an independent predictor of PTMC progression. This is in contrast to what had been observed for clinically apparent PTCs as older age has long been recognized as a poor prognostic factor of PTC [15]. Miyauchi et al. showed that the rate of persistent disease was higher in older (>60 years old) patients than middle-aged patients (40–59 patients) [16]. Our group also showed that even among those who were older (>45 years old), more advanced age (>60 years old) was an independent predictor of disease-specific death [17].

Sugitani et al. also reported a series of 244 patients (with 300 PTMCs) who agreed to undergo active observation after diagnosis of PTMC, with similar inclusion criteria and conversion to surgical treatment as Ito's report [8]. After a mean period of 5 years, 4% of patients developed tumor enlargement and 1% developed lymph node metastasis and so they underwent surgery. No recurrence was identified at 1–12 years after operation [8]. The same group published a more updated report recently [14]. In that report, a total of 415 asymptomatic PTMCs were observed by USG surveillance only. After a mean period of 6.5 ± 4.0 years of observation, 25 PTMCs (6.0%) had tumor size increase while the rest either decreased in size or unchanged. However, unlike Ito et al., [16] Sugitani et al. did not find any significant association between tumor progression and age at diagnosis. Furthermore, serum thyroid-stimulating hormone (TSH) was not a predictor of PTMC progression [14].

Implications from These Trials

Based on the result of these observation trials, one could conclude that despite the lack of treatment or surgery, it was rare for an asymptomatic "low-risk" PTMC to significantly enlarge over time. Under observation, approximately only 1% of patients each year would experience a significant size enlargement (≥3 mm) to warrant immediate surgery. Therefore, using change in size alone as a criterion, surgery was rarely required. Similarly, if new appearance of nodal metastasis was used as a criterion for tumor growth or progression, only around 0.3–0.4% of patients each year would need to undergo immediate surgery (together with neck dissection). Therefore, new development of nodal metastasis as a result of active observation occurred even less commonly than size enlargement. Therefore overall, perhaps less than 2% of patients each year would experience signs of tumor progression during active observation leading to immediate surgery.

The other point worth noting was that delayed surgery (i.e. after a period of active observation) did not appear to compromise the survival or prognosis of those PTMC that progressed over time. In Ito's latest report, of the 191 patients who underwent delayed surgery after a period of observation, none had recurrence except for one patient and also none suffered from distant metastasis or died of PTC after surgery [13]. Similarly, in Sugitani's first report [8], of the 16 patients who had delayed surgery 1–3 years after active observation, no patient had recurrence and death.

Regarding to which patient subgroup benefitted more from active observation rather than surgery, the current data appeared to show the young age (<40) group tended to have greater chance of size enlargement as well as new appearance of lymph node metastasis and therefore, the older age (>60) group should benefit more from active observation [13]. Furthermore, given the shorter life expectancy, it appeared to be logical to offer active observation to older patients with asymptomatic, low-risk PTMC.

Although TSH might be important in the development and progression of PTMC or PTC in general, there is still no evidence to show that TSH suppression should be given during the period of active observation as one study showed that there was no significant correlation between mean TSH during follow-up and change in PTMC size [14]. Therefore, observation alone (without TSH suppression) appeared adequate for low-risk PTMC.

Downsides with Active Observation as Opposed to Immediate Surgery for PTMC

However, despite these findings, there are downsides with active observation. First, as acknowledged by the authors themselves, [11] USG has limitations. For example, it is difficult to image accurately the dorsal part of a PTMC because of the presence of occasional intra-lesional calcifications causing strong echoes behind. Therefore, size determination is less accurate in some cases. Also there is great variability in observers' interpretations of USG images particularly in tumors with a less defined border. Although observation trials so far had dedicated radiologists interpreting USG images throughout the study period, it does raise the question on its applicability in other centers with no dedicated radiologists.

Second, by choosing active observation, it implies a life-long follow-up for the patient. He or she would be committed to at least once or twice yearly USG for the rest of the life. This could be difficult for some who may have not get access to healthcare easily because they live far or in the lower socioeconomic status. Although the cost of USG might be low in some countries, it does vary greatly between countries and so the life-time cumulative cost of USG examinations may be a greater burden for the society than perhaps immediate surgery alone. However, such cost comparison between observation and surgery has never been done.

Third, despite the associated morbidity of thyroidectomy, a hemithyroidectomy by experienced surgeons poses little to no risk to most patients having a low-risk PTMC. A hemi or partial thyroidectomy is a relatively simple operation and could be done as a day or short-stay procedure under general anesthesia. More importantly, it almost cures all patients with an asymptomatic low-risk PTMC without the need for life-long follow-up afterwards.

Fourth, although all of these observation trials demonstrated that few tumors would progress over time, it is unknown how observation itself might affect patient quality of life over time. It could potentially increase patient anxiety and reduce quality of time over time as patients might get increasingly worried despite adequate reassurance. In fact, it was interesting to note that despite such a 2% yearly rate of tumor progression, Ito's latest report showed that after 5 years, 191 or 16% of patients ended up undergoing thyroidectomy for one reason or another. Therefore, a greater proportion of patients would eventually undergo surgery despite the lack of objective tumor progression.

Fifth, there are many practical issues when adapting the observation approach and some of these may cause medico-legal problems. For example, if one patient under observation recurred or died of PTC, the patient's relatives may argue that perhaps surgery could have prevented the recurrence or death [18].

Lastly, since all these observation trials were non-randomized, their findings were prone to selection biases. It is possible that perhaps because most symptomatic and high-risk PTMC were screened out initially, the remaining PTMCs would do well regardless of observation or surgery. Perhaps, the same trial could be applied to larger-sized (>1 cm) PTC and results might be similar because these tumors are known to behave indolently. Therefore, it is important to conduct prospective randomized trials comparing between observation and immediate surgery in the future.

Nevertheless, the Japanese Society of Thyroid Surgeons and the Japan Association of Endocrine Surgeons have endorsed the use of "active observation" as an acceptable alternative to immediate surgery for low-risk PTMC [19].

Conclusions

The fact that the incidence of PTMC in autopsy examination is approximately 500–1000 times higher than that of clinically significant PTC means that the majority of PTMC do not necessarily require surgical treatment over one's lifetime. The "active observation" trials so far from the two Japanese centers have illustrated that in a well-selected group of PTMCs, the rate of significant size enlargement (≥3 mm) and appearance of new nodal metastasis per year without surgery are extremely low (1.0% and 0.3–0.4%, respectively) and patients most likely to benefit from active observation over immediate surgery are those aged >60 years because of lower chance of significant tumor progression. Nevertheless, there are still many uncertainties and controversies with active observation as a treatment option for PTMC and these include its applicability in other less specialized centers, its long-term cost-effectiveness and impact on patients' quality of life and the associated potential medico-legal issues. Larger prospective randomized trials are necessary to resolve some of these controversies.

Recommendation

"PTMC could be safely observed without the need for immediate surgery".

Quality: Moderate	Strength: Weak	Overall grade: C1

References

1. Lang BH, Wong KH, Chan CT. Initial attributable cost and economic burden of clinically-relevant differentiated thyroid cancer: a health care service provider perspective. Eur J Surg Oncol. 2015;41(6):758–65. https://doi.org/10.1016/j.ejso.2015.01.019.
2. Davies L, Welch HG. Increasing incidence of thyroid cancer in the United States, 1973-2002. JAMA. 2006;295:2164–7.
3. Pacini F. Thyroid microcarcinoma. Best Pract Res Clin Endocrinol Metab. 2012;26:421–9.
4. Yokozawa T, Miyauchi A, Kuma K, et al. Accurate and simple method of diagnosing thyroid nodules the modified technique of ultrasound-guided fine needle aspiration biopsy. Thyroid. 1995;5:141–5.
5. Takebe K, Date M, Yamamoto Y, et al. Mass screening for thyroid cancer with ultrasonography. Karkinos. 1994;7:309–17.
6. Cancer incidence and mortality in Hong Kong 1983–2011. Hong Kong Cancer Registry, Hong Kong. http://www3.ha.org.hk/cancereg/. Accessed 12 Mar 2015.
7. Ito Y, Uruno R, Nakano K, et al. An observation trial without surgical treatment in patients with papillary microcarcinoma of the thyroid gland. Thyroid. 2003;13:381–8.
8. Sugitani I, Toda K, Yamada K, et al. Three distinctly different kinds of papillary thyroid microcarcinoma should be recognized: our treatment strategies and outcomes. World J Surg. 2010;34:1222–31.
9. Lo CY, Chan WF, Lang BH, et al. Papillary microcarcinoma: is there any difference between clinically overt and occult tumors? World J Surg. 2006;30:759–66.
10. Yu XM, Wan Y, Sippel RS, et al. Should all papillary thyroid microcarcinomas be aggressively treated? An analysis of 18,445 cases. Ann Surg. 2011;254:653–60.
11. Ito Y, Miyauchi A. Nonoperative management of low-risk differentiated thyroid carcinoma. Curr Opin Oncol. 2015;27:15–20.
12. Ito Y, Miyauchi A, Inoue H, et al. An observational trial for papillary thyroid microcarcinoma in Japanese patients. World J Surg. 2010;34:28–35.
13. Ito Y, Miyauchi A, Kihara M, et al. Patient age is significantly related to the progression of papillary microcarcinoma of the thyroid under observation. Thyroid. 2014;24:27–34.
14. Sugitani I, Fujimoto Y, Yamada K. Association between serum thyrotropin concentration and growth of asymptomatic papillary thyroid microcarcinoma. World J Surg. 2014;38:673–8.
15. Lang BH, Lo CY, Chan WF, Lam KY, Wan KY. Prognostic factors in papillary and follicular thyroid carcinoma: their implications for cancer staging. Ann Surg Oncol. 2007;14(2):730–8.
16. Miyauchi A, Kudo T, Kihara M, et al. Relationship of biochemically persistent disease and thyroglobulin-doubling time to age at surgery in patients with papillary thyroid carcinoma. Endocr J. 2013;60:415–21.
17. Lang BH, Lo CY, Wong KP, Wan KY. Long-term outcomes for older patients with papillary thyroid carcinoma: should another age cutoff beyond 45 years be added? Ann Surg Oncol. 2015;22(2):446–53.
18. Sturgis EM, Sherman SI. Should papillary thyroid carcinoma be observed? A word of caution. Arch Otolaryngol Head Neck Surg. 2010;136:444–6.
19. Takami H, Ito Y, Okamoto T, et al. Revisiting the guidelines issued by the Japanese Society of Thyroid Surgeons and Japan Association of Endocrine Surgeons: a gradual move towards consensus between Japanese and western practice in the management of thyroid carcinoma. World J Surg. 2014;38:2002–10.

First-Line Therapy for Anaplastic Thyroid Cancer: Operation Versus Medical Management

12

Shabirhusain Abadin, Paritosh Suman, Jessica Hwang, Anu Thakrar, and Subhash Patel

Abstract

Anaplastic thyroid cancer (ATC) is a highly lethal disease. First-line therapy for a patient diagnosed with this disease includes surgical resection or chemoradiation. Due to variable treatment and its rarity, there is a paucity of prospective and/or randomized controlled literature studying the initial therapy for patients diagnosed with ATC. To understand which therapy is more appropriate in terms of survival and quality of life, we evaluated the available literature and our own institutional experience with the management of ATC for recommendations regarding this topic. This chapter provides a summary of the pertaining literature and offers recommendations based on these sources for first-line management of a patient with newly diagnosed ATC.

Keywords

Anaplastic thyroid cancer · Carcinoma · Thyroidectomy · Surgery · Chemoradiation · Radiotherapy · Chemotherapy

S. Abadin (✉) · S. Patel
John H. Stroger, Jr. Hospital of Cook County, Department of Surgery, Chicago, IL, USA
e-mail: sabadin@cookcountyhhs.org

P. Suman
NorthShore University HealthSystem/John H. Stroger Hospital of Cook County, Department of Surgery, Evanston, IL, USA

J. Hwang
John H. Stroger, Jr. Hospital of Cook County, Department of Endocrinology and Diabetes, Chicago, IL, USA

A. Thakrar
Department of Radiation Oncology, John H. Stroger, Jr. Hospital of Cook County, Chicago, IL, USA

P. Angelos, R. H. Grogan (eds.), *Difficult Decisions in Endocrine Surgery*, Difficult Decisions in Surgery: An Evidence-Based Approach,
https://doi.org/10.1007/978-3-319-92860-9_12

Introduction

Anaplastic thyroid carcinoma (ATC) is a rare but highly lethal disease. It comprises 1.7% of all newly diagnosed thyroid cancers each year in the United States [1]. In a review article looking at 1771 patients with ATC who were reported in clinical studies, 64% were women, the median survival was 5 months and the 1-year survival was 20% [1]. It typically occurs in the sixth or seventh decade of life. Although there is much scientific research into disease understanding and treatment of ATC, the median overall survival has not changed in recent decades. ATC is poorly differentiated in that it does not produce thyroglobulin, cannot transport iodine and it lacks genetic changes associated with follicular-origin thyroid cancers [2]. Thus, radioactive iodine as an adjuvant therapy is not considered for ATC as it is for the majority of thyroid cancers. In most cases, the prognosis is dismal even with the most aggressive treatment. Clinically, ATC presents most commonly with a rapidly growing neck mass in a short period of time, sometimes days to weeks. Histopathological confirmation is usually obtained by fine needle aspiration but often an open or core needle biopsy is required for diagnosis.

The first-line therapy for a newly diagnosed patient with ATC is controversial. Given the near certain lethality from the disease soon after diagnosis, clinicians have a small window of time to prescribe treatment expeditiously that may improve survival and quality of life. As far as published data and recommendations on management of ATC, the rarity of the tumor forces researchers to utilize multi-institutional data often spanning over several decades during which treatment and dose, and approach has changed. The decision to operate versus chemoradiation therapy at the onset hinges on several patient factors: location(s) and spread of the cancer, proximity and danger to adjacent vital structures, the imminent life-threating concerns from synchronous metastases, comorbidities, and the wishes of the patient. The chapter includes a review of the American Thyroid Association (ATA) guidelines on ATC and published literature to arrive at the most evidence-based approach to first-line therapy (Table 12.1). Overall survival of patients with ATC patients and clinical trials have only lead to small differences in median survival (generally at most 2 months). Depending on an individual patient, the possibility of improving median survival by a few weeks or months may be considered significant or futile [3]. The published clinical trials on ATC have exemplified the challenges for trial design in this very rare and quickly lethal disease. Most trials have been small and often have been terminated early due to poor accrual or inadequate treatment response to justify risks [4].

Table 12.1 PICO table

Population:	Patients with anaplastic thyroid cancer
Intervention:	Surgical resection
Comparator:	Chemoradiation
Outcomes:	Survival, QOL

Early Multidisciplinary Assessment

An early multidisciplinary discussion is integral to the evaluation, workup and treatment of a patient with ATC. Histopathologic diagnosis is necessary. Usually this diagnosis can be made with fine needle aspiration cytology. Infrequently, a surgical incisional biopsy will need to be done to secure the diagnosis. Once the diagnosis is confirmed, an expeditious discussion among primary physician, endocrinologist, medical oncologist, radiation oncologist, surgeon, and palliative care specialist is due in order to form an acceptable mutually agreed upon plan in the patient's best interests. Decisions regarding first-line therapy should be made based on available literature, initial staging, presence of synchronous metastases, comorbidities, and patient's wishes.

Prognostic Factors

Prognostic factors for better suitability and improved outcomes to undergo aggressive treatment include younger age, smaller tumor size, and lack of distant metastases. Existing data suggests a better prognosis for patients less than 70 years old of age. Others have found improved survival outcomes even for those under the age of 60 years [5, 6]. Tumor size less than 5 cm have been associated with a relatively better prognosis [5, 7, 8]. The presence of distant metastases, local tumor extension, rapid tumor growth and poor performance status have all been noted to be poor prognostic factors in a published series from 2005 [9]. In the treatment of ATC, multimodality therapy can be of benefit, however institution of all three modalities, radiation, chemotherapy, and surgery are not always feasible. These prognostic factors should be considered in deciding whether to offer an aggressive tri-modality treatment, but which may have increased complications and significant side effects. Available treatments for ATC are very burdensome for the patient and patients with a reduced performance status or poor prognostic factors may be considered for less aggressive treatment or palliation. Ito et al. demonstrated that patients with a clinically resectable tumor and who underwent multimodal therapy with surgery, chemotherapy and radiation treatment had the longest survival of 13.7 months [10] in comparison to patients who underwent uni or bi-modal treatments.

Determine Resectability

Thyroid ultrasound provides a rapid, non-invasive evaluation of neck mass and regional lymph nodes. Computed tomography (CT) imaging with iodinated contrast can provide important locally invasive structural information and will help determine extent of disease and resectability. If the patient has symptoms or imaging features suggestive of invasion into the recurrent laryngeal nerve, trachea, or esophagus, laryngoscopy for upper airway and larynx, bronchoscopy for trachea, and esophagoscopy for esophagus are warranted as part of the preoperative staging.

Initial resectability requires a detailed evaluation with neck imaging and depends on the presence or absence of local invasion to adjacent structures. Figure 12.1 is a coronal image of a patient with tumor extension into the superior vena cava. This tumor was deemed unresectable due to local invasion into superior vena cava as well into the larynx. Although a decision to resect such aggressive tumors also varies from surgeon to surgeon, it should primarily be dictated by the ability to obtain a R0 or R1 resection with minimal morbidity in the safest way possible.

Metastases with ATC are common. In a series of 41 autopsy cases of ATC, 91% had metastases. The most common sites of metastases were the lungs (78%), intrathoracic lymph nodes (58%), neck lymph nodes (51%), pleura (29%), adrenal glands (24%), liver (20%), brain (18%), heart (18%), and retroperitoneal lymph nodes (18%) [11]. Moreover, up to 50% of patients have distant metastases at presentation [2, 12]. Dedicated imaging of the rest of the body can identify synchronous metastases that may alter first line management. For instance, an impending neurologic crisis either from a growing brain metastasis or a vertebral metastasis compromising the spinal cord, would constitute sufficient cause for delaying primary thyroid surgery until after emergent neurologic care is administered. Similarly, life-threatening pulmonary hemorrhage from metastatic lung disease may demand

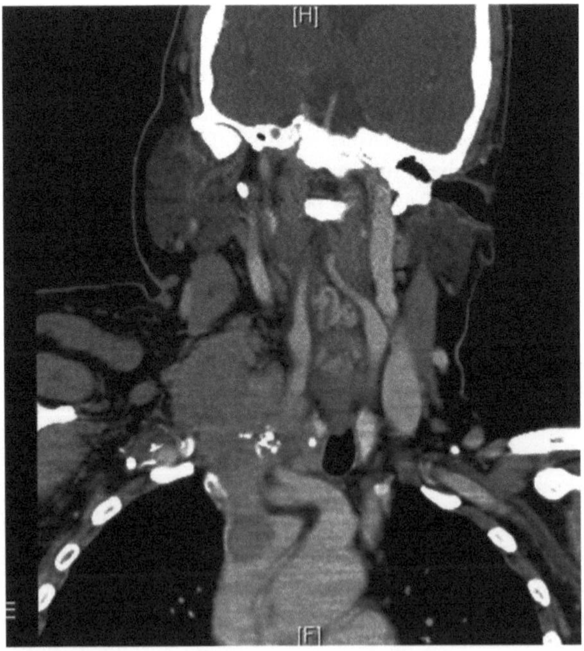

Fig. 12.1 Tumor extension into the superior vena cava in a patient with newly diagnosed anaplastic thyroid carcinoma

priority over neck operation [13, 14]. However, the presence of non-life-threating distant metastases is not a strict contraindication for neck resection. In fact, the workup of distant metastases with biopsy and imaging should not delay the treatment of the primary neck disease often warrants immediate attention [14]. Therefore, in a patient with suspected distant metastases and locally resectable disease in the neck, should be offered a neck resection as first line therapy to obtain local tumor control and prevent airway obstruction. Because ATC frequently invades adjacent organs and tissues, the potential for complete tumor extirpation is not always possible at the time of presentation. Nevertheless, impending airway compromise from primary neck disease will be priority in most cases of ATC.

Operative Resection as First Line Therapy

In patients with newly diagnosed ATC who are deemed resectable, the goal is a gross tumor resection with R0 or R1 margins. Several single center retrospective studies suggest that either an R0 or R1 resection correlates with an improved disease-free and overall survival with or without adjunct therapy. One study of 120 patients examined the utility of restricted radical surgery with the intent to clear as much tumor without removal of vital organs such as the esophagus, larynx, and trachea [15]. Overall survival was poor with median survival time of 3.1 months regardless of approach, nevertheless the patients who had a R0 resection had a 15% 5-year survival whereas no patient survived at 5 years who underwent a R1 or R2 resection [15]. In another study of 33 patients, those patients treated with a potentially curative resection had a median survival of 43 months versus 3 months [16]. The operation should be a total or near-total thyroidectomy. In those with extrathyroidal extension, a more aggressive resection is warranted if gross disease can be safely cleared [10, 17]. In a study of 75 patients that looked at multimodal treatment, the patients that had better locoregional control were those that underwent R0/R1 resection with and without chemoradiation. The survival benefit was minimal but there were three patients who survived for more than 5 years and all of them underwent gross tumor resection [18]. Another retrospective study looking at 40 consecutive patients with ATC evaluated surgical resection followed by chemoradiation and found that patients with less invasive primary tumors that were resected initially and had adjuvant therapy had a survival benefit compared to those with more aggressive and less resectable disease (9.6 months versus 4.0 months) [10].

Patients with locoregional invasion should be offered a resection if gross tumor resection can be achieved with minimal morbidity [14]. Since ATC can spread via direct contiguous invasion and through the lymphatics, adjacent anatomical structures and applicable surgical planes in relation to the tumor must be carefully evaluated. More than 80% of patients with ATC present with primary tumors that have already invaded into surrounding structures including the trachea, esophagus, and carotid artery [19, 20]. Moreover, nearly 40% of patient with ATC taken for resection required extended resections [15]. Operative debulking with gross positive margins should never be a goal as the rate of local recurrence are very high. In a retrospective study with 67 patients, 6-month, 1 year, and 3-year survival rates were reported as 92%, 92%, and 83%, respectively after complete resection. This was much diminished to 53%, 35%, and 0% if the patient underwent debulking surgery [8].

Airway Management

Frequently airway obstruction can be the initial presentation or can develop during the treatment of ATC. Often times, mortality from these aggressive tumors results from airway issues. There is a paucity of literature regarding airway management in ATC.

Historically, prophylactic tracheostomy was employed in many cases of ATC for prevention of airway compromise or suffocation. Current guidelines do not recommend for a routine and elective tracheostomy either with oncological operation or as a prophylactic procedure alone [14]. Tracheostomy is often fraught with inherent issues such as excessive secretions, wound infections and potential local complications including bleeding and tumor overgrowth or tube dislodgement. Furthermore, placement of a tracheostomy usually necessitates an inpatient hospital or nursing facility stay and can delay future treatments. Holting et al. in their experience of 170 patients with ATC showed that tracheostomy resulted in delayed radiation treatments and this was mainly due to tracheostomy related complications [21, 22]. Moreover, tracheostomy resulted in a reduction in median survival from 5 months to 2 months. From a quality or life standpoint, many patients with tracheostomy will lose their voice permanently as decannulation or downsizing with the use of speech valve can rarely be achieved. A potential for future tracheostomy in unstable and unintubatable patients can also lead to a decision to perform prophylactic tracheostomy in a small minority of patients.

A rapidly enlarging central compartment mass, unilateral or bilateral vocal cord paralysis, direct tracheal invasion, bleeding into the trachea, or upper airway edema are the usual causes of airway obstruction [23]. Hoarseness, stridor or dyspnea could indicate impending airway obstruction [24]. Every patient with suspected ATC should undergo evaluation of the vocal cords. The best way to evaluate the vocal cords is with fiberoptic laryngoscopy; however, mirror examination may also be acceptable. Fiberoptic laryngoscopy will also help to assess the opposite vocal cord, mobility of the vocal cords, any endolaryngeal pathology and can also identify any extension of disease in the subglottic or upper tracheal regions [14].

Concerning airway management, a patient's desire and wishes should be taken into consideration in decision-making. A diagnosis of ATC does not necessitate a tracheostomy upfront if the patient is clinically stable from a respiratory standpoint. Medical management with steroids and nebulized epinephrine in conjunction with comfort care measures can be employed. In situations of respiratory distress, securing the airway is the priority. Additionally, management of acute airway issues in the operating room has been advised [23]. Awake intubation in a semirecumbent position, preferably using a flexible laryngoscope should be attempted. The trachea could be almost impossible to reach especially in the presence of a bulky anterior

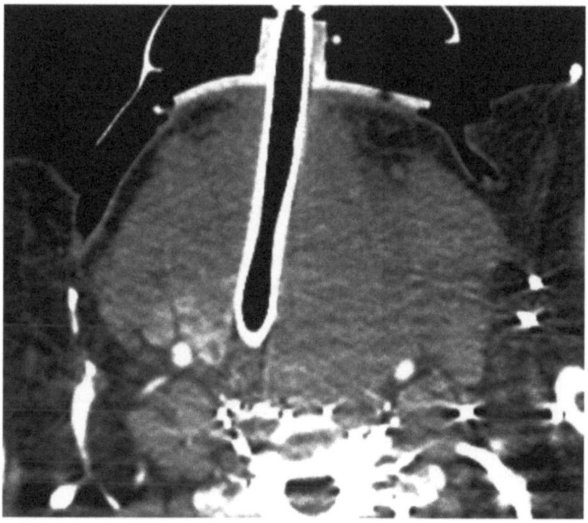

Fig. 12.2 Cricothyroidotomy with long tracheostomy tube placement in a patient with acute airway obstruction from anaplastic thyroid carcinoma

mass requiring the use of a long tracheostomy tube. For long segment tracheal compression, use of airway stents or endotracheal tube via cricothyroidotomy tube have been also described. Figure 12.2 demonstrates a coronal CT image of a patient who had a long tracheostomy tube placed via a cricothyroidotomy for impending airway compromise.

The presence of airway compromise in ATC is almost universally associated with a dismal prognosis. Prophylactic tracheostomy in a patient with a biopsy-proven ATC is not indicated. In contrast to most acute airway situations, a clear and informed discussion about the prognosis and goals of care should be considered prior to any airway interventions as these could be the source of much morbidity in a clinical entity with dismal prognosis.

Medical Management as First-Line Therapy

Two subgroups of patients are candidates for medical therapy as first-line therapy. If a patient who has biopsy-proven ATC is deemed to have a tumor that would not allow for a safe resection, neoadjuvant radiotherapy and/or chemotherapy should be administered. Also, in the case where systemic disease is present upon presentation and the neck disease is confined and does not need immediate resection, initial chemoradiation is indicated. If a patient is truly unresectable from a safety and morbidity standpoint, chemoradiation is the preferred initial management. Patients with ATC who present with locoregionally confined with borderline unresectable disease should consider radiotherapy with or without systemic therapy as these patients may become operable candidates [14] (Fig. 12.3).

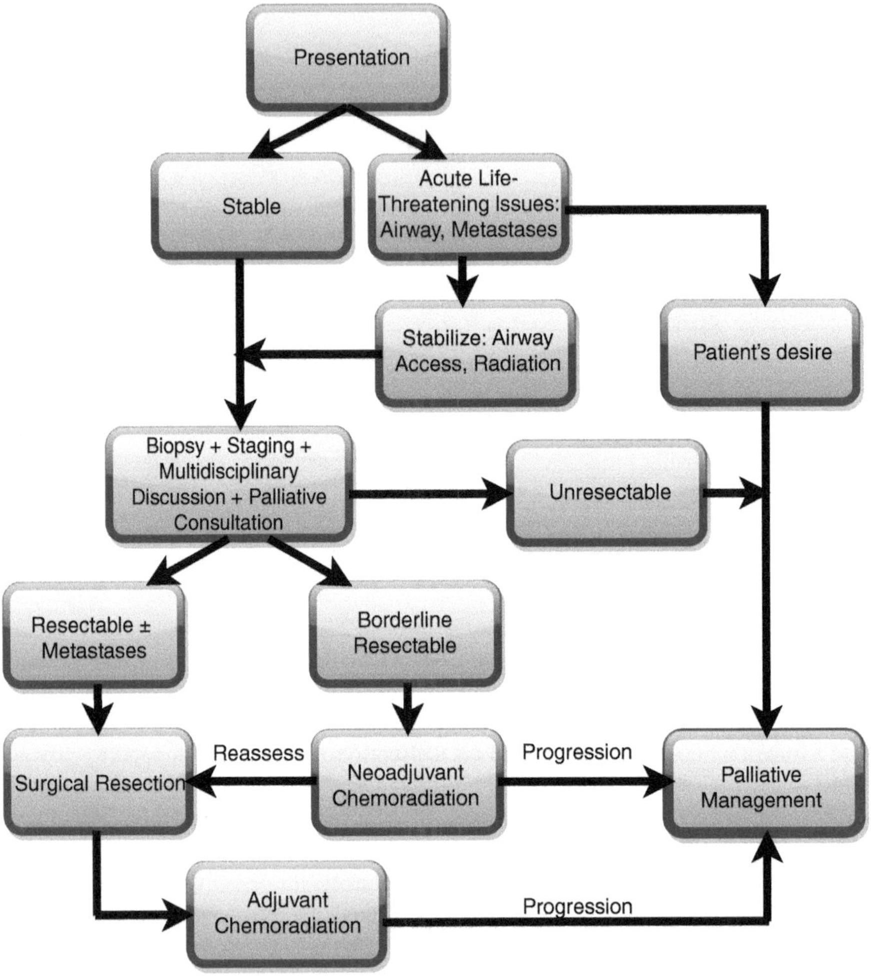

Fig. 12.3 Algorithmic approach for first-line therapy in anaplastic thyroid carcinoma

Radiotherapy

Radiation therapy is delivered with either definitive or palliative intent. Definitive radiotherapy refers to high-dose radiation treatment with the intention to provide long-term local control. Palliative radiotherapy, on the other hand, refers to lower dose treatment in order to alleviate symptoms locally albeit for a shorter duration [14]. In the setting of ATC, external beam radiotherapy (EBRT) is the primary modality of radiation therapy utilized. Intensity-modulated radiotherapy (IMRT) is a type EBRT that allows for radiation to be more conformal to the tumor while sparing adjacent normal tissues. Radiation dose is prescribed in Gray (Gy). Once daily radiation is called standard fractionation. Hyperfractionation is radiation therapy given more than once a day. Hyperfractionated accelerated radiation therapy allows the same total dose to be given in a shorter time frame. This is utilized in ATC with the intent of combatting the rapid repopulation of the tumor.

Dose Benefit

Radiation has been found to prolong survival in ATC, typically by a few months. It is often delivered in conjunction with chemotherapy, but even radiation as a single modality prolongs survival although for a short duration. Radiation dose is a significant prognostic factor. Survival benefit was found in a single institution retrospective review where patients were treated to either a curative dose (>40 Gy) versus a palliative dose of 40 Gy or less [25]. There was a statistically significant improvement in survival for those patients receiving greater than 40 Gy [25] of radiation. Dose is also a significant prognostic factor. Improvements in survival with increasing dose were found to be at 40 Gy in several studies [18, 25, 26]. A higher dose (60 Gy) in some studies demonstrated improvements in survival [26, 27]. In the modern era, higher doses can be delivered with better target coverage and decreased toxicity to normal structures such as the spinal cord utilizing IMRT [28, 29].

Hyperfractionation

However, even though there is a dose response and survival benefit with radiotherapy upfront, survival remains incredibly low. Many institutions have tried to improve survival by altering fractionation. The rationale for the use of hyperfractionation in ATC is due to its rapid doubling time. With hyperfractionation accelerated treatment, the total prescribed dose is delivered over a shorter treatment time. There are several issues with this method, one is patient convenience as the fractions are typically separated by 6 h to decrease toxicity and this involves the patient coming to the radiation center either twice a day or staying for over 6 h at the center. In addition, hyperfractionation typically causes increased acute toxicity such as dysphagia, esophagitis, erythema, and desquamation, but not late side effects [30, 31]. Hyperfractionation has been measured in multiple trials and there is evidence for improved local control, although not always statistically significant, over standard fractionation [7, 25]. Wang et al. treated their radical radiation patients to 60 Gy. Their patients were treated without chemotherapy and a comparison was performed between standard fractionation given in the earlier period of the review (14 patients) vs. twice daily fractionation given in the latter period of the study (9 patients). Standard fractionation was delivered once daily to a total dose of 60 Gy in 30 fractions (6 week course of treatment) or twice daily radiation, most commonly 60 Gy in 40 fractions of 1.5 Gy each (taking 4 weeks to achieve desired dosing) [25]. It was found that there was a trend toward improved overall survival to 13.6 months for patients receiving hyperfractionation vs 10.3 months for standard fractionation, but this difference was not statistically significant ($p = 0.3$). An important caveat here is that hyperfractionation was only offered to patients with good performance status of Eastern Cooperative Oncology Group (ECOG) grade 2 or better [25].

Hyperfractionated accelerated treatment has resulted in improved local control, but not survival. Other studies have looked to further accelerate the radiation treatment, although at times with severe toxicity. One protocol treated with 1 Gy four times daily, with each fraction separated by 3 h and had a 6% rate of radiation myelitis [32]. Other regimens include increasing acceleration by increase in the per fraction dose, as employed by three consecutive protocols run at Lund Hospital [33]. One protocol treated all patients with 46 Gy of radiation. The protocol initially called for treating with 1 Gy twice daily. The second protocol increased the dose per fraction to 1.3 Gy and the third protocol to 1.6 Gy per fraction. Thus each protocol accelerated the time to completion over the previous one. Acceleration showed the benefit of improved local control but did not improve overall survival [33]. The first two protocols had a treatment break after 30 Gy for surgery, but the third protocol was completed without a break. The final radiation protocol had 100% local control, but the shortest survival at 2 months [33]. Given that overall survival has not improved significantly, some institutions have gone back to the standard fractionation [27, 30].

Many patients with ATC are found to be unresectable and can be offered definitive radiation treatment including hyperfractionation if they have good performance status [34, 35]. In one small series of five patients, survival was 13 months with radiotherapy and chemotherapy [34]. Additionally, radiation therapy could also convert an inoperable tumor to an operable one. Besic et al. in 2001 retrospectively divided the eligible patients treated in his institution into 26 patients who received upfront surgery versus those who were treated with upfront chemoradiation (53 patients) [35]. The patients with upfront chemoradiation had a worse prognosis when compared to upfront surgery group likely due to more aggressive tumors, extension outside of the thyroid capsule, and lymph node metastases. There was no difference in overall survival at 1 year between those two groups, 21% chemotherapy and/or radiotherapy first and 25% for surgery first [35]. Of those 53 patients, 12 became operable. The best overall survival of 50% at 1 year was found to be in those 12 patients who first underwent chemoradiation, followed by surgery [35].

Combined Treatment Modalities

Surgery in addition to radiation improves outcomes. A multivariate analysis of the SEER database found that the combination of surgical resection and radiotherapy decreased the cause-specific mortality and was statistically significant [5]. For those patients who can undergo upfront surgery followed by radiotherapy, they may have a better outcome. In another study, there were three patients who had gross tumor resection upfront followed by radiotherapy and survived more than 2 years. Among patients who did not have surgery and only received radiotherapy, none lived greater than 2 years [36]. Another study also found improved survival in those who had a potentially curable resection followed by radiation and chemotherapy had a median survival of 43 months versus 3 months for those who only had a palliative surgery [16].

In patients undergoing surgery first, several studies have found a local control benefit to those who underwent hyperfractionated radiation as opposed to daily treatment [7, 37]. Although not statistically significant, there were no local recurrences for those receiving hyperfractionated radiation [7]. For patients who underwent an R0 or R1 resection, complete locoregional control was 89% in a previously mentioned study [18].

In some cases, chemotherapy is administered concurrently with radiation to act as a radiation sensitizer by making its the anti-tumor properties more effective for local control [14]. Concurrent chemotherapy is now added to most radiation regimens. However, some data suggests that there is no impact on survival [8, 26]. Conversely, there are studies to support improvement in local response [31], local control [3], progression-free survival [27], and overall survival [9, 38]. Regardless, given the high rate of distant metastases and dismal prognosis, a search for better systemic treatment continues.

Systemic Therapy

There are no standard chemotherapy guidelines for ATC and, therefore, there is no clear data on the most appropriate timing of systemic therapy. The importance of performing comprehensive pre-operative staging to address tumor invasiveness to find out whether patients could benefit from neoadjuvant therapy is unfortunately challenged by this tumor's rapid doubling time which often require expeditious therapeutic intervention. Systemic chemotherapy and radiotherapy have been used therapeutically together in the neoadjuvant setting to downstage locally unresectable tumor to enable complete resection. Furthermore, chemoradiation is also used in the adjuvant setting to control locoregional disease and distant metastases, and in the palliative setting [2].

Neoadjuvant Therapy

There have been studies suggesting that neoadjuvant chemoradiation should be considered if disease at presentation is considered unresectable. Besic et al. compared outcomes for a primary surgery group with a primary chemotherapy ± radiation group (16 out of 18 patients had radiotherapy) and found there was no survival difference between the two. Notably, the neoadjuvant therapy group was older, had larger and more rapidly growing disease not confined to the thyroid and had more frequent lymph node metastases [35]. In mouse model studies of ATC, administration of a selective BRAF V600E inhibitor PLX4720 for 1 week in mice with unresectable disease enabled thyroidectomy to be performed and modestly affected lifespan. However, tumor growth resumed after this agent was stopped [39].

Cytotoxic Agents

Doxorubicin is the only FDA-approved drug for systemic therapy that may be used to treat ATC, and, while it has achieved modest effects against advanced ATC, it is often used in multi-modal fashion [2]. Since no single cytotoxic agent or combination of agents has demonstrated a very significant survival advantage especially in stage IVC ATC, systemic chemotherapy is recommended through clinical trials [2]. A randomized trial of patients comparing doxorubicin plus cisplatin (n = 18) to doxorubicin alone (n = 21) concluded with 3 complete responses and 3 partial responses in the combination therapy group (18%) versus 1 partial response in the single agent group (5%) [1]. The sequence of therapy was variable (adjuvant vs. induction) but overall response rate was 50% in this small case series [40]. A phase II trial with paclitaxel demonstrated a longer median survival of 32 weeks compared to only 7 weeks in non-responders [3].

Targeted Therapies

The invasive nature of ATC is in part a result of the accumulation of activated/mutated oncogenes and defective tumor suppressor genes along with the high percentage of patients who have distant metastases at diagnosis [41]. Smallridge et al. reported the prevalence of the following mutations: p53 (55%), RAS (22%), BRAF (26%), PIK3CA (17%) and PTEN (12%) [42]. Liu et al. used polymerase chain reaction (PCR) to analyze the role of the MAPK and PI3K pathway in ATC and found tyrosine kinase receptors like epidermal growth factor receptor (EGFR), platelet-derived growth factor receptor (PDGFR) and vascular endothelial growth factor (VEGFR) are frequently amplified in ATC [43]. Furthermore, mutations in the tumor suppressor gene TP53 which controls cell proliferation and apoptosis have been reported in 50–80% cases [44]. Identifying and targeting specific mutations in ATC has shown promising results in pre-clinical mouse model studies [45]. However, translating what is understood about the molecular pathogenesis of ATC from pre-clinical laboratories to clinical trials has not resulted in large survival benefits in this highly lethal tumor.

Several trials targeting tyrosine kinase inhibitors have demonstrated very limited efficacy. Sorafenib, a BRAF/VEGFR inhibitor is being used in to treat advanced radioiodine refractory thyroid cancer. Since BRAF is also mutated in a quarter of ATC cases, a phase II clinical trial using Sorafenib was conducted involving 20 ATC patients. Only 2 of 20 had a partial response and 5 of 20 had stable disease that was short-lived. Toxicities were manageable and included transient hypertension and rash [4]. Imatinib, a tyrosine kinase inhibitor of Bcr-ABL and PDGF, has been implicated in ATC cell proliferation pre-clinically. A phase II clinical trial (terminated early due to poor accrual) enrolled 11 patients with advanced ATC and overexpressing PDGF receptors or cABL (9 of whom had prior chemoradiation), and were started on imatinib 400 mg BID. There were no complete responses, however 75% of patients either had a partial response or stable disease and 6 month overall survival was 45% which is comparable to other cytotoxic regimens, suggesting some activity in advanced tumors [46]. A trial using Pazopanib also had disappointing results demonstrating no tumor responses among the first 14 patients enrolled such that the trial was closed [47].

Other small molecule inhibitors such as EGFR inhibitors have been studied in radio-resistant advanced thyroid cancer. A phase II trial using EGFR inhibitor Gefitinib in advanced, radio-iodine resistant thyroid cancer (19% of which of were ATC, n = 5) described a single patient who had stable disease for 12 months [13]. A phase II trial evaluating the efficacy and safety of mTOR kinase inhibitor in advanced, radio-resistant thyroid cancer (all histology) included 6 patients (15% of total) with ATC. 63% of total patients, including 1 with ATC experienced tumor shrinkage during the study [48]. Because of this unexpected finding, a non-randomized phase II clinical trial of mTOR kinase inhibitor in metastatic ATC has been designed but has not yet begun enrolling patients.

Preclinical studies demonstrated that peroxisome proliferator-activated receptor (PPAR-γ) agonist therapy inhibits ATC cell proliferation and promotes apoptosis when combined with paclitaxel [49]. Subsequently, a phase I clinical trial (which closed early due to poor accrual) treated 15 ATC patients with paclitaxel and variable doses (0.15 mg BID and 0.3 mg BID) of efatutazone. Dose-dependent biologic activity was observed and median survival was 41% greater with the 0.3 mg BID versus the 0.15 mg BID dosing (138 days vs. 98 days) [49].

Vascular disrupting agents which impact tumor blood supply are another area being actively researched. Most recently, a phase II trial of single-agent fosbretabulin in ATC was performed. Fosbretabulin destabilizes microtubules causing vascular disruption and decreased blood flow/necrosis to tumors [50]. Median survival was 4.7 months in this trial. No patients achieved the primary endpoint of the trial (doubling median survival time), however, the 6-month and 12-month survival rates were 34% and 23%, respectively. The authors concluded that these results were comparable to the aforementioned single-agent study using paclitaxel [51].

Combination Therapy

Results from trials using single selective targeted agents in ATC has been disappointing. Randomized trials using a combination of cytotoxic and targeted therapy hope to achieve improved overall survival. One of the largest randomized prospective trials in ATC (n = 80, enrollment stopped early due to low accrual) investigated the overall survival differences between carboplatin/paclitaxel with or without fosbretabulin. The median survival was 5.2 months in the carboplatin/paclitaxel + fosbretabulin arm versus 4.0 months in the carboplatin/paclitaxel arm. Overall survival rates were greater at 6 months and 1 year in the carboplatin/paclitaxel + fosbretabulin group [50]. A Radiation Therapy Oncology Group (RTOG 0912) randomized phase II clinical trial that is ongoing is evaluating IMRT, paclitaxel and pazopanib in ATC is currently open to accrual. The basis for this trial was preclinical data demonstrating that combination pazopanib with paclitaxel had synergistic anti-tumor effects and part of the mechanism was attributed to possible inhibition of aurora A kinase by pazopanib [52].

Conclusion

Anaplastic thyroid cancer (ATC) is a highly lethal disease even with aggressive multimodal treatment. The debate on initial surgical resection or chemoradiation depends on many factors including the ability to obtain a gross tumor resection with low morbidity, other comorbidities, and the patient's wishes. Historically, palliative measures were the primary treatment options including prophylactic tracheostomy, debulking surgery, and palliative chemoradiation. Although there is a scarcity in prospective literature for ATC treatment, some evidence has suggested that resection is advised in some cases where a RO or R1 resection is possible. Furthermore, airway management has become more tailored to each patient and not the initial and only operation for a patient. Chemoradiation is often the first-line therapy due to the disease extent and invasiveness at presentation. Radiotherapy demonstrates survival benefit and local control but long-term benefit is rare. Systemic therapy has expanded into targeted agents as ATC has been studied and analyzed on a genetic level, but by itself have shown minimal benefit. For many patients who wish to proceed with treatment, chemoradiation is frequently the first-line therapy. Evidence-based literature is low quality as most studies are retrospective and have variable regimens.

Recommendations

Recommendations for Operative Management as First-Line Therapy

- Once the histopathologic diagnosis of anaplastic thyroid cancer is made, if preoperative imaging demonstrates a tumor that can be resected safely and with low morbidity (Strength of Recommendation: Moderate; Quality of Evidence: Low)
- If operative management is selected, it should not be delayed by workup and biopsy of other potential distant tumor sites (Strength of Recommendation: Moderate; Quality of Evidence: Low)
- The presence of distant metastases does not prohibit initial neck resection especially if the neck disease is resectable. If the tumor is confined to the thyroid or can be removed safely with minimal morbidity, neck resection can be performed even in the setting of distant disease, as this may prevent the need for a tracheostomy due to impending airway obstruction. (Strength of Recommendation: Weak; Quality of Evidence: Low)
- Prophylactic tracheostomy is not indicated in all biopsy-proven cases of ATC. Since it is the source of much morbidity, it should be reserved for those patients with impending airway obstruction. If needed, it should be performed in the most controlled setting in the operating room, not as a bedside or intensive care unit (ICU) procedure. (Strength of Recommendation: Weak; Quality of Evidence: Low)

Recommendations for Chemoradiation as First-Line Therapy

- If preoperative staging suggests that initial operation would be unsafe and would cause morbidity, chemoradiation is warranted for local control (Strength of Recommendation: Weak; Quality of Evidence: Low)
- Hyperfractionated radiotherapy may provide local control for locally advanced neck disease and may make the patient a potentially surgical candidate (Strength of Recommendation: Weak; Quality of Evidence: Low)
- In patients receiving definitive radiotherapy, a higher dose of radiation may be used for better local control and survival benefit. (Strength of Recommendation: Weak; Quality of Evidence: Low)
- Chemotherapy should be given in conjunction with radiotherapy for synergistic anti-tumor effects. (Strength of Recommendation: Weak; Quality of Evidence: Low)
- Multiple agents including targeted therapy along with cytotoxic agents may provide greater survival benefit in unresectable patients with distant metastases than single agent therapy. (Strength of Recommendation: Weak; Quality of Evidence: Low)

References

1. Smallridge RC, Copland JA. Anaplastic thyroid carcinoma: pathogenesis and emerging therapies. Clin Oncol (R Coll Radiol). 2010;22(6):486–97.
2. Keutgen XM, Sadowski SM, Kebebew E. Management of anaplastic thyroid cancer. Gland Surg. 2015;4(1):44–51.
3. Derbel O, Limem S, Segura-Ferlay C, Lifante JC, Carrie C, Peix JL, et al. Results of combined treatment of anaplastic thyroid carcinoma (ATC). BMC Cancer. 2011;11:469.
4. Savvides P, Nagaiah G, Lavertu P, Fu P, Wright JJ, Chapman R, et al. Phase II trial of sorafenib in patients with advanced anaplastic carcinoma of the thyroid. Thyroid. 2013;23(5):600–4.
5. Kebebew E, Greenspan FS, Clark OH, Woeber KA, McMillan A. Anaplastic thyroid carcinoma. Treatment outcome and prognostic factors. Cancer. 2005;103(7):1330–5.
6. Kim TY, Kim KW, Jung TS, Kim JM, Kim SW, Chung KW, et al. Prognostic factors for Korean patients with anaplastic thyroid carcinoma. Head Neck. 2007;29(8):765–72.
7. Kobayashi T, Asakawa H, Umeshita K, Takeda T, Maruyama H, Matsuzuka F, et al. Treatment of 37 patients with anaplastic carcinoma of the thyroid. Head Neck. 1996;18(1):36–41.
8. Pierie JP, Muzikansky A, Gaz RD, Faquin WC, Ott MJ. The effect of surgery and radiotherapy on outcome of anaplastic thyroid carcinoma. Ann Surg Oncol. 2002;9(1):57–64.
9. Besic N, Hocevar M, Zgajnar J, Pogacnik A, Grazio-Frkovic S, Auersperg M. Prognostic factors in anaplastic carcinoma of the thyroid-a multivariate survival analysis of 188 patients. Langenbecks Arch Surg. 2005;390(3):203–8.
10. Ito K, Hanamura T, Murayama K, Okada T, Watanabe T, Harada M, et al. Multimodality therapeutic outcomes in anaplastic thyroid carcinoma: improved survival in subgroups of patients with localized primary tumors. Head Neck. 2012;34(2):230–7.
11. Besic N, Gazic B. Sites of metastases of anaplastic thyroid carcinoma: autopsy findings in 45 cases from a single institution. Thyroid. 2013;23(6):709–13.
12. Kihara M, Miyauchi A, Yamauchi A, Yokomise H. Prognostic factors of anaplastic thyroid carcinoma. Surg Today. 2004;34(5):394–8.
13. Smallridge RC. Approach to the patient with anaplastic thyroid carcinoma. J Clin Endocrinol Metab. 2012;97(8):2566–72.

14. Smallridge RC, Ain KB, Asa SL, Bible KC, Brierley JD, Burman KD, et al. American Thyroid Association guidelines for management of patients with anaplastic thyroid cancer. Thyroid. 2012;22(11):1104–39.
15. Passler C, Scheuba C, Prager G, Kaserer K, Flores JA, Vierhapper H, et al. Anaplastic (undifferentiated) thyroid carcinoma (ATC). A retrospective analysis. Langenbecks Arch Surg. 1999;384(3):284–93.
16. Haigh PI, Ituarte PH, Wu HS, Treseler PA, Posner MD, Quivey JM, et al. Completely resected anaplastic thyroid carcinoma combined with adjuvant chemotherapy and irradiation is associated with prolonged survival. Cancer. 2001;91(12):2335–42.
17. Akaishi J, Sugino K, Kitagawa W, Nagahama M, Kameyama K, Shimizu K, et al. Prognostic factors and treatment outcomes of 100 cases of anaplastic thyroid carcinoma. Thyroid. 2011;21(11):1183–9.
18. Swaak-Kragten AT, de Wilt JH, Schmitz PI, Bontenbal M, Levendag PC. Multimodality treatment for anaplastic thyroid carcinoma--treatment outcome in 75 patients. Radiother Oncol. 2009;92(1):100–4.
19. Tan RK, Finley RK 3rd, Driscoll D, Bakamjian V, Hicks WL Jr, Shedd DP. Anaplastic carcinoma of the thyroid: a 24-year experience. Head Neck. 1995;17(1):41–7. discussion 7–8.
20. Zhang ZM, Xu ZG, Tang PZ, Xue LY, Lu N. A retrospective analysis of anaplastic thyroid carcinoma. Zhongguo Yi Xue Ke Xue Yuan Xue Bao. 2006;28(3):322–4.
21. Holting T, Meybier H, Buhr H. Problems of tracheotomy in locally invasive anaplastic thyroid cancer. Langenbecks Arch Chir. 1989;374(2):72–6.
22. Holting T, Meybier H, Buhr H. Status of tracheotomy in treatment of the respiratory emergency in anaplastic thyroid cancer. Wien Klin Wochenschr. 1990;102(9):264–6.
23. Shaha AR. Airway management in anaplastic thyroid carcinoma. Laryngoscope. 2008;118(7):1195–8.
24. Wein RO, Weber RS. Anaplastic thyroid carcinoma: palliation or treatment? Curr Opin Otolaryngol Head Neck Surg. 2011;19(2):113–8.
25. Wang Y, Tsang R, Asa S, Dickson B, Arenovich T, Brierley J. Clinical outcome of anaplastic thyroid carcinoma treated with radiotherapy of once- and twice-daily fractionation regimens. Cancer. 2006;107(8):1786–92.
26. Levendag PC, De Porre PM, van Putten WL. Anaplastic carcinoma of the thyroid gland treated by radiation therapy. Int J Radiat Oncol Biol Phys. 1993;26(1):125–8.
27. Sherman EJ, Lim SH, Ho AL, Ghossein RA, Fury MG, Shaha AR, et al. Concurrent doxorubicin and radiotherapy for anaplastic thyroid cancer: a critical re-evaluation including uniform pathologic review. Radiother Oncol. 2011;101(3):425–30.
28. Nutting CM, Convery DJ, Cosgrove VP, Rowbottom C, Vini L, Harmer C, et al. Improvements in target coverage and reduced spinal cord irradiation using intensity-modulated radiotherapy (IMRT) in patients with carcinoma of the thyroid gland. Radiother Oncol. 2001;60(2):173–80.
29. Posner MD, Quivey JM, Akazawa PF, Xia P, Akazawa C, Verhey LJ. Dose optimization for the treatment of anaplastic thyroid carcinoma: a comparison of treatment planning techniques. Int J Radiat Oncol Biol Phys. 2000;48(2):475–83.
30. Dandekar P, Harmer C, Barbachano Y, Rhys-Evans P, Harrington K, Nutting C, et al. Hyperfractionated Accelerated Radiotherapy (HART) for anaplastic thyroid carcinoma: toxicity and survival analysis. Int J Radiat Oncol Biol Phys. 2009;74(2):518–21.
31. De Crevoisier R, Baudin E, Bachelot A, Leboulleux S, Travagli JP, Caillou B, et al. Combined treatment of anaplastic thyroid carcinoma with surgery, chemotherapy, and hyperfractionated accelerated external radiotherapy. Int J Radiat Oncol Biol Phys. 2004;60(4):1137–43.
32. Wong CS, Van Dyk J, Simpson WJ. Myelopathy following hyperfractionated accelerated radiotherapy for anaplastic thyroid carcinoma. Radiother Oncol. 1991;20(1):3–9.
33. Tennvall J, Lundell G, Wahlberg P, Bergenfelz A, Grimelius L, Akerman M, et al. Anaplastic thyroid carcinoma: three protocols combining doxorubicin, hyperfractionated radiotherapy and surgery. Br J Cancer. 2002;86(12):1848–53.
34. Pudney D, Lau H, Ruether JD, Falck V. Clinical experience of the multimodality management of anaplastic thyroid cancer and literature review. Thyroid. 2007;17(12):1243–50.

35. Besic N, Auersperg M, Us-Krasovec M, Golouh R, Frkovic-Grazio S, Vodnik A. Effect of primary treatment on survival in anaplastic thyroid carcinoma. Eur J Surg Oncol. 2001;27(3):260–4.
36. Sugino K, Ito K, Mimura T, Nagahama M, Fukunari N, Kubo A, et al. The important role of operations in the management of anaplastic thyroid carcinoma. Surgery. 2002;131(3):245–8.
37. Heron DE, Karimpour S, Grigsby PW. Anaplastic thyroid carcinoma: comparison of conventional radiotherapy and hyperfractionation chemoradiotherapy in two groups. Am J Clin Oncol. 2002;25(5):442–6.
38. Troch M, Koperek O, Scheuba C, Dieckmann K, Hoffmann M, Niederle B, et al. High efficacy of concomitant treatment of undifferentiated (anaplastic) thyroid cancer with radiation and docetaxel. J Clin Endocrinol Metab. 2010;95(9):E54–7.
39. Nehs MA, Nagarkatti S, Nucera C, Hodin RA, Parangi S. Thyroidectomy with neoadjuvant PLX4720 extends survival and decreases tumor burden in an orthotopic mouse model of anaplastic thyroid cancer. Surgery. 2010;148(6):1154–62. discussion 62.
40. Seto A, Sugitani I, Toda K, Kawabata K, Takahashi S, Saotome T. Chemotherapy for anaplastic thyroid cancer using docetaxel and cisplatin: report of eight cases. Surg Today. 2015;45(2):221–6.
41. Guerra A, Di Crescenzo V, Garzi A, Cinelli M, Carlomagno C, Tonacchera M, et al. Genetic mutations in the treatment of anaplastic thyroid cancer: a systematic review. BMC Surg. 2013;13(Suppl 2):S44.
42. Smallridge RC, Marlow LA, Copland JA. Anaplastic thyroid cancer: molecular pathogenesis and emerging therapies. Endocr Relat Cancer. 2009;16(1):17–44.
43. Ragazzi M, Ciarrocchi A, Sancisi V, Gandolfi G, Bisagni A, Piana S. Update on anaplastic thyroid carcinoma: morphological, molecular, and genetic features of the most aggressive thyroid cancer. Int J Endocrinol. 2014;2014:790834.
44. Pinto N, Black M, Patel K, Yoo J, Mymryk JS, Barrett JW, et al. Genomically driven precision medicine to improve outcomes in anaplastic thyroid cancer. J Oncol. 2014;2014:936285.
45. Nehs MA, Nucera C, Nagarkatti SS, Sadow PM, Morales-Garcia D, Hodin RA, et al. Late intervention with anti-BRAF(V600E) therapy induces tumor regression in an orthotopic mouse model of human anaplastic thyroid cancer. Endocrinology. 2012;153(2):985–94.
46. Ha HT, Lee JS, Urba S, Koenig RJ, Sisson J, Giordano T, et al. A phase II study of imatinib in patients with advanced anaplastic thyroid cancer. Thyroid. 2010;20(9):975–80.
47. Bible KC, Suman VJ, Menefee ME, Smallridge RC, Molina JR, Maples WJ, et al. A multiinstitutional phase 2 trial of pazopanib monotherapy in advanced anaplastic thyroid cancer. J Clin Endocrinol Metab. 2012;97(9):3179–84.
48. Lim SM, Chang H, Yoon MJ, Hong YK, Kim H, Chung WY, et al. A multicenter, phase II trial of everolimus in locally advanced or metastatic thyroid cancer of all histologic subtypes. Ann Oncol. 2013;24(12):3089–94.
49. Smallridge RC, Copland JA, Brose MS, Wadsworth JT, Houvras Y, Menefee ME, et al. Efatutazone, an oral PPAR-gamma agonist, in combination with paclitaxel in anaplastic thyroid cancer: results of a multicenter phase 1 trial. J Clin Endocrinol Metab. 2013;98(6):2392–400.
50. Sosa JA, Elisei R, Jarzab B, Balkissoon J, Lu SP, Bal C, et al. Randomized safety and efficacy study of fosbretabulin with paclitaxel/carboplatin against anaplastic thyroid carcinoma. Thyroid. 2014;24(2):232–40.
51. Mooney CJ, Nagaiah G, Fu P, Wasman JK, Cooney MM, Savvides PS, et al. A phase II trial of fosbretabulin in advanced anaplastic thyroid carcinoma and correlation of baseline serum-soluble intracellular adhesion molecule-1 with outcome. Thyroid. 2009;19(3):233–40.
52. Isham CR, Bossou AR, Negron V, Fisher KE, Kumar R, Marlow L, et al. Pazopanib enhances paclitaxel-induced mitotic catastrophe in anaplastic thyroid cancer. Sci Transl Med. 2013;5(166):166ra3.

Same-Day Versus Overnight Inpatient Surgery for Total Thyroidectomy

13

Abbas Al-Kurd and Haggi Mazeh

Abstract

Outpatient surgery has gained popularity in recent years, and many procedures that once required prolonged hospitalization are now being performed in a same-day, ambulatory fashion. In spite of patient comfort and cost benefits associated with same-day surgery, the performance of thyroidectomies with same-day discharge has been met with some reservations, namely due to the possible complications that are uniquely inherent to this procedure. These include postoperative hematomas, recurrent laryngeal nerve injury, and hypocalcemia. Those who oppose same-day thyroid surgery claim that the possibility of these complications precludes the safety of this procedure. In this chapter, the authors review the available literature concerning same-day total thyroidectomy. Literature comparing this approach to traditional overnight inpatient surgery is also evaluated and Authors' recommendations regarding same-day thyroidectomy are outlined.

Keywords

Total thyroidectomy · Same-day · Ambulatory · Outpatient · Safety · Complications

A. Al-Kurd (✉)
Department of Surgery, Hadassah-Hebrew University Medical Center, Jerusalem, Israel
e-mail: abbas@hadassah.org.il

H. Mazeh
Endocrine and General Surgery, Department of Surgery, Hadassah-Hebrew University Medical Center, Jerusalem, Israel
e-mail: hmazeh@hadassah.org.il

P. Angelos, R. H. Grogan (eds.), *Difficult Decisions in Endocrine Surgery*, Difficult Decisions in Surgery: An Evidence-Based Approach,
https://doi.org/10.1007/978-3-319-92860-9_13

Introduction

Recent years have shown gradually increasing acceptance of the notion of same-day or out-patient surgery [1]. Several procedures that once required at least 1 day of postoperative hospitalization are now commonly being performed on a same-day, ambulatory basis. This approach has been shown to be safe practice in laparoscopic cholecystectomies, tonsillectomies, hernia repairs, breast surgeries, and in many other procedures [2, 3]. Same-day surgery has been associated with various benefits, including increased patient comfort, decreased iatrogenic complications associated with being in the hospital, and a decreased risk of nosocomial infections. In addition, there is an obvious cost benefit associated with ambulatory, same-day procedures, when compared with those performed on an inpatient basis.

This trend has been slower to catch on in thyroid surgery, a fact that is mainly attributed to the inherent risk of serious, although rare, post-thyroidectomy complications. These complications include hypocalcemia, recurrent laryngeal nerve (RLN) injury, and post-operative hematoma. Although nerve injury can usually be assessed and diagnosed in the immediate postoperative period, the development of hypocalcemia and hematoma formation both take time. For this reason, patients undergoing thyroidectomy were traditionally kept in the hospital for one or more nights, in order to facilitate early diagnosis and swift intervention if these potentially life-threatening complications developed.

The feasibility of same-day thyroidectomy was first reported by Steckler in 1986 [4]. This topic was further advanced in subsequent years by other investigators, including Lo Gerfo, Mowschenson, and Samson [5–7]. Although these initial reports were met with strong opposition, over time more evidence is becoming available to support the theory that same-day thyroidectomy is safe and feasible.

In 2013, the American Thyroid Association published a statement regarding outpatient thyroidectomy [8]. It was concluded that outpatient thyroidectomy is a safe practice in a carefully selected patient population. However, it was recommended that precautionary measures be set in place in order to minimize the likelihood of complications and maximize communication between the patient and the staff.

In this chapter, the available literature concerning same-day total thyroidectomy will be evaluated. Literature comparing this approach to traditional overnight inpatient surgery will also be reviewed (Table 13.1).

Search Strategy

A comprehensive review of the literature was performed, conducted in the PubMed database. Key words that were used included "thyroidectomy", "thyroid surgery", "same-day", "ambulatory", "out-patient", and "complications". Our search returned

Table 13.1 PICO table

*P*opulation	Patients undergoing total thyroidectomy
*I*ntervention	Same-day discharge
*C*omparator	Admission overnight
*O*utcomes	Life-threatening complication

over 200 articles, however after careful review, only a handful were found relevant to this topic. Special emphasis was put on more recently published papers, and those including larger numbers of patient populations.

Complications to Be Considered

Unlike several procedures performed on an outpatient basis, thyroidectomy is unique in the fact that it is associated with a small, but definite risk of life-threatening complications [9]. As previously mentioned, post-thyroidectomy complications relevant to this topic include RLN injury, hypocalcemia, and postoperative hemorrhage or hematoma. When these complications do occur, their rapid recognition and prompt management are essential. Those who oppose same-day thyroidectomy claim that this possible requirement for acute intervention prevents ambulatory thyroidectomy from being a safe procedure. In this section, each of the above-mentioned possible complications will be explored, as will the significance of their occurrence in an ambulatory setting.

Recurrent Laryngeal Nerve Injury

Although the rate of transient RLN injury is reported in the literature to be up to 7% [10], incidence of permanent nerve injury in experienced centers is around 1–2% [11–14]. A unilateral RLN paralysis would unlikely cause airway compromise, and—although unpleasant for the patient—would not prevent early discharge after surgery. Bilateral RLN paralysis, on the other hand, is considered a life-threatening condition. This complication is exceedingly rare, with an incidence reported to be 0.2% in a large study [15]. Bilateral nerve injury would be diagnosed immediately after surgery, far before discharge. Therefore, it could be concluded that the risk of RLN injury in itself cannot be considered a strong argument against performing same-day thyroidectomy.

Hypocalcemia

Some degree of temporary hypocalcemia is common after total thyroidectomy, with incidence rates reported up to 30% in the literature [9]. Hypocalcemia that is clinically significant usually develops 48–72 h post-thyroidectomy, which would be long after discharge in a patient undergoing outpatient surgery. A commonly used method to identify cases likely to develop postoperative hypocalcemia is postoperative parathyroid hormone (PTH) testing, which is routinely used in most centers performing same-day thyroidectomies [16–18]. Prophylactic calcium and vitamin D supplements are routinely utilized in many specialized centers. In addition, adequate patient education and warning regarding the signs of hypocalcemia and its treatment are of utmost importance. In light of these precautionary measures, patients at risk for postoperative hypocalcemia can commonly be identified and accordingly treated. In an educated patient, symptomatic hypocalcemia that occurs outside of the hospital can usually be treated on an ambulatory basis with oral calcium supplementation alone [19]. Therefore, like that of RLN injury, the possibility of postoperative hypocalcemia will not be considered strong evidence against the safety of same-day thyroid surgery.

Hemorrhage

Post-thyroidectomy hemorrhage causing neck hematoma is reported in the literature to occur in 0.25–2.1% of patients [20–22]. It has been shown that this hemorrhage, when it happens, occurs within 6 h from the surgery in 40–50%, within 7–24 h in 40%, and after 24 h in 10–20% of patients [20, 21]. Therefore, due to its delayed presentation in a significant percentage of cases, post-operative hemorrhage seems to be the main risk that must be evaluated when considering the safety of same-day thyroidectomy. The small possibility of a neck hematoma compromising the airway, which may go undiagnosed and untreated at home after discharge, is the primary argument used by those who oppose the notion of same-day thyroidectomy [21]. This point is also the main reason why thyroidectomy has not transformed to be widely performed on an ambulatory basis, as have many other surgeries. However, it is essential to emphasize that although the need for re-operation due to hemorrhage has been reported to be between 0.1 and 1.7% of patients, [19, 21, 23] most endocrine surgeons would agree that the necessity to perform an *emergent* bedside neck decompression is an *extremely rare* occurrence. Therefore it could be concluded that non-life-threatening hemorrhages (which comprise the vast majority of post-thyroidectomy hemorrhages) that occur post-discharge do not form a strong argument against the routine practice of same-day thyroidectomy.

It is clear that the use of modern techniques to facilitate meticulous hemostasis is of great importance and strongly contributes to the minimization of post-operative bleeding. These techniques include the use of energy devices in the ligation of vessels. In addition, loupe-magnification of the operative field allows the identification and control of bleeding from minute vessels. The use of hemostatic materials and pads has also become common practice in many large endocrine surgery centers. In addition, the application of a limited, non-bulky wound dressing can facilitate early identification of postoperative bleeding.

Certain inherent patient risk factors, in addition to events during the operative course must be taken into consideration prior to deciding on same-day discharge. Precaution must be taken when operating patients on anti-platelet or anticoagulant medication, and in this patient group, inpatient thyroidectomy should be strongly considered. Although it seems quite logical that such patients be operated in an inpatient fashion, several large studies have not shown a clear relationship between the use of anti-platelet or anticoagulant treatment and the development of post-operative bleeding in thyroidectomy cases [20, 21].

Review of the Available Literature

Since Steckler reported his institution's experience on same-day discharge after thyroidectomy in 1986 [4], scattered additional studies have appeared in the literature evaluating this issue. The last decade has shown a significant increase in the practice of same-day thyroidectomy; however this still only constitutes a small percentage of thyroidectomy cases performed. According to the British Association of Endocrine and Thyroid Surgeons only 6% of thyroidectomies nationwide were performed as day-case procedures in 2012 [24]. When considering the specific types of thyroidectomies—8% of lobectomies/isthmusectomies and only 1.2% of total thyroidectomies were performed on an ambulatory basis. In a large, New York State based study; it was shown that statewide, 17% of thyroidectomies in general (both partial and total), and approximately 13% of total thyroidectomies were performed as same-day thyroidectomies [25]. Apparently due to the limited number of cases included in most published series, most studies describe both partial and total thyroidectomies as one entity, rarely describing the results and complication rates of total thyroidectomy alone.

One of the largest single series of same-day thyroidectomies was published by Snyder et al. in 2010 [19]. Of 1242 consecutive thyroidectomies, 1136 were planned as outpatient procedures, and of these, 94% were successfully completed in an outpatient (same-day) fashion. Of these operations, 58% constituted total thyroidectomies. In the outpatient surgeries, the median postoperative time to same-day discharge was 2:23 h. Reasons for conversion from outpatient to inpatient surgery included, extensive surgery, extensive intra-operative blood loss, late surgery, and patient health concerns. Conversion to inpatient surgery was more likely to occur in those undergoing total thyroidectomy (66% of those converted). In patients who were planned to undergo outpatient total thyroidectomy, only 7% (48/661) were converted to inpatient procedures. The overall complication rate was found to be significantly less in those undergoing successful outpatient thyroidectomy, when compared to the "converted to inpatient" group and the "previously planned as inpatient" group (26%, 40%, and 44%, respectively, $P < 0.0001$). It should be noted that a wide variety of complications was reported, including asymptomatic and symptomatic hypocalcemia, permanent hypoparathyroidism, transient and permanent RLN injury, postoperative hematoma, seroma, infectious complications and mortality. The rates of postoperative symptomatic hypocalcemia showed no statistically significant difference between the groups (5%, 8%, and 7.6%, respectively), and neither did the rates of permanent hypoparathyroidism (0.2%, 1.4%, 1%, respectively). The rate of overall and transient RLN injury was found to be significantly higher in those converted to inpatient procedures; however, there is an element of bias in this figure, due to the fact that many of those converted to inpatient procedures were done so presumably due to a difficult and possibly complicated operation. The rate of hematoma formation was 0.2% in the outpatient group, 3% in the converted group, and 1% in the inpatient group. It is reported that all of the postoperative hematomas (constituting 0.4% of all patients) required operative drainage, but none—however—needed urgent bedside decompression. The one reported case of mortality in the outpatient group was in an elderly nursing-home patient who died 2 days after the operation from a presumed cardiac event, with no evidence of wound or respiratory problems. No mortalities were described in the "converted to inpatient" group, and three were reported in the "planned as inpatient" group. The conclusion of the authors of this study was that outpatient thyroidectomy is safe and reasonable in experienced hands.

Another large publication exploring the prevalence of same-day thyroidectomy was published by Tuggle et al. in 2011, and presents a New York state-wide database study [25]. Of a total of 6762 thyroidectomies performed, 1168 (17%) were performed on a same-day basis. Those undergoing same-day thyroidectomies had less co-morbidities when compared to the inpatient group. Total thyroidectomies constituted 33% of the outpatient thyroidectomies performed, and most single-day thyroidectomies were performed at high-volume centers by high-volume surgeons. Although a thorough comparative description of the specific complications (RLN injury, hypocalcemia, hematoma, etc.) was not provided—probably due to the fact that this was a database study, no statistically significant difference was shown between the readmission rates of the outpatient and inpatient groups (1.4% and 2.4%, respectively). Risks for readmission included total thyroidectomy, longer length of hospital stay, increased co-morbidities, and less-experienced surgeons.

Mazeh et al. published in 2012 a series of thyroidectomies performed by a single surgeon over a 6-year period [1]. During this time period, 608 thyroidectomies were performed, of which 298 (49%) were same-day cases. Of the patients undergoing total thyroidectomy, 26% were performed on a same-day basis, and approximately 30% of the same-day thyroidectomies performed constituted total thyroidectomies. The overall rate of post-operative complications was found to be significantly higher in the inpatient group (17% vs. 8%, $p = 0.03$), however no statistically significant difference in the individual complication rates was demonstrated between the inpatient and outpatient groups. Transient hypocalcemia occurred in 10% of the inpatient group, and 5% of the same-day thyroidectomy group. Transient RLN injury (as defined by transient hoarseness) occurred in 4% and 2%, respectively. Permanent hypocalcemia occurred in 1% of each group. The rate of postoperative hematoma was 1% in the inpatient group, but occurred in no patients in the same-day thyroidectomy group. None of the same-day thyroidectomy patients required readmission.

Mazeh et al. went further to describe their results after the introduction of postoperative PTH testing [1]. After the initiation of use of this modality, the rate of performing single day surgery in total thyroidectomy increased from 9% to 66% ($p < 0.00001$). When comparing the complication rates for total thyroidectomy in this period, an overall complication rate of 31% was demonstrated for the inpatient group, compared to a mere 6% in the same-day total thyroidectomy group ($p = 0.002$). In addition, when comparing the inpatient and the same-day discharge groups, transient hypocalcemia occurred in 11% and 5% ($p = 0.2$), transient hoarseness in 9% and 2% ($p = 0.03$), and neck hematoma in 6% and 0% ($p = 0.25$), respectively. No patients developed permanent hypocalcemia or permanent RLN injury.

Mazeh et al. proposed recommended criteria that must be fulfilled prior to attempting same-day thyroidectomy (See Table 13.2) [1]. The authors conclude that same-day thyroidectomy is a safe practice and can be routinely performed by highly experienced surgeons in the setting of an adequate support system. The importance of postoperative PTH testing was also strongly emphasized in this study.

Seybt et al. published in 2010 a series of 418 thyroidectomies performed over a period of 4 years, of which 208 (50%) were outpatient procedures [3]. No significant age difference was shown between the outpatient and inpatient groups (45 and 48 years, respectively). Also, no significant difference was shown with regard to ASA (American Society of Anesthesiologists) score or the presence of malignancy. Of all total or completion thyroidectomies 36% were performed on an outpatient basis, and total/completion thyroidectomies constituted 38% of those undergoing outpatient surgery. Transient hypocalcemia was reported in 5% of outpatients and in 16% of inpatients, while permanent hypocalcemia did not occur in any patient. Permanent vocal cord paralysis was reported in none of the outpatients and 0.3% of inpatients. "Other complications" (in which hematomas were included) occurred in none of the outpatients and 2% of inpatients. The readmission rate was also found to be lower in those undergoing outpatient thyroidectomy when compared to inpatient procedures (2% and 6%, respectively).

Seybt et al. also proposed their selection criteria for outpatient thyroidectomy. These included a cooperative patient, the lack of significant medical co-morbidities, the lack of anticoagulant treatment or the need for a drain, the lack of concomitant procedures like lateral neck dissection, and the presence of sufficient patient autonomy and social support [3]. The authors also reported their discharge criteria, which included a stable wound and airway with normal vital signs, an ambulatory patient who can tolerate diet, the control of pain by oral medications, the ability to void, and the availability of a person to accompany the patient home. As in the previously mentioned studies, the authors concluded that ambulatory thyroidectomy could be performed safely in high-volume endocrine centers.

Table 13.2 The recommended criteria that must be fulfilled prior to attempting same-day thyroidectomy, as proposed by Mazeh et al. (modified)

Category	Description
Patient	Consent and preparation for same-day discharge
	Absence of restricting co-morbidities
	Reasonable distance from the patient's residence to the hospital
Surgery	Absence of overt complications
	Absence of extensive lymph node dissection
	Absence of drains
Surgeon	Highly experienced in endocrine surgery
	Previous experience with same-day thyroid lobectomy surgeries
Support system	Availability of postoperative PTH testing
	Allowance of 3–4 h observation before discharge
	Easy conversion to inpatient admission when necessary
	Availability of a dedicated and educated team 24 h per day

The use of local anesthesia in thyroidectomy procedures has been proposed, and may facilitate quicker recovery from anesthesia and therefore shorter post-operative stay, in addition to decreased costs. Spanknebel et al. demonstrated that the use of local anesthesia in 939 out of 1194 thyroidectomy patients enabled them to undergo more outpatient procedures (6 h postoperative observation) when compared with the general anesthesia group (82% vs. 34%, $p < 0.001$) [26].

The American Thyroid Association formed a task-force to investigate the feasibility and safety of outpatient thyroidectomy, and published a statement summarizing its recommendations in 2013 [8]. The proposed eligibility criteria for the performance of such surgeries included: The absence of major co-morbidities, ASA score of less than four, suitable preoperative education, the presence of a team approach to education and clinical care, the availability and willingness of an at-home care giver, the presence of a postoperative social setting that will allow safe postoperative management, and post-discharge proximity to a skilled facility. In addition, a number of relative contraindications for ambulatory surgery were proposed. These included the presence of medical conditions such as uncompensated cardiopulmonary disease, neurological disorders, and end-stage renal failure; use of anticoagulants or antiplatelets; pregnancy; socio-economic factors; and specific surgery-related factors such as the presence of a massive or retrosternal goiter, difficult intraoperative hemostasis, locally-advanced malignancy and a difficult operation in the presence of Hashimoto's thyroiditis or Graves' disease. Also, it was recommended that certain criteria be fulfilled prior to discharge of the patient. These include tolerability of liquids and medications, adequate pain control, ability to void and ambulate, adequate social support and understanding of instructions, and normal vital signs. In addition, before discharge a postoperative examination must be performed, assessing the surgical wound, ruling out neck swelling/hematoma, dysphonia, dyspnea and dysphagia. It was concluded that outpatient thyroidectomy can be safely undertaken in a carefully selection patient population, in the presence of precautionary measures set forth to minimize complications.

Table 13.3 summarizes the results of the largest most recent studies exploring the safety and applicability of same-day thyroid surgery [1, 3, 19, 25, 27–29].

Two explanations can account for the higher complication rate in the inpatient group demonstrated in some of the studies. First, this may simply represent a higher detection rate as these patients were examined and their labs evaluated during their time at the hospital where as outpatients were not as closely monitored. Second, in these retrospective studies a clear selection bias exists as inpatients were excluded from outpatient surgery due to certain characteristics that were for prone for complications such as prolonged surgery, co-morbidities, or any deviance from normal postoperative course at PACU.

Many studies have demonstrated a significant cost benefit from performing same-day thyroidectomies when compared to the performance of these procedures in an inpatient setting. Mowschenson et al. showed a 30% reduction in hospital costs in patients undergoing ambulatory surgery, however stressed that formal hospitalization should still be performed in patients with post-anesthetic complications, in those with serious co-morbid diseases, and when a social reason for

Table 13.3 Summary of the results of the largest most recent studies exploring the safety and applicability of same-day thyroid surgery

Publication	Year	Number of SDT cases	Number of SDTT cases[a]	Comparison to inpatient?	Postoperative complications when compared with inpatients	Hematoma	Transient RLN injury	Symptomatic hypocalcemia	Permanent RLN injury	Permanent hypoparathyroidism	Readmission (SDT vs. inpatient)	Conclusion
Snyder et al. [19]	2010	1064	617	Yes	Less	0.19%	3.7%	5.2%	0.38%	0.28%	NA	SDT safe and reasonable
Tuggle et al. [25]	2011	1168	385	Yes	N/A	N/A	N/A	N/A	N/A	N/A	1.4% (vs 2.4% in inpatients)	Readmission rates are comparable between SDT and inpatient thyroidectomy
Mazeh et al. [1]	2012	298	87	Yes	Less	0%	2%	5%	0%	1%	0%	SDT is safe
Seybt et al. [3]	2010	208	79	Yes	Less	0%	N/A	5.1%	0%	0%	1.9% (vs 5.7% in inpatients)	Outpatient thyroidectomy can be accomplished safely
Trottier et al. [27]	2009	232	61	No	N/A	0.4%	0.4%	2.5%	N/A	N/A	1.7%	Outpatient thyroid surgery is safe
Hessman et al. [28]	2011	138	63	No	N/A	1.4%	N/A	3.6%	N/A	N/A	2.9%	Outpatient thyroidectomy performed by an experienced surgeon is safe and feasible
Sahmkow et al. [29]	2012	176	83	No	N/A	0%	N/A	10%	N/A	N/A	1.7%	Outpatient thyroid surgery is a safe and desirable option

SDT same-day thyroidectomy, *SDTT* same-day total thyroidectomy, *N/A* data not available
[a]This number includes both total and completion thyroidectomies

hospitalization is present [6]. It should be emphasized that the primary factor that should be taken into consideration when an institution decides upon the feasibility of a same-day thyroidectomy program, should be patient safety and comfort, rather than financial benefits.

It is worth noting that some studies in the literature explored the feasibility of an entity termed "short-stay thyroidectomy", in which the patient is hospitalized for less than 23 h [30]. Other studies combine the results of "short-stay" cases with those of same-day cases [7]. In this review short-stay thyroidectomy and inpatients were considered as a combined group and compared to same-day thyroidectomy.

Recommendations

There are currently no available randomized controlled trials comparing same-day thyroidectomy to inpatient thyroidectomy. All recommendations rely on retrospective series or expert opinion and therefore graded as weak evidence and low level of recommendation. Nevertheless, upon reviewing the literature, the majority of the various retrospective and case-control trials support the fact that same-day thyroidectomy is a reasonable and safe practice, with no evidence of increased post-operative complications.

Therefore it is the authors' recommendation that same-day partial or total thyroidectomy may be performed in suitable patient populations. It is recommended that this procedure be performed only by experienced endocrine surgeons in high-volume centers. Preoperative patient selection is essential, as is the development of institutional standards and discharge criteria. Patient education is of utmost importance, with focus on early recognition of complications that may occur at home after discharge vis-à-vis staff availability (physicians/nurse practitioners, physician assistants) over the phone at all times. Lastly, surgeon's discretion must be used to easily convert patients to inpatient surgery when appropriate. It must be stressed that due to the lack of results of randomized controlled trials, the quality of this evidence is low. Our recommendations are in accordance with those proposed in the American Thyroid Association Statement on Outpatient Thyroidectomy.

The authors recommend the use of postoperative PTH testing in order to decrease the occurrence of undiagnosed post-discharge hypocalcemia.

The authors recommend against the performance of same-day total thyroidectomy in patients under anti-platelet or anticoagulant therapy at the time of the operation. Although some studies have not shown clear associations between these treatments and formation of post-operative hematomas, their safety has also not yet been established in this patient population. In addition, there is insufficient data regarding the performance of same-day thyroidectomy associated more extensive procedures (e.g. lateral neck dissection), therefore the authors recommend against same-day discharge in these patients. This is also true for patients requiring a drain in their operation.

The decision of whether or not to perform a same-day surgery is multi-factorial in nature, and although not a topic clearly discussed in the literature, the authors strongly believe that the surgeon should be guided by his or her common sense and best judgment. The surgeon should take into consideration not only medical factors, such as the patient's past illnesses and anticoagulant therapy, but also social factors, such as the proximity to the hospital after discharge and availability by telephone of both the patient and the treating staff. If the surgeon has any doubt regarding the safety of same-day thyroidectomy in a specific patient, then the operation should be performed in an inpatient fashion. Similarly, if at the end of a planned outpatient case the surgeon feels that the patient is at risk, then such patients should be converted to inpatient or short stay admission.

Conclusion

Total thyroidectomy performed on an ambulatory, same-day basis is a safe and feasible practice. Patient selection, in an attempt to decrease post-discharge complications, is important. These operations should only be performed in high-volume centers, by experienced endocrine surgeons. Patient education prior to the operation and prior to discharge is essential to the success of same-day thyroidectomy programs. The use of modern intra-operative hemostatic methods, nerve monitoring, and postoperative PTH testing may decrease the incidence of unrecognized post-discharge complications, and help facilitate the performance of safe ambulatory total thyroidectomies.

References

1. Mazeh H, Khan Q, Schneider DF, Schaefer S, Sippel RS, Chen H. Same-day thyroidectomy program: eligibility and safety evaluation. Surgery. 2012;152(6):1133–41.
2. Gurusamy KS, Junnarkar S, Farouk M, Davidson BR. Day-case versus overnight stay for laparoscopic cholecystectomy. Cochrane Database Syst Rev. 2008;3:CD006798.
3. Seybt MW, Terris DJ. Outpatient thyroidectomy: experience in over 200 patients. Laryngoscope. 2010;120(5):959–63.
4. Steckler RM. Outpatient thyroidectomy: a feasibility study. Am J Surg. 1986;152(4):417–9.
5. Lo Gerfo P, Gates R, Gazetas P. Outpatient and short-stay thyroid surgery. Head Neck 1991;13(2):97–101.
6. Mowschenson PM, Hodin RA. Outpatient thyroid and parathyroid surgery: a prospective study of feasibility, safety, and costs. Surgery. 1995;118(6):1051–3. Discussion 3-4.
7. Samson PS, Reyes FR, Saludares WN, Angeles RP, Francisco RA, EER T Jr. Outpatient thyroidectomy. Am J Surg. 1997;173(6):499–503.
8. Terris DJ, Snyder S, Carneiro-Pla D, Inabnet WB 3rd, Kandil E, Orloff L, et al. American Thyroid Association statement on outpatient thyroidectomy. Thyroid. 2013;23(10):1193–202.
9. Doran HE, Palazzo F. Ambulatory thyroid surgery: do the risks overcome the benefits? Presse Med. 2014;43(3):291–6.
10. Steurer M, Passler C, Denk DM, Schneider B, Niederle B, Bigenzahn W. Advantages of recurrent laryngeal nerve identification in thyroidectomy and parathyroidectomy and the importance of preoperative and postoperative laryngoscopic examination in more than 1000 nerves at risk. Laryngoscope. 2002;112(1):124–33.
11. Enomoto K, Uchino S, Watanabe S, Enomoto Y, Noguchi S. Recurrent laryngeal nerve palsy during surgery for benign thyroid diseases: risk factors and outcome analysis. Surgery. 2014;155(3):522–8.

12. Chiang FY, Wang LF, Huang YF, Lee KW, Kuo WR. Recurrent laryngeal nerve palsy after thyroidectomy with routine identification of the recurrent laryngeal nerve. Surgery. 2005;137(3):342–7.
13. Chan WF, Lang BH, Lo CY. The role of intraoperative neuromonitoring of recurrent laryngeal nerve during thyroidectomy: a comparative study on 1000 nerves at risk. Surgery. 2006;140(6):866–72. Discussion 72-3.
14. Lo CY, Kwok KF, Yuen PW. A prospective evaluation of recurrent laryngeal nerve paralysis during thyroidectomy. Arch Surg. 2000;135(2):204–7.
15. Bergenfelz A, Jansson S, Kristoffersson A, Martensson H, Reihner E, Wallin G, et al. Complications to thyroid surgery: results as reported in a database from a multicenter audit comprising 3,660 patients. Langenbeck's Arch Surg. 2008;393(5):667–73.
16. Grodski S, Lundgren CI, Sidhu S, Sywak M, Delbridge L. Postoperative PTH measurement facilitates day 1 discharge after total thyroidectomy. Clin Endocrinol. 2009;70(2):322–5.
17. Youngwirth L, Benavidez J, Sippel R, Chen H. Postoperative parathyroid hormone testing decreases symptomatic hypocalcemia and associated emergency room visits after total thyroidectomy. Surgery. 2010;148(4):841–4. Discussion 4-6.
18. Houlton JJ, Pechter W, Steward DL. PACU PTH facilitates safe outpatient total thyroidectomy. Otolaryngol Head Neck Surg. 2011;144(1):43–7.
19. Snyder SK, Hamid KS, Roberson CR, Rai SS, Bossen AC, Luh JH, et al. Outpatient thyroidectomy is safe and reasonable: experience with more than 1,000 planned outpatient procedures. J Am Coll Surg. 2010;210(5):575–82. 82-4.
20. Burkey SH, van Heerden JA, Thompson GB, Grant CS, Schleck CD, Farley DR. Reexploration for symptomatic hematomas after cervical exploration. Surgery. 2001;130(6):914–20.
21. Leyre P, Desurmont T, Lacoste L, Odasso C, Bouche G, Beaulieu A, et al. Does the risk of compressive hematoma after thyroidectomy authorize 1-day surgery? Langenbeck's Arch Surg. 2008;393(5):733–7.
22. Bergenfelz A, Jansson S, Martensson H, Reihner E, Wallin G, Kristoffersson A, et al. Scandinavian quality register for thyroid and parathyroid surgery: audit of surgery for primary hyperparathyroidism. Langenbeck's Arch Surg. 2007;392(4):445–51.
23. Promberger R, Ott J, Kober F, Koppitsch C, Seemann R, Freissmuth M, et al. Risk factors for postoperative bleeding after thyroid surgery. Br J Surg. 2012;99(3):373–9.
24. Rajeev P, Sutaria R, Ezzat T, Mihai R, Sadler GP. Changing trends in thyroid and parathyroid surgery over the decade: is same-day discharge feasible in the United Kingdom? World J Surg. 2014;38(11):2825–30.
25. Tuggle CT, Roman S, Udelsman R, Sosa JA. Same-day thyroidectomy: a review of practice patterns and outcomes for 1,168 procedures in New York state. Ann Surg Oncol. 2011;18(4):1035–40.
26. Spanknebel K, Chabot JA, DiGiorgi M, Cheung K, Curty J, Allendorf J, et al. Thyroidectomy using monitored local or conventional general anesthesia: an analysis of outpatient surgery, outcome and cost in 1,194 consecutive cases. World J Surg. 2006;30(5):813–24.
27. Trottier DC, Barron P, Moonje V, Tadros S. Outpatient thyroid surgery: should patients be discharged on the day of their procedures? Can J Surg. 2009;52(3):182–6.
28. Hessman C, Fields J, Schuman E. Outpatient thyroidectomy: is it a safe and reasonable option? Am J Surg. 2011;201(5):565–8.
29. Sahmkow SI, Audet N, Nadeau S, Camire M, Beaudoin D. Outpatient thyroidectomy: safety and patients' satisfaction. J Otolaryngol Head Neck Surg. 2012;41(Suppl 1):S1–12.
30. McHenry CR. "Same-day" thyroid surgery: an analysis of safety, cost savings, and outcome. Am Surg. 1997;63(7):586–9. Discussion 9-90.

Prophylactic Versus Selective Central Neck Dissection in Pediatric Papillary Thyroid Cancer

14

Benjamin James, Raymon H. Grogan, Edwin L. Kaplan, and Peter Angelos

Abstract

The first case of thyroid carcinoma in a child was described in 1902. Following this, Crile published the first case series of pediatric thyroid cancer in 1959, whereby he characterized pediatric thyroid cancer in 18 children. He noted that pediatric thyroid cancer was more commonly metastatic to cervical lymph nodes and to the lungs than was described in the adult population. Despite finding these cancers to be more aggressive than in adults, only one of the patients died of thyroid cancer and four of them were alive with lung metastases. This publication spawned many subsequent studies confirming these findings. As a result, there has been much debate on the appropriate surgical treatment of thyroid cancer in the pediatric population both with respect to the extent of surgery and the use of radioactive iodine.

Keywords

Pediatric thyroid cancer · Adolescent thyroid cancer · Prophylactic neck dissection · Papillary thyroid cancer

B. James (✉)
Section of Endocrine Surgery, Division of Surgical Oncology, Department of Surgery, Beth Israel Deaconess Medical Center, Boston, MA, USA
e-mail: bjames1@bidmc.harvard.edu

R. H. Grogan
Baylor College of Medicine, Michael E. DeBakey Department of Surgery, Endocrine Surgery, Baylor St. Luke's Medical Center, Houston, TX, USA
e-mail: Raymon.Grogan@bcm.edu

E. L. Kaplan
Department of Surgery, The University of Chicago, Chicago, IL, USA

P. Angelos
Department of Surgery and MacLean Center for Clinical Medical Ethics, The University of Chicago, Chicago, IL, USA
e-mail: pangelos@surgery.bsd.uchicago.edu

P. Angelos, R. H. Grogan (eds.), *Difficult Decisions in Endocrine Surgery*, Difficult Decisions in Surgery: An Evidence-Based Approach,
https://doi.org/10.1007/978-3-319-92860-9_14

Introduction

The first case of thyroid carcinoma in a child was described in 1902 [1]. Following this, Crile published the first case series of pediatric thyroid cancer in 1959, whereby he characterized pediatric thyroid cancer in 18 children [1]. He noted that pediatric thyroid cancer was more commonly metastatic to cervical lymph nodes and to the lungs than was described in the adult population. Despite finding these cancers to be more aggressive than in adults, only one of the patients died of thyroid cancer and four of them were alive with lung metastases. This publication spawned many subsequent studies confirming these findings. As a result, there has been much debate on the appropriate surgical treatment of thyroid cancer in the pediatric population both with respect to the extent of surgery and the use of radioactive iodine.

Thyroid cancer represents about 1.4% of all malignancies and has been increasing in incidence [2, 3]. The incidence is significantly higher in adolescents compared to younger children and is five times more common in females than males [2, 4]. As this chapter will detail, childhood thyroid cancer is more aggressive but less lethal than in adults, with a 2% cause-specific mortality [5]. The current surgical treatment of differentiated thyroid cancer in children is a total thyroidectomy for the majority of patients, as a higher rate of recurrence occurs with lobectomy alone [6, 7]. Postoperative radioiodine treatment is generally offered when patients have aggressive features on histologic examination or when cervical nodes are involved.

The chapter will focus will be on prophylactic central neck dissection. We will define a prophylactic neck dissection as performing a central neck dissection in clinically N0 patients (i.e. no evidence of suspicious lymph nodes on physical exam or on imaging). Therapeutic neck dissection should be routinely implemented in clinically N1 patients and will not be discussed further in this chapter. Additionally, while there are clinical and biologic differences between papillary and follicular thyroid carcinoma, we chose to include follicular carcinoma in this chapter as the majority of studies in the pediatric literature did not differentiate papillary from follicular thyroid carcinoma (Table 14.1).

Search Strategy

The literature was searched using the PubMed search engine on June 2nd 2015 to identify all studies evaluating prophylactic central neck dissection in papillary thyroid cancer with respect to complications, recurrence rates and death. There were no limitations placed on language, publication year or publication origin. The search

Table 14.1 PICO table

*P*opulation	Patients under 18 years old with papillary thyroid cancer
*I*ntervention	Routine central lymph node dissection
*C*omparator	Selective central lymph node dissection
*O*utcomes	Recurrence, hypocalcemia, recurrent laryngeal nerve injury

terms included "pediatric", "childhood", "adolescent", "thyroid", "cancer", "carcinoma", "differentiated", "papillary", "prophylactic", "central", "neck", and "dissection". Following this, references from each study found were evaluated to identify other articles not found in the initial search that were relevant to the topic. Studies were excluded if patients under the age of 21 were not evaluated or if the study included histologic subtypes other than differentiated thyroid cancer. Studies were also excluded if the majority of the study cohort was from the Chernobyl accident.

Results

The search yielded 48 articles based on the above search criteria. Two articles evaluated only a radiated cohort and were excluded. One article contained medullary thyroid carcinoma patients in the analysis and was also excluded. This left 45 articles for review. None of the 45 articles specifically evaluated the use of prophylactic central neck dissection. There are no published data on the recurrence or mortality specifically addressing the use of prophylactic central neck dissection in the treatment of pediatric thyroid cancer. Additionally, only two articles stated the percent of central neck lymph nodes involved [8, 9]. Importantly, no studies have been able to ascertain which patients are at a higher risk for locoregional recurrence. As a result, there are no formal guidelines on the use of prophylactic central neck dissection in the pediatric population. When we discuss the benefits of prophylactic central neck dissection, the main outcome being evaluated is recurrence, as mortality from DTC in the pediatric population is near zero. We will therefore discuss the pros and cons of prophylactic central neck dissection.

There are several key arguments for the implementation of prophylactic dissection in the pediatric thyroid cancer population. First, the incidence of lymph node metastases is significantly higher than the adult population. Table 14.2 lists all publications that specifically state the incidence of cervical neck lymph nodes. The incidence ranges from 26.5% to 100%. The publications are extremely heterogeneous in both population studied and in the way the central neck was evaluated. The majority of publications do not differentiate the central from lateral neck dissection. It should also be noted that many of these studies did not differentiate between preoperatively being clinically N0 vs. N1 at the time of surgery. Two studies commented specifically on the incidence of positive central neck lymph nodes. Sugino et al. reported a positive central neck lymph node rate of 62.5% in a population of patients who had undergone both prophylactic and therapeutic central neck dissections [8]. In a retrospective review by Dzepina et al. of 16 patients who underwent varying types of neck dissection without specification of prophylactic neck dissection, a rate of positive central neck lymph nodes of 23% was found [9].

Prior to the early 2000s, "berry-picking", the technique of removing only nodes that appeared grossly abnormal, was routinely used to address the central compartment. Therefore, many of these publications report on central neck lymph nodes based on that technique, which does not assess every lymph node in the central

Table 14.2 Percent of positive cervical lymph nodes: literature review

Author	Publication year	Number of patients[a]	Age (years)	follow up(years)	Percent of lymph nodes
Alessandri [15]	2000	54	12.6 (4.5–16.8)	18.5	60.5
Arici [16]	2002	15	16.8 (8–21)	4.75 (0.4–12.4)	27
Borson-Chazot [17]	2004	74	17 (2–20)	5.1 (0.5–15.4)	88
Ceccarelli [18]	1988	49	6–18	7.7	73
Danese [19]	1997	48	18 (11–20)	4.9 (0.2–15.8)	50
Dottorini [20]	1997	85	15 (5–18)	9.3 (0.1–27)	73
Dzepina [9]	2012	16	16 (10–18)	5	77
Farahati [21]	1998	114	13 (3–18)	1	58
Frankenthaler [22]	1990	117	16 (5–19)	14.5	26
Grigsby [6]	2002	56	15.8 (4–20)	11 (0.6–30.7)	29
Hallwirth [23]	1997	18	16	12.5 (1–26)	83
Harness [24]	1992	89	12.8 (3–18)	[a]	88
Haveman [25]	2003	21	14 (7–17)	11 (2–26)	52
Hay [5]	2010	215	16 (3–20)	29	78
Jarzab [7]	2000	109	13.6 (6–17)	5 (1–23)	59
La Quaglia [26]	1988	93	13.3	20	71
Machens [27]	2010	83	[a]	[a]	84
Massimino [28]	1995	19	11	10	40
Massimino [29]	2006	42	13.5 (6–17)	19.3 (5.7–30.8)	100
Miccoli [30]	2008	346	[a]	[a]	93
Newman [31]	1998	329	15.2 (0.4–20.8)	11.3	74
Robie [32]	1998	67	19	12.6	36
Savio [11]	2005	14	12.5 (5–17)	5.7	41
Schlumberger [33]	1987	72	11 (3–16)	13	90
Sugino [8]	2015	201	18 (7–20)	12.9 (1.3–35.2)	32
Wada [34]	2009	57	13.1 (7–15)	17.4 (0.7–45)	64.9
Wada [35]	2009	120	16.3 (7–19)	11.6 (0.2–29.4)	26.5
Welch Dinauer [36, 37]	1997	170	19 (3–21)	6.6 (0.2–39.5)	38.7
Zimmerman [38]	1988	58	5–16	28 (12.4–40.5)	90

[a]Where the article specified the number that had lymph nodes assessed, the *n* represents this number and not the entire study cohort

neck. This technique is no longer recommended as data suggest that a compartment-based level 6 dissection, removing all lymph nodes in the pretracheal, prelaryngeal and tracheoesophageal regions, has a lower local recurrence rate than "berry-picking" [10].

Jarzab et al. retrospectively evaluated 109 children and found on multivariate analysis that radical surgery was the most significant factor for disease-free survival [7]. The authors describe neck dissection to include a central neck lymph node dissection routinely with biopsy of lateral neck lymph nodes. While this study did not isolate the patients who underwent only a prophylactic central neck dissection, this is the only study that specifically stated they evaluated the outcome with routine prophylactic central neck dissection [7]. Savio et al. performed routine selective neck dissection in 121 pediatric thyroid cancer patients and found at an average follow up of 5.7 years that none of the patients had a recurrence [11]. The authors concluded that there is some evidence for this approach. These are the two sources of evidence suggesting that central neck dissections in the pediatric population decreases the rate of recurrence.

Another argument for an aggressive up front initial surgical approach in pediatric thyroid cancer is that the use of postoperative RAI has decreased in use over the years as a result of concern for second primary malignancies. A recent study by Marti et al. evaluated 1571 patients who received RAI and found a dramatically increased risk for the development of secondary malignancies, most notably in salivary malignancies [12]. Additionally, the majority of deaths in pediatric thyroid cancer survivors is from non-thyroid second primary malignancies [5]. Many of these survivors in this study received post-operative therapeutic radiation. Therefore, if we are utilizing postoperative adjuncts for treatment less, we should make sure our surgical operation is as complete as possible. However, there is a counterargument that routine prophylactic central neck dissection causes excessive upstaging and unnecessary increased use of RAI. This has not been studied in the pediatric population.

The main argument against the implementation of routine prophylactic central neck dissection is the concern for an increased risk of complications. The two most common complications from central neck dissection are injury to the recurrent laryngeal nerve and hypoparathyroidism. The literature search performed was reviewed to find articles that commented on complication rates in their series (Table 14.3). The search yielded 31 articles. Many of the articles did not differentiate temporary from permanent hypoparathyroidism or temporary from permanent nerve injury. Overall, the mean percent of hypoparathyroidism was 15.5% (range 1.4–41.3%). The mean percent of temporary hypoparathyroidism was 11.3%, (range 0–29%). The mean percent of permanent hypoparathyroidism was 10.8% (range 0–36%). The overall voice change percent was 9.2% (range 0–40.1%). The mean percent of temporary voice changes was 18.6% (range 1.1–16.7%). The mean percent of permanent voice changes was 10.9% (range 0–15%). With a permanent rate of hypoparathyroidism and recurrent laryngeal nerve injury of around 11%, surgeons should consider this strongly in their decision to perform aggressive surgery up front. It is imperative that the treatment is not worse than the disease as a lifelong struggle with voice changes and hypoparathyroidism can be debilitating.

While the benefit of prophylactic central neck dissection can be debated, there is no debate that any surgeon operating on a pediatric patient for DTC should be prepared to perform a central neck dissection in every case as in many cases a preoperative N0 patient may convert to a N1 once in the operating room. Certainly, evidence of grossly abnormal lymph nodes should direct the surgeon to convert the operation to a therapeutic neck dissection.

Additionally, it is of critical importance that the operation be performed by an experienced thyroid surgeon. A high volume thyroid surgeon, defined as performing

Table 14.3 Rates of hypoparathyroidism and recurrent laryngeal nerve injury in children with differentiated thyroid carcinoma: literature review

Author	Publication year	Patients, *N*	Age (years)	Follow-up (years)	Hypoparathyroidism (temporary/permanent) %	Voice changes (temporary/permanent) %
Arici [16]	2002	15	12.6 (4.5–16.8)	18.5	13.3 (6.5/6.5)	6.7 (*/6.7)
Bargren [39]	2009	68	15 (5–19)	*	19 (18/1.5)	*
Bingol-Kologlu [40]	1999	18	11.6 (5–16)	7 (4–20)	5.6 (0/5.6)	0
Borson-Chazot [17]	2004	74	17 (2–20)	5.1 (0.5–15.4)	1.4 (*/*)	4 (*/*)
Ceccarelli [18]	1988	49	6–18	7.7	26.5 (*/26.5)	40.1 (*/*)
Danese [19]	1997	48	18 (11–20)	4.9 (0.2–15.8)	20.8 (*/20.8)	8.3 (*/*)
Demidchik [41]	2006	740	11.7 (4.2–14.9)	9.7 (0.13–19.7)	8(1.8/6.2)	23.1 (10.8/12.3)
Dottorini [20]	1997	85	15 (5–18)	9.3 (0.08–27)	8.2 (*/8.2)	3.5 (*/*)
Dzepina [9]	2012	16	16 (10–18)	5	18.8 (12.5/6.3)	0
Frankenthaler [22]	1990	117	16 (5–19)	14.5	*	4
Grigsby [6]	2002	56	15.8 (4–20)	11 (0.6–30.7)	7.1(*/7.1)	5.3 (5.3/*)
Hallwirth [23]	1997	18	16	12.5 (1–26)	16.7 (16.6/0)	16.7 (16.7/0)
Harness [24]	1992	89	12.8 (3–18)	*	4.5 (*/4.5)	4.5 (*/4.5)
Haveman [25]	2003	21	14 (7–17)	11 (2–26)	10 (10/0)	14 (14/0)
Hay [5]	2010	215	16 (3–20)	29	12.8 (0/12.8)	4.6 (*/4.6)
Jarzab [7]	2000	109	13.6 (6–17)	5 (1–23)	5.5 (*/5.5)	9.1 (*/*)
Karnak [42]	2011	16	10.9 (5–16)	*	25 (*/25)	18.8 (*/*)
Kuefer [43]	1997	11	16 (7–25)	*	18.2 (*/*)	*

La Quaglia [26]	1988	93	13.3	20	21.5 (5.4/16.1)	16.1 (1.1/15)
Massimino [28]	1995	19	11	10	36 (*/36)	*
Massimino [29]	2006	42	13.5 (6–17)	19.3 (5.7–30.8)	21 (*/21)	7 (*/*)
Newman [31]	1998	329	15.2 (0.4–20.8)	11.3	31 (29/12)	14 (12/2)
Popovtzer [44]	2006	75	16.1 (6–20)	*	4 (*/4)	9.3 (5.3/4)
Robie [32]	1998	67	19	12.6	17 (*/*)	3 (*/*)
Savio [11]	2005	14	12.5 (5–17)	5.7	21 (14.3/7.1)	*
Schlumberger [33]	1987	72	11 (3–16)	13	6.9 (*/6.9)	25 (*/*)
Spinelli [45]	2004	56	11.5 (4–16)	5.5	7 (*/7)	5 (*/*)
Wada [34]	2009	57	13.1 (7–15)	17.4 (0.7–45)	10.5 (*/10.5)	5.3 (*/*)
Wada [35]	2009	120	16.3 (7–19)	11.6 (0.2–29.4)	18.3 (15.8 /2.5)	2.5 (*/*)
Welch Dinauer [36, 37]	1999	37	19 (9–21)	4.6 (1.3–30.3)	8.1 (*/8.1)	0
Zimmerman [38]	1988	58	5–16	28 (12.4–40.5)	41.3 (17.2/24.1)	0

over 30 thyroid operations per year, reduces the rate of complications [13, 14]. Sosa et al. reviewed 600 pediatric thyroid surgery cases and found a complication rate for high volume surgeons of 8.7% compared to a rate of 13.4% when performed by low volume surgeons [14].

Personal View of the Literature

Unfortunately, the literature on this topic is hard to interpret as there have been many changes over the last 20 years in how a neck dissection is performed. Therefore, interpreting the data as a whole is difficult. The biggest concerns when performing a central neck dissection are the risk of permanent hypoparathyroidism, and recurrent laryngeal nerve injury, and we know that the rate of these complications is lower when performed by high-volume surgeons in adults. In addition there is the theoretical risk of unnecessary upstaging leading to excessive use of RAI. These risks need to be weighed against the benefit of a possible decreased recurrence and subsequent reoperative rate. In light of these observations, the authors advocate for prophylactic central neck dissection in the pediatric population as the limited data suggest that recurrence rates are lower when a neck dissection is performed (level of evidence low, weak recommendation). We know that a significant number of these patients will have positive nodes even when thought to be N0 preoperatively. The one caveat is that the operation should be performed by a high-volume surgeon.

References

1. Crile G Jr. Carcinoma of the thyroid in children. Ann Surg. 1959;150:959.
2. Wu XC, et al. Cancer incidence in adolescents and young adults in the United States, 1992-1997. J Adolesc Health. 2003;32(6):405–15.
3. American Cancer Society. Cancer facts & figures 2009. Atlanta: American Cancer Society; 2009.
4. Waguespack S, et al. In: Bleyer A, et al., editors. Thyroid cancer, in cancer epidemiology in older adolescents and young adults 15 to 29 years of age, including SEER incidence and survival 1975–2000. Bethesda: National Cancer Institute; 2006. p. 143–54.
5. Hay ID, et al. Long-term outcome in 215 children and adolescents with papillary thyroid cancer treated during 1940 through 2008. World J Surg. 2010;34:1192–202.
6. Grigsby PW, et al. Childhood and adolescent thyroid carcinoma. Cancer. 2002;95:724–9.
7. Jarzab B, et al. Multivariate analysis of prognostic factors for differentiated thyroid carcinoma in children. Eur J Nucl Med. 2000;27:833–41.
8. Sugino K, et al. Papillary thyroid carcinoma in children and adolescents: long-term follow-up and clinical characteristics. World J Surg. 2015;39(9):2259–65.
9. Dzepina D. Surgical and pathological characteristics of papillary thyroid cancer in children and adolescents. Coll Antropol. 2012;36(suppl 2):39–45.
10. Musacchio MJ, et al. Greater local recurrence occurs with "berry picking" than neck dissection in thyroid cancer. Am Surg. 2003;69(3):191–6. Discussion 196-7.
11. Savio R, et al. The role of a more extensive surgical approach in the initial multimodality management of papillary thyroid cancer in children. J Pediatr Surg. 2005;40(11):1696–700.

12. Marti JL, et al. Increased risk of second primary malignancy in pediatric and young adult patients treated with radioactive iodine for differentiated thyroid cancer. Thyroid. 2015;25(6):681–7.
13. Sosa JA, et al. Clinical and economic outcomes of thyroid and parathyroid surgery in children. J Clin Endocrinol Metab. 2008;93(8):3058–65.
14. Tuggle CT, et al. Pediatric endocrine surgery: who is operating on our children? Surgery. 2008;144(6):869–77.
15. Alessandri AJ, et al. Age is the major determinant of recurrence in pediatric differentiated thyroid carcinoma. Med Pediatr Oncol. 2000;35(1):41–6.
16. Arici C, et al. Differentiated thyroid carcinoma in children and adolescents. Horm Res. 2002;57:153–6.
17. Borson-Chazot F, et al. Predictive factors for recurrence from a series of 74 children and adolescents with differentiated thyroid cancer. World J Surg. 2004;28:1088–92.
18. Ceccarelli C, et al. Thyroid cancer in children and adolescents. Surgery. 1988;104(6):1143–8.
19. Danese D. Thyroid carcinoma in children and adolescents. Eur J Pediatr. 1997;156:190–4.
20. Dottorini ME, et al. Differentiated thyroid carcinoma in children and adolescents: a 37-year experience in 85 patients. J Nucl Med. 1997;38(5):669–75.
21. Farahati J, et al. Differentiated thyroid cancer in children and adolescents. Langerbeck's Arch Surg. 1998;383(3–4):235–9.
22. Frankenthaler RA, et al. Lymph node metastasis from papillary-follicular thyroid carcinoma in young patients. Am J Surg. 1990;160(4):341–3.
23. Hallwirth U, et al. Differentiated thyroid cancer in children and adolescents: the importance of adequate surgery and review of literature. Eur J Pediatr Surg. 1999;9(6):359–63.
24. Harness JK, et al. Differentiated thyroid carcinoma in children and adolescents. World J Surg. 1992;16(4):547–53.
25. Haveman JW, et al. Surgical experience in children with differentiated thyroid carcinoma. Ann Surg Oncol. 2003;10(1):15–20.
26. La Quaglia MP, et al. Recurrence and morbidity in differentiated thyroid carcinoma in children. Surgery. 1988;104:1149–56.
27. Machens A, et al. Papillary thyroid cancer in children and adolescents does not differ in growth pattern and metastatic behavior. J Pediatr. 2010;157(4):648–52.
28. Massimino M, et al. Primary thyroid carcinoma in children: a retrospective study of 20 patients. Med Pediatr Oncol. 1995;24(1):13–7.
29. Massimino M, et al. Conservative surgical approach for thyroid and lymph-node involvement in papillary thyroid carcinoma in children and adolescents. Pediatr Blood Cancer. 2006;46:307–13.
30. Miccoli P, et al. Papillary thyroid cancer: pathological parameters as prognostic factors in different classes of age. Otolaryngol Head Neck Surg. 2008;138(2):200–3.
31. Newman KD, et al. Differentiated thyroid cancer: determinants of disease progression in patients <21 years of age at diagnosis: a report from the surgical discipline committee of the children's cancer group. Ann Surg. 1998;227(4):533–41.
32. Robie DK, et al. The impact of initial surgical management on outcome in young patients with differentiated thyroid cancer. J Pediatr Surg. 1998;33(7):1134–8.
33. Schlumberger M, et al. Differentiated thyroid carcinoma in childhood: long term follow-up of 72 patients. J Clin Endocrinol Metab. 1987;65(6):1088–94.
34. Wada N, et al. Pediatric differentiated thyroid carcinoma in stage 1: risk factor analysis for disease free survival. BMC Cancer. 2009;9:306.
35. Wada N, et al. Treatment strategy of papillary thyroid carcinoma in children and adolescents: clinical significance of the initial nodal manifestation. Ann Surg Oncol. 2009;16(12):3442–9.
36. Welch Dinauer CA, et al. Clinical features associated with metastasis and recurrence of differentiated thyroid cancer in children, adolescents and young adults. Clin Endocrinol. 1998;49(5):619–28.
37. Welch Dinauer CA, et al. Extensive surgery improves recurrence-free survival for children and young patients with class 1 papillary thyroid carcinoma. J Pediatr Surg. 1999;34(12):1799–804.

38. Zimmerman D, et al. Papillary thyroid carcinoma in children and adults: long-term follow-up of 1039 patients conservatively treated at one institution during three decades. Surgery. 1988;104(6):1157–66.
39. Bargren AE, et al. Outcomes of surgically managed pediatric thyroid cancer. J Surg Res. 2009;156(1):70–3.
40. Bingol-Kologlu M, et al. Surgical treatment of differentiated thyroid carcinoma in children. Eur J Pediatr Surg. 2000;10:347–52.
41. Demidchik YE, et al. Comprehensive clinical assessment of 740 cases of surgically treated thyroid cancer in children of Belarus. Ann Surg. 2006;243(4):525–32.
42. Karnak I, et al. Papillary thyroid carcinoma does not have standard course in children. Pediatr Surg Int. 2011;27:931–6.
43. Kuefer MU, et al. Papillary thyroid carcinoma: demographics, treatment, and outcome in eleven pediatric patients treated at a single institution. Med Pediatr Oncol. 1997;28(6):433–40.
44. Popovtzer A, et al. Thyroid cancer in children: management and outcome experience of a referral center. Otolaryngol Head Neck Surg. 2006;135(4):581–4.
45. Spinelli C, et al. Surgical therapy of the thyroid papillary carcinoma in children: experience with 56 patients ≤16 years old. J Pediatr Surg. 2004;39(10):1500–5.

Subtotal Parathyroidectomy Versus Total Parathyroidectomy with Autotransplantation for Patients with Multiple Endocrine Neoplasia 1 and Primary Hyperparathyroidism

15

Terry C. Lairmore

Abstract

Hyperparathyroidism in patients with MEN 1 is characterized by multiple gland involvement. Two surgical approaches have been advocated in these patients: total parathyroidectomy with heterotopic autotransplantation of parathyroid tissue grafts into skeletal muscle (TP/AT), or subtotal (3 and ½ gland) parathyroidectomy (SP) leaving a vascularized remnant of parathyroid tissue in situ in the neck. Despite the potential advantages and disadvantages of these two commonly practiced operations, previous retrospective studies have demonstrated similar overall rates of recurrent HPT and permanent postoperative hypoparathyroidism in patients undergoing the two operative procedures. Although one of these approaches is often preferred by individual endocrine surgery centers of excellence, improved outcomes or a clear advantage for either operation has not been previously established. The cumulative evidence from prior retrospective studies and a single randomized controlled trail is presented, and recommendations are made based on the available data. The level of evidence and grade for the strength of these recommendations is provided.

Keywords

Multiple endocrine neoplasia type 1 · Parathyroidectomy · Parathyroid transplantation · Persistent and recurrent hyperparathyroidism · Postoperative hypoparathyroidism

T. C. Lairmore
Division of Surgical Oncology, Department of Surgery, Baylor Scott and White Health, Texas A&M University Health Science Center, Temple, TX, USA
e-mail: Terry.Lairmore@BSWHealth.org

P. Angelos, R. H. Grogan (eds.), *Difficult Decisions in Endocrine Surgery*, Difficult Decisions in Surgery: An Evidence-Based Approach,
https://doi.org/10.1007/978-3-319-92860-9_15

Background

The primary hyperparathyroidism (HPT) that occurs in patients with the multiple endocrine neoplasia type 1 (MEN 1) syndrome is associated with unique features that significantly influence treatment decision making. The occurrence of an inactivating DNA mutation [1] in one copy of the *MEN1* tumor suppressor gene in the germline represents a genetic first "hit" that is present in every cell in the body, and subsequent "second hit" events in target cells result in the development of multiple endocrine tumors in involved tissues. The parathyroid neoplasms that occur in patients with MEN 1 are characterized by multiple gland enlargement with synchronous or metachronous development, asymmetrical gland enlargement, and variable age of onset and severity of clinical disease. In strict genetic terms the parathyroid tumors are multiple adenomas (monoclonal) rather than hyperplastic (polyclonal) neoplasms [2]. Essentially all patients who inherit an *MEN1* mutation will develop HPT with an age-dependent onset beginning late in the second decade of life and peaking at approximately 21–30 years of age [3]. Prospective biochemical screening of patients known to be genetically affected results in the diagnosis of HPT at an earlier age [4]. Effective surgical management of this disease requires identification of all four parathyroid glands and a search for supernumerary or ectopic glands. Any operative strategy chosen should be aimed at reducing parathyroid tissue volume sufficiently to achieve parathyroid hormone (PTH) normalization with resulting correction of hypercalcemia, while minimizing postoperative complications. Unique challenges associated with treatment of MEN 1-associated HPT include the risk of recurrent hypersecretion of remaining parathyroid tissue whether preserved in the neck or in a heterotopic site, and the increased risk of permanent postoperative hypoparathyroidism following a 4-gland intervention. Significant controversy exists regarding the optimal timing of intervention and the most appropriate operative procedure to perform. The relative rarity of the condition, variable approaches to management, single surgeon or center biases in screening practices and indications for intervention, and heterogeneity in methods and completeness of clinical follow-up have limited the availability of evidence-based studies to provide solid recommendations.

A number of studies exist that report the results of surgical treatment of HPT in individual series of MEN 1 patients. These retrospective studies are useful in aggregate, but are characterized by their heterogeneity, retrospective analysis, and the limitations described above. A single randomized prospective trial of the two most commonly performed operative procedures for HPT in patients with MEN 1 has been performed [5], but this study is limited by size and statistical power. This chapter examines the controversies associated with the surgical treatment of HPT in patients with the MEN 1 syndrome, with evaluation of available clinical outcomes data. The reported outcomes of subtotal parathyroidectomy (SP) are compared with the outcomes associated with total parathyroidectomy and autotransplantation (TP/AT). The level of clinical evidence and strength of recommendations that can be made from this evidence is discussed (Table 15.1).

Table 15.1 PICO table

*P*opulation	Patients with MEN 1 and primary hyperparathyroidism
*I*ntervention	Total parathyroidectomy with autotransplantation
*C*omparator	Subtotal parathyroidectomy
*O*utcomes	1. Persistent or recurrence of hyperparathyroidism
	2. Permanent postoperative hypoparathyroidism
	3. Disease free interval, period of dependence on supplements

Preoperative Localization Tests

Because the surgical strategies for treatment of HPT in MEN 1 require bilateral neck exploration and identification of all parathyroid glands, preoperative radiographic localizing tests have a diminished role in the preoperative evaluation of these patients [6, 7]. Nilubol and coworkers performed a retrospective analysis of 60 patients undergoing subtotal parathyroidectomy for HPT in MEN 1 and evaluated the utility of preoperative imaging tests including neck ultrasound, sestamibi scan, parathyroid protocol computed tomography scan, and MRI. The imaging tests were performed selectively in variable subsets of the patients. The authors concluded that these preoperative imaging studies altered the operative approach in only 7% of the patients in the study. Further, for patients undergoing routine bilateral neck exploration and transcervical partial thymectomy, routine addition of imaging tests to localize supernumerary or ectopic glands was not useful in the majority of patients.

Four Gland Exploration

Multiple gland involvement characterizes the parathyroid disease in MEN 1. Bilateral cervical exploration and identification of all parathyroid glands has therefore been routinely advocated for treatment of HPT in these patients. In contrast, there has been an evolution of techniques for minimally invasive parathyroidectomy in the treatment of sporadic HPT, and a paradigm shift towards focused unilateral or single gland exploration. A number of important adjuncts have allowed the widespread adoption of concise parathyroidectomy techniques, including improved preoperative localization studies, gamma probe localization of parathyroid adenomas after isotope injection, and importantly, the application of quick intraoperative assays for PTH to confirm biochemical cure. However, sporadic HPT is most commonly caused by a solitary hyperfunctioning parathyroid adenoma, and less frequently by double adenomas or multiple gland disease. The suitability of minimally invasive techniques for the successful treatment of MEN 1-associated HPT requires special consideration.

The role of surgical adjuncts for parathyroidectomy, including gamma probe localization following Tc-99m-Sestamibi injection, quick intraoperative PTH levels [8], and operation using local or regional anesthesia in the ambulatory setting has not been clearly defined in the surgical treatment of patients with MEN 1. The indications for and efficacy of some of these techniques may be altered in the unique circumstance of parathyroid surgery to treat MEN 1 patients. A partial transcervical thymectomy, and a routine search for ectopic parathyroid tissue and supernumerary glands, have been advocated for patients with MEN 1 owing to a suggested increased incidence [6, 7] of extra parathyroid glands in patients with familial HPT. Traditional bilateral neck exploration under general anesthesia and gross identification of all parathyroid glands remains an excellent "gold standard" approach to any patient with primary HPT, and this approach has now been advocated again for all patients by some [9]. Measurement of intraoperative PTH levels represents an assessment of biochemical cure and may provide guidance for the extent of parathyroid resection. Based on the final operative PTH levels, adequacy of subtotal resection as well as the potential need for completion total parathyroidectomy and intramuscular transplantation of additional tissue to maintain parathyroid function may be determined [8].

Less than subtotal parathyroidectomy, or selective removal of only those parathyroid glands that are enlarged at the time of neck exploration is associated with a high incidence of recurrent HPT [10–13]. Nevertheless, one group has advocated minimally invasive parathyroidectomy and selective removal of only enlarged parathyroid glands as an acceptable alternative for patients with MEN 1 to avoid the occurrence of permanent postoperative hypoparathyroidism that can be associated with bilateral cervical exploration and 4-gland interventions [14]. These authors acknowledge the inevitable development of recurrent disease in patients managed by this approach, but have argued that such disease recurrence may take years to develop and can be managed by further focused procedures. When the diagnosis of MEN 1 is not recognized prior to initial neck exploration, selective parathyroidectomy is often performed with a high incidence of recurrent HPT and the need for a second operation.

Subtotal Parathyroidectomy Versus Total Parathyroidectomy with Autotransplantation

The operative management of HPT in patients with MEN 1 requires an attempt to identify and address all four parathyroid glands, as well as a search for ectopic or supernumerary glands. Further, the surgeon must use intraoperative data and judgment to determine the appropriate extent of resection and the manner and location for preservation of the volume of parathyroid tissue intended to function postoperatively and maintain normocalcemia. The unique features and challenges account for a higher rate of permanent hypoparathyroidism and subsequent recurrent HPT in patients undergoing surgical treatment of multiglandular disease in the setting of the MEN 1 syndrome when compared with the results of parathyroidectomy for sporadic HPT.

Two different surgical approaches have been advocated for in the treatment of HPT in patients with MEN 1. The first is total parathyroidectomy with heterotopic autotransplantation of parathyroid tissue grafts into skeletal muscle (TP/AT). The goals of this approach are to reduce the parathyroid tissue volume to an appropriate amount to achieve a normal PTH level and result in normocalcemia, while removing all parathyroid tissue from the neck and creating vascularized autografts in a heterotopic site such as the brachioradialis forearm muscle. The rationale for transplanting the remaining parathyroid tissue to the forearm is to allow reduction of the grafted parathyroid tissue in patients who develop recurrent HPT with a simple and low risk procedure. This procedure may be performed under local anesthesia as an outpatient, without the need cervical re-exploration. Performance of TP/AT requires a high success rate for parathyroid graft function, in order to avoid an unacceptably high incidence of permanent postoperative hypocalcemia. A second frequently employed operation is a subtotal (3 and ½ gland) parathyroidectomy (SP), leaving a vascularized remnant of one parathyroid gland in situ in the neck. This operative strategy seeks to preserve an appropriate volume of vascularized parathyroid tissue to achieve a normal PTH level and maintain normocalcemia, while avoiding a perceived higher rate of permanent hypoparathyroidism associated with heterotopic transplantation of the only remaining parathyroid tissue. In addition, this approach obviates the need for a second incision for parathyroid grafting and may shorten or reduce the severity of the period of transient hypocalcemia requiring supplementation until the grafts function adequately. Despite the potential advantages and disadvantages of these two commonly practiced operations, retrospective studies have demonstrated similar overall rates of recurrent HPT and permanent postoperative hypoparathyroidism in patients undergoing both operations [10, 11, 13, 15–32]. Although one of these approaches is often preferred by individual endocrine surgery centers of excellence, improved outcomes or a clear advantage for either operation has not been established by previous studies.

The available studies collectively provide a large amount of data relating to the epidemiology, presentation, biochemical findings, natural history, and outcome of patients with MEN 1-associated HPT following various surgical treatments. There are significant challenges however, in the interpretation of findings of individual studies, the comparison of reported results between different studies, and an attempt to arrive at a consensus on the specific operative procedure that can be clearly associated with improved outcomes. These difficulties relate to the heterogeneity of the patient populations included in different studies, and the variability in study design and methods of analyzing and interpreting results. In addition, except for a single study [5], all of the available series are retrospective. Most of the studies come from high volume, specialized referral centers that see enough of these unusual patients over time to develop a sufficient experience to standardize the surgical approach and accumulate data on outcomes. The combined results from these studies provides important information for our current understanding of the outcomes of patients with MEN 1-associated HPT following parathyroidectomy and represents our best available evidence. The results from major studies comparing the outcomes of parathyroidectomy in patients with primary hyperplasia and MEN 1 are depicted in Table 15.2. The postoperative outcomes separated for SP and TP/AT are shown in summary form in Tables 15.3 and 15.4, respectively.

There are notable limitations in interpreting the data from these studies that should be recognized. Some studies included patients with multiglandular disease

Table 15.2 Results of surgical treatments for multiglandular hyperparathyroidism

Year	Study	Patients (no.)	Design	Associated condition (s)	Operative procedure	Persistent or recurrent HPT	Permanent HypoCa	Mean F/U (year)
1979	Edis et al. [15]	55	R	PHP	SP	13% (7/55)	5% (3/55)	3.9
1980	Wells et al. [16]	36	R	PHP	TP/AT[a]	31% (11/36)	5.6% (2/36)	ns
1981	Prinz et al. [17]	12	R	MEN 1	SP	33% (4/12)	25% (3/12)	9.5
1983	Van Heerden et al. [18]	43	R	MEN 1/2	SP	14% (6/43)	14% (6/43)	>3.25
		2			TP/AT	ns	ns	
1986	Malmaeus et al. [19]	21	R	MEN 1	LSP	88% (18/21)	5% (1/21)	>4
		6			SP	33% (2/6)	0% (0/21)	
		18			TP/AT[a]	0% (0/18)	28% (5/18)	
1991	Goretzki et al. [20]	18	R	MGD	SP	11% (2/18)	0% (0/18)	ns
1992	Hellman et al. [11]	23	R	MEN 1	LSP	53%	3%	11.9
		11			SP	9%	9%	
		23			TP/AT[a]	22%	30%	6.1
1992	Kraimps et al. [21]	14	R	MEN 1/2	SP[a]	50% (7/14)	10% (4/40)	8
		26			LSP	15% (4/26)		
1993	O'Riordain et al. [22]	84	R	MEN 1	SP (54)	0% pHPT (0/54) 17% pHPT(5/30)	8% (7/84)	6.7
					LSP (30)	16% rHPT @ 10y		
2001	Dotzenrath et al. [24]	39	R	MEN 1	SP (25)	12% (3/25)	12% (3/25)	4.5
					LSP (13)	23% (3/13)	15% (2/13)	
					TP/AT (1)	–	–	
2002	Arnalsteen et al. [26]	79	R	MEN 1	SP (66)	7.6% (6/79)	13% (10/79)	4.2
					LSP (13)	Combined	Combined	3.1
2003	Elaraj et al. [27]	92	R	MEN 1	LSP (13)	46% (6/13)	15% (2/13)	5.3
					SP (63)	31% (22/71)-	26% (15/58)	6.1
					TP/AT (16)	All ≥3-gland (SP + TP/AT)	46% (6/13)	–

2006	Hubbard et al. [28]	29	R	MEN 1	SP (21)	5% (1/21)	10% (2/21)	5.1 (7.4 overall)
					LSP (4)	25% (1/4)	0% (0/4)	
					TP/AT (4)	50% (2/4)	25% (1/4)	
2007	Tonelli et al. [31]	51	R	MEN 1	TP/AT[a]	10% (5/51)	25% (13/51)	7
2011	Schreinemakers et al. [13]	52	R	MEN 1	SP (17)	71% (12/17)	24% (4/17)	12
					LSP (29)	90% (26/29)	7% (2/29)	8.25
					TP/AT (6)	0% (0/6)	67% (4/6)	1.3
2012	Pieterman et al. [32]	73[a]	R	MEN 1	SP (23)	17% (4/23)	39% (9/23)	4.25 overall
					LSP (17)	53% (9/17)	24% (4/17)	
					TP/AT(32)	19% (6/32)	66% (21/32)	
2014	Lairmore et al. [5]	32	RPT	MEN 1	SP	24% (4/17)	12% (2/17)	7.5 ± 5.7
					TP/AT	13% (2/15)	7% (1/15)	
2016	Fyrsten et al. [10]	69[a]	R	MEN 1	SP (30)	7% (2/30)	10% (2/20)	20.6 year overall
					LSP (31)	23% (7/31)	25% (5/20)	
					TP/AT (8)	13% (1/8)	80% (4/5)	

HPT hyperparathyroidism, *rHPT* recurrent hyperparathyroidism, *pHPT* persistent hyperparathyroidism, *HypoCa* hypocalcemia, *ns* not specified, *R* retrospective, *RPT* randomized, prospective trial, *PHP* primary (chief cell) hyperplasia, *MGD* multiple gland disease, *MEN 1/2* multiple endocrine neoplasia types 1 and 2, *LSP* less than subtotal parathyroidectomy (<3 glands), *SP* subtotal parathyroidectomy (3 or 3 ½ gland), *TP/AT* total parathyroidectomy with autotransplantation

[a]Includes both primary operations and reoperative procedures

Table 15.3 Outcomes for subtotal parathyroidectomy (SP)

Year	Study	Patients (no.)	Studyperiod	Associated condition(s)	Persistent HPT (%)	Recurrent HPT (%)	Permanent HypoCa (%)	Mean F/U (year)
1979	Edis et al. [15]	55	1959–76	PHP	13	0	5	3.9
1981	Prinz et al. [17]	12	1955–76	MEN 1	33	0	25	9.5
1983	Van Heerden et al. [18]	43	1960–83	MEN 1/2	6.6	6.6	14	>3.25
1986	Malmaeus et al. [19]	27	1961–85	MEN 1	19	56	4	>4
1991	Goretzki et al. [20]	18	1986–90	MGD	11	0	0	ns
1992	Hellman et al. [11]	11	1982–91	MEN 1	0	27.3	27.3	11.9
1992	Kraimps et al. [21]	14 26	1966–88	MEN 1/2	14	36	10	8
1993	O'Riordain et al. [22]	54	1970–91	MEN 1	0	16[a]	8	6.7
2001	Dotzenrath et al. [24]	25	1986–98	MEN 1	ns	12	12	4.5
2002	Arnalsteen et al. [26]	66	1992–2001	MEN 1	ns	33[a]	13	4.2
2003	Elaraj et al. [27]	63	1960–2002	MEN 1	ns	51[a]	26[a]	6.1
2006	Hubbard et al. [28]	21	1974–2002	MEN 1	0	5	10	5.1
2011	Schreinemakers et al. [13]	17	1967–2008	MEN 1	7	65	24	12
2012	Pieterman et al. [32]	23	1990–2009	MEN 1	(17) combined	(17) combined	39	4.25
2014	Lairmore et al. [5]	17	1996–2014	MEN 1	6	24%	12	7.5
2016	Fyrsten et al. [10]	30	1963–2012	MEN 1	(7) combined	(7) combined	10	21

ns not specified, *HPT* hyperparathyroidism, *PHP* primary (chief cell) hyperplasia, *MGD* multiple gland disease, *MEN 1/2* multiple endocrine neoplasia types 1 and 2
[a]Estimated

Table 15.4 Outcomes for total parathyroidectomy and parathyroid autotransplantation (TP/AT)

Year	Study	Patients (no.)	Study period	Associated condition(s)	Persistent HPT (%)	Recurrent HPT (%)	Permanent HypoCa (%)	MeanF/U (yr)
1980	Wells et al. [16]	36	1973–80	PHP	3	30	5.6	ns
1986	Malmaeus et al. [19]	18	1961–85	MEN 1	0	0	28	>4
1992	Hellman et al. [11]	23	1982–91	MEN 1	0	22	30	6.1
2003	Elaraj et al. [27]	16	1960–2002	MEN 1	ns	16[a]	46	6.1
2006	Hubbard et al. [28]	4	1974–2002	MEN 1	0	50	25	7.4
2007	Tonelli et al. [31]	51	1990–2006	MEN 1	0	10	25	7
2011	Schreinemakers et al. [13]	6	1967–2008	MEN 1	0	0	67	1.3
2012	Pieterman et al. [32]	32	1990–2009	MEN 1	ns	19	66	4.25
2014	Lairmore et al. [5]	15	1996–2014	MEN 1	0	13	7	7.5
2016	Fyrsten et al. [10]	8	1963–2012	MEN 1	0	13	80	20.6

ns not specified, *HPT* hyperparathyroidism, *PHP* primary (chief cell) hyperplasia, *MEN 1* multiple endocrine neoplasia type 1
[a]Estimated

or "primary chief cell hyperplasia", with or without a clear familial association. There were varying definitions for establishing a diagnosis of MEN 1. For those studies that included both MEN 1 and MEN 2 patients, only the results for the MEN 1 patients are shown. The study cohort for each of these studies includes patients treated over several decades, necessarily spanning different treatment eras. Differences in the availability of informative preoperative imaging, as well as surgical adjuncts to guide intraoperative parathyroid gland identification and appropriate extent of resection exist between patients treated in early versus late time periods. Further, the recent understanding of the genetic basis for disease has facilitated diagnosis and earlier intervention with an operation tailored to address disease affecting all 4 glands, with a resulting increase in the proportion of patients treated with a disease-specific operation as the first procedure. Finally, in some studies the results of patients undergoing a primary procedure and those undergoing a second procedure after a failed initial operation (either elsewhere or at the study institution), were reported in aggregate. Some studies include patients that underwent a primary operation prior to recognition of the associated MEN 1 diagnosis. These patients may have been treated with a selective parathyroidectomy, but outcomes are included with the patients that were treated with a strategy intended to address all 4 parathyroid glands. There is great potential for selection and treatment biases within individual institutions, as well as widely differing treatment protocols and level of experience with specific operative techniques (e.g. parathyroid autotransplantation) between the surgeon(s) performing the operations in any particular study.

Despite these limitations, some important observations can be made when carefully reviewing the reported outcomes in aggregate. Persistent or recurrent HPT occurs very frequently following any operative procedure for HPT in patients with MEN 1. Because these patients harbor a genetic mutation present in every parathyroid cell, there is an inherent predisposition to recurrent disease-associated proliferation and hyperfunction of parathyroid tissue whether it is left as a vascularized remnant in the neck, or transplanted to a heterotopic site in the forearm muscle. If patients are followed long enough, it is not surprising that recurrent disease can be expected in a significant percentage of patients. The general rates of recurrent HPT after parathyroidectomy for MEN 1 reported in the available studies range from approximately 15–50% after 5–10 years of follow-up (see Table 15.2).

Similarly, the reported rates of permanent postoperative hypoparathyroidism following parathyroidectomy for MEN 1-associated HPT are higher when compared with the results for patients with sporadic HPT. In the collected studies the frequency of hypoparathyroidism is approximately 5–30% after 5–10-year follow-up, with rates up to 60–80% depending on the specific operative procedure (see Table 15.2). In general, these rates are highest for patients undergoing parathyroid autotransplantation, and concern over avoiding this unfavorable outcome underlies the opinion of many surgeons that total parathyroidectomy with transplant of the only remaining parathyroid tissue to a heterotopic site is associated with an unacceptable risk of graft failure. This potential conclusion deserves further discussion with careful analysis of the results in all available studies.

For the purposes of this chapter, it is the intention of this author to present the whole of available evidence, and as unbiased an evaluation of the validity of the conclusions made based on the data presented as possible. In keeping with this pledge, I will endeavor to clearly delineate where statements provided are supported by available data, and where they represent best expert opinion. The following arguments regarding the results of TP/AT represent the observations and *opinion* of the author. The success rate of transplantation of immediate, fresh parathyroid autografts is highly technique dependent. Numerous variables including the manner of preparing the fragments for grafting, the technique for creating pockets, choice of anatomic site and ideal portion of skeletal muscle, and the number and distribution of parathyroid fragments transplanted can significantly affect the likelihood of neovascularization and ultimate graft function. The widely disparate results reported following autotransplantation likely reflects the varying levels of surgeon experience. Surgeons invested in performing a meticulous technique and with extensive experience report very good results with immediate parathyroid autotransplantation [5, 16, 31]. Nevertheless, the significant dependence of parathyroid transplantation on operator technique and experience arguably represents a basis for caution in advocating this strategy for all surgeons.

The premise that preserving a vascularized gland or portion of a gland in the neck provides better protection against hypocalcemia also deserves further comment. It is well recognized by endocrine surgeons that a parathyroid gland or remnant preserved in situ on its vascular supply may nevertheless fail to have sufficient function to maintain a normal calcium level without dependence on postoperative supplementation long-term. Inadequate function can occur even when the surgeon is confident a sufficient volume of tissue remains and appears to have excellent perfusion by visual inspection. The intraoperative PTH level following the maximum parathyroid tissue reduction can be used to guide appropriate resection, but does not always accurately predict postoperative hypoparathyroidism [8]. This observation represents not only the opinion of the author, but is also supported by the results of SP in the available studies, with reported rates of permanent hypoparathyroidism following SP of 12–39% [5, 13, 24, 26, 27, 32]. A recent study [33] showed very high success with transplantation of parathyroid tissue to subcutaneous fat, highlighting the potential importance of local factors to promote angiogenesis and neovascularization of grafted parathyroid tissue.

Routine cryopreservation of a portion of the parathyroid tissue resected during either SP or TP/AT can allow salvage of a subset of patients that develop postoperative hypoparathyroidism. Cohen et al. [34] reported their 13-year experience with the results of transplantation of cryopreserved parathyroid tissue. The study included 26 patients undergoing 30 procedures for cryopreserved heterotopic parathyroid autotransplantation (CHPA). Approximately 60% of delayed CHPA grafts were functional, and 40% of the autografts functioned sufficiently to maintain normal calcium levels without supplementation. The duration of cryopreservation was a significant predictor of graft function, and no functional autograft was observed after 22 months of preservation. Optimal care may be provided by specialized centers with the capability to perform routine cryopreservation of parathyroid tissue and delayed grafting when needed.

If an exercise is taken to determine the relative number of studies advocating one surgical approach to provide support for the best operation, it is evident that most studies have concluded that SP is the preferred treatment. Considering the 18 major studies included in Table 15.2, 12 recommend SP [10, 13, 15, 17, 18, 21, 22, 24, 26–28, 32], three recommend TP/AT [16, 19, 31], and three find the two operative procedures to provide similar results [5, 11, 20]. For an individual study, this conclusion may be based on the authors' best opinion, with variable strength of support from the data presented and with the numerous limitations itemized above. It is fair to say that the predominant opinion of "experts" appears to favor SP. As is the case for many controversies and difficult decisions in endocrine surgery, the relative infrequency of this disease and variability in surgical techniques and study design make the performance of a well-controlled, multicenter randomized prospective trial very difficult. In fact, probably less than 10% of all current surgical practices are supported by data from randomized controlled trials (RCT) [35, 36] highlighting the need for more such studies [37, 38]. Clearly, additional study is needed to adequately address the important issues for the optimal surgical treatment of HPT in patients with MEN 1. However, much can still be learned from the large volume of results reported in the available studies over an approximately 35-year period.

A multicenter study has also been reported including analysis of 245 patients with HPT and MEN 1 retrieved through the French and Belgian GENEM study group's database [25]. In this study, the patients were divided into three groups: those treated before 1986, 1986–1990, and after 1990. The authors followed trends in surgical treatment and outcomes over different treatment eras, and noted that 20% of patients were still hypercalcemic immediately after primary surgery in the most recent treatment era, with increasing rates of recurrent disease over time. Their results highlight the challenges in managing the multiple gland disease in patients with MEN 1. The overall conclusion of this study was that subtotal parathyroidectomy should be advocated, and is best performed in specialized high-volume centers.

In 2014, Lairmore et al. [5] reported the results of the first randomized prospective trial of operative treatments for HPT in patients with MEN 1. The study population included 32 MEN 1 patients randomized to receive either SP or TP/AT with a mean follow-up of 7.5 years. The overall rate of recurrent HPT was 19% (6/32). Recurrent HPT occurred in 4 of 17 patients (24%) treated with SP, and 2 of 15 patients (13%) treated with TP/AT (P = 0.66). Permanent hypoparathyroidism occurred in 3 of 32 patients (9%) overall. The incidence of permanent hypoparathyroidism was 12% (2/17) in the SP group and 7% (1/15) in the TP/AT group. A second operation was performed in 4 of 17 patients initially treated with SP (24%), compared with 1 of 15 patients undergoing TP/AT (7%). Although the need for reoperation was higher in the SP group, the difference did not meet statistical significance (P = 0.34). The study concluded that no difference could be demonstrated when comparing the outcomes of SP and TP/AT, and that both procedures were associated with acceptable results. However, SP may be associated advantages in that it involves only one incision and avoids an obligate period of transient postoperative hypocalcemia.

It is important to also consider the severity and duration of hypocalcemic symptoms associated with the two procedures, as well as other factors relating to patient discomfort, cosmetic concerns, and transient functional limitations during convalescence. TP/AT requires two surgical incision sites compared with one for SP. In addition, patients undergoing TP/AT can be expected to have an obligate period of transient hypoparathyroidism and dependence on oral supplementation that may be associated with greater severity and duration compared with patients that have preservation of a native vascularized parathyroid remnant. These considerations may confer mild incremental advantages to SP beyond achievement of equivalent surgical outcomes. Although not studied, the longer duration of this supplementation period may result in the potential need for interventions or hospital readmissions to manage complications. Cost differences have not been demonstrated. On the other hand, some studies suggest that the need for a second operative procedure occurs more frequently following SP compared with TP/AT [5, 19], with attendant significant potential for increase in costs and resource utilization. Finally, it is important to consider the time interval to recurrence based on extent of resection. Limited data exist, but where this metric has been evaluated more extended resections have been associated with a longer disease-free interval. Elaraj et al. [27] found that mean recurrence-free interval was not significantly different between SP versus TP/AT, but it was longer for SP and TP/AT combined compared with lesser resection (16.5 versus 7.0 years; $P = 0.03$). In the study of 52 MEN 1 patients by Schreinemakers et al. [13], time to recurrence was 61 months longer after SP than after less that subtotal resection, and recurrent HPT was not seen after TP/AT. Therefore, even with equivalent rates of recurrent HPT, patients undergoing more extensive resection (e.g. TP/AT) may take longer to recur.

Conclusions

The outcomes of surgical treatment for HPT in patients with MEN 1 syndrome are strongly influenced by (1) preoperative recognition of the diagnosis of MEN 1, (2) performance of an adequate operative procedure to address all four parathyroid glands, (3) appropriate timing of intervention and selection of procedure based on surgeon experience, and (4) the employment of meticulous surgical technique and adjuncts to determine optimal extent of parathyroid resection. Selective or less than subtotal parathyroidectomy can be expected to result in persistent or recurrent HPT in the majority of patients. The outcomes and curative potential of the specific surgical procedure should be guided by surgeon experience and understanding of the natural history and reported results of the two commonly performed operative treatments. The available evidence provides useful guidance, but a clear advantage of one operative procedure over the other is not provided.

In summary, the outcomes of SP and TP/AT in patients with MEN 1 are similar in the available retrospective studies, and a single randomized prospective trial failed to show significant differences in the overall incidence of recurrent HPT and permanent hypoparathyroidism between the two operations. In individual studies, SP is associated with lower hypoparathyroidism compared with TP/AT [19, 27], and in some a higher persistent/recurrent HPT [19] and more frequent requirement for a second operation [5]. The results of TP/AT are surgeon and technique dependent, but in centers with experience and expertise in performing this procedure, is associated with similar outcomes compared with SP [5, 19]. The time interval to recurrence may be prolonged after TP/AT [10, 28]. TP/AT is a good operation with good outcomes in selected centers, but may not be appropriate for all surgeons.

Recommendations

1. Depending on the expertise and experience of individual surgeons, subtotal parathyroidectomy (SP) *may* be the preferred operative treatment for HPT associated with the MEN 1 syndrome for many clinicians who care for these patients. Rates of recurrent/persistent HPT and permanent hypoparathyroidism vary considerably in available retrospective studies, but overall are similar to those following total parathyroidectomy and autotransplantation (TP/AT). SP may have minor incremental advantages because it involves only one surgical incision and avoids a longer obligate period of postoperative transient hypoparathyroidism and dependence on oral calcium and/or vitamin D supplementation.

   Level of evidence [39], *3*: multiple comparative retrospective studies

   GRADE strength of recommendation, B, moderate: Further research is likely to have an important impact on the outcome studies.
2. Less than subtotal (selective) parathyroidectomy of only grossly enlarged glands will result in almost uniform recurrence and is not recommended for patients with a known diagnosis of MEN 1.

   Level of evidence, 3: multiple comparative retrospective studies with uniform outcome

   GRADE strength of recommendation, A, high: Further research is very unlikely to change this recommendation.
3. Total parathyroidectomy with autotransplantation (TP/AT) results in similar outcomes when compared with SP. Therefore, TP/AT represents a good and acceptable treatment for MEN 1-associated HPT when performed by experienced surgeons. The interval to recurrence may be longer after TP/AT compared with SP.

Level of evidence, 2: lesser quality randomized controlled trial (single RCT with small numbers and low statistical power)

GRADE strength of recommendation, B, moderate: Further research is likely to have an important impact on the outcome studies.

References

1. Chandrasekharappa SC, Guru SC, Manickamp P, Olufemi S, Collins FS, Emmert-Buck M, et al. Positional cloning of the gene for multiple endocrine neoplasia-type 1. Science. 1997;276:404–7.
2. Doherty GM, Lairmore TC, DeBenedetti MK. Multiple endocrine neoplasia type 1 parathyroid adenoma development over time. World J Surg. 2004;28(11):1139–42.
3. Marx S, Spiegel AM, Skarulis MC, Doppman JL, Collins FS, Liotta LA. Multiple endocrine neoplasia type 1: clinical and genetic topics. Ann Intern Med. 1998;129:484–94.
4. Lairmore TC, Piersall LD, DeBenedetti MK, Dilley WG, Mutch MG, Whelan AJ, et al. Clinical genetic testing and early surgical intervention in patients with multiple endocrine neoplasia type 1 (MEN 1). Ann Surg. 2004;239(5):637–45. Discussion 45-7.
5. Lairmore TC, Govednik CM, Quinn CE, Sigmond BR, Lee CY, Jupiter DC. A randomized, prospective trial of operative treatments for hyperparathyroidism in patients with multiple endocrine neoplasia type 1. Surgery. 2014;156(6):1326–34. Discussion 34-5.
6. d'Alessandro AF, Montenegro FL, Brandao LG, Lourenco DM Jr, Toledo Sde A, Cordeiro AC. Supernumerary parathyroid glands in hyperparathyroidism associated with multiple endocrine neoplasia type 1. Rev Assoc Med Bras. 2012;58(3):323–7.
7. Nilubol N, Weinstein L, Simonds WF, Jensen RT, Phan GQ, Hughes MS, et al. Preoperative localizing studies for initial parathyroidectomy in MEN1 syndrome: is there any benefit? World J Surg. 2012;36(6):1368–74.
8. Nilubol N, Weisbrod AB, Weinstein LS, Simonds WF, Jensen RT, Phan GQ, et al. Utility of intraoperative parathyroid hormone monitoring in patients with multiple endocrine neoplasia type 1-associated primary hyperparathyroidism undergoing initial parathyroidectomy. World J Surg. 2013;37(8):1966–72.
9. Norman J, Lopez J, Politz D. Abandoning unilateral parathyroidectomy: why we reversed our position after 15,000 parathyroid operations. J Am Coll Surg. 2012;214(3):260–9.
10. Fyrsten E, Norlen O, Hessman O, Stalberg P, Hellman P. Long-term surveillance of treated hyperparathyroidism for multiple endocrine neoplasia type 1: recurrence or hypoparathyroidism? World J Surg. 2016;40(3):615–21.
11. Hellman P, Skogseid B, Juhlin C, Akerstrom G, Rastad J. Findings and long term results of parathyroid surgery in multiple endocrine neoplasia type 1. World J Surg. 1992;16:718–23.
12. Nilubol N, Weinstein LS, Simonds WF, Jensen RT, Marx SJ, Kebebew E. Limited parathyroidectomy in multiple endocrine neoplasia type 1-associated primary hyperparathyroidism: a setup for failure. Ann Surg Oncol. 2016;23(2):416–23.
13. Schreinemakers JM, Pieterman CR, Scholten A, Vriens MR, Valk GD, Rinkes IH. The optimal surgical treatment for primary hyperparathyroidism in MEN1 patients: a systematic review. World J Surg. 2011;35(9):1993–2005.
14. Versnick M, Popadich A, Sidhu S, Sywak M, Robinson B, Delbridge L. Minimally invasive parathyroidectomy provides a conservative surgical option for multiple endocrine neoplasia type 1-primary hyperparathyroidism. Surgery. 2013;154(1):101–5.
15. Edis AJ, van Heerden JA, Scholz DA. Results of subtotal parathyroidectomy for primary chief cell hyperplasia. Surgery. 1979;86(3):462–9.
16. Wells SA Jr, Farndon JR, Dale JK, Leight GS, Dilley WG. Long term evaluation of patients with primary parathyroid hyperplasia managed by total parathyroidectomy and heterotopic autotransplantation. Ann Surg. 1980;192:451–8.
17. Prinz RA, Gamvros DI, Selly D, Lynn JA. Subtotal parathyroidectomy for primary chief cell hyperplasia in the multiple endocrine neoplasia type I syndrome. Ann Surg. 1981;193:26.
18. van Heerden JA, Kent RB, Sizemore GW, Grant CS, ReMine WM. Primary hyperparathyroidism in patients with multiple endocrine neoplasia syndromes: surgical experience. Arch Surg. 1983;118:533–6.
19. Malmaeus J, Benson L, Johansson H, Ljunghall S, Rastad J, Akerstrom G, et al. Parathyroid surgery in the multiple endocrine neoplasia type I syndrome: choice of surgical procedure. World J Surg. 1986;10(4):668–72.

20. Goretzki PE, Dotzenrath C, Roeher HD. Management of primary hyperparathyroidism caused by multiple gland disease. World J Surg. 1991;15(6):693–7.
21. Kraimps JL, Duh Q-Y, Demeure M, Clark OH. Hyperparathyroidism in multiple endocrine neoplasia syndrome. Surgery. 1992;112:1080–8.
22. O'Riordain DS, O'Brien T, Grant CS, Weaver A, Gharib H, van Heerden JA. Surgical management of primary hyperparathyroidism in multiple endocrine neoplasia types 1 and 2. Surgery. 1993;114:1031–9.
23. Hellman P, Skogseid B, Oberg K, Juhlin C, Akerstrom G, Rastad J. Primary and reoperative parathyroid operations in hyperparathyroidism of multiple endocrine neoplasia type 1. Surgery. 1998;124(6):993–9.
24. Dotzenrath C, Cupisti K, Goretzki PE, Yang Q, Simon D, Ohmann C, et al. Long-term biochemical results after operative treatment of primary hyperparathyroidism associated with multiple endocrine neoplasia types I and IIa: is a more or less extended operation essential? Eur J Surg. 2001;167(3):173–8.
25. Goudet P, Cougard P, Verges B, Murat A, Carnaille B, Calender A, et al. Hyperparathyroidism in multiple endocrine neoplasia type I: surgical trends and results of a 256-patient series from Groupe D'etude des Neoplasies Endocriniennes Multiples Study Group. World J Surg. 2001;25(7):886–90.
26. Arnalsteen LC, Alesina PF, Quiereux JL, Farrel SG, Patton FN, Carnaille BM, et al. Long-term results of less than total parathyroidectomy for hyperparathyroidism in multiple endocrine neoplasia type 1. Surgery. 2002;132(6):1119–24. Discussion 24-5.
27. Elaraj DM, Skarulis MC, Libutti SK, Norton JA, Bartlett DL, Pingpank JF, et al. Results of initial operation for hyperparathyroidism in patients with multiple endocrine neoplasia type 1. Surgery. 2003;134(6):858–64. Discussion 64-5.
28. Hubbard JG, Sebag F, Maweja S, Henry JF. Subtotal parathyroidectomy as an adequate treatment for primary hyperparathyroidism in multiple endocrine neoplasia type 1. Arch Surg. 2006;141(3):235–9.
29. Norton JA, Venzon DJ, Berna MJ, Alexander HR, Fraker DL, Libutti SK, et al. Prospective study of surgery for primary hyperparathyroidism (HPT) in multiple endocrine neoplasia-type 1 and Zollinger-Ellison syndrome: long-term outcome of a more virulent form of HPT. Ann Surg. 2008;247(3):501–10.
30. Tonelli F, Giudici F, Cavalli T, Brandi ML. Surgical approach in patients with hyperparathyroidism in multiple endocrine neoplasia type 1: total versus partial parathyroidectomy. Clinics (Sao Paulo). 2012;67(Suppl 1):155–60.
31. Tonelli F, Marcucci T, Fratini G, Tommasi MS, Falchetti A, Brandi ML. Is total parathyroidectomy the treatment of choice for hyperparathyroidism in multiple endocrine neoplasia type 1? Ann Surg. 2007;246(6):1075–82.
32. Pieterman CR, van Hulsteijn LT, den Heijer M, van der Luijt RB, Bonenkamp JJ, Hermus AR, et al. Primary hyperparathyroidism in MEN1 patients: a cohort study with longterm follow-up on preferred surgical procedure and the relation with genotype. Ann Surg. 2012;255(6):1171–8.
33. Jansson S, Tisell LE. Autotransplantation of diseased parathyroid glands into subcutaneous abdominal adipose tissue. Surgery. 1987;101(5):549–56.
34. Cohen MS, Dilley WG, Wells SA Jr, Moley JF, Doherty GM, Sicard GA, et al. Long-term functionality of cryopreserved parathyroid autografts: a 13-year prospective analysis. Surgery. 2005;138(6):1033–40. Discussion 40-1.
35. McCulloch P, Taylor I, Sasako M, Lovett B, Griffin D. Randomised trials in surgery: problems and possible solutions. BMJ. 2002;324(7351):1448–51.
36. Pollock AV. Surgical evaluation at the crossroads. Br J Surg. 1993;80(8):964–6.
37. Solomon MJ, McLeod RS. Should we be performing more randomized controlled trials evaluating surgical operations? Surgery. 1995;118(3):459–67.
38. Wells SA Jr. Surgeons and surgical trials-why we must assume a leadership role. Surgery. 2002;132(3):519–20.
39. Howick J, Chalmers I, Glasziou P, Greenhalgh T, Heneghan C, Liberati A, Moschetti I, Phillips B, Thornton H. The 2011 Oxford CEBM levels of evidence (introductory document). Oxford: Oxford Centre for Evidence-Based Medicine; 2011. http://www.cebm.net/index.aspx?o=5653.

16 Four-Gland Exploration Versus Four-Dimensional Computed Tomography in Patients with Nonlocalized Primary Hyperparathyroidism

Courtney E. Quinn and Tobias Carling

Abstract

The surgical management of patients with primary hyperparathyroidism (PHPT) varies greatly among parathyroid surgeons, as well as across institutions. Four gland exploration, or bilateral neck exploration (BNE) has long been the "gold standard" operation for PHPT; it involves direct visualization of all parathyroid glands, with removal of enlarged parathyroid tissue, and has yielded excellent cure and complication rates, when performed by experienced surgeons. However, given that approximately 85% of patients with PHPT have single-gland disease, unilateral, minimally-invasive approaches have been advocated. The latter approaches require preoperative localization studies to identify the abnormal gland(s). While non-invasive imaging studies are routinely employed before index parathyroid surgery, negative, discordant or equivocal non-invasive localization studies are not uncommon, even in the unexplored patient. In this setting, an experienced parathyroid surgeon will still find and cure PHPT in the vast majority of patients. While bilateral neck exploration remains an excellent operation, controversy has developed in recent years, regarding the potential superiority of more focused, minimally invasive approaches. To address this issue, we evaluated the available literature for recommendations regarding the use of preoperative four-dimensional computed tomography (4DCT) versus direct, four gland exploration in patients

C. E. Quinn (✉) · T. Carling
Section of Endocrine Surgery, Department of Surgery, Yale University School of Medicine, New Haven, CT, USA
e-mail: courtney.quinn@yale.edu

P. Angelos, R. H. Grogan (eds.), *Difficult Decisions in Endocrine Surgery*, Difficult Decisions in Surgery: An Evidence-Based Approach,
https://doi.org/10.1007/978-3-319-92860-9_16

with negative sestamibi and/or neck ultrasound studies. We summarize the available data and provide recommendations on how to surgically treat patients undergoing parathyroidectomy for PHPT.

Keywords
Primary hyperparathyroidism · Parathyroid adenoma · 4D CT · Four-gland exploration · Bilateral neck exploration · Sestamibi · Neck ultrasound · Non-invasive imaging · Parathyroidectomy · Minimally invasive parathyroidectomy

Introduction

Approximately 85% of patients with PHPT have single parathyroid gland enlargement, referred to as a parathyroid adenoma. A subset of patients with sporadic disease have multi-gland disease, in which all parathyroid glands are involved. Once the diagnosis of PHPT is made and patients meet surgical criteria, imaging studies are often undertaken to localize abnormal gland(s). Preoperative localization studies help identify patients who are candidates for minimally invasive approaches. While non-invasive imaging studies are routinely employed before index parathyroid surgery, negative, discordant or equivocal sestamibi and ultrasound studies are not uncommon, even in the unexplored patient. In recent years, four-dimensional computed tomography (4DCT) has been employed for parathyroid localization. The fourth dimension, time, accounts for differences in perfusion characteristics between the hyperfunctioning parathyroid gland and surrounding structures, such as the thyroid gland. Proponents of 4DCT hypothesize that routine institution of this preoperative localization study may lead to decreased operative time, shorter length of hospital stay, and improved cure rates. However, since BNE remains an excellent operation and avoids the increased radiation exposure associated with 4DCT, controversy has developed in recent years, regarding the optimal surgical approach for patients with PHPT. We evaluated the available literature for recommendations regarding the use of preoperative four-dimensional CT (4DCT) versus direct, four gland exploration in patients with negative sestamibi and/or neck ultrasound studies. To date, few large-scale studies have been performed to address this issue. Many of the recommendations in the literature have been based on the practices of single institutions. We summarize the available data and provide recommendations on how to surgically treat patients with non-localized PHPT (Table 16.1).

Table 16.1 PICO table

*P*opulation	Primary hyperparathyroidism with negative (non-localized) ultrasound and sestamibi
*I*ntervention	4DCT (preop)
*C*omparator	4-gland exploration
*O*utcome	Cure rates, cost benefit, complications

Search Strategy

We conducted a focused review of the current guidelines related to preoperative localization studies for parathyroid adenomas/hyperplasia. We then performed a comprehensive review of the literature related to non-invasive imaging and parathyroid surgery. Literature searches were conducted in the PubMed database using the key words: primary hyperparathyroidism, parathyroid adenoma, 4D CT, four-gland exploration, bilateral neck exploration, sestamibi, non-invasive imaging, parathyroidectomy, and minimally invasive parathyroidectomy. Searches were limited to the English language, human subjects, and literature published in the last 15 years. Our search returned 618 articles; we critically reviewed 38 articles related to parathyroid surgery, as well as international guidelines from the Fourth International Workshop for the management of asymptomatic primary hyperparathyroidism. Emphasis was made on current national guidelines and recommendations.

Preoperative Localization of Abnormal Parathyroid Glands in Primary Hyperparathyroidism

The purpose of preoperative imaging in parathyroid surgery is to assist the surgeon in planning and performing an appropriate operation; such imaging should not be used for diagnosis, as PHPT is a biochemical diagnosis. Preoperative localization studies can help identify patients who may be candidates for a minimally invasive approach. An additional advantage is the potential for identification of concurrent thyroid disease, which may allow for a combined endocrine surgical procedure. A variety of non-invasive imaging options exist, including: neck ultrasound (U/S), sestamibi (SeS) ± single-photon emission computed tomography (SPECT), 4DCT, MRI, and positron emission tomography computed tomography (PET-CT).

The most commonly used non-invasive imaging for preoperative localization in PHPT are neck U/S, SeS ± SPECT, and 4DCT. Each imaging modality has its own advantages, as well as its own limitations. Parathyroid U/S has the best safety profile because it does not use ionizing radiation. Additionally, it is particularly sensitive in the detection of concurrent thyroid disease, and is relatively inexpensive. However, it requires a skilled technician to adequately demonstrate an abnormal parathyroid gland. It is also has very limited ability to identify ectopically-located parathyroid adenomas, such as in the retroesophageal or mediastinal location.

There exists a variety of nuclear scintigraphic agents and techniques. Currently, the most preferred non-invasive imaging study for parathyroid disease uses ^{99m}Tc-SeS with SPECT. This modality's improved spatial resolution allows for detection of smaller parathyroid lesions than those found with sestamibi alone. However, similar to neck U/S, the sensitivity of SeS is greatly diminished by multiglandular parathyroid disease and concurrent thyroid pathology. More recently, 4DCT has been utilized for parathyroid localization; the fourth dimension (time) accounts for differences in perfusion characteristics between parathyroid adenomas/hyperplastic glands, and surrounding structures, such as the thyroid gland. Of note, because of the use of intravenous contrast, 4DCT should not be utilized in patients with known contrast allergy, renal insufficiency or known or suspected thyroid carcinoma.

In an effort to determine which non-invasive preoperative imaging modality is best for localizing abnormal parathyroid glands, several studies in the literature have been performed, most of which are retrospective analyses or case series (Table 16.2). Rodgers et al. [1] compared the results of preoperative imaging studies in 75 patients undergoing parathyroidectomy for PHPT. These investigators found that compared to neck U/S or SeS, 4DCT had significantly higher sensitivity and specificity for lateralization of the aberrant gland(s). Additionally, 4DCT localized the aberrant gland to the correct quadrant in 70% of cases, which was a significant improvement over neck U/S or SeS. Starker et al. [2] performed a retrospective analysis of a prospective database of patients undergoing parathyroidectomy for PHPT by a single experienced endocrine surgeon. Similar to the prior study, the researchers found 4DCT to be superior to neck U/S and SeS-SPECT, for both localization and lateralization of abnormal parathyroid tissue. A meta-analysis of 32 studies on preoperative localization techniques for patients with PHPT found that ultrasound and SeS were similar in their ability to preoperatively localize abnormal parathyroid glands, with pooled sensitivities of 76.1% and 78.9%, respectively [3]. Since an insufficient number of preoperative 4DCT studies were available for inclusion in this meta-analysis, the authors could not definitively demonstrate an advantage of 4DCT over U/S or SeS. However, results of those two studies suggested increased sensitivity of 4DCT. Recently, Suh et al. [4] carried out a prospective case series to compare 4DCT, U/S and SeS as methods of preoperative localization for patients undergoing parathyroidectomy. Thirty-eight patients underwent all three imaging modalities prior to surgery. All imaging studies were reviewed independently and in a blinded fashion. Once again, 4D CT proved superior in terms of sensitivity and specificity. In a most recent retrospective analysis, comparisons were made between the three aforementioned non-invasive imaging modalities for preoperative localization rate and accuracy in 200 patients who underwent parathyroidectomy for PHPT [5]. Results showed that in patients with single-gland disease, the sensitivity of 4DCT, SeS and U/S were 96%, 65.4% and 57.7%, respectively. Furthermore, these investigators used a modified 4DCT that decreased the effective radiation dose compared to standard 4DCT, noting an average radiation dose of 11–13 mSv, which is comparable to that of SeS. This was an important finding, as one criticism of the routine use of 4DCT has been the higher level of radiation dose given to patients, with its inherent increased risk of subsequent malignancy.

Recommendations

- 4DCT has higher sensitivity and specificity over U/S or SeS in the preoperative localization of abnormal parathyroid glands, and therefore may be considered as a first-line imaging choice for patients undergoing MIP, in centers/institutions where this modality is readily available.

Table 16.2 Studies on preoperative non-invasive imaging for primary hyperparathyroidism

Study/Year	Study type	N	Imaging modality (% Sensitivity) lateralization			Imaging modality (% Specificity) lateralization			Imaging modality (% Sensitivity) localization			Strength of evidence
			4DCT	U/S	SeS	4DCT	U/S	SeS	4DCT	U/S	SeS	
Rodgers 2006 [1]	Retrospective	75	88[a]	57	65	88	94	88	70[b]	29	33	Strong
Starker 2010 [2]	Retrospective	87	93.9[c]	71.2	61.5	–	–	–	85.7[c]	48.0	40.4	Strong
Cheung 2012 [3]	Meta-analysis	[d]32	–	76.1	78.9	–	–	–	–	–	–	Low
Suh 2014 [4]	Case series	38	92.1[e]	84.2	84.2	95.6[e]	86.8	90.4	94.7[e]	86.2	88.8	Moderate
Kukar 2015 [5]	Retrospective	200	96.1[f]	57.7	65.5	97.2[e]	96.3	93.4	–	–	–	Moderate

[a] $P < 0.0001$
[b] $P < 0.05$
[c] $P < 0.005$
[d] N = number of studies evaluated
[e] $P < 0.01$
[f] $P < 0.001$

- 4DCT should not be used in patients with suspected or definitive thyroid carcinoma, renal insufficiency, or in those allergic to intravenous contrast
- The combination of U/S + SeS, when studies are concordant, serve as adequate localization prior to surgical intervention.
- In cases of known multigland disease, or genetic causes of PHPT preoperative imaging for localization purposes are not necessary.

Because MIP requires preoperative imaging for localization of abnormal parathyroid glands, some surgeons question the cost-effectiveness of such a strategy, in comparison to the costs associated with BNE. In an effort to comprehensively evaluate the short-terms costs associated with various preoperative parathyroid localization strategies, cost-utility analysis models have been developed (Table 16.3). Wang et al. [6] described five different preoperative imaging algorithms to determine their incremental cost-utility ratio in patients with PHPT. They found that although U/S alone was the least expensive imaging modality ($6666), sestamibi-SPECT + U/S ± 4DCT was the most cost effective method. These savings are likely attributed to the decreased amount of BNE performed when this preoperative localization strategy is instituted. Lubitz et al. [7] developed a cost-analysis model to evaluate the short-term costs of preoperative localization strategies for patients with PHPT. In this model, U/S + 4DCT was the most cost effective strategy. However, both studies found that the most expensive strategy was direct BNE.

Recommendations

- A combined imaging strategy of either U/S + sestamibi, U/S + 4DCT, or U/S + sestamibi ± 4DCT are the most cost effective strategies for preoperative localization in patients with PHPT.
- Direct BNE is the most expensive approach, and should be limited to patients with known multigland disease, including those with genetic endocrine disorders (Table 16.3).

Unilateral Versus Bilateral Neck Exploration for Primary Hyperparathyroidism

Bilateral neck exploration (BNE) has long been the "gold standard" for the surgical management of primary hyperparathyroidism. However, in recent years, more focused, minimally invasive approaches have been promoted. This is largely due to the finding that a vast majority of patients with PHPT (85%) have single-gland disease. Therefore, a limited, unilateral approach could lead to curative rates comparable to BNE.

Data comparing BNE to minimally invasive parathyroidectomy (MIP) in patients with PHPT are limited. While several small to moderate-scale randomized clinical trials (RCTs) have been reported in the literature, the methods for BNE and MIP are

Table 16.3 Cost-effectiveness of various preoperative localization strategies

Study/Year	Cost (US dollars)								Strength of evidence
	SeS-SPECT	U/S	4DCT	SeS-SPECT + U/S	SeS-SPECT + U/S ± 4DCT	U/S ± 4DCT	SeS ± 4DCT	BNE	
Wang 2011 [6]	$7330	$6666	$6773	$7371	$7214	–	–	$7662	Moderate
Lubitz 2012 [7]	$6374	$6028	$6110	$6329	$6319	$5901	$6266	$6824	Moderate

extremely variable, making it somewhat challenging to compare across studies. The first RCT compared a video-assisted MIP approach to BNE in 38 patients undergoing surgery for PHPT [8]. While the authors found no difference in cure rate between the two groups, they reported shorter operative time, less pain and improved cosmesis in the MIP cohort. Several years later the same group of investigators compared a video-assisted MIP approach to an endoscopic BNE approach and found no differences in operative time, cure or complication rates between the two groups [9].

In 2002 Bergenfelz et al. [10] randomized 91 patients with PHPT to unilateral or bilateral neck exploration; preoperative scintigraphy and intraoperative parathyroid hormone (PTH) measurement guided the unilateral exploration. They found no differences in cost, transient recurrent laryngeal nerve (RLN) injury or short-term cure rates between the two groups. A five-year follow-up study confirmed comparable long-term cure rates between the two groups [11]. Another study by Bergenfelz et al. [12] looked specifically at the incidence of transient, post-operative hypocalcemia in 50 patients randomized to either MIP or BNE. The authors found a higher rate of transient hypocalcemia in the latter group. The remaining RCTs found no differences in cure or complication rates between MIP and BNE; variable differences in operative time and overall lower cost with BNE were reported [13–16].

In 2011, Udelsman et al. [17] compared the results of MIP with conventional BNE in a retrospective cohort of 1650 consecutive patients with PHPT. Interestingly, these authors found statistically significant higher curative rates, lower complication rates, as well as lower costs in the MIP group. To date, this study represents one of the largest series of patients who underwent parathyroidectomy for treatment of PHPT by a single, experienced endocrine surgeon.

Recommendations

A Surgical Taskforce, in connection with the Fourth International Workshop on the Management of Asymptomatic Primary Hyperparathyroidism developed evidence-based guidelines regarding surgery for PHPT [18]. They are as follows:

- Both bilateral, or four-gland exploration, and minimally invasive parathyroidectomy yield excellent cure rates and minimal complication rates, when performed by an experienced surgeon.
- Bilateral cervical exploration is the ideal operation for most patients with multigland disease, including those with genetic disease.
- Minimally invasive parathyroidectomy procedures are not recommended in centers that do not have sophisticated imaging, intraoperative PTH assays, and experienced endocrine surgeons.
- Intraoperative PTH assays are useful adjuncts during parathyroid surgery, and are essential, if focused approaches are employed.
- Although minimally invasive techniques have become increasingly adopted, all parathyroid surgeons must be able to perform a standard bilateral cervical exploration, in the event that occult multigland disease is present (Table 16.4).

Table 16.4 Studies on focused versus conventional parathyroidectomy for primary hyperparathyroidism

Study/Year	Study type	N		Overall complication rate (%)		Mortality	Cure rate (%)		Cost		Strength of evidence
		MIP	Standard	MIP	Standard		MIP	Standard	MIP	Standard	
Miccoli 1999 [8]	RCT	20	18	n/a	n/a	None	100	100	$1720	$1910	Moderate
Bergenfelz 2002 [9]	RCT	47	44	4	11	None	96	98	$2258	$2097	Moderate
Bergenfelz 2005 [10]	RCT	25	25	4	4	None	98	100	n/a	n/a	Moderate
Sozio 2005 [11]	RCT	34	35	0	0	None	100	100	n/a	n/a	Moderate
Russell 2006 [12]	RCT	54	46	0	4		100	100			
Westerdahl 2007 [13][a]	RCT (5 year f/u)	38	33	0	3	None	89	94	n/a	n/a	Moderate
Aarum 2007 [14]	RCT	50	50	2	0	None	96	94	82200EU	67800EU	Low
Miccoli 2008 [14]	RCT	20	20	0	0	None	100	100	–	–	Low
Slepavicius 2008 [16]	RCT	24	24	4	4	None	100	100	1428EU[b]	1166EU	Moderate
Udelsman 2011 [17]	Retrospective	986	478	1.45[b]	3.10	None	MIP: 99.4[b]	Standard: 97.9	$6 K[c]	$7.4 K	Moderate

RCT randomized, controlled trial
[a]Five year follow-up study of 2002 Bergenfelz RCT
[b]$P < 0.05$
[c]$P < 0.0001$

Four-Gland Exploration Versus 4D CT in Patients with Non-localized Primary Hyperparathyroidism

As mentioned earlier, four-gland exploration has long been the standard of care for the surgical treatment of PHPT. Recent data suggest that a more focused, or minimally invasive approach is fast becoming the "new standard". Success of the latter approach requires adequate preoperative localization on radiologic evaluation, whereas the former approach does not require such imaging. While the choice between MIP and BNE remains a matter of debate, most parathyroid surgeons would likely proceed with MIP for patients with concordant positive imaging, while reserving BNE for cases with discordant imaging. However, there exists a subset of patients with discordant imaging (U/S and SeS)—to date, the management of such patients is not standardized.

Given that up to 70% of cases with discordant imaging still have single-gland disease [19], there is the possibility that a focused approach could be undertaken in many patients, pending some other means of preoperative localization (i.e. 4DCT). The other option would be to proceed straight to BNE to identify and remove the culprit gland. To date, there are no randomized trials comparing MIP to BNE in patients with PHPT and non-localized or discordant imaging. In an effort to assess the role of 4DCT in patients with negative or discordant preoperative U/S and SeS studies, Lubitz et al. [20] retrospectively reviewed 60 patients with PHPT and discordant preoperative U/S and SeS who underwent both localization with 4DCT and operative intervention by an experienced endocrine surgeon. These authors found that 4DCT correctly lateralized and localized the abnormal parathyroid gland(s) in 76 and 60% of cases, respectively. Although the majority of these patients underwent bilateral neck exploration (as per convention for non-localizing imaging), 4DCT imaging allowed for a focused approach in 34% of patients who would have otherwise undergone BNE. The authors concluded that 4DCT identifies patients amenable to focused intervention in more than half of the patients with negative (or discordant) U/S and SeS.

Summary of Recommendations

Preoperative Localization of Abnormal Parathyroid Glands in Primary Hyperparathyroidism

4DCT has higher sensitivity and specificity over U/S or SeS in the preoperative localization of abnormal parathyroid glands, and therefore may be considered as a first-line imaging choice for patients undergoing MIP, in centers/institutions where this modality is readily available (evidence quality strong; strong recommendation). The combination of U/S + SeS, when studies are concordant, serve as adequate localization prior to surgical intervention (evidence quality strong; strong recommendation). In cases of known multigland disease, or genetic causes of PHPT preoperative imaging for localization purposes are not necessary (evidence quality moderate; moderate recommendation) (Table 16.4).

Unilateral Versus Bilateral Neck Exploration for Primary Hyperparathyroidism

A combined imaging strategy of either U/S + sestamibi, U/S + 4DCT, or U/S + sestamibi ± 4DCT are the most cost effective strategies for preoperative localization in patients with PHPT (evidence quality moderate; moderate recommendation). Direct BNE is the most expensive approach, and should be limited to patients with known multigland disease, including those with genetic endocrine disorders (evidence quality moderate; moderate recommendation).

Four-Gland Exploration Versus 4D CT in Patients with Non-localized Primary Hyperparathyroidism

There are no randomized clinical trials comparing 4DCT as a third imaging study prior to parathyroidectomy, versus direct four-gland exploration without further imaging in patients with PHPT and negative or discordant preoperative U/S and SeS scanning. However 4DCT imaging may be beneficial in the subset of patients with PHPT and negative or discordant U/S and SeS. Future studies on the comparative effectiveness of these two surgical strategies are warranted.

Conclusion

We discuss the perioperative management of patients with PHPT and discordant preoperative imaging, specifically the use of preoperative four-dimensional computed tomography (4DCT) versus direct, four gland exploration in patients with negative sestamibi and/or neck ultrasound studies. While there are no prospective, randomized clinical trials comparing these two surgical strategies, a substantial amount of useful information can inferred from the current literature on this topic. The recommendations for preoperative localization strategies prior to focused parathyroidectomy are largely straightforward. Controversy remains regarding the best approach to operative management in patients with PHPT and discordant or negative U/S and SeS. Because this issue is of both clinical and economic significance, future randomized trials are necessary to determine how to best manage these patients.

A Personal View of the Data

We routinely use 4DCT as a preoperative imaging strategy for patients undergoing parathyroidectomy for PHPT. If referred patients have already undergone U/S and SeS, with positive concordant studies, then such patients proceed to MIP (in the absence of concomitant thyroid disease). However, if imaging is discordant, or if referral patients have only undergone one prior non-invasive imaging study (either U/S or SeS), then those patients undergo 4DCT prior to surgical intervention. Exceptions to this strategy include patients with either renal insufficiency, known or suspected well-differentiated thyroid cancer, or contrast allergy (in the latter case, pretreatment prior to 4DCT can allow for some studies to be carried out).

If 4DCT localized the abnormal parathyroid gland, then patients undergo a MIP; in cases of non-localization with 4DCT, or concern for multigland disease, patients either undergo a focused approach with the possibility to conversion to bilateral neck exploration, or proceed directly with BNE. The operative strategy for this subset of patients is made on a case-by-case basis, and involves several factors including (but not limited to) preoperative serum calcium and intact PTH (iPTH) levels, as well as a thorough review of all imaging studies undertaken. Additionally, we use intraoperative PTH monitoring as an adjunct to surgery for all cases, both MIP and four-gland exploratory procedures.

The major criticism of the routine use of 4DCT is its relatively high radiation dose and risk of subsequent cancer. However many authors have demonstrated radiation doses that are comparable to that obtained with SeS. Furthermore, reductions in radiation dose with modified 4DCT imaging may be attainable as more refined reconstruction techniques become available (Tables 16.5, 16.6, and 16.7).

Table 16.5 Recommendations for preoperative localization of abnormal parathyroid glands in primary hyperparathyroidism

• 4DCT has higher sensitivity and specificity over U/S or SeS in the preoperative localization of abnormal parathyroid glands, and therefore may be considered as a first-line imaging choice for patients undergoing MIP, in centers/institutions where this modality is readily available
• 4DCT should not be used in patients with suspected or definitive thyroid carcinoma, renal insufficiency, or in those allergic to intravenous contrast
• The combination of U/S + SeS, when studies are concordant, serve as adequate localization prior to surgical intervention
• In cases of known multigland disease, or genetic causes of PHPT preoperative imaging for localization purposes are not necessary
• A combined imaging strategy of either U/S + sestamibi, U/S + 4DCT, or U/S + sestamibi ± 4DCT are the most cost effective strategies for preoperative localization in patients with PHPT

Table 16.6 Recommendations for unilateral versus bilateral neck exploration for primary hyperparathyroidism

• Both bilateral, or four-gland exploration, and minimally invasive parathyroidectomy yield excellent cure rates and minimal complication rates, when performed by an experienced surgeon
• Bilateral cervical exploration is the ideal operation for most patients with multigland disease, including those with genetic disease
• Minimally invasive parathyroidectomy procedures are not recommended in centers that do not have sophisticated imaging, intraoperative PTH assays, and experienced endocrine surgeons
• Intraoperative PTH assays are useful adjuncts during parathyroid surgery, and are essential, if focused approaches are employed
• Although minimally invasive techniques have become increasingly adopted, all parathyroid surgeons must be able to perform a standard bilateral cervical exploration, in the event that occult multigland disease is present

Table 16.7 Recommendations for Four-gland exploration versus 4D CT in patients with non-localized primary hyperparathyroidism

• 4DCT imaging may be beneficial in the subset of patients with PHPT and negative or discordant U/S and SeS
• Future studies on the comparative effectiveness of these two surgical strategies are warranted

References

1. Rodgers SE, Hunter GJ, Hamberg LM, Schellingerhout D, Doherty DB, Ayers GD, et al. Improved preoperative planning for directed parathyroidectomy with 4-dimensional computed tomography. Surgery. 2006;140(6):932–40. Discussion 40-1.
2. Starker LF, Mahajan A, Bjorklund P, Sze G, Udelsman R, Carling T. 4D parathyroid CT as the initial localization study for patients with de novo primary hyperparathyroidism. Ann Surg Oncol. 2011;18(6):1723–8.
3. Cheung K, Wang TS, Farrokhyar F, Roman SA, Sosa JA. A meta-analysis of preoperative localization techniques for patients with primary hyperparathyroidism. Ann Surg Oncol. 2012;19(2):577–83.
4. Suh YJ, Choi JY, Kim SJ, Chun IK, Yun TJ, Lee KE, et al. Comparison of 4D CT, ultrasonography, and 99mTc Sestamibi SPECT/CT in localizing single-gland primary hyperparathyroidism. Otolaryngol Head Neck Surg. 2014;18:1723–8.
5. Kukar M, Platz TA, Schaffner TJ, Elmarzouky R, Groman A, Kumar S, et al. The use of modified four-dimensional computed tomography in patients with primary hyperparathyroidism: an argument for the abandonment of routine sestamibi single-positron emission computed tomography (SPECT). Ann Surg Oncol. 2015;22(1):139–45.
6. Wang TS, Cheung K, Farrokhyar F, Roman SA, Sosa JA. Would scan, but which scan? A cost-utility analysis to optimize preoperative imaging for primary hyperparathyroidism. Surgery. 2011;150(6):1286–94.
7. Lubitz CC, Stephen AE, Hodin RA, Pandharipande P. Preoperative localization strategies for primary hyperparathyroidism: an economic analysis. Ann Surg Oncol. 2012;19(13):4202–9.
8. Miccoli P, Bendinelli C, Berti P, Vignali E, Pinchera A, Marcocci C. Video-assisted versus conventional parathyroidectomy in primary hyperparathyroidism: a prospective randomized study. Surgery. 1999;126(6):1117–21. Discussion 21-2.
9. Miccoli P, Berti P, Materazzi G, Ambrosini CE, Fregoli L, Donatini G. Endoscopic bilateral neck exploration versus quick intraoperative parathormone assay (qPTHa) during endoscopic parathyroidectomy: a prospective randomized trial. Surg Endosc. 2008;22(2):398–400.
10. Bergenfelz A, Lindblom P, Tibblin S, Westerdahl J. Unilateral versus bilateral neck exploration for primary hyperparathyroidism: a prospective randomized controlled trial. Ann Surg. 2002;236(5):543–51.
11. Westerdahl J, Bergenfelz A. Unilateral versus bilateral neck exploration for primary hyperparathyroidism: five-year follow-up of a randomized controlled trial. Ann Surg. 2007;246(6):976–80. Discussion 80-1.
12. Bergenfelz A, Kanngiesser V, Zielke A, Nies C, Rothmund M. Conventional bilateral cervical exploration versus open minimally invasive parathyroidectomy under local anaesthesia for primary hyperparathyroidism. Br J Surg. 2005;92(2):190–7.
13. Slepavicius A, Beisa V, Janusonis V, Strupas K. Focused versus conventional parathyroidectomy for primary hyperparathyroidism: a prospective, randomized, blinded trial. Langenbeck's Arch Surg. 2008;393(5):659–66.
14. Aarum S, Nordenstrom J, Reihner E, Zedenius J, Jacobsson H, Danielsson R, et al. Operation for primary hyperparathyroidism: the new versus the old order. A randomised controlled trial of preoperative localisation. Scand J Surg. 2007;96(1):26–30.
15. Sozio A, Schietroma M, Franchi L, Mazzotta C, Cappelli S, Amicucci G. Parathyroidectomy: bilateral exploration of the neck vs minimally invasive radioguided treatment. Minerva Chir. 2005;60(2):83–9.

16. Russell CF, Dolan SJ, Laird JD. Randomized clinical trial comparing scan-directed unilateral versus bilateral cervical exploration for primary hyperparathyroidism due to solitary adenoma. Br J Surg. 2006;93(4):418–21.
17. Udelsman R, Lin Z, Donovan P. The superiority of minimally invasive parathyroidectomy based on 1650 consecutive patients with primary hyperparathyroidism. Ann Surg. 2011;253(3):585–91.
18. Udelsman R, Akerstrom G, Biagini C, Duh QY, Miccoli P, Niederle B, et al. The surgical management of asymptomatic primary hyperparathyroidism: proceedings of the fourth international workshop. J Clin Endocrinol Metab. 2014;99(10):3595–606.
19. Philippon M, Guerin C, Taieb D, Vaillant J, Morange I, Brue T, et al. Bilateral neck exploration in patients with primary hyperparathyroidism and discordant imaging results: a single-centre study. Eur J Endocrinol. 2014;170(5):719–25.
20. Lubitz CC, Hunter GJ, Hamberg LM, Parangi S, Ruan D, Gawande A, et al. Accuracy of 4-dimensional computed tomography in poorly localized patients with primary hyperparathyroidism. Surgery. 2010;148(6):1129–37. Discussion 37-8.

Lymph Node Dissection Versus No Lymph Node Dissection for Parathyroid Cancer

17

Reese W. Randle and David F. Schneider

Abstract

Surgery is the primary treatment for parathyroid carcinoma, but no consensus statement exists regarding the optimal extent of the initial resection. Given the rare nature of the disease, the literature is almost entirely limited to retrospective reviews, but was used in an attempt to determine the impact a routine central neck dissection has on recurrence, survival, and complications in patients being treated for parathyroid carcinoma. Nodal metastases do seem to predict recurrence but not worse survival. However, no clear difference was observed in recurrence or survival based on whether or not a lymph node dissection was performed indicating that there is minimal value in a nodal dissection as a routine procedure in all patients. While the addition of a central neck dissection does not increase rates of vocal cord palsies or hematomas, it does carry a significant risk of permanent hypoparathyroidism. Therefore, because there is no definitive benefit in patients with parathyroid carcinoma, the added risk of a routine central node dissection is not justified for all patients.

Keywords

Parathyroid cancer · Central compartment lymph node dissection · Lymph node metastases · Parathyroidectomy · Neck exploration

R. W. Randle
Section of Endocrine Surgery, Department of Surgery, University of Kentucky, Lexington, KY, USA

D. F. Schneider (✉)
Section of Endocrine Surgery, Department of Surgery, University of Wisconsin, Madison, WI, USA
e-mail: schneiderd@surgery.wisc.edu

P. Angelos, R. H. Grogan (eds.), *Difficult Decisions in Endocrine Surgery*, Difficult Decisions in Surgery: An Evidence-Based Approach,
https://doi.org/10.1007/978-3-319-92860-9_17

Introduction

Parathyroid carcinoma is rare affecting less than one person per million people, and accounting for merely 0.005% of all malignancies diagnosed in the United States each year [1, 2]. However, the incidence is increasing, and for patients undergoing parathyroidectomy for primary hyperparathyroidism the reported incidence of parathyroid cancer has ranged from 0.5 to 5.3% [1, 3–17]. The treatment for parathyroid carcinoma is primarily surgical, but the optimal extent of resection is controversial. Retrospective reviews have failed to demonstrate a consistent link between lymph node metastases and survival, and as a result, some investigators question whether central neck dissection is necessary in the treatment of patients with parathyroid cancer and clinically negative nodes. A PICO format question, designed to address this controversy, is the focus of the current chapter [18] (Table 17.1). In other words, this chapter aims to review the impact routine central lymph node dissection has on disease recurrence, long-term survival, and complication rates for patients with parathyroid carcinoma.

Current Recommendations

In order to more fully understand the controversy at hand, a general knowledge of the current treatment strategies for parathyroid carcinoma is necessary. Surgery is the mainstay of treatment for patients with parathyroid carcinoma. Chemotherapy has added little to no benefit in terms of disease control, biochemical response, or survival [15, 19–23]. Radiotherapy has also been employed without a clear improvement in outcomes [1, 24–28]. This leaves surgery as the best and only hope for cure in patients with parathyroid cancer. No consensus exists, however, as to the ideal extent of surgery. Certainly, en bloc resection of the tumor keeps with sound oncologic principles and avoids tumor rupture. Furthermore, local excision is more likely to result in positive margins [26]. Unfortunately, many parathyroid cancers are locally excised when the surgeon believes it to be an adenoma and only realizes the tumor was malignant upon receiving the final pathology report. Some retrospective studies have demonstrated a link between the extent of the initial surgery and survival [23, 29], yet others have failed to identify a survival difference based on the initial surgery [1, 3, 5, 20, 24, 26]. Without a clear answer in the literature, prevailing opinions and institutional preferences are considered to be among the main influences determining the extent of the initial surgery [20]. In general, en bloc resection of the tumor with the ipsilateral thyroid, isthmus, involved strap muscles,

Table 17.1 PICO table

Population	Patients with parathyroid carcinoma
Intervention	Routine central lymph node dissection
Comparator	No lymph node dissection
Outcome	Recurrence, survival, and complications

and central lymph node compartment is recommended [2, 14, 28, 30–32]. A modified radical lymph node dissection is not merited as a routine [9, 32, 33]. However, the value of routine central compartment node dissection in patients with clinically negative nodes remains unclear.

Furthermore, the reported prognostic importance of lymph node metastases has varied [1–3, 24–26, 31]. Due at least in part to the paucity of clear prognosticators, the American Joint Committee on Cancer nor the National Comprehensive Cancer Network have developed a staging system for parathyroid cancer. At least two proposed TNM staging systems include lymph node status as a component, but their correlation with recurrence and survival has varied [3, 26, 31, 34]. Neither has been universally adopted. Thus recommendations for the optimal surgical treatment of parathyroid carcinoma remain ambiguous especially concerning the central lymph nodes.

Difficulty in Diagnosis

Regardless of the recommended surgical treatment, proper handling of parathyroid carcinoma requires pre- and intra-operative recognition. An accurate and timely diagnosis may prevent a simple excision as would be the preferred treatment for the majority of benign parathyroid pathology. Imaging is not consistently reliable, and no specific tumor marker exists. Markedly elevated parathyroid hormone and calcium levels may suggest a diagnosis preoperatively. Tumor adherence to surrounding tissue is a helpful sign and may allow proper recognition [28]. Also, parathyroid cancers may be gray and hard. While vocal cord paralysis and a palpable cervical mass in a patient with presumed primary hyperparathyroidism are concerning signs that make a diagnosis of cancer highly likely, the rate of patients presenting with a neck mass is decreasing [6, 8, 20, 23, 27, 33, 35, 36]. Large tumor size is another concerning feature. In one study, carcinomas were 3.8 cm on average compared with 1.7 cm for adenomas or hyperplastic glands ($P = 0.03$) [37]. However, tumor size is also decreasing [1, 37]. Earlier detection of parathyroid cancer with calcium screening and parathyroid hormone assays may be responsible for these trends [8, 35]. There is no question that timely recognition of parathyroid cancer affects the procedure that is ultimately undertaken [2, 20, 25, 28, 29]. Therefore, a high index of suspicion is key in treating patients with hyperparathyroidism so that the appropriate operation is performed.

Current Practice

The very low incidence of parathyroid cancer, the ambiguity of current recommendations, and the difficulty in obtaining a timely diagnosis are reflected in the great variability with which patients are currently being treated. The proportion of patients receiving an en bloc resection as their initial operation has ranged from 5 to 78%, however, population based data indicates this number is actually closer to the lower end (5–11%) [1, 3, 22, 25, 26, 29, 31, 38]. Although institutional rates of central node dissection vary greatly (Table 17.2), only about a third of patients receive a lymph node evaluation as a part of their initial surgery [1–3, 5, 6, 8, 10, 25, 26, 28, 31, 32, 36]. The rate of node positivity is also quite variable, yet overall, lymph node metastases are an uncommon feature of parathyroid carcinoma. Taken as a whole, lymph node involvement is identified in less than one-sixth of patients with a node dissection. When considering the fact that most patients being treated for parathyroid cancer do not get a nodal evaluation, the rate of known lymph node metastases in all patients is less than 5%, although this value does not capture patients with lymph node metastases who did not get a lymph node dissection at their initial operation (Table 17.2).

Another important consideration involves the trouble in defining parathyroid carcinoma. The definition of parathyroid cancer has not only been difficult to develop but also has changed over time [17, 34, 39]. The validity of findings derived from population-based datasets depends on the accuracy of coding "parathyroid cancer." For example, inclusion of atypical adenomas or parathyromatosis could falsely decrease the overall incidence of lymph node metastases. On the other hand, calculating rates of nodal metastases from a collection of case reports might potentially falsely increase the incidence given that surgeons may be less likely to report early, unremarkable cancers diagnosed and treated appropriately [31].

Overall Outcomes

Despite the discrepancies in what is recommended and what is actually being done, disease specific survival is relatively good at 91–94% at 5 years and 69–90% at 10 years [1, 3, 25]. Because many patients with parathyroid carcinoma do not actually die from tumor burden but from the metabolic effects of hypercalcemia, they may not always get properly coded as having died from parathyroid carcinoma. Overall survival may capture more cancer-specific deaths, but this obviously becomes difficult to distinguish in large datasets. Overall survival has ranged from 78 to 86% at 5 years and 49–70% at 10 years [2, 21, 24, 25, 29]. Recurrence is quite variable, ranging from 33 to 86%, although some of the institutions reporting the higher rates may be influenced by referral bias [15, 19, 21, 22, 24, 29, 31, 38]. Reoperations in the neck for recurrence are common as locoregional recurrence constitutes 58–92% of the overall recurrence rates in larger studies [3, 15, 29, 31, 32].

Complication rates for the treatment of parathyroid carcinoma are also considerable. Nearly 45–60% of patients will experience a complication during their treatment including vocal cord paralysis in 18–38%, temporary hypocalcemia in 22–34%, and permanent hypocalcemia in 5.4% [24, 32]. Perioperative mortality can be as high as 1.8% [24]. Less frequently observed but important perioperative complications include hematoma, jugular venous thrombosis, esophageal injury, fluid collection, and wound infections [24, 32].

Table 17.2 Incidence of lymph node dissections and lymph node metastases in patients with parathyroid carcinoma

Study	Patient population	Total No. of patients	No. (%) of patients with LN dissection	No. of patients with LN metastases	% of patients with LND that have LN metastases	% of all patients that have known LN metastases[a]
Hsu et al. [25]	SEER, 1988–2010	405	114 (28.1)	12	10.5	3.0
Sadler et al. [26]	NCDB, 1998–2011	1022	295 (28.9)	23	7.8	2.3
Villar del Moral et al. [3]	Spain- multicenter 1980–2013	62	20 (32.3)	8	40.0	12.9
Schulteet al. [38]	International- multicenter	82	64 (78.0)	8	12.5	9.8
Schulteet al. [32]	United Kingdom-single institution, 2005–2009	11	11 (100)	1	9.1	9.0
Talat and Schulte [31]	Collection of case reviews, 1961–2009	330	43 (13.0)	27	62.8	8.2
Fernandez-Ranvieret al. [36]	United States- single institution, 1966–2005	28	3 (10.7)	5	100.0	17.9
Iihara et al. [5]	Japan- single institution, 1981–2005	38	22 (57.9)	3	13.6	7.9
Ippolito et al. [8]	France- single institution, 1974–2005	11	7 (63.6)	0	0	0
Lee et al. [1]	SEER, 1988–2003	224	150 (67.0)	9	6.0	4.0
Pelizzo et al. [10]	Italy- single institution, 1980–2000	17	2 (11.8)	0	0	0
Hundahl et al. [2]	NCDB, 1985–1995	286	105 (36.7)	16	15.2	5.6
Cordeiroet al. [28]	Brazil- single institution, 1970–1995	9	2 (18.2)	1	50.0	11.1
Wang andGaz [6]	United States- single institution, 1948–1983	28	4 (14.3)	1	25.0	3.6
Totals[b]		2553	842 (33.0)	114	13.5	4.5

LN Lymph Node, *LND* Lymph Node Dissection, *SEER* Surveillance, Epidemiology and End Results Registry, *NCDB* National Cancer Database

[a]Does not capture patients with LN metastases that did not get a LND

[b]Some patient data may be duplicated in the totals

The impact a central lymph node dissection has on recurrence, survival, and complications becomes difficult to discern especially considering the variations in the treatment of patients with parathyroid cancer. Nevertheless, a careful appraisal of the literature within the context of its limitations is important in order to understand the value of a central compartment node dissection in this disease.

Outcomes with and Without Central Lymph Node Dissection

All available data regarding lymph node dissections in patients with parathyroid carcinoma is retrospective in nature. Given this fact, one might expect a selection bias to be a major determining factor in which patients did and did not get a central lymph node dissection as a component of their operation for parathyroid carcinoma. Perhaps more concerning disease may have alerted the surgeon pre- or intraoperatively to proceed with a more extensive initial operation. However, using population based data to compare patients that did and did not receive a lymph node dissection, Hsu et al. were unable to identify any differences between the two groups in terms of age, gender, diagnostic period, tumor size, the presence of local invasion, or the presence of metastases [25]. Similarly, Talat and Schulte did not observe any difference in pathologic features based on the type of procedure performed [31]. Even though patients receiving and not receiving a central lymph node dissection appear to be similar cohorts in terms of demographics and tumor characteristics, the presence of a significant selection bias cannot be entirely ruled out. Retrospective data does not capture the operating surgeon's thought process, degree of suspicion, or threshold to perform a lymph node dissection. Nor do retrospective databases have variables describing the extent of local invasion or dense adherence to surrounding tissue. Therefore, comparisons between these two groups must be made allowing the possibility that more extensive disease might be clustered in the lymph node dissection group.

Recurrence

Both locoregional and distant recurrence are independent predictors of worse survival in patients with parathyroid carcinoma [3]. Survival worsens as the number of cervical recurrences increases [24]. While it stands to reason that a more extensive initial resection would decrease recurrence, actual reports vary. Many studies show higher recurrence after parathyroidectomy alone compared with en bloc resection [5, 23, 31], but not all [24]. En bloc resection resulted in fewer reoperations (32% versus 65%) when compared with local excision according data from cases gathered by Talat and Schulte [31]. Few studies specifically evaluated the impact of nodal dissection on recurrence. Villar del Moral et al. [3] found that performing a nodal dissection had no discernable effect on disease recurrence in a multicenter review of 62 patients [3]. In their review of 330 case reports, Talat and Schulte [31] did observe higher recurrence at 5 years and overall in patients who did not receive a systematic lymph node dissection, although this latter group included both patients that received an en bloc resection without a node dissection as well as patients who simply underwent local excision. They suggest that high locoregional recurrence rates in patients following a resection with negative margins may be explained by the presence of occult nodal disease. In comparing patients getting an en bloc resection with or without node dissection, however, the number of reoperations for recurrence appeared similar, possibly indicating that the addition of a lymph node dissection did not decrease recurrence relative to an en bloc resection alone [31]. Additionally, patterns of initial recurrence indicate that recurrence in the cervical lymph nodes occurs infrequently (Table 17.3). For example, in a review of 95 cases of parathyroid cancer, Sandelin et al. [29] observed a recurrence rate of 42% requiring a range of reoperations from 1 to 9 in 36 patients. Lymph node metastases only accounted for three of these initial recurrences with the majority occurring elsewhere in the neck (n = 30) or the lungs (n = 9) [29]. These data suggest that occult nodal disease is not a major contributor to the high recurrence rates experienced by patients with parathyroid carcinoma.

While it does seem that lymph node metastases do predict higher recurrence rates, the evidence is not overwhelming. Unfortunately, population-based data generally lacks reliable recurrence information. In a single institution review of 37 patients, Harari et al. [24] found that lymph node metastases were a significant predictor of recurrence as did Talat and Schulte in their collection of case reports [31]. In a multicenter retrospective review by Villar del Moral et al. [3] nodal metastases were associated with recurrence on univariate analysis but not after controlling for other significant predictors of recurrence [3]. Given that the later review included only eight patients with lymph node metastases compared with the 27 in the review by Talat and Schulte, it seems that Villar del Moral et al. may have lacked the numbers necessary to identify higher recurrence in patients with lymph node metastases [3, 31]. Several even smaller studies have implicated lymph node metastases as a marker for recurrence. Fernandez-Ranvier et al. [36] reported recurrence in 5 out of 5 patients that presented with lymph node metastases [36]. In a review by Iihara et al. [5] 3 of 3 patients with lymph node metastases recurred and eventually died of disease [5]. Schulte et al. [32] found that 1 of 11 patients who underwent lymph node dissections had positive lymph nodes, and this same patient recurred [32].

Overall, lymph node metastases do seem to predict recurrence, yet it remains unclear if nodal disease contributes to the mechanism of recurrence or if it simply serves as a marker for more aggressive biologic behavior. In a review of 11 patients, Schulte et al. [32] found two lymph nodes that contained metastatic parathyroid cancer but only one was distinct from the large inflammatory mass that contained the primary tumor. They also observed that surgeons harvest fewer nodes from the central compartment in lymph node dissections for parathyroid cancer compared to thyroid cancer, and they suggest it may be because the contents of the central compartment were replaced by the tumor itself [32]. Thus, nodal disease likely reflects locoregional spread of disease rather than true lymphatic metastases. Given that the majority of locoregional recurrence does not involve the lymph nodes

Table 17.3 Initial recurrence patterns in patients with parathyroid carcinoma

Study	No. ofpatients, n	Lymph nodedissection, n (%)	Positivenodes, n (%)	Overallrecurrence, n (%)	Locoregional recurrence			Distant recurrence			
					Overall	Cervical	Lymphnodes	Overall	Lung	Bone	Other
Villar del Moralet al. [3]	62	20	8	14 (18.6)	13	10	3	3	0	3	0
Lee et al. [16]	7	NR	NR	1 (14.3)	0	0	0	1	1	0	0
Schulte et al. [32]	11	11	1	1 (9.1)	1	1	0	0	0	0	0
Talat and Schulte[31, 32]	330	43	27	207[a] (62.7)	97	26	19	100	67	16	27
Agarwal et al. [7]	4	NR	NR	3 (75.0)	2	2	1	1	0	0	1
Cordeiro et al. [28]	9	2	1	5 (55.6)	5	5	0	3	3	1	0
Sandelin et al. [29]	95	2	NR	40 (42.1)	–	30	3	–	9	2	0
Wynne et al. [15]	43	NR	NR	29[b] (67.4)	19	–	–	9	2	0	7

NR not reported
[a]Sites of recurrence only known for 166 (80%)
[b]Sites of recurrence only known in 25

(Table 17.3), the role lymphatic dissemination plays in recurrence is questionable. Tumor rupture may result in dissemination throughout the operative field and is likely responsible for many local recurrences [2, 22, 29]. Direct or discontinuous extensions of the cancer may be another mechanism responsible for locoregional recurrence [32]. Vascular invasion is another independent predictor of recurrence and likely a predominant mechanism of cancer dissemination [31, 38]. Hematogenous spread from vascular invasion may explain reports of distant metastases in patients without documented nodal disease. These data, together with the fact that nodal recurrence is uncommon, suggest that lymphatic spread is not a major contributor in the dissemination of parathyroid carcinoma but simply an important marker for recurrence.

Survival

As with recurrence, the available literature is somewhat contradictory regarding the impact of a nodal dissection on survival in patients with parathyroid carcinoma. Villar del Moral et al. [3] found that a lymph node dissection did not affect survival. Similarly, Lee et al. [1] and Sadler et al. [26] using the Surveillance, Epidemiology, and End Results (SEER) registry and National Cancer Database (NCDB), respectively, found that unknown nodal disease did not predict worse survival when compared to patients with known negative nodes [1, 26]. In fact, survival was similar between patients with no nodal dissection and those with known negative nodes after adjusting for other significant predictors of survival [26]. Hsu et al. [25], who also used SEER data, did not find any difference in rates of metastases and death between patients who did and did not have lymph nodes examined [25]. In an earlier NCDB study, Hundhal et al. reported generally similar 5-year overall survival between patients with negative nodes (83.3%) and unknown nodal status (86.7%). In contrast, Talat and Schulte [31] identified the omission of a systematic lymph node dissection as a significant predictor of 5-year mortality but not overall mortality. The reason for the discrepancies between Talat and Schultes' systematic review and population-based data from the United States is not immediately apparent. Talat and Schulte [31] used data from previously published case reports to construct their cohort of 330 cases of parathyroid carcinoma. A lymph node dissection was performed in 13% of the entire cohort, and lymph node metastases were observed in 62% of those undergoing lymph node dissection [31]. This is in contrast to the studies using population based data by Sadler and Hsu which both reported lymph node dissections in about 28%, and rates of nodal metastases nearly one-sixth that reported by Talat and Schulte [25, 26, 31]. In light of their unique method of collecting data, Talat and Schulte [31] suggest that a reporting bias may have skewed their results [31]. While all of the studies may be biased by the nonrandom selection of those who received a central node dissection, similar tumor size and similar rates of local invasion and metastases in the groups with and without lymph node evaluations would argue against a significant selection bias [25].

Even if a lymph node dissection does not have a clear impact on survival, it is important to investigate if lymph node metastases predict worse survival in patients with parathyroid carcinoma. While some investigators found that positive lymph nodes confer worse survival [3, 23, 24, 26, 31] others found this not to be the case [1, 2, 25]. However, due to the infrequency of lymph node metastases, small numbers were an unavoidable limitation in all reports (Table 17.4). The reported hazard ratios comparing mortality in patients with positive lymph nodes to those with known negative nodes ranged from 2.8 to 16.3. In addition to the wide range in risk, the confidence intervals also were quite large indicating the wide variability and imprecision that exists within the literature for this disease [1, 3, 24–26, 31]. This makes it difficult to really indicate the magnitude of risk lymph node metastases have on disease-specific mortality. Taken as a whole, it seems that the presence of lymph node metastases is a marker of more advanced disease and recurrence, but there is not sufficient evidence to consider it a marker of worse survival in all patients presenting with parathyroid cancer. There may be a subset of patients, however, for whom lymph node metastases may confer worse survival. Hsu et al. [25] reported a 7.5 times greater incidence in lymph node metastases in patients with tumors measuring over 3 cm (21% versus 2.8%, $p = 0.02$) [25]. Their findings indicate that it may be possible to identify patients who would be more likely to benefit from the prognostic value of a central neck lymphadenectomy as a component of their initial resection. Besides size, there may be other variables that would aid in the risk stratification of patients who would benefit from a more aggressive resection and allow surgeons to tailor a patient specific approach to the optimal extent of surgery.

Due to the conflicting data regarding the prognostic importance of nodal metastases, attempts to incorporate lymph node status into a staging system are not widely accepted. Lee et al. [1] compared survival based on SEER historic stage and found that unstaged patients (presumably for lack of lymph node or other metastatic data) experienced similar survival to patients with localized disease [1]. Both Shaha and Shah [34] and Talat and Schulte [31] proposed TNM staging systems. In Shaha and Shah's system lymph node metastases equated to stage IIIc [34]. In an attempt to validate Shaha and Shah's system, Talat and Schulte found that higher stages (III and IV) did not reliably correlate with worse survival than lower stages (I and II) where lymph nodes were uninvolved. In light of this, they introduced their own TNM staging system where both lymph node metastases and invasion of vital organs were considered stage III disease [31, 38]. They reported that unstagable patients, often due to lack of a lymph node evaluation, experienced survival worse those assigned stage III but better than stage IV, and suggested that unstaged patients are likely being under treated. In a more simplified risk classification system also developed by Talat and Schulte [31], patients are categorized into low or high risk categories with the presence of lymph node metastases placing patients in the high risk category even in the absence of other prognostic features [31]. In contrast to the findings by Talat and Schulte, Sadler et al. [26], reported that patients with unknown lymph node status experienced survival that was more akin to that seen in Shulte's low risk category. They

Table 17.4 Impact of lymph node metastases on survival in patients with parathyroid carcinoma

Study	Patient population	No. of patients with node dissection	No. of patients with negative nodes	No. of patients with positive nodes	Hazard ratio (95% confidence interval) Positive nodes versus Negative nodes	P
Hsu et al. [25]	SEER, 1988–2010	114	102	12	3.72[a] (0.5–26.4)	0.19
Sadler et al. [26]	NCDB, 1998–2011	295	272	23	6.47[b] (1.8–23.1)	0.004
Villar del Moral et al. [3]	Spain- multicenter1980–2013	20	12	8	16.3[a] (1.7–87.4)	0.01
Harari et al. [24]	United States- single institution, 1966–2009	NR	NR	NR	4.27[b] (1.2–15.3)	<0.05
Talat and Schulte [31]	Collection of case reviews, 1961–2009	43	16	27	6.16[b,c] (0.9–42.9)	<0.01
Lee et al. [1]	SEER, 1988–2003	150	141	9	2.84[b] (NR)	0.23
Koea and Shaw [23]	Collection of case reviews, 1933–1999	NR	NR	10	NR	<0.001

SEER Surveillance Epidemiology and End Results Registry, *NCDB* National Cancer Database, *NR* Not Reported
[a]Risk of disease specific mortality
[b]Risk of overall mortality
[c]Derived from a univariate analysis

suggest that there is insufficient evidence to recommend a prophylactic central node dissection for patients with clinically negative nodes [26]. Because lymph node metastases are not a common feature in patients with parathyroid carcinoma, it is possible that the impact patients with retained occult nodal metastases have on prognosis is negligible within the large cohort of patients without a lymph node evaluation. This further emphasizes the importance of targeting a select high-risk cohort who may benefit from the added node dissection. Taken as a whole however, the population of patients with parathyroid carcinoma and clinically negative nodes stands to benefit very little from a central node dissection. Therefore, in the absence of a therapeutic benefit and with prognostic value limited to predicting recurrence, routine central compartment lymphadenectomy must be considered within the context of its risks.

Complications

Any potential benefit achieved with a central node dissection in patients with parathyroid carcinoma must be carefully weighed against the risk of en bloc resection of the mass alone. There is a general lack of data comparing complications in patients with parathyroid carcinoma receiving en bloc resection with or without central neck dissection, but a relative wealth of retrospective data concerning the risks of a central neck dissection exists in patients with thyroid cancer. Analyzing retrospective data, many investigators have failed to identify a significant difference in vocal cord palsies or hypoparathyroidism based on the addition or omission of a central node dissection in patients receiving thyroidectomies [40–42]. In a comparison of 113 patients receiving a total thyroidectomy to 119 patients receiving a total thyroidectomy with central lymph node dissection reported by So et al. [42], the addition of a node dissection did not significantly increase vocal cord palsies, hematoma, or chyle leaks. Even though their observed rate of permanent hypocalcemia was three times greater in the group that received a lymph node dissection, this difference was not statistically significant [42]. Palestini et al. [43] reported significantly higher rates of transient hypocalcemia in patients who had the addition of a node dissection to their total thyroidectomy, but long term complications were comparable between groups [43]. On the other hand, the first prospective randomized controlled trial comparing central node dissection to its omission in patients with clinically node negative papillary thyroid cancer reported a higher rate of permanent hypoparathyroidism in patients who had the central neck dissection (19.4% versus 8.0%, $p = 0.02$) indicating that routine central node dissections are not without added risk [44]. In patients with thyroid cancer getting a central compartment neck dissection, hypoparathyroidism presumably occurs from the inadvertent removal of one or more inferior parathyroid glands within the nodal tissue. In extrapolating these data to patients with parathyroid carcinoma, it is logical to expect that the risk of permanent hypoparathyroidism is equal or greater. For parathyroid cancer, one gland is already being removed. If another is removed with the nodal dissection, and the others are injured during exploration of the contralateral neck, permanent hypoparathyroidism becomes a strong possibility. However, this scenario may not occur in all parathyroid cancer cases, depending on preoperative localization studies. Therefore, total thyroidectomy is not universally comparable to operations for parathyroid cancer. Nonetheless, the most abundant data on central neck dissection comes from the thyroid cancer literature.

The risk of a central compartment dissection at the initial surgery must also be weighed within the context of reoperating for nodal disease that might later become apparent either as a recurrence or as progression of occult disease. In a study looking at complications from a central nodal dissection in a reoperative field compared to those from a central node dissection at the initial surgery, Alvarado et al. reported similar rates of vocal cord palsies, hypoparathyroidism, and wound infections [45]. These data indicate that waiting until a patient recurs before removing their central nodes is safe and spares patients who will not recur the added risk at the first operation. Furthermore, because locoregional recurrence and reoperations for such are common in patients with nodal metastases, it is unlikely that removing occult nodal disease at the first operation will spare a cervical reoperation.

Summary

Due to the retrospective nature of all of the available data, there are substantial limitations to the strength of conclusions derived in this chapter. A prospective trial comparing lymph node dissection to no lymph node dissection in patients with parathyroid carcinoma is impractical given the rarity of the disease. Data collaboratives such as the Collaborative Endocrine Surgery Quality Improvement Program will provide more abundant and uniform data on this type of rare endocrine tumor and may help direct future recommendations.

Parathyroid cancer is difficult to recognize partly due to its rare nature and similarity to benign parathyroid pathology. Surgery is the mainstay of therapy and offers the only hope for cure. A timely diagnosis affects the operation performed requiring surgeons to have a high clinical suspicion. The historically recommended operative approach is en bloc resection with adjacent tissues and the ipsilateral thyroid along with the lymph nodes of the central neck. Nodal metastases seem to be an important marker of aggressive biologic behavior and recurrence. Yet even though lymph node metastases predict higher recurrence, positive lymph nodes in parathyroid carcinoma are uncommon occurring in only 13.5% of patients with a lymph node evaluation. Furthermore, the current literature fails to identify a substantial therapeutic benefit of the inclusion of a central node dissection to an en bloc resection for parathyroid carcinoma in terms of disease recurrence or survival. The risk of permanent hypoparathyroidism is increased when a central node dissection is performed, and that risk must be weighed against the anticipated benefit of more extensive surgery. Tumor size is one factor, although there are likely other factors, that may allow surgeons to risk stratify who might benefit from a central node dissection, facilitate patient-specific treatment, and spare low-risk patients an unnecessary procedure.

Recommendations

The following recommendations are rated according to the GRADE format which takes the quality of evidence into account and assigns a grade according to the strength of the recommendation [18].

- Lymph node metastases in parathyroid carcinoma likely predict recurrence but do not definitively predict survival. Given that most patients will be enrolled in surveillance, predicting recurrence is not a sufficient indication for routine central node dissection (evidence quality low; weak recommendation).
- There is not a clear therapeutic benefit to adding a central node dissection to an en bloc resection in patients with clinically node negative parathyroid cancer as a whole, therefore routine central node dissection should not be performed. Certain patient subsets may benefit from central neck dissection, but further study is required to help surgeons risk stratify patients. (evidence quality low; weak recommendation).
- Locoregional recurrence is common and dominated by soft tissue involvement rather than nodal involvement. A central neck dissection performed during a cervical reoperation for recurrence may be performed safely if indicated (evidence quality low; weak recommendation).
- Patients with parathyroid cancers greater than 3 cm are more likely to have lymph node metastases and may benefit from a central node dissection (evidence quality low; weak recommendation).

Conclusions

Parathyroid carcinoma is rare but its incidence is increasing. Although lymph node metastases predict recurrence, nodal involvement is rare and routine central node dissections are not without complications. Furthermore, patients who do not receive a central node dissection as a component of their initial resection seem to have similar recurrence and survival compared with those that do. Subjecting all patients with parathyroid carcinoma to the risks of a routine central node dissection when the available literature cannot identify a therapeutic benefit is not justified. Future investigations may however, identify a more targeted cohort of patients with parathyroid carcinoma for which a central node dissection is indicated.

References

1. Lee PK, Jarosek SL, Virnig BA, Evasovich M, Tuttle TM. Trends in the incidence and treatment of parathyroid cancer in the United States. Cancer. 2007;109(9):1736–41.
2. Hundahl SA, Fleming ID, Fremgen AM, Menck HR. Two hundred eighty-six cases of parathyroid carcinoma treated in the U.S. between 1985–1995: a National Cancer Data Base Report. The American College of Surgeons Commission on cancer and the American Cancer Society. Cancer. 1999;86(3):538–44.

3. Villar-Del-Moral J, Jimenez-Garcia A, Salvador-Egea P, Martos-Martinez JM, Nuno-Vazquez-Garza JM, Serradilla-Martin M, et al. Prognostic factors and staging systems in parathyroid cancer: a multicenter cohort study. Surgery. 2014;156(5):1132–44.
4. Ruda JM, Hollenbeak CS, Stack BC Jr. A systematic review of the diagnosis and treatment of primary hyperparathyroidism from 1995 to 2003. Otolaryngol Head Neck Surg. 2005;132(3):359–72.
5. Iihara M, Okamoto T, Suzuki R, Kawamata A, Nishikawa T, Kobayashi M, et al. Functional parathyroid carcinoma: long-term treatment outcome and risk factor analysis. Surgery. 2007;142(6):936–43.
6. Wang CA, Gaz RD. Natural history of parathyroid carcinoma. Diagnosis, treatment, and results. Am J Surg. 1985;149(4):522–7.
7. Agarwal G, Prasad KK, Kar DK, Krishnani N, Pandey R, Mishra SK. Indian primary hyperparathyroidism patients with parathyroid carcinoma do not differ in clinicoinvestigative characteristics from those with benign parathyroid pathology. World J Surg. 2006;30(5):732–42.
8. Ippolito G, Palazzo FF, Sebag F, De MC, Henry JF. Intraoperative diagnosis and treatment of parathyroid cancer and atypical parathyroid adenoma. Br J Surg. 2007;94(5):566–70.
9. Cohn K, Silverman M, Corrado J, Sedgewick C. Parathyroid carcinoma: the Lahey clinic experience. Surgery. 1985;98(6):1095–100.
10. Pelizzo MR, Piotto A, Bergamasco A, Rubello D, Casara D. Parathyroid carcinoma. Therapeutic strategies derived from 20 years of experience. Minerva Endocrinol. 2001;26(1):23–9.
11. Trigonis C, Cedermark B, Willems J, Hamberger B, Granberg PO. Parathyroid carcinoma--problems in diagnosis and treatment. Clin Oncol. 1984;10(1):11–9.
12. Smith JF, Coombs RR. Histological diagnosis of carcinoma of the parathyroid gland. J Clin Pathol. 1984;37(12):1370–8.
13. McKeown PP, McGarity WC, Sewell CW. Carcinoma of the parathyroid gland: is it overdiagnosed?A report of three cases. Am J Surg. 1984;147(2):292–8.
14. Obara T, Fujimoto Y. Diagnosis and treatment of patients with parathyroid carcinoma: an update and review. World J Surg. 1991;15(6):738–44.
15. Wynne AG, van HJ, Carney JA, Fitzpatrick LA. Parathyroid carcinoma: clinical and pathologic features in 43 patients. Medicine (Baltimore). 1992;71(4):197–205.
16. Lee YS, Hong SW, Jeong JJ, Nam KH, Chung WY, Chang HS, et al. Parathyroid carcinoma: a 16-year experience in a single institution. Endocr J. 2010;57(6):493–7.
17. Favia G, Lumachi F, Polistina F, D'Amico DF. Parathyroid carcinoma: sixteen new cases and suggestions for correct management. World J Surg. 1998;22(12):1225–30.
18. Chandar AK, Falck-Ytter Y. Evidence based medicine: quality of evidence and evaluation systems. In: Ferguson MK, editor. Difficult decisions in thoracic surgery, difficult decisions in surgery: an evidence-based approach 1. 3rd ed. London: Springer; 2014. p. 17–33.
19. Anderson BJ, Samaan NA, Vassilopoulou Sellin R, Ordonez NG, Hickey RC. Parathyroid carcinoma: features and difficulties in diagnosis and management. Surgery. 1983;94(6):906–15.
20. Busaidy NL, Jimenez C, Habra MA, Schultz PN, El-Naggar AK, Clayman GL, et al. Parathyroid carcinoma: a 22-year experience. Head Neck. 2004;26(8):716–26.
21. Hakaim AG, Esselstyn CB Jr. Parathyroid carcinoma: 50-year experience at the Cleveland Clinic Foundation. Cleve Clin J Med. 1993;60(4):331–5.
22. Kebebew E, Arici C, Duh QY, Clark OH. Localization and reoperation results for persistent and recurrent parathyroid carcinoma. Arch Surg. 2001;136(8):878–85.
23. Koea JB, Shaw JH. Parathyroid cancer: biology and management. Surg Oncol. 1999;8(3):155–65.
24. Harari A, Waring A, Fernandez-Ranvier G, Hwang J, Suh I, Mitmaker E, et al. Parathyroid carcinoma: a 43-year outcome and survival analysis. J Clin Endocrinol Metab. 2011;96(12):3679–86.
25. Hsu KT, Sippel RS, Chen H, Schneider DF. Is central lymph node dissection necessary for parathyroid carcinoma? Surgery. 2014;156(6):1336–41.
26. Sadler C, Gow KW, Beierle EA, Doski JJ, Langer M, Nuchtern JG, et al. Parathyroid carcinoma in more than 1,000 patients: a population-level analysis. Surgery. 2014;156(6):1622–30.

27. Holmes EC, Morton DL, Ketcham AS. Parathyroid carcinoma: a collective review. Ann Surg. 1969;169(4):631–40.
28. Cordeiro AC, Montenegro FL, Kulcsar MA, Dellanegra LA, Tavares MR, Michaluart P Jr, et al. Parathyroid carcinoma. Am J Surg. 1998;175(1):52–5.
29. Sandelin K, Auer G, Bondeson L, Grimelius L, Farnebo LO. Prognostic factors in parathyroid cancer: a review of 95 cases. World J Surg. 1992;16(4):724–31.
30. Clayman GL, Gonzalez HE, El-Naggar A, Vassilopoulou-Sellin R. Parathyroid carcinoma: evaluation and interdisciplinary management. Cancer. 2004;100(5):900–5.
31. Talat N, Schulte KM. Clinical presentation, staging and long-term evolution of parathyroid cancer. Ann Surg Oncol. 2010;17(8):2156–74.
32. Schulte KM, Talat N, Miell J, Moniz C, Sinha P, Diaz-Cano S. Lymph node involvement and surgical approach in parathyroid cancer. World J Surg. 2010;34(11):2611–20.
33. Schantz A, Castleman B. Parathyroid carcinoma. A study of 70 cases. Cancer. 1973; 31(3):600–5.
34. Shaha AR, Shah JP. Parathyroid carcinoma: a diagnostic and therapeutic challenge. Cancer. 1999;86(3):378–80.
35. Owen RP, Silver CE, Pellitteri PK, Shaha AR, Devaney KO, Werner JA, et al. Parathyroid carcinoma: a review. Head Neck. 2011;33(3):429–36.
36. Fernandez-Ranvier GG, Khanafshar E, Jensen K, Zarnegar R, Lee J, Kebebew E, et al. Parathyroid carcinoma, atypical parathyroid adenoma, or parathyromatosis? Cancer. 2007;110(2):255–64.
37. Bae JH, Choi HJ, Lee Y, Moon MK, Park YJ, Shin CS, et al. Preoperative predictive factors for parathyroid carcinoma in patients with primary hyperparathyroidism. J Korean Med Sci. 2012;27(8):890–5.
38. Schulte KM, Gill AJ, Barczynski M, Karakas E, Miyauchi A, Knoefel WT, et al. Classification of parathyroid cancer. Ann Surg Oncol. 2012;19(8):2620–8.
39. LiVolsi VA, Hamilton R. Intraoperative assessment of parathyroid gland pathology. A common view from the surgeon and the pathologist. Am J Clin Pathol. 1994;102(3):365–73.
40. Kwan WY, Chow TL, Choi CY, Lam SH. Complication rates of central compartment dissection in papillary thyroid cancer. ANZ J Surg. 2013;85(4):274–8.
41. Sadowski BM, Snyder SK, Lairmore TC. Routine bilateral central lymph node clearance for papillary thyroid cancer. Surgery. 2009;146(4):696–703.
42. So YK, Seo MY, Son YI. Prophylactic central lymph node dissection for clinically node-negative papillary thyroid microcarcinoma: influence on serum thyroglobulin level, recurrence rate, and postoperative complications. Surgery. 2012;151(2):192–8.
43. Palestini N, Borasi A, Cestino L, Freddi M, Odasso C, Robecchi A. Is central neck dissection a safe procedure in the treatment of papillary thyroid cancer? Our experience. Langenbeck's Arch Surg. 2008;393(5):693–8.
44. Viola D, Materazzi G, Valerio L, Molinaro E, Agate L, Faviana P, et al. Prophylactic central compartment lymph node dissection in papillary thyroid carcinoma: clinical implications derived from the first prospective randomized controlled single institution study. J Clin Endocrinol Metab. 2015;100(4):1316–24. https://doi.org/10.1210/jc.2014-3825.
45. Alvarado R, Sywak MS, Delbridge L, Sidhu SB. Central lymph node dissection as a secondary procedure for papillary thyroid cancer: is there added morbidity? Surgery. 2009;145(5):514–8.

Early Versus Late Parathyroidectomy for Tertiary (Posttransplant) Hyperparathyroidism

18

Jyotirmay Sharma and Collin Weber

Abstract

Tertiary hyperparathyroidism is hypercalcemia after kidney transplantation. A near-total parathyroidectomy is curative for tertiary hyperparathyroidism and should be considered within the first year of kidney transplantation if hypercalcemia does not resolve. Cure rates of hypercalcemia after a parathyroidectomy for tertiary hyperparathyroidism are >95%.

Keywords

Tertiary hyperparathyroidism · Parathyroidectomy · Kidney transplant

Introduction

Tertiary hyperparathyroidism (3HPT) is described as persistent hyperparathyroidism with hypercalcemia despite correction of secondary hyperparathyroidism (from chronic renal failure) with renal transplantation. The reported incidence of post renal transplant hyperparathyroidism ranges from 25–50% at 1 year after transplant and about 17% at 4 years after transplant [1, 2]. The average time for parathyroid levels to return to normal post transplant varies between three to 6 months [3]. Calcium levels post renal transplant are also highly variable. The natural history of post transplant calcium levels can be categorized into three distinct groups: eucalcemia, hypercalcemia, and fluctuating calcium levels. These varying calcium levels present an obstacle to identifying patients with true tertiary hyperparathyroidism as opposed to patients who are still undergoing gland involution. Resolution of hypercalcemia >1 year

J. Sharma (✉) · C. Weber
Department of Surgery, Emory University School of Medicine, Atlanta, GA, USA
e-mail: jsharm3@emory.edu; cweber@emory.edu

P. Angelos, R. H. Grogan (eds.), *Difficult Decisions in Endocrine Surgery*, Difficult Decisions in Surgery: An Evidence-Based Approach,
https://doi.org/10.1007/978-3-319-92860-9_18

post-transplant is highly unlikely. The incidence of "true" 3HPT with hypercalcemia post renal transplant ranges from 0.5% to 5.6% [4–9] (Table 18.1).

Indications for Parathyroidectomy in Tertiary Hyperparathyroidism

Tertiary hyperparathyroidism leads to decreased bone mineral density, changes in mental status, myopathies, and; importantly, volume depletion and calcification of the renal allograft, which may affect allograft function [10–12]. Parathyroidectomy (PTX) is the only definitive treatment option for 3HPT. Current indications for PTX include highly increased and persistent hypercalcemia, symptomatic hypercalcemia, increased parathyroid hormone levels, hypophosphatemia, decreased bone mineral density, or kidney function decline associated with hyperparathyroidism; however, it is unclear as to what calcium or parathyroid hormone level and at what time point after renal transplantation one should refer a patient for PTX [5]. At our institution and many others, patients are referred for PTX by the transplant nephrology department, and their criteria for referral are based on the level and persistence (greater than 6 months) of serum calcium and increases in PTH. Pharmaceutical therapy for hypercalcemia management is often initiated in these patients with a varied response. The role and timing of implementation of calcimimetics is controversial and it can be associated with worsening allograft function with a paucity of long term outcomes data. The decision to initiate calcimimetic therapy or to proceed with parathyroidectomy is often individual and institution dependent with a paucity of consensus derived guidelines. Studies have shown similar renal graft survival between patients who undergo PTX and control groups even though some studies report a decrease in GFR in patients who have undergone PTX. Benefits of PTX may include improved patient survival, improved bone mineral density, and alleviation of symptoms [13–17].

The optimal timing of PTX post-kidney transplant in patients with 3HPT is also difficult and the decision to proceed with PTX is based upon expectation of resolution of hypercalcemia, risks of surgery, cure rates and improvement in symptomology. Near-total or total PTX with autograft are both effective in curing 3HPT with numerous series documenting a cure rate >95% when resolution of hypercalcemia is used as a marker for cure [18]. However, up to 20% of patients will have elevated PTH levels and this is likely due to vitamin D deficiency, fluctuations in GFR and remaining hyperplastic tissue [19, 20]. Although, the rate of reoperations is low; patients with persistent marked elevations in PTH should be followed closely for hypercalcemia and some require a reoperation. The risks of parathyroidectomy are related to anesthesia and neck surgery. Permanent voice alteration from recurrent laryngeal nerve injury rates vary between 0–8% and are relatively uncommon in the hands of experienced endocrine surgeons [16]. Transient and permanent hypoparathyroidism is a known complication of any parathyroidectomy and the rates are low after PTX for 3HPT. Bone hunger and vitamin D deficiency should be assessed during the postoperative course and invariably patients will require calcium supplementation and vitamin D repletion. Permanent hypoparathyroidism is an extremely rare and avoidable complication. Careful assessment of the remnant parathyroid and its vascular viability should be routine in the operation and an

Table 18.1 Review of studies associated with 3HPT

Study	Population	Study type	Number of Patients with PTX	Mean Follow-up (years)	Mean Time from Tx to PTX (months)	Post-PTX kidney function assessed	Cure Rate (normocalcemia)	Quality of Evidence
Dewberry et al. [23]	Kidney transplant alone + PTX	Retrospective Case-control	105	3.1	62	Y	97%	Medium
Kandil et al. [6]	Kidney transplant alone + PTX	Retrospective Case-control	19	3	13.8	Y	NA	Low
Somnay et al. [24]	PTX	Retrospective	80	0.5	NA	N	96%	Low
Hseih et al. [25]	PTX	Retrospective	14	5.8	33	N	100%	Low
Park et al. [26]	PTX	Retrospective	15	4.5	43	N	93%	Low
Pitt et al. [11]	PTX	Retrospective	140	5.3	28	N	94%	Low
Sadideen et al. [27]	PTX	Retrospective	26	>5	49	N	85%	Low
Schlosser et al. [28]	PTX	Retrospective	69	1	43.3	Y	100%	Low
Triponez et al. [29]	PTX	Retrospective	74	5.4	50	Y	100%	Low
Yang et al. [30]	Kidney transplant + PTX	Retrospective Case-control	18	1	20	Y	100%	Medium
Milas et al. [16]	PTX	Retrospective	49	2	48	N	96%	Low

immediate autograft of parathyroid fragments should be performed if the remnant is ischemic. Cryopreservation of parathyroid fragments should be performed in all patients with storage of fragments for at least 3–6 months. Intraoperative parathyroid hormone (IOPTH) monitoring can not only help assess the adequacy and completeness of a PTX, and IOPTH also helps assess parathyroid remnant function.

Effect on allograft function from 3HPT and PTX is an area of controversy with conflicting data on outcomes [6, 12]. Hypercalcemia and hyperparathyroidism can cause vasoconstriction, renal arterial calcification and tubulointerstitial calcification which can lead to decrease allograft function and lead to graft failure [20]. There are direct effects of PTH on vascular contractility and vascular calcifications which can lead to decrease allograft blood flow [21, 22]. Increasing GFR without evidence of rejection can serve as a marker for consideration of PTX. There are conflicting reports on improvement in GFR and a decrease in rejection episodes after PTX in 3HPT. In case-controlled series an increase in GFR was noted in patients undergoing PTX when compared to patients with medical management, however, this group also had a higher rate of eventual graft failure.

Uncontrolled 3HPT is associated with increased mortality, myocardial disease, vascular calcification, worsening bone disease, calciphylaxis, neuropsychiatric symptoms, generalized malaise and fatigue [4–9]. Improvements in all of these are well documented in literature from PTX and calcimimetic therapy. In the past few years calcimimetic therapy is more readily available and therefore more likely to be utilized. However, PTX results in immediate and the most profound control of hypercalcemia and symptoms and it is also cost-effective.

Early intervention may improve outcomes in patients with 3HPT. Kidney transplantation results in normal urinary excretion of phosphorus and restores calcium and vitamin D homeostasis, which in >95% patients is curative for hyperparathyroidism. However up to 5% of patients will develop 3HPT. In patients undergoing PTX for 3HPT there are pre-transplant and post-transplant factors associated with an increased risk for 3HPT [23]. Pre-transplant factors with increased risk of the development of 3HPT were elevated serum calcium, very high PTH levels (>1000 pg/mL), longer vintage of dialysis, failed parathyroidectomy and use of calcimimetics (Table 18.2). Hypercalcemia immediately after kidney transplantation is observed in many patients with resolution seen in the majority of patients.

Table 18.2 Patient factors associated with increased risk of 3HPT and PTX

	PTX	Control
Age, years*	41.8 ± 11.5	46.5 ± 11.5
Gender (M:F ratio)	1.1:1	1.46:1
Race (%AA)	58.1%	48.3%
Dialysis duration, years*	6 ± 4.9	2.8 ± 2.8
Cause of renal failure (%HTN)*	43.3%	22.8%
Cinacalcet use*	24.7%	8.3%
Pre-transplant PTH at 1 year prior to transplant*	745 ± 84 pg/dL	245 ± 92 pg/dL
Pre-transplant calcium at 6 months prior to transplant*	9.9 ± 0.9 mg/d	9.1 ± 0.9 mg/d
Post-transplant calcium at 1 month*	10.4 ± 1.0 mg/dL	9.4 ± 1.0 mg/dL
Post-transplant PTH at 1 month*	351 ± 187 pg/dL	112 ± 73 pg/dL

*p < 0.05

However, when patients are hypercalcemic at 1 or 3 months they are 11 and 15 times more likely to require PTX, respectively. When PTH and serum calcium are used concurrently at 1 month post-kidney transplant they are strong predictors of the development of 3HPT. We believe that an early PTX (within the first year of transplant) is cost-effective and likely to offer a greater benefit to the patient and further waiting is unlikely to be curative for 3HPT.

Techniques of Parathyroidectomy in Tertiary Hyperparathyroidism

The technique described here is as a near-total parathyroidectomy is a more precise variant of subtotal parathyroidectomy. In 3HPT parathyroid glands are hyperplastic, three and three fourths are removed, leaving a vascularized remnant of one gland which approximates the size of 2 normal parathyroids; and the fragment which are equivalent of 8–10 normal glands are cryopreserved. The in-situ gland remnant may be marked with a permanent suture for future identification (Fig. 18.1). Alternately,

Time	IOPTH*	Procedure
08:20	915	
08:40		LL – NTPTX
08:53		LU – Rx
09:03	435	
09:08		RU – Rx
09:13		RU – Rx
09:18	82	
09:24	68	
Cryopreservation		

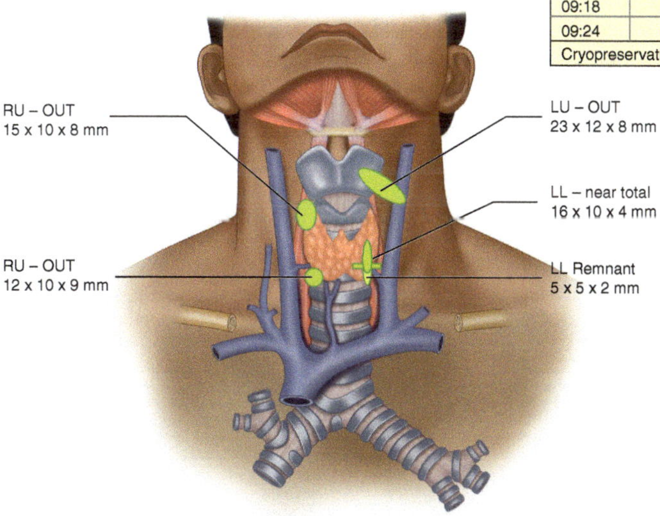

Preoperative Data
(42yo; dialysis vintage: 4 year; kidney transplant 1 year ago)
PTH = 1074, Serum Ca = 10.7 mg/dL, GFR = 53

Follow-up @ 5 years
PTH = 89, Serum Ca = 8.2 mg/dL
GFR = 49

Fig. 18.1 Schema of patient undergoing parathyroidectomy for tertiary hyperparathyroidism

all parathyroids may be removed from the neck, and the equivalent of 1–2 normal parathyroids may be minced into 1–2 mm fragments and autografted into either the sterno-cleidomastoid or nondominant forearm muscle. Autografted fragments should not be prepared from nodular parathyroids but from the more uniform parathyroids. In this instance, additional fragments should be cryopreserved as a safeguard in case the autografted tissue is insufficient. Total parathyroidectomy and autotransplantation has the advantage that recurrent parathyroid hyperfunction may be treated by partial autograft excision under local anesthesia. However, some autografts fail to function. In these patients a vascularized parathyroid remnant often functions better, and patients may be discharged sooner. Furthermore, in our experience, vascularized remnant regrowth is distinctly uncommon if the size of the remnant is small (the equivalent of 2 normal parathyroids in mass, approximately 80 mg). In some institutions, a small group of patients undergo a less than subtotal or near-total parathyroidectomy due to variation in appearance, size and vascularity of the observed parathyroid glands. Outcomes of this type of "limited" parathyroidectomy in 3HPT have been good in some series by experienced surgeons. Although this practice may be efficacious for some patients, we believe there are pitfalls in such an approach and this has led to referrals to many endocrine surgeons for reoperations in patients for persistent 3HPT. Also the pathophysiology of 3HPT is of renal insufficiency triggered hyperplasia leading to abnormality in all glands. This may play role in recurrence of hyperparathyroidism for patients after a kidney transplant since a significant number of patients develop chronic renal insufficiency with decrease graft function and up to 20% of patients also progress to failure of the transplanted kidney and resumption of dialysis. Leaving as small an amount of parathyroid tissue as possible without leading to hypoparathyroidism with cryopreservation of parathyroid fragments is the ideal approach.

References

1. Apaydin S, Sariyar M, Erek E, Ataman R, Yiğitbaş R, Hamzaoğlu I, Serdengeçti K, Ulkü U. Hypercalcemia and hyperparathyroidism after renal transplantation. Nephron. 1999;81(3):364–5.
2. Evenepoel P, Claes K, Kuypers D, Maes B, Bammens B, Vanrenterghem Y. Natural history of parathyroid function and calcium metabolism after kidney transplantation: a single-centre study. Nephrol Dial Transplant. 2004;19(5):1281–7.
3. Triponez F, Clark OH, Vanrenthergem Y, Evenepoel P. Surgical treatment of persistent hyperparathyroidism after renal transplantation. Ann Surg. 2008;248(1):18–30. https://doi.org/10.1097/SLA.0b013e3181728a2d.
4. Gwinner W, Suppa S, Mengel M, Hoy L, Kreipe HH, Haller H, Schwarz A. Early calcification of renal allografts detected by protocol biopsies: causes and clinical implications. Am J Transplant. 2005;5(8):1934–41.
5. D'Alessandro AM, Melzer JS, Pirsch JD, Sollinger HW, Kalayoglu M, Vernon WB, Belzer FO, Starling JR. Tertiary hyperparathyroidism after renal transplantation: operative indications. Surgery. 1989;106(6):1049–55. discussion 1055–6.
6. Kandil E, Florman S, Alabbas H, Abdullah O, McGee J, Noureldine S, Slakey D, Zhang R. Exploring the effect of parathyroidectomy for tertiary hyperparathyroidism after

kidney transplantation. Am J Med Sci. 2010;339(5):420–4. https://doi.org/10.1097/MAJ.0b013e3181d8b6ff.

7. Kinnaert P, Nagy N, Decoster-Gervy C, De Pauw L, Salmon I, Vereerstraeten P. Persistent hyperparathyroidism requiring surgical treatment after kidney transplantation. World J Surg. 2000;24(11):1391–5.
8. Kerby JD, Rue LW, Blair H, Hudson S, Sellers MT, Diethelm AG. Operative treatment of tertiary hyperparathyroidism: a single-center experience. Ann Surg. 1998;227(6):878–86.
9. Evenepoel P, Claes K, Kuypers DR, Debruyne F, Vanrenterghem Y. Parathyroidectomy after successful kidney transplantation: a single Centre study. Nephrol Dial Transplant. 2007;22(6):1730–7.
10. Rix M, Lewin E, Olgaard K. Posttransplant bone disease. Transplant Rev. 2003;17:176–86.
11. Pitt SC, Sippel RS, Chen H. Secondary and tertiary hyperparathyroidism, state of the art surgical management. Surg Clin North Am. 2009;89(5):1227–39. https://doi.org/10.1016/j.suc.2009.06.011.
12. Schwarz A, Rustien G, Merkel S, et al. Decreased renal transplant function after parathyroidectomy. Nephrol Dial Transplant. 2007;22:584–91.
13. Madorin C, Owen RP, Fraser WD, Pellitteri PK, Radbill B, Rinaldo A, Seethala RR, Shaha AR, Silver CE, Suh MY, Weinstein B, Ferlito A. The surgical management of renal hyperparathyroidism. Eur Arch Otorhinolaryngol. 2012;269(6):1565–76. https://doi.org/10.1007/s00405-011-1833-2.
14. Sharma J, Raggi P, Kutner N, Bailey J, Zhang R, Huang Y, Herzog CA, Weber C. Improved long-term survival of dialysis patients after near-total parathyroidectomy. J Am Coll Surg. 2012;214(4):400–7 discussion 407–8. https://doi.org/10.1016/j.jamcollsurg.2011.12.046.
15. Heyliger A, Tangpricha V, Weber C, Sharma J. Parathyroidectomy decreases systolic and diastolic blood pressure in hypertensive patients with primary hyperparathyroidism. Surgery. 2009;146(6):1042–7. https://doi.org/10.1016/j.surg.2009.09.024.
16. Milas M, Weber CJ. Near-total parathyroidectomy is beneficial for patients with secondary and tertiary hyperparathyroidism. Surgery. 2004;136(6):1252–60.
17. Daniel WT, Weber C, Bailey JA, Raggi P, Sharma J. Prospective analysis of coronary calcium in patients on dialysis undergoing a near-total parathyroidectomy. Surgery. 2013;154(6):1315–21 discussion 1321–2. https://doi.org/10.1016/j.surg.2013.06.030.
18. McPhaul JJ, McIntosh DA, Hammond WS, Park OK. Autonomous secondary (renal) parathyroid hyperplasia. N Engl J Med. 1964;271:1342–5.
19. Evenepoel P, Van Den Bergh B, Naesens M, De Jonge H, Bammens B, Claes K, Kuypers D, Vanrenterghem Y. Calcium metabolism in the early posttransplantation period. Clin J Am Soc Nephrol. 2009;4(3):665–72. https://doi.org/10.2215/CJN.03920808.
20. Torres A, Lorenzo V, Salido E. Calcium metabolism and skeletal problems after transplantation. J Am Soc Nephrol. 2002;13(2):551–8.
21. Sutliff RL, Weber CS, Qian J, Miller ML, Clemens TL, Paul RJ. Vasorelaxant properties of parathyroid hormone-related protein in the mouse: evidence for endothelium involvement independent of nitric oxide formation. Endocrinology. 1999;140(5):2077–83.
22. Massfelder T, Parekh N, Endlich K, Saussine C, Steinhausen M, Helwig JJ. Effect of intrarenally infused parathyroid hormone-related protein on renal blood flow and glomerular filtration rate in the anaesthetized rate. Br J Pharmacol. 1996;118(8):1995–2000.
23. Dewberry L, Tata S, Graves S, Weber C, Sharma J. Predictors of tertiary hyperparathyroidism: who will benefit from parathyroidectomy? Surgery. 2014;156:1631–7.
24. Somnay Y, Weinlander E, Alfhedi A, Schneider D, Sippel R, Chen H. Radioguided parathyroidectomy for tertiary hyperparathyroidism. J Surg Res. 2015;195:406–11.
25. Hsieh TM, Sun CK, Chen YT, Chou FF. Total parathyroidectomy versus subtotal parathyroidectomy in the treatment of tertiary hyperparathyroidism. Am Surg. 2012;78:600–6.
26. Park JH, Kang S-W, Jeong JJ, Nam K-H, Chang HS, Chung WY, et al. Surgical treatment of tertiary hyperparathyroidism after renal transplantation: a 31-year experience in a single institution. Endocr J. 2011;58:827–33.

27. Sadideen HM, Taylor JD, Goldsmith DJ. Total parathyroidectomy without autotransplantation after renal transplantation for tertiary hyperparathyroidism: long-term follow-up. Int Urol Nephrol. 2012;44:275–81.
28. Schlosser K, Endres N, Celik I, Fendrich V, Rothmund M, Fernández ED. Surgical treatment of tertiary hyperparathyroidism: the choice of procedure matters! World J Surg. 2007;31:1947–53.
29. Triponez F, Kebebew E, Dosseh D, Duh QY, Hazzan M, Noel C, et al. Less-than-subtotal parathyroidectomy increases the risk of persistent/recurrent hyperparathyroidism after parathyroidectomy in tertiary hyperparathyroidism after renal transplantation. Surgery. 2006;140:990–7.
30. Yang RL, Freeman K, Reinke CE, Fraker DL, Karakousis GC, Kelz RR, Doyle AM. Tertiary hyperparathyroidism in kidney transplant recipients: characteristics of patients selected for different treatment strategies. Transplantation. 2012;15(94):70–6.

Observation Versus Surgery for Pregnant Patients with Primary Hyperparathyroidism

19

James Y. Lim and James A. Lee

Abstract

Primary hyperparathyroidism (PHP) in the pregnant patient can pose significant risks to the mother and fetus. The actual incidence of PHP in the pregnant population is unknown as the subtle symptoms and findings can often be masked by the physical and physiologic changes that occur with pregnancy. The range of presentations runs from the asymptomatic to severely symptomatic. Symptoms in the mother can include all of the typical symptoms of PHP such as nephrolithiasis, dehydration, pancreatitis, bone disease, and hypercalcemic crisis as well as hyperemesis gravidarum. Symptoms manifested by the developing fetus can include spontaneous abortion, preterm delivery, postpartum neonatal tetany, and permanent hypoparathyroidism. The prompt diagnosis of this condition can prevent many of these complications. The following chapter will discuss the physiology of calcium homeostasis between the mother and fetus, diagnosis of PHP, as well as the surgical and medical treatment options.

Keywords

Primary hyperparathyroidism · Pregnancy · Complications · Parathyroidectomy

J. Y. Lim
Division of Surgical Oncology, Oregon Health and Science University, Portland, OR, USA
e-mail: ljam@ohsu.edu

J. A. Lee (✉)
Department of Surgery, Columbia University Medical Center, New York, NY, USA
e-mail: jal74@cumc.columbia.edu

P. Angelos, R. H. Grogan (eds.), *Difficult Decisions in Endocrine Surgery*, Difficult Decisions in Surgery: An Evidence-Based Approach,
https://doi.org/10.1007/978-3-319-92860-9_19

Evidence Summary

The literature consists of case reports, case series, and reviews of the literature, with most papers describing a single case only. The total number of pregnant patients with primary hyperparathyroidism described in the literature amounts to less than 200 cases. At earlier time points, patients tended to be managed medically, however with high associated maternal and fetal complication rates, the more recent trend has been towards surgical management. This move towards surgical management has led to a dramatic decrease in maternal and fetal complications. As the surgical and anesthetic techniques have become safer for, both, mother and fetus, the benefits of surgery appear to outweigh the risks. From the period from 1992 to 2014, there were no case reports describing infant or maternal deaths in the peri-operative and peri-partum periods.

Quality of Evidence

Numerous case reports and case series provide consistent results when comparing outcomes after surgical treatment versus medical treatment. The lack of any statistical measures or controls across the different case reports leads to evidence that is low in quality (Grade C).

Best Estimates

There appear to be improved outcomes after surgery in pregnant patients with PHP for both the mother and fetus as compared to patients managed medically.

Judgment of Benefits Versus Risks, Burden, and Cost

Given the reduction in maternal and fetal complications after parathyroidectomy, the benefits of surgery outweigh the minimal risks of surgery and general anesthesia as well as medical therapy alone. No cost analyses have been performed.

Grade of Recommendation

Although the quality of evidence is low, the consistent demonstration of improved outcomes and lower maternal and fetal complications with surgical management are striking when compared to the potential complications including fetal demise if the mother's hypercalcemic state is inadequately treated medically. The limited number of medications that can be safely used during pregnancy to aggressively treat hypercalcemia further limits the safety of medical management (Grade 1C).

Introduction

Primary hyperparathyroidism (PHP) is one of the most common endocrine disorders in the general population with an incidence of 0.15% [1]. Within this population, the disease is more common in women and it is estimated that the incidence within the childbearing population is up to 25% [2]. The actual reported incidence within the pregnant population is unknown with much of the medical literature limited to case reports and small case series. It is suspected that an estimated 80% of pregnant women with primary hyperparathyroidism are either asymptomatic, or the physiologic and physical changes of pregnancy leads to the masking of symptoms. PHP may also be underdiagnosed since current prenatal screening guidelines, according to the American Congress of Obstetricians and Gynecologists, do not recommend routine testing for calcium levels or parathyroid hormone (PTH) levels during pregnancy [3]. Since the first report of PHP in the pregnant patient was reported in 1939, the considerable morbidity associated with this condition has been well-recognized [4]. Undiagnosed, PHP during pregnancy is associated with significant risks of severe complications for both mother and fetus. The incidence of maternal and fetal complications is as high as 67% and 80% respectively, with maternal and fetal deaths the most serious of those complications. [5] However, with an appropriate level of suspicion and proper screening, management strategies have improved to make maternal and fetal complications preventable events (Table 19.1).

Methods

A search of the Medline database from 1962 to 2014 with keywords related to primary hyperparathyroidism, pregnancy and its complications was performed. Letters, communications and non-English language papers were excluded. Papers were excluded if no medical treatment was instituted prior to childbirth and if the diagnosis of hyperparathyroidism occurred postnatal. References from all articles retrieved were also reviewed to identify any further additional articles.

Calcium Homeostasis During Pregnancy

Over the course of a pregnancy, the developing fetus requires a total of 25–30 g of calcium which is obtained from the maternal circulation [6]. The majority of the calcium is transferred during the last trimester as bone mineralization of the

Table 19.1 PICO table

Population	Pregnant patients with PHP
Intervention	Parathyroidectomy
Comparator	Observation, medical treatment
Outcomes	Reduce maternal and fetal complications

fetal skeleton accelerates. The transfer of calcium occurs across the placental barrier throughout gestation and the calcium pumps are thought to be maintained by parathyroid hormone–related peptide (PTHrP) secreted by the fetal parathyroid glands and placenta [5, 7]. PTHrP is consistently elevated during pregnancy as opposed to PTH levels which are often depressed [8]. Other physiologic changes that occur are an increase in extracellular fluid volume and increased renal clearance of calcium due to an increase in glomerular filtration rate. Pregnant women excrete twice the amount of calcium in their urine as compared to non-pregnant women. These changes lead to a decreased level of total serum calcium while ionized calcium levels remain unchanged. Despite these increased demands on maternal calcium stores, there is no evidence that pregnant women suffer from skeletal demineralization during a normal gestation. The primary compensatory adjustment that occurs in pregnant women are increased levels of 1,25-dihydroxyvitamin D, nearly two to three times the levels seen in non-pregnant women, resulting in an increased intestinal absorption rate of 0.8–1.5 g/day [9]. It was thought in the past that there was a physiological compensatory increase in parathyroid hormone but these levels are normally decreased during pregnancy. The mechanism behind the increase in 1, 25-dihydroxyvitamin D levels in pregnant women is unclear, but these increased levels likely also explain the normal depression seen in parathyroid hormone levels in pregnant women due to inhibition at the level of gene transcription.

Diagnosis of Primary Hyperparathyroidism During Pregnancy

Making the diagnosis of PHP in the pregnant population can be difficult. Subtle symptoms such as fatigue, lethargy, and proximal muscle weakness that might prompt an evaluation for PHP in the general population, can easily be overlooked in pregnant women [5]. One review looking at 70 cases, found the most common symptoms to be nausea/vomiting/anorexia (36%), fatigue/weakness (34%), mental symptoms (26%), asymptomatic (24%) and renal colic (17%) [10]. As a result, although women of childbearing age make up 25% of the total number of cases of PHP, PHP during pregnancy is rarely reported in the literature. It is presumed that the prevalence is underreported due to the nonspecific symptoms of presentation and, in addition, shunting of high levels of calcium to the fetus, especially in the third trimester, may also be protective against maternal hypercalcemia. The degree of maternal hypercalcemia can also be masked on laboratory tests by the changes in calcium homeostasis. These changes include calcium being shunted to the placenta, increased maternal hypercalciuria, as well as the physiologic hypoalbuminemia that develops during pregnancy. In the past, the diagnosis was most commonly made postpartum with the newborn presenting with tetany. An evaluation should also be prompted when patients have a history of, or present with, nephrolithiasis, peptic ulcer disease, pancreatitis, osteoporosis, severe nausea and vomiting, or a history of spontaneous abortions/stillbirths or neonatal death.

The workup of PHP during pregnancy is the same as for non-pregnant patients and should start with serum calcium, parathyroid hormone, and vitamin D levels.

However, different threshold values, especially for calcium should be considered. Elevated calcium levels may differ based on the trimester of the pregnancy. For example, one study stated that total serum calcium concentration greater than 10.1 mg/dL (2.52 mmol/L) or 8.8 mg/dL (2.2 mmol/L) during the second or third trimester, respectively, should prompt the clinician to suspect possible hyperparathyroidism [10]. Ionized calcium may also be useful in the pregnant patient as total calcium may be blunted by physiologic changes while ionized levels should remain unchanged. Elevated calcium levels in the setting of normal to elevated PTH levels confirm the diagnosis of PHP. During the evaluation of PHP, the possibility of hereditary syndromes such as multiple endocrine neoplasia 1 and 2A should be considered, as well as familial hypocalciuric hypercalcemia. Once a diagnosis of PHP is made, parathyroidectomy should be considered for all pregnant patients in order to avoid the complications of the disease in both the mother and fetus.

Fetal Complications

Untreated, PHP in the mother can cause significant morbidity to the fetus with an incidence of complications as high as 80% [11]. The major complications ranged from stillbirth, neonatal death, neonatal tetany, and permanent hypoparathyroidism. Of mothers that have been managed conservatively with medications, neonatal complications have been cited as high as 53% with one-third of those cases resulting in neonatal death [5, 12]. One study found that the rate of miscarriage was 3.5 times higher in women with primary hyperparathyroidism, and fetal losses typically occurred in the late first or early second trimester [13]. The risk of fetal death was proportional to the elevation in the calcium levels within this study. Maternal calcium levels above 11.5 mg/dL was associated with a 50% risk of fetal death and increased to 85% when calcium levels reached 13 mg/dL [13]. Other studies have found that maternal calcium levels do not correlate with the likelihood of complications [14]. More studies are necessary to identify at what elevated calcium levels, non-operative management may be safe for the fetus and mother.

Post-partum, neonatal tetany is the most common presentation of maternal PHP. This is due to the lack of development of the fetal parathyroid glands due to the chronically high levels of calcium provided by the maternal circulatory system during pregnancy. Up to 50% of infants born to untreated mothers will demonstrate tetany, most often from day of life 2 to 14 [12, 15]. When this complication is anticipated and calcium supplementation is begun early, infant outcomes are generally good. In the most severe cases, hypocalcemia can persist in the infant for several months and several cases of permanent hypoparathyroidism in infants have been described due to persistently high levels of calcium during the first and second trimesters of pregnancy [16]. Other fetal complications can include intrauterine growth restriction, low birth weight, and the risk of preterm delivery [5, 14, 17]. With proper interventions to treat the maternal hyperparathyroidism, fetal complications have been reduced by a factor of four [18]. The goal of treatment should be to bring the mother and fetus back to a eucalcemic state prior to delivery.

Maternal Complications

Studies indicate that the complication rate for pregnant women with uncontrolled PHP is as high as 67% and mirror complications seen in the non-pregnant patient [19, 20]. Although rare, one of the most feared complications is that of acute hypercalcemic crisis. This condition is typically accompanied by elevations in serum calcium greater than 14 mg/dL and has the potential for rapid deterioration. Symptoms of this condition include severe muscle weakness, fatigue, nausea, vomiting, dehydration, uremia, confusion and mental status changes that can lead to coma and death. In particular, the postpartum period can lead to worsening hypercalcemia since the fetus is no longer present to divert calcium stores [20, 21]. Six cases of hypercalcemic crisis have been identified in the literature in pregnant patients. Three cases occurred during pregnancy and three cases occurred immediately postpartum. Each of these cases was associated with significant complications including maternal death (two cases), fetal demise (two cases), or neonatal tetany (two cases) [10].

Nephrolithiasis is the most common complication seen in pregnant patients with PHP [2, 10, 22]. Recent studies looking at primary hyperparathyroidism have identified an incidence of nephrolithiasis in the pregnant population of 24–36% [10]. The risk of pancreatitis is also significantly elevated in pregnant patients with PHP with the prevalence in this specific population quoted at 7–13% as compared to a prevalence of 1–2% in the non-pregnant population. In patients with PHP and pancreatitis, the maternal mortality rate has been reported to be as high as 37% and premature labor rates are up to 60% when diagnosed in the third trimester [23].

Other complications that can occur in the mother include bone disease, hyperemesis gravidarum, urinary tract infections as well as the muscle weakness, constitutional symptoms and mental status changes generally associated with hyperparathyroidism. Radiographically demonstrated bone disease has been reported in 13–19% of pregnant patients [24]. Hyperemesis gravidarum has also been found to be significantly increased in patients with PHP [5]. Finally, there have also been increased associations with preeclampsia and polyhydramnios in mothers with PHP [25, 26] (Table 19.2).

Table 19.2 List of maternal and fetal complications due to PHP in pregnancy

Maternal complications	Fetal complications
• Dehydration	• Stillbirth
• Cardiac arrhythmias	• Spontaneous abortion
• Nephrolithiasis	• Preterm delivery
• Pancreatitis	• Intrauterine growth retardation
• Bone disease	• Neonatal tetany
• Urinary tract infections	• Permanent hypoparathyroidism
• Mental status changes	• Hypotonia
• Hyperemesis gravidarum	• Respiratory distress
• Preeclampsia	• Neonatal death
• Coma	
• Death	

Management of Primary Hyperparathyroidism in the Pregnant Patient

Once the diagnosis of PHP has been confirmed, parathyroidectomy should be considered for all pregnant patients. Although there are no specific guidelines for surgery in pregnant patients with PHP, guidance can be obtained by looking at current guidelines for the non-pregnant population. Indications for surgery in the general population include anyone who is symptomatic from PHP. In the asymptomatic population, indications for surgery include serum calcium concentration of 1.0 mg/dL or more above the upper limit of normal, creatinine clearance that is reduced to <60 mL/min, bone density at the hip, lumbar spine, or distal radius that is more than 2.5 standard deviations below peak bone mass, and age less than 50 years [27]. Based on these criteria, parathyroidectomy for PHP will almost always be recommended in the pregnant population either due to symptoms or on the basis that most women will be under the age of 50.

One of the largest reviews written on the topic demonstrated the benefits of parathyroidectomy in this patient population with improved outcomes in the surgical group as compared to the medically managed group. The review looked at 39 surgically treated cases and 70 medically treated cases of PHP during pregnancy and found the rate of neonatal complications and death in the medical group to be 53% and 16% respectively, while the rate of neonatal complications and death in the surgical group was 12.5% and 2.5%, respectively [12, 17]. Due to the significant maternal, fetal, and neonatal risks associated with primary hyperparathyroidism, surgery has become the recommended therapy for PHP in pregnant patients.

If possible, parathyroidectomy should be performed in the second trimester, when the risks of anesthesia-induced preterm labor are the least and the organogenesis that occurs in the first trimester is complete. For cases that are diagnosed in the third trimester, there is an increasing number of case reports in which parathyroidectomy was performed safely during that period without an increase in preterm labor. These reports are in stark contrast to an earlier review that associated third trimester parathyroidectomy with a 58% perinatal complication rate and so surgery should still be given consideration, even in advanced gestation [10, 28–30].

Although parathyroidectomy is the definitive management of maternal PHP, medications can be used to stabilize patients and treat hypercalcemia if non-operative management is chosen. Pregnant patients with severe PHP are generally volume depleted and require rapid intravenous resuscitation with normal saline in a monitored setting in addition to medications to treat the hypercalcemia. Calcium wasting diuretics such as Lasix (category C medication) can be started. Calcitonin (category B), an inhibitor of osteoclast function, and oral phosphate (category C), have both been used safely in pregnancies although they are known to cross the placental barrier. Bisphosphonates, such as Pamidronate (category C), have been shown to be teratogenic in extremely high doses in rabbits and mice, and its safety in pregnancy is unclear. Mithramycin (category X) has been discontinued, and was never recommended due to severe hepatic, renal and marrow toxicity [5]. Cinacalcet (category C), a calcimimetic agent that lowers calcium by acting at the extracellular calcium sensing receptor, is another medication that is known to cross the placental barrier and must be used with caution in the pregnant patient. There have been isolated case reports where Cinacalcet has been used in pregnant patients with no adverse effects on the fetus reported [31]. These medications are particularly important when a pregnant patient is admitted in hypercalcemic crisis and needs to be initially stabilized medically. The safety profiles of these medications have not been well studied in the developing human fetus and caution must be exercised when using any of these medications in the pregnant patient.

Conclusion

Primary hyperparathyroidism in pregnant women can carry high rates of morbidity and mortality to both the mother and fetus when left untreated. Once diagnosed, parathyroidectomy, ideally in the second trimester, is recommended for definitive treatment. More studies are required to validate this recommendation in both the symptomatic and asymptomatic pregnant PHP populations given that the only available data consists of case reports and case series.

References

1. Jesudason WV, Murphy J, England RJ. Primary hyperparathyroidism in pregnancy. J Laryngol Otol. 2004;118(11):891–2. https://doi.org/10.1258/0022215042703714.
2. Purnell DC, Smith LH, Scholz DA, Elveback LR, Arnaud CD. Primary hyperparathyroidism: a prospective clinical study. Am J Med. 1971;50(5):670–8.
3. American Academy of Pediatrics, American College of Obstetricians and Gynecologists. Guidelines for perinatal care. 7th ed. Washington, DC: American Academy of Pediatrics; American College of Obstetricians and Gynecologists; 2012.
4. Mestman JH. Parathyroid disorders of pregnancy. Semin Perinatol. 1998;22(6):485–96.
5. Schnatz PF, Curry SL. Primary hyperparathyroidism in pregnancy: evidence-based management. Obstet Gynecol Surv. 2002;57(6):365–76. https://doi.org/10.1097/01.OGX.0000017377.65823.CA.
6. Mahadevan S, Kumaravel V, Bharath R. Calcium and bone disorders in pregnancy. Indian J Endocrinol Metab. 2012;16(3):358–63. https://doi.org/10.4103/2230-8210.95665.
7. Lafond J, Goyer-O'Reilly I, Laramee M, Simoneau L. Hormonal regulation and implication of cell signaling in calcium transfer by placenta. Endocrine. 2001;14(3):285–94. https://doi.org/10.1385/ENDO:14:3:285.
8. Davis OK, Hawkins DS, Rubin LP, Posillico JT, Brown EM, Schiff I. Serum parathyroid hormone (PTH) in pregnant women determined by an immunoradiometric assay for intact PTH. J Clin Endocrinol Metab. 1988;67(4):850–2. https://doi.org/10.1210/jcem-67-4-850.
9. Kovacs CS. Calcium and bone metabolism disorders during pregnancy and lactation. Endocrinol Metab Clin N Am. 2011;40(4):795–826. https://doi.org/10.1016/j.ecl.2011.08.002.
10. Carella MJ, Gossain VV. Hyperparathyroidism and pregnancy: case report and review. J Gen Intern Med. 1992;7(4):448–53.
11. Delmonico FL, Neer RM, Cosimi AB, Barnes AB, Russell PS. Hyperparathyroidism during pregnancy. Am J Surg. 1976;131(3):328–37.
12. Truong MT, Lalakea ML, Robbins P, Friduss M. Primary hyperparathyroidism in pregnancy: a case series and review. Laryngoscope. 2008;118(11):1966–9. https://doi.org/10.1097/MLG.0b013e318180276f.

13. Norman J, Politz D, Politz L. Hyperparathyroidism during pregnancy and the effect of rising calcium on pregnancy loss: a call for earlier intervention. Clin Endocrinol. 2009;71(1):104–9. https://doi.org/10.1111/j.1365-2265.2008.03495.x.
14. McMullen TP, Learoyd DL, Williams DC, Sywak MS, Sidhu SB, Delbridge LW. Hyperparathyroidism in pregnancy: options for localization and surgical therapy. World J Surg. 2010;34(8):1811–6. https://doi.org/10.1007/s00268-010-0569-2.
15. Wagner G, Transbol I, Melchior JC. Hyperparathyroidism and Pregnancy. Acta Endocrinol. 1964;47:549–64.
16. Bruce J, Strong JA. Maternal hyperparathyroidism and parathyroid deficiency in the child; with an account of the effect of parathyroidectomy on renal function, and of an attempt to transplant part of the tumour. Q J Med. 1955;24(96):307–19.
17. Kelly TR. Primary hyperparathyroidism during pregnancy. Surgery. 1991;110(6):1028–33. Discussion 1033-1024.
18. Shangold MM, Dor N, Welt SI, Fleischman AR, Crenshaw MC Jr. Hyperparathyroidism and pregnancy: a review. Obstet Gynecol Surv. 1982;37(4):217–28.
19. Kort KC, Schiller HJ, Numann PJ. Hyperparathyroidism and pregnancy. Am J Surg. 1999;177(1):66–8.
20. Pothiwala P, Levine SN. Parathyroid surgery in pregnancy: review of the literature and localization by aspiration for parathyroid hormone levels. J Perinatol. 2009;29(12):779–84. https://doi.org/10.1038/jp.2009.84.
21. Sato K. Hypercalcemia during pregnancy, puerperium, and lactation: review and a case report of hypercalcemic crisis after delivery due to excessive production of PTH-related protein (PTHrP) without malignancy (humoral hypercalcemia of pregnancy). Endocr J. 2008;55(6):959–66.
22. Silverberg SJ. Natural history of primary hyperparathyroidism. Endocrinol Metab Clin N Am. 2000;29(3):451–64.
23. Inabnet WB, Baldwin D, Daniel RO, Staren ED. Hyperparathyroidism and pancreatitis during pregnancy. Surgery. 1996;119(6):710–3.
24. Kristoffersson A, Dahlgren S, Lithner F, Jarhult J. Primary hyperparathyroidism in pregnancy. Surgery. 1985;97(3):326–30.
25. Hultin H, Hellman P, Lundgren E, Olovsson M, Ekbom A, Rastad J, Montgomery SM. Association of parathyroid adenoma and pregnancy with preeclampsia. J Clin Endocrinol Metab. 2009;94(9):3394–9. https://doi.org/10.1210/jc.2009-0012.
26. Shani H, Sivan E, Cassif E, Simchen MJ. Maternal hypercalcemia as a possible cause of unexplained fetal polyhydramnion: a case series. Am J Obstet Gynecol. 2008;199(4):410.e411–5. https://doi.org/10.1016/j.ajog.2008.06.092.
27. Udelsman R, Akerstrom G, Biagini C, Duh QY, Miccoli P, Niederle B, Tonelli F. The surgical management of asymptomatic primary hyperparathyroidism: proceedings of the Fourth International Workshop. J Clin Endocrinol Metab. 2014;99(10):3595–606. https://doi.org/10.1210/jc.2014-2000.
28. Petousis S, Kourtis A, Anastasilakis CD, Makedou K, Giomisi A, Kalogiannidis I, Margioula-Siarkou C, Xanthopoulou E, Rousso D. Successful surgical treatment of primary hyperparathyroidism during the third trimester of pregnancy. J Musculoskelet Neuronal Interact. 2012;12(1):43–4. Quiz 45.
29. Hong MK, Hsieh CT, Chen BH, Tu ST, Chou PH. Primary hyperparathyroidism and acute pancreatitis during the third trimester of pregnancy. J Matern Fetal Med. 2001;10(3):214–8.
30. Schnatz PF. Surgical treatment of primary hyperparathyroidism during the third trimester. Obstet Gynecol. 2002;99(5 Pt 2):961–3.
31. Horjus C, Groot I, Telting D, van Setten P, van Sorge A, Kovacs CS, Hermus A, de Boer H. Cinacalcet for hyperparathyroidism in pregnancy and puerperium. J Pediatric Endocrinol Metab. 2009;22(8):741–9.

Four-Gland Exploration Versus Focused Parathyroidectomy for Hyperparathyroidism Jaw Tumor Syndrome

20

Dhaval Patel and Electron Kebebew

Abstract

Primary hyperparathyroidism, a common endocrine disorder, is associated with familial disease in about 10% of cases. These syndromes include multiple endocrine neoplasia types 1, 2A and 4 (MEN1, MEN2A, MEN4), familial isolated hyperparathyroidism (FIHP), and the hyperparathyroidism jaw tumor (HPT-JT) syndrome. HPT-JT syndrome, an autosomal dominant disease with incomplete penetrance, results from a germline inactivating mutation in the *HRPT2* gene. HPT-JT manifests with about 20% of patients having multiple enlarged parathyroid glands and/or parathyroid carcinoma. Furthermore, 28% of patients will have a recurrence during follow-up. Since these patients have a high rate of multiple enlarged parathyroid glands, parathyroid carcinoma, and recurrence, it is controversial as to what is the optimal initial surgical approach for parathyroidectomy. Clinical evidence for the optimal initial surgical approach for HPT-JT syndrome is limited to case series and retrospective small cohort studies. Furthermore, there is scant data on the clinical utility of localization studies to select the optimal operative approach. Only one study reported the results of localization studies and showed a lack of benefit due to high rates of multigland disease that would have been missed if a focused parathyroidectomy approach was used. Given the high rates of multigland disease, parathyroid carcinoma, risk of recurrence, and the possibility of missing additional enlarged glands not seen on preoperative localizing studies, bilateral neck exploration with identification of all four glands and removal of enlarged glands would be the best surgical approach given our current knowledge.

D. Patel
Endocrine Oncology Branch, National Cancer Institute, National Institutes of Health, Bethesda, MD, USA

E. Kebebew (✉)
Department of Surgery, School of Medicine, Stanford University, Stanford, CA, USA
e-mail: kebebew@stanford.edu

P. Angelos, R. H. Grogan (eds.), *Difficult Decisions in Endocrine Surgery*, Difficult Decisions in Surgery: An Evidence-Based Approach,
https://doi.org/10.1007/978-3-319-92860-9_20

Keywords
Hyperparathyroidism · HRPT2 · Parathyroid carcinoma · Focused single gland parathyroidectomy · Bilateral exploration · Multiglandular disease

Introduction

Primary hyperparathyroidism (PHPT) is a common endocrine disease that results from parathyroid adenoma(s) (single or multiple enlarged glands), or parathyroid carcinoma. In about 10% of cases, PHPT is associated with hereditary syndromes. These syndromes include multiple endocrine neoplasia types 1, 2A and 4 (MEN1, MEN2A, MEN4), familial isolated hyperparathyroidism (FIHP), and the hyperparathyroidism jaw tumor (HPT-JT) syndrome [1].

HPT-JT syndrome is an autosomal dominant inherited syndrome with incomplete penetrance and variable expression. In approximately 90% of carriers, PHPT will develop due to single or multiple parathyroid tumors. About 35% of patients may also develop ossifying fibromas of the mandible and/or maxilla [2]. Albeit less common, patients with HPT-JT syndrome also manifest with renal lesions (Wilm's tumors, polycystic disease, hamartomas, and adenocarcinomas) and uterine tumors [1, 2]. A recent report also indicated that there may be an association with thoracic aneurysms and HPT-JT syndrome [3].

HPT-JT syndrome is due to inactivating mutations in *HRPT2/CDC73*, a tumor suppressor gene, located on chromosome 1q31.2. The *HRPT2/CDC73* gene encodes the ubiquitously expressed nuclear protein parafibromin [4]. The function of parafibromin is believed to be inhibition of cellular proliferation through cell cycle arrest, and it is believed to act as a transcriptional regulator through interactions with the RNA polymerase II–associated factor 1 (PAF1) complex [5]. The identification of the *HRPT2/CDC73* as a susceptibility gene for HPT-JT and its presence as a somatic mutation in parathyroid carcinoma has provided additional information that should be considered when evaluating patients suspected or known to have HPT-JT. One controversial issue is what the optimal surgical approach is in patients with HPT-JT? Variable approaches have been advocated in the literature ranging from a focused parathyroidectomy approach based on preoperative localization results versus routine bilateral neck exploration with four gland identification and removal of enlarged parathyroid gland(s). The controversy exists because of the high rates of multiglandular disease, parathyroid carcinoma, and recurrence in patients with HPT-JT.

Search Strategy

A comprehensive review of the literature related to HPT-JT syndrome was performed. Literature searches were conducted in the PubMed database using the key words: hyperparathyroidism jaw-tumor syndrome, familial isolated hyperparathyroidism, *CDC73*, and *HRPT2*. Searches were limited to the English language and human subjects. Our search returned 476 articles. Thirty-seven articles related to HPT-JT syndrome with clinical and surgical data were reviewed. When families were reported in multiple articles, either the most current article related to that family or the article reporting the largest number of kindred was included in the analysis.

Intervention

Approximately 90% of individuals with germline *HRPT2/CDC73* inactivating mutations will develop biochemical evidence of PHPT [2]. Given the genetic predisposition, these patients pose a clinical question as to what is the optimal surgical approach. The standard surgical approach for these patients has been bilateral neck exploration with four gland identification. A recent study by Iacobone et al. questioned whether a focused parathyroidectomy may be a superior approach compared to a bilateral neck exploration in order to reduce morbidity. Iacobone et al. reported retrospective results of parathyroidectomy in 17 affected members in three large families. In this study, 23 out of 44 patients who underwent clinical examination were found to be carriers. Of the 23 patients, one patient was excluded due to death from metastatic renal cell carcinoma and lack of clinical data regarding parathyroid pathology. Six patients were asymptomatic, and in the remaining 16 patients, the authors reported biochemical evidence of PHPT. All 16 patients underwent bilateral neck exploration with identification of all four parathyroid glands. At the time of surgery, all patients had only a single parathyroid adenoma. Final pathology showed parathyroid adenoma for fifteen patients, and one patient had an atypical parathyroid adenoma (classified as parathyroid carcinoma by the authors).

Based on these results and a review of the literature, the authors proposed a focused parathyroidectomy should be considered in patients with HPT-JT syndrome who have localizing studies suggesting single gland disease. In their analysis of the literature, they found that there was single gland involvement in 89.0% of patients and synchronous multiglandular involvement in only 13.2% of patients [1, 2, 6–28]. In addition, the authors reported that the rate of parathyroid carcinoma in their series was only 11.8%, compared to data in the literature showing 24.3% of patients with HPT-JT syndrome have parathyroid carcinoma. The theoretical advantage of such an approach would be to avoid tissue trauma, leading to less scar tissue in reoperative cases, and possibly lower rate of recurrent laryngeal nerve injury and hypoparathyroidism as only one side of the neck would be explored. However, a major weakness in this study was that preoperative localization data was not reported. A recommendation of using a focused approach for parathyroidectomy in patients with HPT-JT syndrome should be based on data on the clinical utility of localizing studies similar to what has been done in patients with sporadic PHPT. Thus, the data presented by the authors can only speculate as to whether this approach would have been possible [29].

Comparator

As in other familial PHPT syndromes, bilateral neck exploration and the identification of four glands has been the gold standard surgical approach given the high rate of multigland disease in patients with germline mutations of *HRPT2/CDC73*. A comprehensive review of the literature showed a nearly one in five chance of having multigland disease at the initial neck exploration (Table 20.1). The rate of multiglandular disease in these patients is higher as compared to sporadic PHPT. Sarquis et al. reported their findings in three families [26]. The largest family had nine members affected, and six out of the nine patients who had neck exploration and parathyroidectomy had multigland disease. Preoperative localization data was not reported [26]. The evidence in this case series provides a strong case for bilateral neck exploration and four gland identification due to the rate of synchronous multigland involvement.

In another large cohort of patients, Mehta et al. examined the rate of multigland disease and parathyroid carcinoma. In that cohort, there were 16 affected family members, and the rate of synchronous multigland disease was 31.3%, or five out of 16 patients. Most strikingly, however, was the rate of parathyroid carcinoma, which was 37.5%. Given the rate of synchronous multigland disease and the risk of parathyroid carcinoma, the authors recommended a bilateral neck exploration and four-gland identification in all patients. Furthermore, in a thorough analysis of the literature, this study was the only study to report preoperative localization data with surgical approach and pathology with long term follow up. The authors found that preoperative localization was not always accurate for patients with synchronous multigland involvement with only two out of three patients being correctly identified with synchronous multigland involvement with preoperative localization studies [30].

The high risk of multigland disease and parathyroid carcinoma is also underscored by an affected patient reported by Korpi-Hyovalti et al.. In their series of patients, there were seven patients with HTP-JT and one patient had synchronous multigland disease. The patient underwent bilateral neck exploration and was found to have a 1.5 cm enlarged upper right parathyroid gland and a 1.4 cm enlarged upper left parathyroid gland. On final pathology, the authors reported that the right gland was parathyroid carcinoma based on histology showing vascular invasion and a Ki-67 proliferation index of 5%. The left parathyroid gland was reported as an atypical adenoma. Preoperative localization studies were, unfortunately, not reported in this study [3].

Outcome

In the literature, nearly all studies have defined cure as postoperative normalization of serum calcium and intact PTH levels for at least 6 months. Persistent disease has been defined as biochemical evidence of PHPT recurring within 6 months. Recurrent disease has been defined as biochemical evidence of PHPT occurring 6 months after

Table 20.1 Review of the literature focusing on HRPT2-related HPT (period 2002–2015)

Reference	Family (n)	Affected patients (n)	Patients with PHPT (n)	Single-gland involvement (n)	Synchronous multiglandular involvement (n)	Recurrences (n)	Follow-up (average years)	Jaw-tumor (n)	Parathyroid carcinoma (n)	Renal lesions (n)	Uterine lesions (n)
Carpten [1]	14	66	66/66	NA	NA	NA	NA	30/66	11/66	18/66	NA
Shattuck [6]	3	3	3/3	NA	NA	NA	NA	NA	3/3	NA	NA
Howell [7]	3	7	7/7	NA	NA	0/7	NA	0/7	3/7	0/7	NA
Simonds [8]	1	4	4/4	4/4	0/4	0/4	NA[a]	0/4	1/4	0/4	NA
Cetani [9]	2	4	4/4	3/4	1/4	NA	NA	0/4	0/4	0/4	NA
Villablanca [10]	2	9	9/9	7/9	2/9	3/9	7.44	0/9	0/9	0/9	NA
Cavaco [11]	6	11	9/11	5/9[b]	1/9[b]	0/9	5.56	2/11	0/11	2/11	NA
Howell [12]	1	2	2/2	2/2	0/2	0/2	NA	1/2	0/2	NA	NA
Gimm [32]	1	3	3/3	NA	NA	1/3	NA	NA	1/3	NA	NA
Bradley [2]	2	11	9/11	NA	NA	NA	NA	0/11	2/11	0/11	6/7
Moon [14]	1	2	2/2	2/2	0/2	NA	NA	1/2	2/2	NA	NA
Mizusawa [15]	3	7	7/7	6/7[c]	NA[c]	1/7	5.43	1/7	1/7	0/7	0/3
Aldred [16]	1	3	3/3	3/3	0/3	0/3	NA	2/3	0/3	NA	NA
Bradley [17]	5	5	5/5	4/5	1/5	NA	NA	2/5	0/5	0/5	1/4
Juhlin [18]	1	1	1/1	1/1	0/1	NA	NA	NA	0/1	NA	NA
Guarnieri [19]	1	5	4/5	4/4	0/4	1/4	2	NA	1/5	0/4	2/3
Kelly [20]	1	2	2/2	1/2	1/2	2/2	1.25	NA	2/2	NA	NA
Yamashita [21]	1	1	1/1	1/1	0/1	0/1	2	1/1	0/1	NA	NA
Cetani [22]	1	1	1/1	1/1	0/1	1/1	19	0/1	0/1	0/1	NA
Cetani [23]	2	3	3/3	NA	NA	NA	NA	NA	3/3	NA	NA
Raue [24]	1	2	2/2	1/2	1/2	NA	NA	1/2	1/2	NA	NA
Cetani [25]	1	1	1/1	1/1	0/1	NA	10	0/1	1/1	NA	NA

(continued)

Table 20.1 (continued)

Reference	Family (n)	Affected patients (n)	Patients with PHPT (n)	Single-gland involvement (n)	Synchronous multiglandular involvement (n)	Recurrences (n)	Follow-up (average years)	Jaw-tumor (n)	Parathyroid carcinoma (n)	Renal lesions (n)	Uterine lesions (n)
Sarquis [26]	3	11	11/11	5/11	6/11	8/11[d]	6.54	1/11	1/11	4/11	5/6
Guarnieri [27]	4	9	6/9	6/6	0/6	3/6	NA[e]	0/9	3/9	3/9	NA
Howell [28]	1	1	1/1	1/1	0/1	0/1	1	NA	NA	NA	NA
Iacobone [29]	3	17	16/17	15/16[f]	0/16[f]	3/16	8.60	1/17	1/17	1/17	8/13
Rekik [33]	1	1	1/1	1/1	0/1	0/1	NA	1/1	0/1	0/1	1/1
Panicker [34]	1	6	5/6	NA	NA	0/5	6	1/6	0/6	0/6	1/2
Cavaco [35]	2	2	2/2	2/2	0/2	1/2	NA	0/2	2/2	0/2	0/2
Pichardo-Lowden [36]	1	1	1/1	1/1	0/1	1/1	7	0/1	0/1	1/1	NA
Domingues [37]	1	1	1/1	1/1	0/1	0/1	1	0/1	0/1	0/1	NA
Bricaire [38]	15	13	12/13	NA	NA	NA	NA	3/15	2/15	2/15	2/6
Mehta [30]	7	16	16/16	11/16	5/16	4/16	5.12	2/16	6/16	3/16	2/6
Kong [39]	4	12	10/12	7/9	2/9	5/9	13.76	1/9	1/9	0/9	3/5
Korpi-Hyövälti [3]	1	8	8/8	6/7	1/7	NA	NA	0/7	2/7	2/7	NA
Total	98	251	238/251	79.7%	17.4%	28.0%	–	22.2%	20.0%	16.3%	53.5%

[a]A range of 3–29 years of normocalcemia was reported. No median follow-up time provided
[b]Three patients with known PHPT were not operated on; pathology (number of glands, histology) unknown
[c]Information concerning gland involvement not available for the patient with PHPT and parathyroid carcinoma
[d]Two of the patients had persistent disease after surgical intervention
[e]Individual data, not available. Each family had 2–4 years of follow-up
[f]One patient with known PHPT was not operated on; pathology (number of glands, histology) unknown

curative surgery. Iacobone et al. achieved cure by selective parathyroidectomy in 93.3% of patients. One patient had persistent disease after en-bloc parathyroidectomy and thyroid lobectomy. This patient was suspected and later diagnosed with parathyroid carcinoma. Aside from the patient with parathyroid carcinoma, the remaining patients were cured for an average of 12.3 years. Three patients had recurrent PHPT and were found to have metachronous single parathyroid tumors [29]. In another large series, Sarquis et al. had a higher rate of recurrence compared to the literature with eight out of 11 patients recurring after parathyroidectomy with an average disease free interval of 5 years. In the largest family, two out of the nine patients had persistent disease, and four out of the nine patients had recurrent disease. The average time to recurrence was 4.6 years for the six patients who had recurrence. One out of the nine patients had a second recurrence 30 years after her initial surgery [26]. Mehta et al. reported that one patient had persistent disease and three patients had recurrent disease. All four of these patients were found to have parathyroid carcinoma at either initial operation or subsequent operations. The average time to recurrence was 3.3 years for the three patients who were cured with their initial surgery [30]. In patients with HPT-JT, the rate of persistent/recurrent disease is approximately 28% based on review of the literature (Table 20.1).

In order to maximize the success of focused parathyroidectomy, preoperative localization studies should be reliable and accurate for demonstrating single gland disease. The evidence for the accuracy of localization in HPT-JT syndrome has not been reported extensively. To our knowledge, the study by Mehta et al. is the only study that analyzed preoperative imaging study results, surgical approaches, final pathology and patient outcome. Eleven patients with single gland disease and two patients with synchronous multigland disease were identified accurately by preoperative imaging and confirmed after bilateral neck exploration and on pathology. One patient was thought to have single gland involvement by preoperative localizing studies, but was found to have synchronous multigland disease intraoperatively [30]. Given the paucity of preoperative localization data in HPT-JT syndrome, evaluating preoperative localization data in other familial PHPT syndromes such as MEN1 may be helpful. Nilubol et al. analyzed the accuracy of neck ultrasonography, sestamibi parathyroid scan, parathyroid protocol CT scan, and neck MRI relative to the total number of enlarged parathyroid glands found intraoperatively in patients with MEN1. Preoperative imaging was found to be not helpful in this cohort of patients, who like HPT-JT syndrome, had a high rate of synchronous multigland involvement [31].

The main risks of parathyroidectomy are bleeding, recurrent laryngeal nerve injury and hypoparathyroidism. Unfortunately, due to the rarity of the disease and lack of uniformity in reporting of case series, there is minimal data regarding complications specifically in patients with HPT-JT. Mehta et al. did report that two out of 16 patients had postoperative permanent hypoparathyroidism. In their series, although there were no permanent recurrent laryngeal nerve injuries and/or hematomas at initial operation, one patient did have a recurrent laryngeal nerve injury during their second operation. Many of these patients will have recurrent disease, and the risk of recurrent laryngeal nerve injury in reoperative parathyroid surgery is higher [30]. This fact emphasizes the importance of patients with HPT-JT being treated by an experienced endocrine surgeon. The importance of reporting complications and outcome data cannot be over emphasized and evaluation of this information by surgeons is important in determining what the optimal surgical approach is for parathyroidectomy in patients with HPT-JT.

Recommendations

The evidence for selecting focused parathyroidectomy or bilateral neck exploration with four gland identification and removal of enlarged parathyroid gland(s) in patients with HPT-JT syndrome is based on limited retrospective data. There are no prospective or randomized controlled trials and they are unlikely to be conducted given the rarity of HPT-JT syndrome, even at referral centers. Thus, the recommendation on the optimal surgical approach is based on the high rates of synchronous multigland disease, higher rate of parathyroid carcinoma at initial presentation or at the time of recurrent disease, and the overall higher rate of recurrence. In our own series of patients where we reported localizing data, surgical approach and final pathology, and follow up data, we believe that bilateral neck exploration with identification of all parathyroid glands and removal of enlarged glands is the optimal approach. In selected subjects a focused approach may be considered if (1) multiple localizing studies suggest single gland disease, (2) the biochemical profile and imaging studies are not suspicious for parathyroid carcinoma, (3) intraoperative PTH monitoring will be used as an adjunct to confirm biochemical cure, (4) the patient is young with no family members who had parathyroid carcinoma, and (5) the patient prefers a focused approach, or has had a previous thyroid or parathyroid operation and presents with persistent/recurrent disease. In our opinion, the morbidity of parathyroid carcinoma and the high rate of synchronous multigland disease outweigh the morbidity of bilateral neck exploration, especially when done by specialized endocrine surgeons.

References

1. Carpten JD, Robbins CM, Villablanca A, Forsberg L, Presciuttini S, Bailey-Wilson J, et al. HRPT2, encoding parafibromin, is mutated in hyperparathyroidism-jaw tumor syndrome. Nat Genet. 2002;32(4):676–80. PMID: 12434154.
2. Bradley KJ, Hobbs MR, Buley ID, Carpten JD, Cavaco BM, Fares JE, et al. Uterine tumours are a phenotypic manifestation of the hyperparathyroidism-jaw tumour syndrome. J Intern Med. 2005;257(1):18–26. PMID: 15606373.
3. Korpi-Hyovalti E, Cranston T, Ryhanen E, Arola J, Aittomaki K, Sane T, et al. CDC73 intragenic deletion in familial primary hyperparathyroidism associated with parathyroid carcinoma. J Clin Endocrinol Metab. 2014;99(9):3044–8. PMID: 24823466. PMCID: 4207936.
4. Yart A, Gstaiger M, Wirbelauer C, Pecnik M, Anastasiou D, Hess D, et al. The HRPT2 tumor suppressor gene product parafibromin associates with human PAF1 and RNA polymerase II. Mol Cell Biol. 2005;25(12):5052–60. PMID: 15923622. PMCID: 1140601.
5. Masi G, Barzon L, Iacobone M, Viel G, Porzionato A, Macchi V, et al. Clinical, genetic, and histopathologic investigation of CDC73-related familial hyperparathyroidism. Endocr Relat Carcinoma. 2008;15(4):1115–26. PMID: 18755853.

6. Shattuck TM, Valimaki S, Obara T, Gaz RD, Clark OH, Shoback D, et al. Somatic and germ-line mutations of the HRPT2 gene in sporadic parathyroid carcinoma. N Engl J Med. 2003;349(18):1722–9. PMID: 14585940.
7. Howell VM, Haven CJ, Kahnoski K, Khoo SK, Petillo D, Chen J, et al. HRPT2 mutations are associated with malignancy in sporadic parathyroid tumours. J Med Genet. 2003;40(9):657–63. PMID: 12960210. PMCID: 1735580.
8. Simonds WF, Robbins CM, Agarwal SK, Hendy GN, Carpten JD, Marx SJ. Familial isolated hyperparathyroidism is rarely caused by germline mutation in HRPT2, the gene for the hyperparathyroidism-jaw tumor syndrome. J Clin Endocrinol Metab. 2004;89(1):96–102. PMID: 14715834.
9. Cetani F, Pardi E, Borsari S, Viacava P, Dipollina G, Cianferotti L, et al. Genetic analyses of the HRPT2 gene in primary hyperparathyroidism: germline and somatic mutations in familial and sporadic parathyroid tumors. J Clin Endocrinol Metab. 2004;89(11):5583–91. PMID: 15531515.
10. Villablanca A, Calender A, Forsberg L, Hoog A, Cheng JD, Petillo D, et al. Germline and de novo mutations in the HRPT2 tumour suppressor gene in familial isolated hyperparathyroidism (FIHP). J Med Genet. 2004;41(3):e32. PMID: 14985403. PMCID: 1735713.
11. Cavaco BM, Guerra L, Bradley KJ, Carvalho D, Harding B, Oliveira A, et al. Hyperparathyroidism-jaw tumor syndrome in Roma families from Portugal is due to a founder mutation of the HRPT2 gene. J Clin Endocrinol Metab. 2004;89(4):1747–52. PMID: 15070940.
12. Howell VM, Zori RT, Stalker HJ, Williams C, Jesse N, Nelson AE, et al. A molecular diagnosis of hyperparathyroidism-jaw tumor syndrome in an adolescent with recurrent kidney stones. J Pediatr. 2004;145(4):567. PMID: 15480389.
13. Gimm O, Lorenz K, Nguyen Thanh P, Schneyer U, Bloching M, Howell VM, et al. Das familiare Nebenschilddrusenkarzinom Indikation zur prophylaktischen Parathyreoidektomie? [Prophylactic parathyroidectomy for familial parathyroid carcinoma]. Chirurg. 2006;77(1):15–24. PMID: 16418876.
14. Moon SD, Park JH, Kim EM, Kim JH, Han JH, Yoo SJ, et al. A Novel IVS2-1G>A mutation causes aberrant splicing of the HRPT2 gene in a family with hyperparathyroidism-jaw tumor syndrome. J Clin Endocrinol Metab. 2005;90(2):878–83. PMID: 15613436.
15. Mizusawa N, Uchino S, Iwata T, Tsuyuguchi M, Suzuki Y, Mizukoshi T, et al. Genetic analyses in patients with familial isolated hyperparathyroidism and hyperparathyroidism-jaw tumour syndrome. Clin Endocrinol. 2006;65(1):9–16. PMID: 16817812.
16. Aldred MJ, Talacko AA, Savarirayan R, Murdolo V, Mills AE, Radden BG, et al. Dental findings in a family with hyperparathyroidism-jaw tumor syndrome and a novel HRPT2 gene mutation. Oral Surg Oral Med Oral Pathol Oral Radiol Endod. 2006;101(2):212–8. PMID: 16448924.
17. Bradley KJ, Cavaco BM, Bowl MR, Harding B, Cranston T, Fratter C, et al. Parafibromin mutations in hereditary hyperparathyroidism syndromes and parathyroid tumours. Clin Endocrinol. 2006;64(3):299–306. PMID: 16487440.
18. Juhlin C, Larsson C, Yakoleva T, Leibiger I, Leibiger B, Alimov A, et al. Loss of parafibromin expression in a subset of parathyroid adenomas. Endocr Relat Carcinoma. 2006;13(2):509–23. PMID: 16728578.
19. Guarnieri V, Scillitani A, Muscarella LA, Battista C, Bonfitto N, Bisceglia M, et al. Diagnosis of parathyroid tumors in familial isolated hyperparathyroidism with HRPT2 mutation: implications for carcinoma surveillance. J Clin Endocrinol Metab. 2006;91(8):2827–32. PMID: 16720667.
20. Kelly TG, Shattuck TM, Reyes-Mugica M, Stewart AF, Simonds WF, Udelsman R, et al. Surveillance for early detection of aggressive parathyroid disease: carcinoma and atypical adenoma in familial isolated hyperparathyroidism associated with a germline HRPT2 mutation. J Bone Miner Res. 2006;21(10):1666–71. PMID: 16995822.
21. Yamashita Y, Akiyama T, Mizusawa N, Yoshimoto K, Goto M. A case of hyperparathyroidism-jaw tumour syndrome found in the treatment of an ossifying fibroma in the maxillary bone. Int J Oral Maxillofac Surg. 2007;36(4):365–9. PMID: 17052894.

22. Cetani F, Pardi E, Ambrogini E, Viacava P, Borsari S, Lemmi M, et al. Different somatic alterations of the HRPT2 gene in a patient with recurrent sporadic primary hyperparathyroidism carrying an HRPT2 germline mutation. Endocr Relat Carcinoma. 2007;14(2):493–9. PMID: 17639062.
23. Cetani F, Ambrogini E, Viacava P, Pardi E, Fanelli G, Naccarato AG, et al. Should parafibromin staining replace HRTP2 gene analysis as an additional tool for histologic diagnosis of parathyroid carcinoma? Eur J Endocrinol. 2007;156(5):547–54. PMID: 17468190.
24. Raue F, Haag C, Frank-Raue K. Hyperparathyreoidismus-Kiefertumor-Syndrom. Eine hereditare Form des primaren Hyperparathyreoidismus mit Nebenschilddrusenkarzinom [Hyperparathyroidism-jaw tumor syndrome. A hereditary form of primary hyperparathyroidism with parathyroid carcinoma]. Dtsch Med Wochenschr. 2007;132(27):1459–62. PMID: 17583828.
25. Cetani F, Pardi E, Ambrogini E, Banti C, Viacava P, Borsari S, et al. Hyperparathyroidism 2 gene (HRPT2, CDC73) and parafibromin studies in two patients with primary hyperparathyroidism and uncertain pathological assessment. J Endocrinol Investig. 2008;31(10):900–4. PMID: 19092296.
26. Sarquis MS, Silveira LG, Pimenta FJ, Dias EP, Teh BT, Friedman E, et al. Familial hyperparathyroidism: surgical outcome after 30 years of follow-up in three families with germline HRPT2 mutations. Surgery. 2008;143(5):630–40. PMID: 18436011.
27. Guarnieri V, Bisceglia M, Bonfitto N, Cetani F, Marcocci C, Minisola S, et al. Re: Familial hyperparathyroidism: surgical outcome after 30 years of follow-up in three families with germline HRPT2 mutations. Surgery. 2008;144(5):839–40. PMID: 19081034.
28. Howell VM, Gill A, Clarkson A, Nelson AE, Dunne R, Delbridge LW, et al. Accuracy of combined protein gene product 9.5 and parafibromin markers for immunohistochemical diagnosis of parathyroid carcinoma. J Clin Endocrinol Metab. 2009;94(2):434–41. PMID: 19017757.
29. Iacobone M, Masi G, Barzon L, Porzionato A, Macchi V, Ciarleglio FA, et al. Hyperparathyroidism-jaw tumor syndrome: a report of three large kindred. Langenbeck's Arch Surg. 2009;394(5):817–25. PMID: 19529956.
30. Mehta A, Patel D, Rosenberg A, Boufraqech M, Ellis RJ, Nilubol N, et al. Hyperparathyroidism-jaw tumor syndrome: Results of operative management. Surgery. 2014;156(6):1315–24. Discussion 24–5. PMID: 25444225. PMCID: 4255585.
31. Nilubol N, Weinstein L, Simonds WF, Jensen RT, Phan GQ, Hughes MS, et al. Preoperative localizing studies for initial parathyroidectomy in MEN1 syndrome: is there any benefit? World J Surg. 2012;36(6):1368–74. PMID: 22350475.
32. Gimm O, Lorenz K, Nguyen Thanh P, et al. Das Familiäre Nebenschilddrüsenkarzinom. Indikation zur prophylaktischen Parathyreoidektomie? Chirurg. 2006;77:15–24. PMID: 16418876.
33. Rekik N, Ben Naceur B, Mnif M, Mnif F, Mnif H, Boudawara T, et al. Hyperparathyroidism-jaw tumor syndrome: a case report. Ann Endocrinol (Paris). 2010;71(2):121–6. PMID: 19942209. Epub 2009/11/28. eng.
34. Panicker LM, Zhang JH, Dagur PK, Gastinger MJ, Simonds WF. Defective nucleolar localization and dominant interfering properties of a parafibromin L95P missense mutant causing the hyperparathyroidism-jaw tumor syndrome. Endocr Relat Carcinoma. 2010;17(2):513–24. PMID: 20304979. PMCID: 3098453. Epub 2010/03/23. eng.
35. Cavaco BM, Santos R, Felix A, Carvalho D, Lopes JM, Domingues R, et al. Identification of de novo germline mutations in the HRPT2 gene in two apparently sporadic cases with challenging parathyroid tumor diagnoses. Endocr Pathol. 2011;22(1):44–52. PMID: 21360064. Epub 2011/03/02. eng.
36. Pichardo-Lowden AR, Manni A, Saunders BD, Baker MJ. Familial hyperparathyroidism due to a germline mutation of the CDC73 gene: implications for management and age-appropriate testing of relatives at risk. Endocr Pract. 2011;17(4):602–9. PMID: 21324824. Epub 2011/02/18. eng.
37. Domingues R, Tomaz RA, Martins C, Nunes C, Bugalho MJ, Cavaco BM. Identification of the first germline HRPT2 whole-gene deletion in a patient with primary hyperparathyroidism. Clin Endocrinol. 2012;76(1):33–8. PMID: 21790700. Epub 2011/07/28. eng.

38. Bricaire L, Odou MF, Cardot-Bauters C, Delemer B, North MO, Salenave S, et al. Frequent large germline HRPT2 deletions in a French National cohort of patients with primary hyperparathyroidism. J Clin Endocrinol Metab. 2013;98(2):E403–8. PMID: 23293331. Epub 2013/01/08. eng.
39. Kong J, Wang O, Nie M, Shi J, Hu Y, Jiang Y, et al. Familial isolated primary hyperparathyroidism/hyperparathyroidism-jaw tumour syndrome caused by germline gross deletion or point mutations of CDC73 gene in Chinese. Clin Endocrinol. 2014;81(2):222–30. PMID: 24716902.

21 Long-Term Success of Surgery for Primary Hyperparathyroidism: Focused Exploration using Intraoperative Parathyroid Hormone Monitoring Versus Four-Gland Exploration

Wesley Barnes, Peter F. Czako, and Sapna Nagar

Abstract

Primary hyperparathyroidism is a common problem that is a result of the excessive secretion of parathyroid hormone (PTH) from the parathyroid glands. This is most commonly caused by a single hypersecreting adenomatous gland. Most all patients with primary hyperparathyroidism meet criteria for surgery. The best operation should provide the highest rate of cure with the lowest rate of complications. The standard surgical approach has traditionally been a four-gland exploration. Though this method has endured many years of excellent cure rates, it has been challenged because a long-lasting cure is possible with the removal of a single adenoma in the majority of cases. Thus, a focused exploration via an image-guided, open unilateral exploration employing intraoperative PTH (ioPTH) monitoring has gained popularity over the last two decades. Specifically, ioPTH monitoring has been shown to be paramount to this approach, enabling a more limited exploration by accurately guiding gland excision and predicting postoperative cure. Several large series of focused parathyroid operations have shown excellent, durable cure rates similar to standard four-gland exploration. Focused exploration guided by ioPTH is a safe, effective technique that is recommended for most patients with sporadic primary hyperparathyroidism.

Keywords

Primary hyperparathyroidism · Hypercalcemia · Four-gland exploration · Bilateral neck exploration · Focused parathyroidectomy · Minimally invasive parathyroidectomy(MIP) · Limited parathyroidectomy · Intraoperative parathyroid hormone monitoring (IOPTH)

W. Barnes · P. F. Czako · S. Nagar (✉)
Department of Surgery, Oakland University William Beaumont School of Medicine, Beaumont Hospitals, Royal Oak, MI, USA
e-mail: Sapna.Nagar@beaumont.edu

P. Angelos, R. H. Grogan (eds.), *Difficult Decisions in Endocrine Surgery*, Difficult Decisions in Surgery: An Evidence-Based Approach,
https://doi.org/10.1007/978-3-319-92860-9_21

Population: Patients with Primary Hyperparathyroidism Undergoing Surgery

Epidemiology

Primary hyperparathyroidism is a common problem with 100,000 new cases detected annually in the United States [1]. It is the third most common endocrine disorder, and the most common cause of hypercalcemia in the nonhospitalized patient [2]. It is more common in women than men. Prevalence depends on the age of the population being studied. It is present in about 1 out of every 500 women and 1 out of every 2000 men over the age of 40 [3]. The typical patient is a postmenopausal female.

For decades after its initial description as a medical disorder, primary hyperparathyroidism was diagnosed after bone or renal complications produced symptoms. However, as routine calcium screening became more common with the advent of automated multichannel analysis in the early 1970s, there was a significant increase in its incidence. As an example, the annual incidence rose from 15 per 100,000 person-years before 1974 (prescreening) to a peak of 112 per 100,000 person-years in 1975 following the introduction of calcium screening in the population of Rochester, Minnesota [4]. This was attributed to the identification of previously unrecognized patients with asymptomatic hypercalcemia and primary hyperparathyroidism [5]. Furthermore, in this Rochester population, the proportion of patients presenting with classical symptoms or complications of primary hyperparathyroidism decreased from 22% in the prescreening era to 6% thereafter [4]. A more recent study from a racially mixed population in Southern California showed that the incidence of primary hyperparathyroidism tripled during the study period from 1995 to 2010, increasing from 76 to 233 per 100,000 female-years and from 30 to 85 per 100,000 male-years [6].

Pathophysiology

Primary hyperparathyroidism is the result of excessive secretion of parathyroid hormone (PTH) from one or more parathyroid glands. Chief cells in the parathyroid gland release PTH mainly in response to low extracellular calcium detected by a calcium-sensing receptor (CaSR) on their cell membranes. Other stimuli of PTH secretion include low levels of 1,25-dihydroxyvitamin D and hypomagnesemia. PTH along with vitamin D and calcitonin regulate serum calcium and phosphorus levels through their interactions with three target organ systems—the skeleton, the kidneys, and the gastrointestinal tract. In the bone, PTH stimulates bone resorption via increased osteoclastic activity. In the kidney, PTH promotes tubular reabsorption of calcium and the hydroxylation of 25-hydroxyvitamin D but inhibits phosphorus absorption. Finally, PTH indirectly stimulates calcium absorption from the gut by increasing 1,25-dihydroxyvitamin D production. As a result of these interactions, PTH serves to increase serum calcium and reduce serum phosphorus. With rising calcium levels, feedback inhibition of the CaSR on chief cells normally results in a decrease in PTH secretion.

Failure of this feedback regulation permits inappropriately high levels of PTH release. Primary hyperparathyroidism results from the autonomous production of PTH from one of three different pathologic lesions: parathyroid adenoma, parathyroid hyperplasia, or parathyroid carcinoma. Single gland adenomas are the most common cause (accounting for 75–85% of cases); double adenomas are seen in 2–12% of cases, and three gland adenomas represent less than 1–2% of cases. Four-gland hyperplasia is seen in up to 15% of patients with primary hyperparathyroidism, and parathyroid carcinoma is rare—accounting for approximately 1% of cases [2]. In the majority of patients, primary hyperparathyroidism arises spontaneously, and no known cause is identified to explain the loss of calcium sensitivity at the glandular level. Some authors have found an association between exposure of the head and neck to ionizing radiation and the future development of hyperparathyroidism [7]. Although the etiology of sporadic primary hyperparathyroidism is unclear, it is certainly different from secondary or tertiary hyperparathyroidism caused by chronic renal insufficiency and from familial disorders like multiple endocrine neoplasia (MEN) with identifiable genetic abnormalities.

Diagnosis

Clinical Manifestations

In the United States, most patients lack the classic clinical manifestations described by Fuller Albright such as osteitis fibrosa cystica, nephrolithiasis, peptic ulcer disease, pancreatitis, gout and neuromuscular weakness [8]. At first, primary hyperparathyroidism was a disease of the bones, but it soon became evident that kidney stones were more common. Historically, the classic pentad of symptoms included painful bones, kidney stones, abdominal groans, psychic moans, and fatigue overtones. Constipation, anorexia, polyuria, depression, fatigue, and weakness are manifestations of hypercalcemia in general. Only symptoms of fatigue, bone pain, and weight loss seem to correlate with the severity of hypercalcemia [9]. It is estimated that approximately 20% of patients with primary hyperparathyroidism present with symptoms from kidney stones, bone disease, or proximal neuromuscular weakness [10–12]. Nephrolithiasis is the most common complication (15–20%) and less than 5% of patients present with osteitis fibrosa cystica. The clinical presentation often differs drastically in developing countries that do not have access to routine calcium screening. In these situations, the search for classic symptoms unveils the disease [13]. Perhaps these geographical differences in presentation can be explained to some degree by evidence suggesting the disease is more severe in countries where hypovitaminosis D is more widespread [14–16].

Today, the classic skeletal consequence of primary hyperparathyroidism is really only seen in parts of the world where symptomatic disease predominates. Advanced primary hyperparathyroidism is characterized by osteitis fibrosa cystica (generalized bone pain, fragility fractures, "brown" tumors; radiologic features include salt-and-pepper appearance of the skull, subperiosteal bone resorption of the phalanges, and tapering of the distal third of the clavicle). Although this classic feature is now rare in most places, skeletal involvement remains a critical aspect of the disease. Today, bone mineral density (BMD) testing has become a suitable method for the detection of skeletal complications of asymptomatic primary hyperparathyroidism. BMD measurement is now a standard of care for the evaluation of this disease [17]. Usually, bone loss is most prominent in the distal one-third of the radius (comprised mostly of cortical bone) and least evident at the lumbar spine (comprised mostly of trabecular bone) [18]. Despite data suggesting that the spine is relatively preserved, most studies have demonstrated an increased risk of fractures at all sites—trabecular bone of the spine as well as cortical sites (forearm, hip)—in patients with primary hyperparathyroidism [19–22]. A longitudinal 15-year study out of Columbia revealed progressive BMD losses from cortical sites in 37% of asymptomatic patients over the entire study period [23].

Nephrolithiasis is a key component of the classic pentad of clinical features described previously, and the kidney remains a principal target of primary hyperparathyroidism. The kidney is the organ most likely to demonstrate overt clinical manifestations as a result of the effects of the disease today. Approximately 15% to 20% of patients with primary hyperparathyroidism experience nephrolithiasis. About 3% of patients with stone disease have primary hyperparathyroidism [24]. Kidney stone disease is multifactorial and cannot be explained purely by hypercalciuria. Nevertheless, hypercalciuria is a significant urinary risk factor for the development of calcium oxalate and phosphate stones. Nephrocalcinosis (mineralization of the renal parenchyma) seems to be much less common and not present until disease becomes severe. Primary hyperparathyroidism is associated with renal insufficiency as well; this is demonstrated by a decline in estimated glomerular filtration rate below 60 mL/min in up to 17% of patients suffering from asymptomatic disease [25].

Currently many authors believe that primary hyperparathyroidism is associated with cardiovascular disease, including hypertension, coronary artery disease, heart failure, left ventricular hypertrophy, atherosclerosis, valvular calcifications, and cerebrovascular accidents. Cardiovascular morbidity and mortality were increased in classical primary hyperparathyroidism, but the cardiovascular outcomes from mild or asymptomatic disease continue to be less clear [17]. Studies out of Scotland found increased cardiovascular mortality in primary hyperparathyroidism [26, 27]. Hypertension is frequently associated with this disease, even among those with mild disease [28, 29]. Some studies have found that left ventricular mass [30] and aortic valve calcification area [31, 32] correlate with PTH levels but do not seem to improve following parathyroidectomy. A recent study suggested that the carotid artery may be more affected than the heart, indicating that primary hyperparathyroidism may not initiate but could propagate intimal medial thickness and plaque thickness [32]. However, the degree to which these relationships exist along with the reversibility of such manifestations following surgical correction remains a topic of considerable debate as most available data are observational. Thus, at this time, there is no evidence to suggest that cardiovascular function or structure should be routinely evaluated in the workup of primary hyperparathyroidism [14].

Today, around 80% of patients diagnosed in the United States are asymptomatic with mild hypercalcemia. Because a biochemical diagnosis is often made incidentally in an asymptomatic patient, the history and physical seldom provide any insight into the diagnosis of primary hyperparathyroidism. However, vague or non-specific effects on fatigue, cognition, and depression may be more common than previously thought [33].

Initial Investigations

Primary hyperparathyroidism is often initially suspected after an incidental finding of elevated calcium on routine serum chemistry. The total serum calcium should be adjusted for any albumin abnormality. Although ionized calcium can be measured, most centers use total serum calcium concentration. For the hypercalcemic patient, a serum calcium should be repeated in conjunction with intact PTH (iPTH). A diagnosis of primary hyperparathyroidism is established by an elevated PTH concentration in a hypercalcemic patient or by a PTH concentration that is within the mid to upper end of normal range but inappropriately high for a patient's degree of hypercalcemia. The second most common cause of hypercalcemia is malignancy, which can generally be ruled out by an elevated PTH level.

Other laboratory values that are useful in confirming the diagnosis of primary hyperparathyroidism include 24-h urine calcium excretion (elevated in approximately 25% to 35% of patients) and 25-hydroxyvitamin D levels (usually low-normal range) [13]. Patients with primary hyperparathyroidism have a low or low-normal serum phosphorus level and an increased serum chloride-to-phosphorus ratio. Also, these patients exhibit a mild hyperchloremic metabolic acidosis from renal bicarbonate wasting. Differential diagnosis of the hypercalcemic patient with an elevated PTH also includes familial hypocalciuric hypercalcemia (FHH), hyperparathyroidism secondary to lithium or thiazide diuretic administration, and tertiary hyperparathyroidism seen with end-stage renal disease.

Formally recognized in 2008, normocalcemic hyperparathyroidism has been detected most often through the evaluation of individuals with osteoporosis and recurrent nephrolithiasis [34, 35]. The diagnosis of normocalcemic hyperparathyroidism is a challenge. In order to make a diagnosis, all secondary causes of hyperparathyroidism must be ruled out, ionized calcium levels should be normal, and the serum 25-hydroxyvitamin D level should not be below the lower limit of normal. It is not yet clear whether patients with this normocalcemic variant in fact have an early form of primary hyperparathyroidism, and thus their calcium levels, if followed long enough, would be expected to rise [36, 37]. However, this variant remains incompletely described with regard to its epidemiology, natural history, and management [17].

Natural History of Asymptomatic Primary Hyperparathyroidism Without Surgery

As mentioned previously, prior to the introduction of automated equipment for analyzing routine serum calcium levels, primary hyperparathyroidism was a symptomatic disorder in which debilitating bone disease, kidney stones, and muscular weakness were common. Throughout history, symptomatic patients have continued to undergo parathyroidectomy for prevention of disease progression and relief of symptoms. However, the majority of patients today seem to have a milder form of the disease and, thus, treatment decisions that are rooted in risk-benefit analyses hinge largely on the natural history of the disease. A prospective 10-year follow-up study was begun at the Mayo Clinic in 1968, and it showed that the majority of asymptomatic patients who were followed without surgery did well with no significant disease progression [38]. Later, Rao et al. examined the course of 80 untreated asymptomatic patients for up to 11 years; there were no episodes of worsening hypercalcemia, renal function, nephrolithiasis, or densitometric indices during this period [39]. These studies and others like them validated the nonoperative surveillance of mild asymptomatic primary hyperparathyroidism by reporting that rapid progression of biochemistry, symptoms, or metabolic complications is uncommon with borderline hypercalcemia.

However, a longitudinal 15-year follow-up study out of Columbia University Medical Center published in 2008 demonstrated that BMD in cortical sites (distal radius, femoral neck) declines over time in asymptomatic patients who do not undergo surgery regardless of administration of antiresorptive therapy, but BMD improves following parathyroidectomy [23]. Furthermore, 37% of asymptomatic patients in this study showed disease progression (i.e., developing one or more new indication for surgery during the study period) [23]. In another study, patients younger than 50 years of age were about three times more likely to have disease progression [40]. Several studies have provided more data on the natural history of untreated asymptomatic primary hyperparathyroidism [41–43]. Biochemistries may remain largely unchanged for up to 12 years, and BMD is stable for up to 8 years [23]. However, long-term observation seems suboptimal for skeletal outcomes. These data led to the consensus response that surgery is appropriate in the majority of patients with asymptomatic primary hyperparathyroidism despite evidence for biochemical and densitometric stability with nonsurgical surveillance because current data suggests that this stability is not indefinite [44].

Surgical Management of Primary Hyperparathyroidism

The approach to managing patients with primary hyperparathyroidism has undergone several changes over the last few decades. Yet, parathyroidectomy remains the only definitive cure [45]. There is universal agreement that all symptomatic patients should undergo surgery. However, the optimal treatment strategy for asymptomatic patients is less clear. In order to provide an evidence-based consensus on the management of asymptomatic primary hyperparathyroidism, the National Institutes of Health (NIH) met in 1990, 2002, and 2013 to develop guidelines for the surgical treatment of this disease (Table 21.1). Surgery is also indicated in patients who refuse to undergo medical surveillance and in patients opting for an operation even if they do not meet any guidelines [14]. Following successful parathyroidectomy, kidney stone formation is reduced in those with a history of stones, bone density improves, fracture incidence decreases, and subjective improvements in

Table 21.1 PICO table

P	Population	Patients with primary hyperparathyroidism undergoing surgery: • Symptomatic primary hyperparathyroidism • Asymptomatic primary hyperparathyroidism with following indications [14]: – Age <50 years – Serum calcium 1.0 mg/dL above the upper limit of normal – BMD by DXA: T-score <−2.5 at lumbar spine, total hip, femoral neck, or distal 1/3 of radius – Vertebral fracture by radiograph, CT, MRI, or VFA – Creatinine clearance <60 mL/min – 24-h urinary calcium >400 mg/day and increased calcium-containing stone risk by biochemical analysis – Presence of nephrolithiasis or nephrocalcinosis by radiograph, ultrasound, or CT
I	Intervention	Four-gland exploration has served as the gold standard for several decades, demonstrating cure rates that range from 95 to 99% and a low risk of permanent recurrent laryngeal nerve injury (<1%) and permanent hypoparathyroidism (<0.5%)
C	Comparator	Focused exploration via an image-guided, open unilateral exploration employing ioPTH. With ioPTH monitoring, the surgeon can: • Make an objective determination of cure in the operating room • Often perform a more limited procedure with a potential to decrease risk of injuring the recurrent laryngeal nerves and other normal parathyroid glands
O	Outcome	A review of the literature comparing focused exploration using ioPTH monitoring to traditional four-gland exploration demonstrates the following: • No statistically significant difference in persistent primary hyperparathyroidism, which ranged from 0% to 4% for focused exploration • No statistically significant difference in recurrent primary hyperparathyroidism, which ranged from 0% to 4% for focused exploration • No statistically significant difference in complications (recurrent laryngeal nerve injury, permanent hypoparathyroidism, cervical hematoma, wound infection, etc.) Focused exploration guided by ioPTH is a safe, effective technique that is recommended for most patients with sporadic primary hyperparathyroidism (moderate quality GRADE recommendation)

BMD bone mineral density, *CT* computed tomography, *DXA* dual-energy X-ray absorptiometry, *MRI* magnetic resonance imaging, *VFA* vertebral fracture assessment, *ioPTH* intraoperative parathyroid hormone

neurocognitive elements as well as quality of life are noted [14]. Cardiovascular disease is one of the most common causes of mortality in patients with both treated and untreated primary hyperparathyroidism [46–51]. However, at this time, parathyroidectomy should not be performed for improvement of cardiovascular endpoints [14]. Even with these guidelines in place, there still remains no true agreement among practicing endocrinologists and endocrine surgeons about whether most patients should be referred for parathyroidectomy or surveyed while administering medical therapy. Furthermore, the majority of patients who meet surgical criteria are not undergoing surgery [52].

Intervention: Four-Gland Exploration

When surgery is indicated, the surgeon must choose the appropriate operative approach. The best operation among these choices should give the highest rate of cure with the lowest rate of complications. Traditionally, since Felix Mandel's report of the first successful parathyroidectomy in 1925, the surgical management of primary hyperparathyroidism involved a bilateral neck exploration with visualization of all four glands and removal of one or more enlarged glands [53]. However, minimally invasive parathyroidectomy (MIP) has gained popularity with improvements in preoperative localization techniques and the development of intraoperative parathyroid hormone (ioPTH) monitoring. The definition of "minimally invasive" encompasses procedures that use open, endoscopic, and robotic-assisted techniques. This chapter will focus on comparing a bilateral exploration with an image-guided, open unilateral exploration employing ioPTH, which will be referred to as a "focused exploration."

Technique of Four-Gland Exploration

This procedure relies on an expert understanding of parathyroid embryology as well as normal and variant anatomy of the glands. Upon establishing a diagnosis of primary hyperparathyroidism, preoperative workup should include risk stratification of undergoing anesthesia and possible endoscopic evaluation of the vocal cords.

At our institution, the patient is placed under general anesthesia and positioned with a roll beneath the shoulders and the neck extended. The neck is open via a symmetrical transverse collar incision overlying the thyroid isthmus, which is typically about two fingerbreadths above the suprasternal notch. The platysma is divided, and a skin-platysma flap is developed within a relatively avascular plane just deep this muscle. The cervical fascia is divided in the midline and strap muscles separated from the underlying thyroid as well as thymus. Next, the thyroid lobe on the side to be explored is rotated anteriorly and medially. Sometimes the ipsilateral middle thyroid vein must be divided to allow this maneuver. In order to facilitate identification of the parathyroid glands, the surgical field should remain bloodless if possible because blood staining of the tissues can make exploration quite difficult.

The right upper parathyroid gland is sought first, followed by identification of the right lower gland. With the thyroid rotated anteromedially, the surgeon examines the tissues posterior to the lobe. A thorough understanding of the relationships seen with both normal and aberrant parathyroid anatomy is critical. A delicate dissection is carried out in the usual locations first. However, when a gland is unable to be identified in its normal location, the search is continued for an ectopic gland. Any abnormalities should be investigated. Normal parathyroid glands are a light yellow-brown color, whereas adenomatous glands take on a reddish-brown color. Suspicious fat lobules should be inspected and opened because the inferior parathyroid glands are often surrounded by thymic fat. The recurrent laryngeal nerve is not exposed routinely, but the surgeon must be familiar with its course so as to protect it from harm at all times. After both right-sided glands have been identified, the contralateral neck should then be explored in a similar manner. In general, all four glands should be discovered before any gland is removed. When a solitary adenoma is found, the vascular pedicle of the gland is ligated and then resected. If more than one parathyroid gland is enlarged, they are resected, and normal glands are marked with a metallic clip to facilitate identification should re-operation be necessary. At least one of these normal-appearing glands should be biopsied and sent as frozen section to rule out parathyroid hyperplasia. A subtotal parathyroidectomy is performed when all four glands are abnormal.

Outcomes Following Four-Gland Exploration

The goal of parathyroid surgery is the excision of all hyperfunctioning glands so as to cure the patient's disease, achieve normocalcemia, reverse metabolic complications, and relieve symptoms. The results for bilateral cervical exploration are outstanding.

Cure Rates

Bilateral parathyroid exploration has served as the standard operation for a successful cure of hyperparathyroidism for 90 years. The ultimate goal of parathyroidectomy for primary hyperparathyroidism is to achieve postoperative eucalcemia that is both immediate and long-lasting. Although persistent and recurrent primary hyperparathyroidism are often presented as combined surgical outcomes, they are two very different entities. If elevated serum calcium is seen within the first 6 months postoperatively, then that patient is said to have persistent hyperparathyroidism. A failed initial operation is most often the result of surgeon inexperience, missed parathyroid adenoma (either in a normal or ectopic location), undiagnosed second adenoma, or misdiagnosis of parathyroid hyperplasia [54–57]. On the other hand, if hypercalcemia returns after 6 months of normocalcemia postoperatively, this is considered recurrent hyperparathyroidism. Whether this results from metachronous postoperative autonomous hypersecretion of a previously normally functioning gland or from a synchronous additional latent abnormal gland that was previously unrecognized is a matter of debate. Multiple studies have demonstrated high surgical cure rates, ranging from 95% to 99%, with bilateral neck exploration and excision of all macroscopically enlarged parathyroid glands or histologically abnormal glands [58–65]. Recurrence following the traditional approach ranges from 0.4% to 5% [58, 60, 62, 66–70]. The importance of an experienced surgeon cannot be overstated. In a 1988 study out of Scandinavia, it is clearly demonstrated that up to 70% of patients may fail to become normocalcemic in the hands of less experienced surgeons performing fewer than ten operations for primary hyperparathyroidism annually [71].

Complications

Major complications following bilateral neck exploration and parathyroidectomy are rare. The overall combined perioperative morbidity is less than 4% in most reported series [45]. This rate may be slightly higher in the elderly patient undergoing general anesthesia. Mortality is rare if not nonexistent in the majority of studies.

Hoarseness is a postoperative finding that is often indicative of a recurrent laryngeal nerve injury, which may be transient or permanent. Injury may be a result of crushing or traction as opposed to actual transection of the nerve [72]. However, this hoarseness may be the result of endotracheal intubation, which can have an incidence up to 40% [73]. Permanent recurrent nerve injuries are generally reported to be less than 1% at the time of initial exploration [62–65]. Injuries involving the external branch of the superior laryngeal nerve are often subtle clinically and less likely to be reported [45]. Meticulous dissection by a surgeon well versed in the possible variations of the course of these nerves helps to avoid injury.

Postoperative hypocalcemia to some degree occurs relatively frequently, especially in patients who are severely hypercalcemic or chronically vitamin D deficient preoperatively. This is usually transient in nature and managed on an outpatient basis with oral calcium and vitamin D supplementation. Symptoms of hypocalcemia include perioral or digital paresthesias, anxiety, tetany, and seizures. Mild hypocalcemia is often caused by a transient relative hypoparathyroidism, resulting from a delay of normal parathyroid glands in returning to their baseline functional status after a period of suppression by hyperactive tissue. Permanent hypoparathyroidism is much less common but can occur secondary to ischemia from a failure to preserve the blood supply to normal parathyroid glands or following subtotal parathyroidectomy for multigland disease with nonviable remnant tissue. In a study of 1112 patients undergoing bilateral neck explorations for primary hyperparathyroidism, transient hypocalcemia was seen in 1.8% of patients with no patients suffering permanent hypoparathyroidism [63]. Other studies demonstrate similar results with permanent hypocalcemia rates less than 0.5% [60, 65].

Wound infections and neck hematomas are rare (<1%), but a potentially fatal airway obstruction can occur from a rapidly expanding hematoma that should be managed emergently with evacuation if encountered. Despite the observed success and limited morbidity of this approach, there has been a steady worldwide trend toward a more focused, unilateral exploration.

Comparator: Focused Exploration Using Intraoperative Parathyroid Hormone Monitoring

Historical Perspective of Unilateral Exploration

The operative approach to parathyroid exploration has undergone a major shift over the past three decades. Although the bilateral neck exploration has endured many years of excellent cure rates, it has been challenged because a long-lasting cure is quite often possible with the removal of a single adenoma—accounting for up to 85% of cases of sporadic primary hyperparathyroidism.

Unilateral neck exploration was initially advocated by Wang [74] and later by Tibblin [75] in the 1970s when an adenoma and a normal gland were found on the same side. The Lund University surgeons advocated for intraoperative oil red O staining of frozen sections of the macroscopically normal ipsilateral gland to exclude the possibility of multiglandular disease [75]. In principle, the goal was to restrict the neck exploration to the side with the solitary adenoma. At first, surgeons did not use localization studies, and so approximately half of patients had the correct side explored originally. If the wrong side was explored initially, an adenoma was sought on the opposite side. Then, there was a surge of interest in parathyroid localization with preoperative imaging. Early efforts often were of limited value leading to the often quoted remark by Doppman, an interventional radiologist, who said the "only localizing study necessary for primary hyperparathyroidism is to locate an experienced parathyroid surgeon." [76, 77] However, over the following decades, we have seen a trend toward a focused exploration. This paradigm shift is primarily attributable to the advancements made in the accuracy of preoperative localization tests and availability of ioPTH monitoring.

Preoperative Localization Tests

In an effort to improve the surgeon's likelihood of initially exploring the correct side beyond that of mere random chance, preoperative imaging studies have been developed to guide the surgeon to the side with the adenoma. The strategy involves knowledge of and dissection on the side of the adenoma, thus reducing the operating time, cost, and possibly some of the morbidity associated with the procedure. No localization study should be regarded as diagnostic. These tests are meant for operative planning, and so it follows that they are unnecessary if a patient is not an operative candidate [78]. Thus, the surgeon in collaboration with the radiologist or nuclear medicine physician should be making the decisions regarding parathyroid localization [45]. Preoperative imaging is not required for bilateral neck exploration in the "virgin neck" because all four glands will be investigated intraoperatively. Consequently, localization is most appropriate when a focused approach or a reoperative neck case is planned.

Multiple imaging modalities are available for identifying the offending parathyroid gland(s). They can be divided into invasive and noninvasive tests. Noninvasive imaging studies include ultrasonography, technetium 99m (^{99m}Tc)-sestamibi scintigraphy, computed tomography (CT), and magnetic resonance imaging (MRI). Invasive options consist mainly of selective venous sampling and parathyroid arteriography.

Ultrasound

Cervical ultrasonography for the evaluation of parathyroid glands was first described in the late 1970s [79, 80]. Preoperative parathyroid ultrasonography was introduced at our institution a few years later, and we reported on our initial experiences with this technique between 1979 and 1988 [81]. Normal glands are uncommonly visualized with this modality. Retroesophageal lesions are infrequently visible, and ultrasound cannot be used to locate mediastinal glands because it cannot penetrate the sternum. Parathyroid adenomas are characteristically homogeneous, hypoechoic structures with a peripheral rim of vascularity on ultrasonography employing grayscale and color Doppler imaging [82]. A meta-analysis that included 19 studies reporting results on parathyroid ultrasound demonstrated a pooled sensitivity and positive predictive value (PPV) of 76% and 93%, respectively [83]. This study included only patients at the time of initial presentation with primary hyperparathyroidism regardless of etiology, but another review of the literature [84] showed that sensitivity diminishes for patients with double adenomas (16%) and multiglandular hyperplasia (35%). Smaller gland size, ectopic gland location under the sternum or behind clavicles, and patient obesity have also been shown to limit the detection of abnormal glands [85].

Ultrasound is attractive because it is widely available, it is inexpensive, it does not expose the patient to ionizing radiation, and it can be performed by the surgeon. Also, concomitant thyroid pathology is seen in approximately 20% to 30% of patients with primary hyperparathyroidism [86]. Cervical ultrasound is a sensitive technique for evaluating the thyroid for synchronous nodules and preparing for the possibility of simultaneous parathyroid-thyroid surgery [87–89]. Although ultrasound has been successful in the localization of larger adenomas found within the neck in the absence of concurrent thyroid pathology, the accuracy of this modality is highly dependent on skilled sonographers performing and interpreting the study [81, 90–93].

Sestamibi Scintigraphy

Young et al. initially described the ability to reliably locate parathyroid adenomas utilizing thallium-201 (^{201}Tl) and ^{99m}Tc subtraction scintigraphy in 1983 [94]. In 1989, Coakley et al. reported that ^{99m}Tc-sestamibi, which was being used for cardiac imaging at the time, also was concentrating within parathyroid tissue [95]. A variety of nuclear scintigraphic agents have been employed, but ^{99m}Tc remains the agent of choice today. Mitochondrial uptake of ^{99m}Tc-sestamibi occurs in both the thyroid and parathyroid glands, but the radioisotope is retained longer by the mitochondria-rich parathyroid glands. Normal parathyroid glands are not seen on sestamibi scintigraphy, but hyperfunctioning tissue more avidly concentrates ^{99m}Tc-sestamibi. A review of the literature demonstrates a wide range of sensitivities for sestamibi scanning. One meta-analysis of 52 studies reported sensitivities from 39% to greater than 90% [96]. Parathyroid hyperplasia and multiple adenomas can cause false negative results [97], and concurrent thyroid disease, particularly follicular and Hurthle cell thyroid neoplasms, may result in false positive results [98, 99]. Another meta-analysis found an overall sensitivity of 88% for single adenomas, 30% for double adenomas, and 44% for multiple gland hyperplasia [84].

Similar to ultrasonography, the advantages of ^{99m}Tc-sestamibi include widespread availability and relatively low cost. Sestamibi scanning is less operator dependent than ultrasound, and its wider field of view facilitates the evaluation of ectopic glands, namely those in the mediastinum or retroesophageal locations [95]. Also, like ultrasound, sestamibi scintigraphy is more accurate in predicting the side rather than the quadrant of a single adenoma [100]. Scintigraphy does result in a modest dose of radiation.

Sestamibi scanning can be enhanced by three-dimensional imaging through its fusion with single-photon emission computed tomography (^{99m}Tc-SPECT or SPECT) and with CT (^{99m}Tc-SPECT/CT or SPECT/CT) to yield more readily interpretable images as well as provide better anatomic detail. The additional dimension improves detection of ectopic glands and multiglandular disease along with overall sensitivity compared to planar imaging. A meta-analysis of 9 SPECT studies reports a pooled sensitivity and PPV of 79% and 91%, respectively, for this modality [83]. Another meta-analysis reviewing 24 studies showed a pooled sensitivity of 86% for SPECT/CT, which was superior to the sensitivities of SPECT (74%) and planar (70%) techniques [101]. Although these results are encouraging, SPECT/CT results in both increased cost and radiation exposure [78]. Also, by adding delayed sestamibi scans (so called dual-phase imaging) or subtraction techniques to planar, SPECT, or SPECT/CT, even higher accuracy may be obtained by decreasing false positives that result from concurrent thyroid lesions or lymph nodes [102]. However, multiglandular disease remains difficult to image whether employing SPECT or SPECT/CT. Based on this data, dual-phase SPECT or SPECT/CT is often the preferred imaging modality for parathyroid localization prior to initial exploration by most surgeons.

Computed Tomography

Although standard CT with intravenous contrast has been used in the evaluation of parathyroid adenomas, its sensitivity has been inferior to that of other techniques, and it exposes the patient to more radiation than other modalities. Yet CT can be helpful in visualizing mediastinal tumors as well as those in a retroesophageal location. Four-dimensional CT (4D-CT) is an imaging modality that relies upon the characteristic rapid uptake and washout of contrast from parathyroid adenomas. The fourth dimension is time. 4D-CT seems particularly useful in reoperative neck cases where other initial imaging studies (sestamibi and ultrasound) fail to localize a tumor. In a study of 45 patients with primary hyperparathyroidism who had undergone previous neck exploration, 4D-CT demonstrated 88% sensitivity for abnormal parathyroid glands compared to SPECT or neck US (54% and 21%, respectively) [103]. 4D-CT also seems highly effective in detecting the presence of multiglandular disease and the location of ectopic glands [104]. Compared to SPECT, 4D-CT results in a modest increase in total radiation dose; however, the radiation dose to the thyroid with 4D-CT is 57 times that of SPECT [105]. This must be considered particularly in young patients, who tend to have a higher risk of thyroid cancer [105]. In addition to the radiation exposure, 4D-CT is not widely available, and it is difficult to interpret.

Invasive Localization

Venous catheterization with sampling for PTH, referred to as selective venous sampling (SVS), as well as parathyroid arteriography have largely been replaced by the above described noninvasive imaging modalities. However, these more invasive options still may play a role in lateralizing the side of disease in difficult reoperative cases with inconclusive, contradictory, or nondiagnostic noninvasive localization studies [78].

In summary, ultrasound, sestamibi scintigraphy, and CT scans are the most commonly utilized localization studies today [90]. The most preferred approach to localizing abnormal parathyroid glands in a patient with an initial diagnosis of primary hyperparathyroidism is combining ^{99m}Tc-SPECT with cervical ultrasound. Four-dimensional CT is reserved for equivocal or discordant initial imaging results. Preoperative localization is most commonly utilized today when a focused exploration is planned or in patients with prior history of a neck operation. With experienced sonographers and nuclear medicine physicians, the combination of SPECT and ultrasonography can accurately localize greater than 90% of single parathyroid adenomas preoperatively [106]. However, as discussed above, these localization studies may fail to recognize double adenomas and multiple gland hyperplasia. Moreover, nonlocalizing studies seem to be more common in patients with multiglandular disease [107]. Traditionally in cases of multigland disease, one-third of patients will have a negative scan, one-third will have a scan consistent with a single adenoma, and one-third will have a scan showing more than one abnormal gland [108, 109]. It should be emphasized that negative or discordant imaging studies should not discourage physicians from referring a patient to an endocrine surgeon [78]. Because the incidence of multiglandular disease is reported between 4% and 30% [110–119], reliance on imaging alone appears to increase the operative failure rate [107, 120, 121]. Thus, other adjuncts have been applied to rule out multiglandular disease intraoperatively.

Intraoperative Localization Tests

Intraoperative Gamma Probe

Some surgeons have promoted utilization of an intraoperative gamma probe as a useful aid in parathyroid exploration [122, 123]. Following the intravenous administration of ^{99m}Tc-sestamibi preoperatively, hyperfunctioning parathyroid glands are identified by a handheld gamma probe that assesses sestamibi uptake. However, the expert panel constituted by the Committee of the Fourth International Workshop on the Surgical Management of Asymptomatic Primary Hyperparathyroidism does not advocate routine use of this technique [45]. It is an adjunct that may be employed in reoperative cases.

Intraoperative Parathyroid Hormone Monitoring

A focused parathyroidectomy utilizes preoperative localization (where to start) and intraoperative PTH monitoring (when to stop) to guide operative success as well as to minimize dissection and time in the operating theater. Theoretically, once all hyperfunctioning tissue has been resected, the circulating levels of PTH should decline. If levels fail to decline, then additional hyperfunctioning tissue needs to be removed. Because of the short half-life of PTH (mean half-life of 3.5 to 4 min), it is ideal for monitoring intraoperatively in order to prove that surgical cure has been accomplished. Nussbaum and coworkers first described intraoperative measurement of intact PTH in 1988 using a two-site antibody technique that proved more sensitive and specific than previous assays [124]. In 1991, Irvin et al. modified Nussbaum's technique and reported on a quick method for intraoperative PTH (ioPTH) monitoring as a "biochemical frozen section" that would provide feedback within 15 min [125]. A rapid PTH assay then became commercially available in 1996, facilitating its widespread utilization in the operating room. Since this time, ioPTH has been employed more and more frequently during parathyroid surgery, particularly with focused exploration.

There are numerous assays available for intraoperative use today, but the principles underlying their use in the operating room are similar for all. The ioPTH assay confirms the resection of all hyperfunctioning parathyroid glands, helps to direct decisions regarding need for further cervical exploration, and allows for a focused unilateral parathyroid exploration. Furthermore, PTH levels can be analyzed from fine-needle aspirates or frozen sections to determine if suspicious tissue is indeed a parathyroid gland in the operating room rather than a lymph node or thyroid nodule [126]. Lastly, the assay can also be used to lateralize the side of the neck that is harboring hypersecreting tissue through the measurement of a jugular venous gradient in patients with equivocal preoperative imaging studies.

A considerable amount of controversy surrounds the criterion that should be used to predict operative success, as the accuracy of this surgical adjunct seems to depend on the timing and frequency of ioPTH measurements as well as the percentage drop in PTH levels from baseline values. An optimal algorithm for ioPTH monitoring is one that accurately validates cure—particularly for multiglandular disease—as well as minimizes unnecessary cervical exploration, resection of normally functioning parathyroid glands, operative time, and number of blood draws. In 1993, Irvin first described the "Miami criterion" that could be used to predict a postoperative return to normocalcemia [127]. This criterion is defined as a 50% or more drop in ioPTH from the highest of either the pre-incision or pre-excision level at 10 min after resection of all hyperfunctioning tissue [110, 127]. Since this criterion was established, a significant amount of work has gone into defining the optimal interpretation strategy of ioPTH values. Several other authors have developed protocols for monitoring changes in ioPTH dynamics in an attempt to better confirm operative cure (Table 21.2). Furthermore, scoring models that utilize either pre- or intra- operative variables are available to predict the likelihood of multiglandular disease and thus those most likely to benefit from further neck exploration [128, 129].

In the operating room, peripheral vein cannulation is most commonly used for collection of blood samples. Jugular venous sampling often demonstrates higher overall absolute ioPTH values when compared to peripheral samples, thus increasing the time it takes ioPTH levels to decline adequately and possibly leading to unnecessary neck explorations. Vein access is kept open with saline infusion throughout the procedure. Only 2–3 mL of whole blood is needed for ioPTH measurement, but prior to taking this sample 10 mL of blood is discarded to avoid sample dilution by saline infusion. The blood sample is placed in an ethylenediaminetetra-acetic acid (EDTA) coated glass tube. Routinely performing blood draws at specific intervals during parathyroidectomy allows for reliable analysis of intraoperative hormone dynamics. When following the Miami criterion, samples are most commonly taken at the following times: (1) before skin incision is made (pre-incision); (2) just before dividing the blood supply to the suspicious parathyroid gland (pre-excision); (3) at 5 min after excision of the suspected gland; and (4) at 10 min post-excision. During the 8 to 15 min of turnaround time for ioPTH assays, the surgeon can close the incision. Manipulation of the remaining normal parathyroid glands can falsely elevate PTH levels and delay hormone decline, thus manipulation should be avoided when closing. If the assumed criterion is not met with the 10-min level, then the surgeon should pursue further neck exploration by finding the other ipsilateral gland before moving to the contralateral side and employ the same protocol for each additional hyperfunctioning gland removed.

Table 21.2 Criteria for intraoperative parathyroid hormone (ioPTH) decline to predict cure

Miami criterion [110]	An ioPTH drop by 50% or more from the highest of either pre-incision or pre-excision level at 10 min post-excision
Vienna criterion [113]	An ioPTH drop by 50% or more from the baseline (pre-incision) within 10 min post-excision
Halle criterion [113]	An ioPTH drop into the low-normal range (≤35 pg/mL) within 15 min post-excision
Rome criterion [134]	An ioPTH drop by greater than 50% from the highest pre-excision level, and/or ioPTH concentration within the reference range at 20 min post-excision, and/or ioPTH less than or equal to 7.5 pg/mL lower than the value at 10 min post-excision
Wisconsin rule [132]	An ioPTH drop by 50% or more from the baseline (pre-incision) at 5, 10, or 15 min post-excision • If the 5-min post-excision value is elevated above the baseline pre-incision value, then the "baseline" should be reset to this peak (5-min) value, and curative resection is then predicted by a 50% fall in the ioPTH level from the redefined 5-min ioPTH peak within 15 min of this peak (approximately 20 min after resection of the initial gland)
Mayo protocol [140]	An ioPTH drop by 50% or more from baseline (pre-excision) to a normal (or near normal) level at 10 min post-excision

The PTH level measured for diagnosis of primary hyperparathyroidism should not be used as the pre-incision sample. All values should be collected under the same conditions and using the same assay that will be utilized in the operating room. The second or pre-excision sample will help to capture any decrease or increase in circulating PTH that may have occurred during gland dissection. Refer to Table 21.3 regarding definitions used to calculate the accuracy of ioPTH. Carniero et al. proposed that inadvertent premature devascularization of the hyperfunctioning gland during dissection may result in a pre-excision value that has already fallen below the pre-incision value [110]. Riss et al. reported that PTH spikes, defined as an increase in PTH exceeding 50 pg/mL before excision of the gland, resulting from the manipulation of hypersecreting glands may occur in 15% to 50% of patients [130]. For example, the Miami criterion could incorrectly predict a cure (i.e., false positive) before removal of any tissue if the highest ioPTH value was to be obtained during one of these spikes. Also, one can debate whether this elevated ioPTH level is a true reflection of the patient's PTH level, and so it follows that a 50% drop from this falsely elevated level might result in increased failure rates. Chiu and colleagues reported that always using the pre-incision level as baseline may actually detect more abnormal glands by reducing false positives [131]. On the other hand, spikes occurring at the time of adenoma removal might result in a delayed decay of ioPTH and incorrectly predict the presence of additional hyperfunctioning tissue (i.e., false negative), thus leading to unnecessary bilateral explorations [130]. To cut costs incurred by multiple measurements, some surgeons employ a protocol that does not include a pre-excision value. However, when a pre-excision level is not obtained, a 50% drop may not be obtained at 10 min post-excision because of the aforementioned PTH spike that may occur. A criticism of this method is that it results in too many unnecessary continued neck explorations [110]. Because this PTH stimulation may be the result of surgical manipulation as opposed to multigland disease, a few studies [45, 130, 132] recommend that the surgeon should attempt to wait for the ioPTH to fall below 50% of the pre-incision baseline value, especially if the suspicious gland was correctly located by preoperative imaging. The Wisconsin rule was developed to help obviate this potential pitfall and avoid any unnecessary exploration [132]. Barczynski et al. showed that using the Miami criterion without adding 15 and 20 min post-excision samples may contribute to a higher number of false negative explorations [115]. In addition, prolonged PTH clearance in patients with subclinical renal insufficiency may contribute to false negatives [130].

Table 21.3 Definitions used to calculate the accuracy of intraoperative parathyroid hormone (ioPTH) with the Miami criterion in predicting postoperative calcium levels

	Operative success (normal or low calcium for ≥6 months postoperatively)	Operative failure (high calcium within 6 months postoperatively)
ioPTH drop by ≥50%	True positive	False positive
ioPTH drop by <50%	False negative	True positive

The Miami criterion is the most commonly employed algorithm today [45]. In 2004, Irvin et al. reported that this criterion predicted postoperative calcium levels with a false negative rate of 2%, a false positive rate of 1%, a sensitivity of 98%, a specificity of 96%, and an overall accuracy of 98% [133]. However, there have been variable success rates reported in the literature utilizing this algorithm to predict cure, largely attributed to missed double adenomas or multiglandular hyperplasia [109, 114, 134–137]. For example, Siperstein et al. published a large study to evaluate the prevalence of additional parathyroid pathology following focused parathyroidectomy by continuing with bilateral exploration with excision of additional enlarged glands despite a significant drop of ioPTH levels [114]. In this study, the authors suggest that unrecognized enlarged glands may be left in situ in at least 16% of patients, risking future recurrent hyperparathyroidism [114]. However, the Miami group claims that ioPTH monitoring does not miss multiglandular disease in a review of its 10-year outcomes with a mean follow-up of 83 months where the recurrence rate was 3% [138]. In fact, the main cause of operative failures in another study by the Miami group was the surgeon's inability to find the abnormal gland rather than missed multiglandular disease [139]. Other investigators have suggested stricter criteria or alternative interpretations so as to reduce the reported incidence of false positives (i.e., failure to recognize multigland disease and achieve cure despite a sufficient drop in hormone levels) [113, 134, 135, 140]. Richards and colleagues reported on the Mayo protocol, stating that it had the highest sensitivity (96%), PPV (99%), and accuracy (95%) compared with other strategies, including a 50% drop from baseline at 10 min post-excision [140]. Specifically, with respect to multiglandular disease, the Mayo protocol [141] may have a higher sensitivity (95%), specificity (100%), and accuracy (97%) compared to that reported by the Miami group—90%, 94%, and 92%, respectively [110]. Another study suggests that even stricter criteria (post-excision ioPTH level that is ≥75% lower than baseline and within normal range) should be used to predict success when multiglandular disease is recognized [142]. However, stricter criteria than the Miami criterion were estimated to increase operative success by only 0.3% but significantly increase unnecessary bilateral explorations to 20% in one study [143]. In general, attempts at improving detection of multiglandular disease by lowering the number of false positive outcomes have resulted in an increased specificity but at the cost of further unnecessary neck explorations with prolongation of operative time through an increase in false negatives, lower sensitivity and lower overall accuracy [115].

Because the various criteria for ioPTH monitoring were not found to be equivalent in predicting cure or detecting multiglandular disease, there have been multiple studies comparing these strategies [110, 113, 115, 131]. Barczynski et al. performed a retrospective review of the Miami, Vienna, Halle, and Rome ioPTH criteria [115]. This study found that the Miami criterion followed by the Vienna criterion had the highest overall accuracy in predicting cure (97% and 92%, respectively) while the Rome criterion followed by the Halle criterion was most useful in the intraoperative detection of multiglandular disease. In contrast, another study by Riss et al. found that the Vienna and Halle criteria correctly detected multiglandular disease in 91% of patients, whereas the Miami criterion did so in only 57% of patients [113]. A criticism of some of these comparison studies is that the incidence of multiglandular disease ranged from only 4% to 7% [110, 113, 115, 117–119, 144, 145], whereas a rate of 15% to 30% is reported by other groups [111, 112, 114]. It is possible that these higher rates may overestimate the true incidence of multiglandular disease as these unrecognized enlarged glands are not necessarily hyperfunctioning, thus may not be contributing to hyperparathyroidism. Long-term follow-up data is needed to determine whether these are in fact "latent" adenomas increasing the chance for recurrence or just enlarged "nonsecreting" glands. Variations in multiglandular disease may also be associated with regional differences in vitamin D deficiency, familial disease, and referral patterns [140].

Another point of contention regards the role of ioPTH for the patient with concordant imaging studies. In up to two-thirds of cases, both sestamibi and ultrasound imaging identify the same, solitary adenoma in patients with sporadic primary hyperparathyroidism. In this setting, a focused exploration without ioPTH monitoring has been shown to be successful in 96% of patients [108], and so some authors will not perform ioPTH monitoring for these patients with concordant imaging studies because they feel it would be of little value [146, 147]. However, as discussed above, all hyperfunctioning glands cannot be accurately localized preoperatively in the majority of patients with multiglandular disease. Thus, ioPTH monitoring can help to solve this issue and improve operative success [107, 109, 121].

The quick intraoperative measurement of PTH dynamics has significantly altered the approach to parathyroidectomy in the management of primary hyperparathyroidism. In theory, not having to locate the remaining parathyroid glands after identification of an adenoma minimizes the extent of dissection, shortens the operating time, and lowers the risk of inadvertently injuring the recurrent laryngeal nerve or the other normal glands. With piqued patient interest in any surgical technique that can be converted to minimally invasive and with increased surgeon experience utilizing ioPTH, focused parathyroidectomy has rapidly become an attractive alternative to bilateral neck exploration.

Outcome: Comparison of Cure Rates and Complications Following Focused Versus Four-Gland Exploration

Since the mid-1990s, ioPTH has effectively guided an increasing number of surgeons who perform parathyroidectomy. Its popularity has continued to grow with 90% of surgeons practicing a focused parathyroidectomy and 95% of high-volume surgeons using ioPTH monitoring today [140]. It seems that the focused approach with ioPTH monitoring has successfully replaced traditional bilateral cervical exploration in the surgical management of most patients with sporadic primary hyperparathyroidism and positive localization studies. As with any change in tradition, an evaluation of the long-term outcomes is necessary.

Cure Rates

In most studies, operative success is defined as continuous eucalcemia for at least 6 months postoperatively. As mentioned previously, there is an important difference between persistent hyperparathyroidism (i.e., operative failure) and recurrent hyperparathyroidism. Many surgeons believe that focused parathyroidectomy is equally effective in immediately restoring normocalcemia as bilateral neck exploration. Table 21.4 summarizes the results of several studies comparing the operative success of focused exploration using ioPTH with a bilateral approach in the management of primary hyperparathyroidism. Cure rates exceeding 95% are possible with a focused exploration, and these data compare favorably to the reported cure rates after traditional bilateral neck exploration, which also typically range from 95% to 99% [58–65, 70, 133]. When these two operative approaches are compared, there is generally no significant increase in operative success offered by a bilateral approach over a focused one [58, 61, 62, 70, 139, 144, 148, 149]. In fact, a few studies demonstrated a marginally, but significantly, lower rate of persistent hyperparathyroidism in patients undergoing focused parathyroidectomy [60, 133].

The most feared potential problem of the focused exploration is failure to identify multiglandular disease (i.e., a second adenoma or hyperplasia). This risk depends on the percentage of patients with multiglandular disease, the accuracy of localization studies in identifying multiglandular disease, and the accuracy of the ioPTH assay in detecting a residual pathologic parathyroid gland [150]. Studies involving traditional bilateral neck exploration, where parathyroidectomy is guided by surgeon experience and subjective interpretation of gland size as well as gross appearance, have consistently documented an incidence of multiglandular disease ranging from 15% to 30% [111, 112, 114]. However, when gland excision is guided by ioPTH, fewer parathyroid glands are resected with the incidence of multiglandular disease ranging from 4% to 7% [110, 113, 115]. If limitations in localization studies and ioPTH truly miss multiglandular disease in at least 16% of cases at the time of surgery [114], then we would expect focused parathyroidectomy to demonstrate higher rates of persistent hyperparathyroidism. In theory, multiglandular disease should not lead to recurrence because it represents the presence of more than one hypersecreting gland responsible for hypercalcemia at the time of parathyroidectomy. Thus, if all of these glands are not removed, then persistent (not recurrent) hyperparathyroidism will result within 6 months postoperatively [144]. However, as demonstrated in Table 21.4, similar operative failure rates are seen with both techniques.

Despite excellent short-term results with utilization of ioPTH, which are challenging what the incidence of multiglandular disease truly is, some authors that espouse the bilateral approach argue that the low recurrence rates reported for a focused approach are due to a lack of long-term follow-up data. In fact, a concern over focused exploration leaving latent disease behind has led some surgeons to abandon it altogether in favor of a bilateral approach, which has proven durable historically [59]. Now that ioPTH monitoring has been commercially available for nearly 20 years, we have gained more insight into the recurrence rates to be expected from focused parathyroidectomy with this

Table 21.4 Outcomes comparing focused exploration (FE) with ioPTH versus bilateral neck exploration (BNE) for primary hyperparathyroidism (pHPT)

Study [source #]	Procedure	Criterion	Total number of patients	Single gland disease	Multigland disease	Persistent pHPT/ operative failure	Follow-up	Recurrence	Time to recurrence
Irvin et al. [133]	FE with ioPTH	Miami	421	409 (97%)	12 (2.9%)[a]	11 (3%)[a]	n/a	n/a	n/a
	BNE	n/a	340	308 (91%)	32 (9%)[a]	20 (6%)[a]	n/a	n/a	n/a
Grant et al. [70]	FE with ioPTH	Mayo	601	87%[b]	13%[b]	15 (3%)	Mean 25 months[b]	1 (0.2%)	n/a
	BNE	n/a	760	87%[b]	13%[b]	26 (3%)	Mean 25 months[b]	0 (0%)	n/a
Westerdahl et al. [62][c]	FE with ioPTH	≥60% decline from pre-excision value at 15 min post-excisicn	47	41 (87%)	5 (11%)	2 (4%)	45 (96%) at 1 year 38 (81%) at 5 years	2 (4%)	1 at a year 1 at 5 y
	BNE	n/a	44	40 (91%)	4 (9%)	1 (2%)	43 (97%) at 1 year 33 (75%) at 5 years	1 (2%)	1 at a year
McGill et al. [61]	FE with ioPTH	Miami	405	360 (89%)	45 (11%)[a]	15 (4%)	n/a	n/a	n/a
	BNE	n/a	395	330 (84%)	65 (16%)[a]	9 (2%)	n/a	n/a	n/a
Slepavicius et al. [151][c]	FE with ioPTH	≥50% decline from pre-incision value at 15 mins post-excision	24	21 (87.5%)	3 (12.5%)	0 (0%)	n/a	n/a	n/a
	BNE	n/a	23	21 (91%)	2 (9%)	0 (0%)	n/a	n/a	n/a

(continued)

Table 21.4 (continued)

Study [source #]	Procedure	Criterion	Total number of patients	Single gland disease	Multigland disease	Persistent pHPT/ operative failure	Follow-up	Recurrence	Time to recurrence
Udelsman [60]	FE with ioPTH	Miami	1037	934 (90%)	100 (10%)[a]	6 (0.6%)[a]	Mean 15 months	4 (0.4%)	6.5, 10, 33, 46 months
	BNE	n/a	613	515 (84.0%)	86 (14%)[a]	18 (2.9%)[a]	Mean 36 months	1 (0.2%)	1 at 70 months
Schneider et al. [58]	FE with ioPTH	Wisconsin	1006	– (80.6% overall)	– (19.4% overall)	4 (0.4%)	Median 9 months	25 (2.5%)	Mean 28.1 months
	BNE	n/a	380	– (80.6% overall)	– (19.4% overall)	3 (0.8%)	Median 9 months	8 (2.1%)	Mean 27.2 months

[a]Statistically significant difference
[b]Study did not report single gland disease or multigland disease or follow-up time independently based on the type of procedure performed
[c]Prospective randomized controlled trial

surgical adjunct. Table 21.4 details several reports on recurrent disease following focused parathyroidectomy. The majority of these studies are retrospective in nature as very few prospective randomized control trials [62, 151] have been published specifically comparing focused exploration with ioPTH against bilateral exploration. A review of this data indicates that any "missed" glands, if they were truly undiscovered, require a long period of time (several years in some studies) to become physiologically active. In 2011, Udelsman [60] published his series on 1650 consecutive patients undergoing parathyroidectomy (of which 613 were performed in the standard fashion and 1037 were focused with ioPTH) for sporadic primary hyperparathyroidism. He concluded that a focused parathyroidectomy employing ioPTH is a superior technique offering significant improvements in the cure rate compared to conventional surgery (99.4% vs 97.1%). Schneider et al. [58] recently reported on the long-term results of 1386 parathyroid operations for primary hyperparathyroidism in an attempt to determine whether operative approach (focused exploration with ioPTH or bilateral exploration) influenced disease recurrence. Their conclusion was that neither technique independently predicted recurrence. Age, sex, preoperative PTH level, nonlocalizing sestamibi scan, and the number of glands removed were included in the multivariate analysis but did not independently predict recurrence. However, the percentage decrease in ioPTH was protective against recurrent hyperparathyroidism with the optimal threshold determined to be a decline greater than 63%. Although many surgeons attribute failure to ioPTH, these data underscore the importance of this adjunct, as it was the only factor protective against recurrence for both the entire cohort (which included those undergoing four-gland exploration) and those specifically undergoing a focused exploration [58].

Complications

The routine use of bilateral exploration is not without risk. In theory, when a surgeon does not have to explore the contralateral neck because ioPTH predicts operative success, potential advantages include a lower risk of inadvertently injuring the remaining normal parathyroid glands or the recurrent nerves as well as a decrease in operative time. Although it seems intuitive that complications should occur less frequently with a unilateral approach, this remains a matter of debate. The mortality risk of parathyroidectomy is essentially zero, regardless of which technique is employed. The overall combined perioperative morbidity rate is less than 4% in most reported series, but this rate may be higher in elderly patients receiving general anesthesia [45]. If a single parathyroid gland is explored and resected, then there is no risk of permanent hypoparathyroidism. However, this no longer holds when ioPTH monitoring guides the surgeon to pursue dissection of the contralateral neck. A few studies [60, 64, 152] report a higher incidence of transient hypocalcemia with traditional surgery. Lund University surgeons reported that patients who underwent unilateral neck exploration had a lower incidence of early postoperative hypocalcemia that necessitated calcium supplementation than did those who underwent a bilateral approach. However, there were no significant differences with respect to complication rates between the two groups [64]. Udelsman demonstrated a trend toward lower rates of postoperative hypocalcemia and recurrent nerve injury with a significant decrease in the overall perioperative complication rate, favoring a focused over a bilateral exploration [60]. Schneider et al. showed that more transient hypocalcemia occurred with a bilateral approach than with focused exploration (1.9% vs 0.1%, respectively). Furthermore, although there was no statistical significance, there was documentation of bleeding and recurrent laryngeal nerve injury within the group that had a bilateral exploration but none of these complications were seen in the group that underwent a focused approach [152].

None of the prospective randomized controlled trials [64, 151, 153] have found a significant difference between focused and bilateral exploration for recurrent nerve injury. Unless specifically documented by postoperative serum calcium levels or progress notes, retrospective reviews relying on patient recall alone may be more likely to miss transient postoperative hypocalcemia and recurrent nerve deficits than randomized prospective controlled trials. Many surgeons also routinely prescribe oral calcium supplementation in the early postoperative period to limit the incidence of symptomatic hypocalcemia, which also minimizes the documentation of this complication. It seems that both approaches are safe and demonstrate minimal, but similar, overall complication rates with the vast majority experiencing an uncomplicated perioperative course.

Other Advantages of a Focused Exploration

Some authors report on the potential benefits of improved cosmesis [151], less pain [151], decreased operative time [154], decreased costs [60, 133, 155], a decreased length of stay [60, 155, 156], and an improved quality of life [156] offered by a focused exploration. Finally, the rare patient who is not cured after a focused exploration can generally undergo a simple, and technically less challenging, second operation that is performed in virgin tissue planes.

Recommendations

Although surgeon judgment and experience remain critical to success in parathyroid surgery, enhancements in preoperative localization techniques along with ioPTH assays have facilitated the treatment of patients with sporadic primary hyperparathyroidism. Specifically, the intraoperative measurement of PTH has been shown to be a valuable tool available to the surgeon during parathyroidectomy and has largely supplanted the subjective evaluation of parathyroid hypersecretion based on gland size. It has enabled a more limited exploration by accurately guiding gland excision and minimizing tissue trauma. There are many large series of focused parathyroid operations guided by ioPTH that have shown excellent, durable cure rates similar to standard four-gland exploration. In fact, some studies have documented the superiority of the focused approach.

When making an evidence-based recommendation regarding the approach to parathyroidectomy based on the literature in Table 21.4, one important criticism is that the overwhelming majority of the data comes from retrospective reviews. This lack of randomization introduces some selection bias. The patients who are undergoing focused exploration in these studies are highly selected and include mainly patients with a positive localization study, no prior neck operations, and no familial component to their primary hyperparathyroidism. On the other hand, series involving the traditional four-gland exploration routinely include complex reoperative cases and multiglandular hyperplasia.

After employing the GRADE method for evaluating the quality of available evidence, we found a lack of high quality data. More long-term data from prospective, randomized controlled trials are necessary to provide even higher-grade evidence in favor of one approach over another. The strength of a recommendation, however, is not necessarily determined by quality of evidence alone. It also relies on other factors, such as risk-benefit ratios, costs, and patient preferences. Thus, we are moderately confident that a focused exploration is a safe, effective technique that is appropriate for most patients with sporadic primary hyperparathyroidism and likely to be comparable to four-gland exploration with regard to cure rates and risk of complications. A specific algorithm for monitoring hormone dynamics so as to accurately predict postoperative eucalcemia is essential. Also, the use of this technique generally requires adequate preoperative imaging and an experienced surgeon. Nevertheless, four-gland exploration remains a valuable technique, especially for those who have familial forms of primary hyperparathyroidism.

References

1. Coker LH, Rorie K, Cantley L, Kirkland K, Stump D, Burbank N, et al. Primary hyperparathyroidism, cognition, and health-related quality of life. Ann Surg. 2005;242(5):642–50.
2. Fraser WD. Hyperparathyroidism. Lancet. 2009;374(9684):145–58.
3. Clark OH, Duh QY. Primary hyperparathyroidism. A surgical perspective. Endocrinol Metab Clin N Am. 1989;18(3):701–14.
4. Wermers RA, Khosla S, Atkinson EJ, Hodgson SF, O'Fallon WM, Melton LJ 3rd. The rise and fall of primary hyperparathyroidism: a population-based study in Rochester, Minnesota, 1965–1992. Ann Intern Med. 1997;126(6):433–40.
5. Heath H 3rd, Hodgson SF, Kennedy MA. Primary hyperparathyroidism. Incidence, morbidity, and potential economic impact in a community. N Engl J Med. 1980;302(4):189–93.
6. Yeh MW, Ituarte PH, Zhou HC, Nishimoto S, Liu IL, Harari A, et al. Incidence and prevalence of primary hyperparathyroidism in a racially mixed population. J Clin Endocrinol Metab. 2013;98(3):1122–9.
7. Beard CM, Heath H 3rd, O'Fallon WM, Anderson JA, Earle JD, Melton LJ 3rd. Therapeutic radiation and hyperparathyroidism. A case-control study in Rochester, Minn. Arch Intern Med. 1989;149(8):1887–90.
8. Albright F. A page out of the history of hyperparathyroidism. J Clin Endocrinol Metab. 1948;8(8):637–57.
9. Clark OH, Wilkes W, Siperstein AE, Duh QY. Diagnosis and management of asymptomatic hyperparathyroidism: safety, efficacy, and deficiencies in our knowledge. J Bone Miner Res. 1991;6(Suppl 2):S135–42. discussion 51–2.

10. Turken SA, Cafferty M, Silverberg SJ, De La Cruz L, Cimino C, Lange DJ, et al. Neuromuscular involvement in mild, asymptomatic primary hyperparathyroidism. Am J Med. 1989;87(5):553–7.
11. Bilezikian JP, Brandi ML, Rubin M, Silverberg SJ. Primary hyperparathyroidism: new concepts in clinical, densitometric and biochemical features. J Intern Med. 2005;257(1):6–17.
12. Silverberg SJ, Shane E, Jacobs TP, Siris ES, Gartenberg F, Seldin D, et al. Nephrolithiasis and bone involvement in primary hyperparathyroidism. Am J Med. 1990;89(3):327–34.
13. Silverberg SJ, Bilezikian JP. Asymptomatic primary hyperparathyroidism: a medical perspective. Surg Clin North Am. 2004;84(3):787–801.
14. Bilezikian JP, Brandi ML, Eastell R, Silverberg SJ, Udelsman R, Marcocci C, et al. Guidelines for the management of asymptomatic primary hyperparathyroidism: summary statement from the Fourth International Workshop. J Clin Endocrinol Metab. 2014;99(10):3561–9.
15. Rao DS, Honasoge M, Divine GW, Phillips ER, Lee MW, Ansari MR, et al. Effect of vitamin D nutrition on parathyroid adenoma weight: pathogenetic and clinical implications. J Clin Endocrinol Metab. 2000;85(3):1054–8.
16. Kandil E, Tufaro AP, Carson KA, Lin F, Somervell H, Farrag T, et al. Correlation of plasma 25-hydroxyvitamin D levels with severity of primary hyperparathyroidism and likelihood of parathyroid adenoma localization on sestamibi scan. Arch Otolaryngol Head Neck Surg. 2008;134(10):1071–5.
17. Silverberg SJ, Clarke BL, Peacock M, Bandeira F, Boutroy S, Cusano NE, et al. Current issues in the presentation of asymptomatic primary hyperparathyroidism: proceedings of the Fourth International Workshop. J Clin Endocrinol Metab. 2014;99(10):3580–94.
18. Silverberg SJ, Shane E, de la Cruz L, Dempster DW, Feldman F, Seldin D, et al. Skeletal disease in primary hyperparathyroidism. J Bone Miner Res. 1989;4(3):283–91.
19. De Geronimo S, Romagnoli E, Diacinti D, D'Erasmo E, Minisola S. The risk of fractures in postmenopausal women with primary hyperparathyroidism. Eur J Endocrinol. 2006;155(3):415–20.
20. Khosla S, Melton LJ 3rd, Wermers RA, Crowson CS, O'Fallon W, Riggs B. Primary hyperparathyroidism and the risk of fracture: a population-based study. J Bone Miner Res. 1999;14(10):1700–7.
21. Larsson K, Ljunghall S, Krusemo UB, Naessen T, Lindh E, Persson I. The risk of hip fractures in patients with primary hyperparathyroidism: a population-based cohort study with a follow-up of 19 years. J Intern Med. 1993;234(6):585–93.
22. Khosla S, Melton J 3rd. Fracture risk in primary hyperparathyroidism. J Bone Miner Res. 2002;17(Suppl 2):N103–7.
23. Rubin MR, Bilezikian JP, McMahon DJ, Jacobs T, Shane E, Siris E, et al. The natural history of primary hyperparathyroidism with or without parathyroid surgery after 15 years. J Clin Endocrinol Metab. 2008;93(9):3462–70.
24. Sorensen MD, Duh QY, Grogan RH, Tran TC, Stoller ML. Urinary parameters as predictors of primary hyperparathyroidism in patients with nephrolithiasis. J Urol. 2012;187(2):516–21.
25. Tassone F, Gianotti L, Emmolo I, Ghio M, Borretta G. Glomerular filtration rate and parathyroid hormone secretion in primary hyperparathyroidism. J Clin Endocrinol Metab. 2009;94(11):4458–61.
26. Yu N, Donnan PT, Flynn RW, Murphy MJ, Smith D, Rudman A, et al. Increased mortality and morbidity in mild primary hyperparathyroid patients. The Parathyroid Epidemiology and Audit Research Study (PEARS). Clin Endocrinol. 2010;73(1):30–4.
27. Yu N, Leese GP, Donnan PT. What predicts adverse outcomes in untreated primary hyperparathyroidism? The Parathyroid Epidemiology and Audit Research Study (PEARS). Clin Endocrinol. 2013;79(1):27–34.
28. Lind L, Hvarfner A, Palmer M, Grimelius L, Akerstrom G, Ljunghall S. Hypertension in primary hyperparathyroidism in relation to histopathology. Eur J Surg. 1991;157(8):457–9.
29. Lind L, Jacobsson S, Palmer M, Lithell H, Wengle B, Ljunghall S. Cardiovascular risk factors in primary hyperparathyroidism: a 15-year follow-up of operated and unoperated cases. J Intern Med. 1991;230(1):29–35.

30. Persson A, Bollerslev J, Rosen T, Mollerup CL, Franco C, Isaksen GA, et al. Effect of surgery on cardiac structure and function in mild primary hyperparathyroidism. Clin Endocrinol. 2011;74(2):174–80.
31. Iwata S, Walker MD, Di Tullio MR, Hyodo E, Jin Z, Liu R, et al. Aortic valve calcification in mild primary hyperparathyroidism. J Clin Endocrinol Metab. 2012;97(1):132–7.
32. Walker MD, Rundek T, Homma S, DiTullio M, Iwata S, Lee JA, et al. Effect of parathyroidectomy on subclinical cardiovascular disease in mild primary hyperparathyroidism. Eur J Endocrinol. 2012;167(2):277–85.
33. Adler JT, Sippel RS, Schaefer S, Chen H. Preserving function and quality of life after thyroid and parathyroid surgery. Lancet Oncol. 2008;9(11):1069–75.
34. Bilezikian JP, Khan AA, Potts JT Jr, Third International Workshop on the Management of Asymptomatic Primary Hyperthyroidism. Guidelines for the management of asymptomatic primary hyperparathyroidism: summary statement from the third international workshop. J Clin Endocrinol Metab. 2009;94(2):335–9.
35. Siperstein AE, Shen W, Chan AK, Duh QY, Clark OH. Normocalcemic hyperparathyroidism. Biochemical and symptom profiles before and after surgery. Arch Surg. 1992;127(10):1157–6. discussion 61–3.
36. Silverberg SJ, Bilezikian JP. "Incipient" primary hyperparathyroidism: a "forme fruste" of an old disease. J Clin Endocrinol Metab. 2003;88(11):5348–52.
37. Tordjman KM, Greenman Y, Osher E, Shenkerman G, Stern N. Characterization of normocalcemic primary hyperparathyroidism. Am J Med. 2004;117(11):861–3.
38. Scholz DA, Purnell DC. Asymptomatic primary hyperparathyroidism. 10-year prospective study. Mayo Clin Proc. 1981;56(8):473–8.
39. Rao DS, Wilson RJ, Kleerekoper M, Parfitt AM. Lack of biochemical progression or continuation of accelerated bone loss in mild asymptomatic primary hyperparathyroidism: evidence for biphasic disease course. J Clin Endocrinol Metab. 1988;67(6):1294–8.
40. Silverberg SJ, Brown I, Bilezikian JP. Age as a criterion for surgery in primary hyperparathyroidism. Am J Med. 2002;113(8):681–4.
41. Ambrogini E, Cetani F, Cianferotti L, Vignali E, Banti C, Viccica G, et al. Surgery or surveillance for mild asymptomatic primary hyperparathyroidism: a prospective, randomized clinical trial. J Clin Endocrinol Metab. 2007;92(8):3114–21.
42. Bollerslev J, Jansson S, Mollerup CL, Nordenstrom J, Lundgren E, Torring O, et al. Medical observation, compared with parathyroidectomy, for asymptomatic primary hyperparathyroidism: a prospective, randomized trial. J Clin Endocrinol Metab. 2007; 92(5):1687–92.
43. Rao DS, Phillips ER, Divine GW, Talpos GB. Randomized controlled clinical trial of surgery versus no surgery in patients with mild asymptomatic primary hyperparathyroidism. J Clin Endocrinol Metab. 2004;89(11):5415–22.
44. Silverberg SJ, Lewiecki EM, Mosekilde L, Peacock M, Rubin MR. Presentation of asymptomatic primary hyperparathyroidism: proceedings of the third international workshop. J Clin Endocrinol Metab. 2009;94(2):351–65.
45. Udelsman R, Akerstrom G, Biagini C, Duh QY, Miccoli P, Niederle B, et al. The surgical management of asymptomatic primary hyperparathyroidism: proceedings of the Fourth International Workshop. J Clin Endocrinol Metab. 2014;99(10):3595–606.
46. Hedback G, Tisell LE, Bengtsson BA, Hedman I, Oden A. Premature death in patients operated on for primary hyperparathyroidism. World J Surg. 1990;14(6):829–35. discussion 36.
47. Ogard CG, Engholm G, Almdal TP, Vestergaard H. Increased mortality in patients hospitalized with primary hyperparathyroidism during the period 1977–1993 in Denmark. World J Surg. 2004;28(1):108–11.
48. Sivula A, Pelkonen R. Long-term health risk of primary hyperparathyroidism: the effect of surgery. Ann Med. 1996;28(2):95–100.
49. Ronni-Sivula H. Causes of death in patients previously operated on for primary hyperparathyroidism. Ann Chir Gynaecol. 1985;74(1):13–8.
50. Bostrom H, Alveryd A. Stroke in hyperparathyroidism. Acta Med Scand. 1972;192(4):299–308.

51. Palmer M, Adami HO, Bergstrom R, Akerstrom G, Ljunghall S. Mortality after surgery for primary hyperparathyroidism: a follow-up of 441 patients operated on from 1956 to 1979. Surgery. 1987;102(1):1–7.
52. Yeh MW, Wiseman JE, Ituarte PH, Pasternak JD, Hwang RS, Wu B, et al. Surgery for primary hyperparathyroidism: are the consensus guidelines being followed? Ann Surg. 2012;255(6):1179–83.
53. Mandel F. Therapeutisher Versuch bein Einem Falls von Ostitis Fibrosa Generalisata Mittles: Extirpation eins Epithelkorperchen Tumors. Wein Klin Wochenshr Zentral. 1926; 143:245–84.
54. Kebebew E, Arici C, Duh QY, Clark OH. Localization and reoperation results for persistent and recurrent parathyroid carcinoma. Arch Surg. 2001;136(8):878–85.
55. Jaskowiak N, Norton JA, Alexander HR, Doppman JL, Shawker T, Skarulis M, et al. A prospective trial evaluating a standard approach to reoperation for missed parathyroid adenoma. Ann Surg. 1996;224(3):308–20. discussion 20–1.
56. Shen W, Duren M, Morita E, Higgins C, Duh QY, Siperstein AE, et al. Reoperation for persistent or recurrent primary hyperparathyroidism. Arch Surg. 1996;131(8):861–7. discussion 7–9.
57. Bruining HA, Birkenhager JC, Ong GL, Lamberts SW. Causes of failure in operations for hyperparathyroidism. Surgery. 1987;101(5):562–5.
58. Schneider DF, Mazeh H, Chen H, Sippel RS. Predictors of recurrence in primary hyperparathyroidism: an analysis of 1386 cases. Ann Surg. 2014;259(3):563–8.
59. Norman J, Lopez J, Politz D. Abandoning unilateral parathyroidectomy: why we reversed our position after 15,000 parathyroid operations. J Am Coll Surg. 2012;214(3):260–9.
60. Udelsman R, Lin Z, Donovan P. The superiority of minimally invasive parathyroidectomy based on 1650 consecutive patients with primary hyperparathyroidism. Ann Surg. 2011;253(3):585–91.
61. McGill J, Sturgeon C, Kaplan SP, Chiu B, Kaplan EL, Angelos P. How does the operative strategy for primary hyperparathyroidism impact the findings and cure rate? A comparison of 800 parathyroidectomies. J Am Coll Surg. 2008;207(2):246–9.
62. Westerdahl J, Bergenfelz A. Unilateral versus bilateral neck exploration for primary hyperparathyroidism: five-year follow-up of a randomized controlled trial. Ann Surg. 2007;246(6):976–80. discussion 80–1.
63. Allendorf J, DiGorgi M, Spanknebel K, Inabnet W, Chabot J, Logerfo P. 1112 consecutive bilateral neck explorations for primary hyperparathyroidism. World J Surg. 2007;31(11):2075–80.
64. Bergenfelz A, Lindblom P, Tibblin S, Westerdahl J. Unilateral versus bilateral neck exploration for primary hyperparathyroidism: a prospective randomized controlled trial. Ann Surg. 2002;236(5):543–51.
65. van Heerden JA, Grant CS. Surgical treatment of primary hyperparathyroidism: an institutional perspective. World J Surg. 1991;15(6):688–92.
66. Clark OH, Way LW, Hunt TK. Recurrent hyperparathyroidism. Ann Surg. 1976;184(4):391–402.
67. Cooke TJ, Boey JH, Sweeney EC, Gilbert JM, Taylor S. Parathyroidectomy: extent of resection and late results. Br J Surg. 1977;64(3):153–7.
68. Rudberg C, Akerstrom G, Palmer M, Ljunghall S, Adami HO, Johansson H, et al. Late results of operation for primary hyperparathyroidism in 441 patients. Surgery. 1986;99(6):643–51.
69. Tibblin S, Bizard JP, Bondeson AG, Bonjer J, Bruining HA, Meier F, et al. Primary hyperparathyroidism due to solitary adenoma. A comparative multicentre study of early and long-term results of different surgical regimens. Eur J Surg. 1991;157(9):511–5.
70. Grant CS, Thompson G, Farley D, van Heerden J. Primary hyperparathyroidism surgical management since the introduction of minimally invasive parathyroidectomy: Mayo Clinic experience. Arch Surg. 2005;140(5):472–8. discussion 8–9.
71. Malmaeus J, Granberg PO, Halvorsen J, Akerstrom G, Johansson H. Parathyroid surgery in Scandinavia. Acta Chir Scand. 1988;154(7–8):409–13.

72. Snyder SK, Lairmore TC, Hendricks JC, Roberts JW. Elucidating mechanisms of recurrent laryngeal nerve injury during thyroidectomy and parathyroidectomy. J Am Coll Surg. 2008;206(1):123–30.
73. Chen H. Radioguided parathyroid surgery. Adv Surg. 2004;38:377–92.
74. Wang CA. Surgical management of primary hyperparathyroidism. Curr Probl Surg. 1985;22(11):1–50.
75. Tibblin S, Bondeson AG, Ljungberg O. Unilateral parathyroidectomy in hyperparathyroidism due to single adenoma. Ann Surg. 1982;195(3):245–52.
76. Doppman JL. Reoperative parathyroid surgery; localization procedures. Prog Surg. 1986;18:117–32.
77. Clark OH. Surgical treatment of primary hyperparathyroidism. Adv Endocrinol Metab. 1995;6:1–16.
78. Kunstman JW, Kirsch JD, Mahajan A, Udelsman R. Clinical review: parathyroid localization and implications for clinical management. J Clin Endocrinol Metab. 2013;98(3):902–12.
79. Sample WF, Mitchell SP, Bledsoe RC. Parathyroid ultrasonography. Radiology. 1978;127(2):485–90.
80. Arima M, Yokoi H, Sonoda T. Preoperative identification of tumor of the parathyroid by ultrasonotomography. Surg Gynecol Obstet. 1975;141(2):242–4.
81. Lucas RJ, Welsh RJ, Glover JL. Unilateral neck exploration for primary hyperparathyroidism. Arch Surg. 1990;125(8):982–4. discussion 4–5.
82. Rickes S, Sitzy J, Neye H, Ocran KW, Wermke W. High-resolution ultrasound in combination with colour-Doppler sonography for preoperative localization of parathyroid adenomas in patients with primary hyperparathyroidism. Ultraschall Med. 2003;24(2):85–9.
83. Cheung K, Wang TS, Farrokhyar F, Roman SA, Sosa JA. A meta-analysis of preoperative localization techniques for patients with primary hyperparathyroidism. Ann Surg Oncol. 2012;19(2):577–83.
84. Ruda JM, Hollenbeak CS, Stack BC Jr. A systematic review of the diagnosis and treatment of primary hyperparathyroidism from 1995 to 2003. Otolaryngol Head Neck Surg. 2005;132(3):359–72.
85. Berber E, Parikh RT, Ballem N, Garner CN, Milas M, Siperstein AE. Factors contributing to negative parathyroid localization: an analysis of 1000 patients. Surgery. 2008;144(1):74–9.
86. Bentrem DJ, Angelos P, Talamonti MS, Nayar R. Is preoperative investigation of the thyroid justified in patients undergoing parathyroidectomy for hyperparathyroidism? Thyroid. 2002;12(12):1109–12.
87. Prager G, Czerny C, Ofluoglu S, Kurtaran A, Passler C, Kaczirek K, et al. Impact of localization studies on feasibility of minimally invasive parathyroidectomy in an endemic goiter region. J Am Coll Surg. 2003;196(4):541–8.
88. Milas M, Mensah A, Alghoul M, Berber E, Stephen A, Siperstein A, et al. The impact of office neck ultrasonography on reducing unnecessary thyroid surgery in patients undergoing parathyroidectomy. Thyroid. 2005;15(9):1055–9.
89. Morita SY, Somervell H, Umbricht CB, Dackiw AP, Zeiger MA. Evaluation for concomitant thyroid nodules and primary hyperparathyroidism in patients undergoing parathyroidectomy or thyroidectomy. Surgery. 2008;144(6):862–6. discussion 6–8.
90. De Feo ML, Colagrande S, Biagini C, Tonarelli A, Bisi G, Vaggelli L, et al. Parathyroid glands: combination of (99m)Tc MIBI scintigraphy and US for demonstration of parathyroid glands and nodules. Radiology. 2000;214(2):393–402.
91. Haber RS, Kim CK, Inabnet WB. Ultrasonography for preoperative localization of enlarged parathyroid glands in primary hyperparathyroidism: comparison with (99m)technetium sestamibi scintigraphy. Clin Endocrinol. 2002;57(2):241–9.
92. Reeder SB, Desser TS, Weigel RJ, Jeffrey RB. Sonography in primary hyperparathyroidism: review with emphasis on scanning technique. J Ultrasound Med. 2002;21(5):539–52. quiz 53–4.
93. Gilat H, Cohen M, Feinmesser R, Benzion J, Shvero J, Segal K, et al. Minimally invasive procedure for resection of a parathyroid adenoma: the role of preoperative high-resolution ultrasonography. J Clin Ultrasound. 2005;33(6):283–7.

94. Young AE, Gaunt JI, Croft DN, Collins RE, Wells CP, Coakley AJ. Location of parathyroid adenomas by thallium-201 and technetium-99m subtraction scanning. Br Med J. 1983;286(6375):1384–6.
95. Coakley AJ, Kettle AG, Wells CP, O'Doherty MJ, Collins RE. 99Tcm sestamibi—a new agent for parathyroid imaging. Nucl Med Commun. 1989;10(11):791–4.
96. Gotthardt M, Lohmann B, Behr TM, Bauhofer A, Franzius C, Schipper ML, et al. Clinical value of parathyroid scintigraphy with technetium-99m methoxyisobutylisonitrile: discrepancies in clinical data and a systematic metaanalysis of the literature. World J Surg. 2004;28(1):100–7.
97. Mihai R, Gleeson F, Buley ID, Roskell DE, Sadler GP. Negative imaging studies for primary hyperparathyroidism are unavoidable: correlation of sestamibi and high-resolution ultrasound scanning with histological analysis in 150 patients. World J Surg. 2006;30(5):697–704.
98. Erbil Y, Barbaros U, Yanik BT, Salmaslioglu A, Tunaci M, Adalet I, et al. Impact of gland morphology and concomitant thyroid nodules on preoperative localization of parathyroid adenomas. Laryngoscope. 2006;116(4):580–5.
99. Vattimo A, Bertelli P, Cintorino M, Burroni L, Volterrani D, Vella A, et al. Hurthle cell tumor dwelling in hot thyroid nodules: preoperative detection with technetium-99m-MIBI dual-phase scintigraphy. Journal of nuclear medicine : official publication. Soc Nucl Med. 1998;39(5):822–5.
100. Siperstein A, Berber E, Mackey R, Alghoul M, Wagner K, Milas M. Prospective evaluation of sestamibi scan, ultrasonography, and rapid PTH to predict the success of limited exploration for sporadic primary hyperparathyroidism. Surgery. 2004;136(4):872–80.
101. Wong KK, Fig LM, Gross MD, Dwamena BA. Parathyroid adenoma localization with 99mTc-sestamibi SPECT/CT: a meta-analysis. Nucl Med Commun. 2015;36(4):363–75.
102. Lavely WC, Goetze S, Friedman KP, Leal JP, Zhang Z, Garret-Mayer E, et al. Comparison of SPECT/CT, SPECT, and planar imaging with single- and dual-phase (99m)Tc-sestamibi parathyroid scintigraphy. Journal of nuclear medicine : official publication. Soc Nucl Med. 2007;48(7):1084–9.
103. Mortenson MM, Evans DB, Lee JE, Hunter GJ, Shellingerhout D, Vu T, et al. Parathyroid exploration in the reoperative neck: improved preoperative localization with 4D-computed tomography. J Am Coll Surg. 2008;206(5):888–95. discussion 95–6.
104. Starker LF, Mahajan A, Bjorklund P, Sze G, Udelsman R, Carling T. 4D parathyroid CT as the initial localization study for patients with de novo primary hyperparathyroidism. Ann Surg Oncol. 2011;18(6):1723–8.
105. Mahajan A, Starker LF, Ghita M, Udelsman R, Brink JA, Carling T. Parathyroid four-dimensional computed tomography: evaluation of radiation dose exposure during preoperative localization of parathyroid tumors in primary hyperparathyroidism. World J Surg. 2012;36(6):1335–9.
106. Patel CN, Salahudeen HM, Lansdown M, Scarsbrook AF. Clinical utility of ultrasound and 99mTc sestamibi SPECT/CT for preoperative localization of parathyroid adenoma in patients with primary hyperparathyroidism. Clin Radiol. 2010;65(4):278–87.
107. Chiu B, Sturgeon C, Angelos P. What is the link between nonlocalizing sestamibi scans, multigland disease, and persistent hypercalcemia? A study of 401 consecutive patients undergoing parathyroidectomy. Surgery. 2006;140(3):418–22.
108. Arici C, Cheah WK, Ituarte PH, Morita E, Lynch TC, Siperstein AE, et al. Can localization studies be used to direct focused parathyroid operations? Surgery. 2001;129(6):720–9.
109. Sugg SL, Krzywda EA, Demeure MJ, Wilson SD. Detection of multiple gland primary hyperparathyroidism in the era of minimally invasive parathyroidectomy. Surgery. 2004;136(6):1303–9.
110. Carneiro DM, Solorzano CC, Nader MC, Ramirez M, Irvin GL 3rd. Comparison of intraoperative iPTH assay (QPTH) criteria in guiding parathyroidectomy: which criterion is the most accurate? Surgery. 2003;134(6):973–9. discussion 9–81.
111. Haciyanli M, Lal G, Morita E, Duh QY, Kebebew E, Clark OH. Accuracy of preoperative localization studies and intraoperative parathyroid hormone assay in patients with primary hyperparathyroidism and double adenoma. J Am Coll Surg. 2003;197(5):739–46.

112. Clerici T, Brandle M, Lange J, Doherty GM, Gauger PG. Impact of intraoperative parathyroid hormone monitoring on the prediction of multiglandular parathyroid disease. World J Surg. 2004;28(2):187–92.
113. Riss P, Kaczirek K, Heinz G, Bieglmayer C, Niederle B. A "defined baseline" in PTH monitoring increases surgical success in patients with multiple gland disease. Surgery. 2007;142(3):398–404.
114. Siperstein A, Berber E, Barbosa GF, Tsinberg M, Greene AB, Mitchell J, et al. Predicting the success of limited exploration for primary hyperparathyroidism using ultrasound, sestamibi, and intraoperative parathyroid hormone: analysis of 1158 cases. Ann Surg. 2008;248(3):420–8.
115. Barczynski M, Konturek A, Hubalewska-Dydejczyk A, Cichon S, Nowak W. Evaluation of Halle, Miami, Rome, and Vienna intraoperative iPTH assay criteria in guiding minimally invasive parathyroidectomy. Langenbeck's Arch Surg. 2009;394(5):843–9.
116. Kaplan EL, Yashiro T, Salti G. Primary hyperparathyroidism in the 1990s. Choice of surgical procedures for this disease. Ann Surg. 1992;215(4):300–17.
117. Molinari AS, Irvin GL 3rd, Deriso GT, Bott L. Incidence of multiglandular disease in primary hyperparathyroidism determined by parathyroid hormone secretion. Surgery. 1996;120(6):934–6. discussion 6–7.
118. Westerdahl J, Lindblom P, Bergenfelz A. Measurement of intraoperative parathyroid hormone predicts long-term operative success. Arch Surg. 2002;137(2):186–90.
119. Vignali E, Picone A, Materazzi G, Steffe S, Berti P, Cianferotti L, et al. A quick intraoperative parathyroid hormone assay in the surgical management of patients with primary hyperparathyroidism: a study of 206 consecutive cases. Eur J Endocrinol. 2002; 146(6):783–8.
120. Westerdahl J, Bergenfelz A. Sestamibi scan-directed parathyroid surgery: potentially high failure rate without measurement of intraoperative parathyroid hormone. World J Surg. 2004;28(11):1132–8.
121. Carneiro-Pla DM, Solorzano CC, Irvin GL 3rd. Consequences of targeted parathyroidectomy guided by localization studies without intraoperative parathyroid hormone monitoring. J Am Coll Surg. 2006;202(5):715–22.
122. Norman J. Recent trends becoming standard of care yielding smaller, more successful operations at a lower cost. Otolaryngol Clin N Am. 2004;37(4):683–8. vii.
123. Chen H, Mack E, Starling JR. Radioguided parathyroidectomy is equally effective for both adenomatous and hyperplastic glands. Ann Surg. 2003;238(3):332–7. discussion 7–8.
124. Nussbaum SR, Thompson AR, Hutcheson KA, Gaz RD, Wang CA. Intraoperative measurement of parathyroid hormone in the surgical management of hyperparathyroidism. Surgery. 1988;104(6):1121–7.
125. Irvin GL 3rd, Dembrow VD, Prudhomme DL. Operative monitoring of parathyroid gland hyperfunction. Am J Surg. 1991;162(4):299–302.
126. James BC, Nagar S, Tracy M, Kaplan EL, Angelos P, Scherberg NH, et al. A novel, ultrarapid parathyroid hormone assay to distinguish parathyroid from nonparathyroid tissue. Surgery. 2014;156(6):1638–43.
127. Irvin GL 3rd, Dembrow VD, Prudhomme DL. Clinical usefulness of an intraoperative "quick parathyroid hormone" assay. Surgery. 1993;114(6):1019–22. discussion 22–3.
128. Mazeh H, Chen H, Leverson G, Sippel RS. Creation of a "Wisconsin index" nomogram to predict the likelihood of additional hyperfunctioning parathyroid glands during parathyroidectomy. Ann Surg. 2013;257(1):138–41.
129. Kebebew E, Hwang J, Reiff E, Duh QY, Clark OH. Predictors of single-gland vs multigland parathyroid disease in primary hyperparathyroidism: a simple and accurate scoring model. Arch Surg. 2006;141(8):777–82. discussion 82.
130. Riss P, Kaczirek K, Bieglmayer C, Niederle B. PTH spikes during parathyroid exploration--a possible pitfall during PTH monitoring? Langenbeck's Arch Surg. 2007;392(4):427–30.
131. Chiu B, Sturgeon C, Angelos P. Which intraoperative parathyroid hormone assay criterion best predicts operative success? A study of 352 consecutive patients. Arch Surg. 2006;141(5):483–7. discussion 7–8.

132. Cook MR, Pitt SC, Schaefer S, Sippel R, Chen H. A rising ioPTH level immediately after parathyroid resection: are additional hyperfunctioning glands always present? An application of the Wisconsin criteria. Ann Surg. 2010;251(6):1127–30.
133. Irvin GL 3rd, Solorzano CC, Carneiro DM. Quick intraoperative parathyroid hormone assay: surgical adjunct to allow limited parathyroidectomy, improve success rate, and predict outcome. World J Surg. 2004;28(12):1287–92.
134. Lombardi CP, Raffaelli M, Traini E, Di Stasio E, Carrozza C, De Crea C, et al. Intraoperative PTH monitoring during parathyroidectomy: the need for stricter criteria to detect multiglandular disease. Langenbeck's Arch Surg. 2008;393(5):639–45.
135. Weber KJ, Misra S, Lee JK, Wilhelm SW, DeCresce R, Prinz RA. Intraoperative PTH monitoring in parathyroid hyperplasia requires stricter criteria for success. Surgery. 2004;136(6):1154–9.
136. Jaskowiak NT, Sugg SL, Helke J, Koka MR, Kaplan EL. Pitfalls of intraoperative quick parathyroid hormone monitoring and gamma probe localization in surgery for primary hyperparathyroidism. Arch Surg. 2002;137(6):659–68. discussion 68–9.
137. Gauger PG, Agarwal G, England BG, Delbridge LW, Matz KA, Wilkinson M, et al. Intraoperative parathyroid hormone monitoring fails to detect double parathyroid adenomas: a 2-institution experience. Surgery. 2001;130(6):1005–10.
138. Lew JI, Irvin GL 3rd. Focused parathyroidectomy guided by intra-operative parathormone monitoring does not miss multiglandular disease in patients with sporadic primary hyperparathyroidism: a 10-year outcome. Surgery. 2009;146(6):1021–7.
139. Lew JI, Rivera M, Irvin GL 3rd, Solorzano CC. Operative failure in the era of focused parathyroidectomy: a contemporary series of 845 patients. Arch Surg. 2010;145(7):628–33.
140. Richards ML, Thompson GB, Farley DR, Grant CS. An optimal algorithm for intraoperative parathyroid hormone monitoring. Arch Surg. 2011;146(3):280–5.
141. Richards ML, Grant CS. Current applications of the intraoperative parathyroid hormone assay in parathyroid surgery. Am Surg. 2007;73(4):311–7.
142. Hughes DT, Miller BS, Doherty GM, Gauger PG. Intraoperative parathyroid hormone monitoring in patients with recognized multiglandular primary hyperparathyroidism. World J Surg. 2011;35(2):336–41.
143. Carneiro-Pla DM, Solorzano CC, Lew JI, Irvin GL 3rd. Long-term outcome of patients with intraoperative parathyroid level remaining above the normal range during parathyroidectomy. Surgery. 2008;144(6):989–93. discussion 93–4.
144. Carneiro DM, Solorzano CC, Irvin GL 3rd. Recurrent disease after limited parathyroidectomy for sporadic primary hyperparathyroidism. J Am Coll Surg. 2004;199(6):849–53. discussion 53–5.
145. Carneiro DM, Irvin GL 3rd. Late parathyroid function after successful parathyroidectomy guided by intraoperative hormone assay (QPTH) compared with the standard bilateral neck exploration. Surgery. 2000;128(6):925–9. discussion 35–6.
146. Barczynski M, Golkowski F, Nawrot I. The current status of intraoperative iPTH assay in surgery for primary hyperparathyroidism. Gland Surg. 2015;4(1):36–43.
147. Stalberg P, Sidhu S, Sywak M, Robinson B, Wilkinson M, Delbridge L. Intraoperative parathyroid hormone measurement during minimally invasive parathyroidectomy: does it "value-add" to decision-making? J Am Coll Surg. 2006;203(1):1–6.
148. Chen H, Pruhs Z, Starling JR, Mack E. Intraoperative parathyroid hormone testing improves cure rates in patients undergoing minimally invasive parathyroidectomy. Surgery. 2005;138(4):583–7. discussion 7–90.
149. Venkat R, Kouniavsky G, Tufano RP, Schneider EB, Dackiw AP, Zeiger MA. Long-term outcome in patients with primary hyperparathyroidism who underwent minimally invasive parathyroidectomy. World J Surg. 2012;36(1):55–60.
150. Proye CA, Carnaille B, Bizard JP, Quievreux JL, Lecomte-Houcke M. Multiglandular disease in seemingly sporadic primary hyperparathyroidism revisited: where are we in the early 1990s? A plea against unilateral parathyroid exploration. Surgery. 1992;112(6):1118–22.

151. Slepavicius A, Beisa V, Janusonis V, Strupas K. Focused versus conventional parathyroidectomy for primary hyperparathyroidism: a prospective, randomized, blinded trial. Langenbeck's Arch Surg. 2008;393(5):659–66.
152. Schneider DF, Mazeh H, Sippel RS, Chen H. Is minimally invasive parathyroidectomy associated with greater recurrence compared to bilateral exploration? Analysis of more than 1,000 cases. Surgery. 2012;152(6):1008–15.
153. Miccoli P, Bendinelli C, Berti P, Vignali E, Pinchera A, Marcocci C. Video-assisted versus conventional parathyroidectomy in primary hyperparathyroidism: a prospective randomized study. Surgery. 1999;126(6):1117–21. discussion 21–2.
154. Irvin GL 3rd, Sfakianakis G, Yeung L, Deriso GT, Fishman LM, Molinari AS, et al. Ambulatory parathyroidectomy for primary hyperparathyroidism. Arch Surg. 1996;131(10):1074–8.
155. Chen H, Sokoll LJ, Udelsman R. Outpatient minimally invasive parathyroidectomy: a combination of sestamibi-SPECT localization, cervical block anesthesia, and intraoperative parathyroid hormone assay. Surgery. 1999;126(6):1016–21. discussion 21–2.
156. Adler JT, Sippel RS, Chen H. The influence of surgical approach on quality of life after parathyroid surgery. Ann Surg Oncol. 2008;15(6):1559–65.

The Evidence for and Against Parathyroid Cryopreservation: Should We Continue to Promote Parathyroid Cryopreservation?

22

Selyne Samuel and Marlon A. Guerrero

Abstract

Permanent hypoparathyroidism is a rare, yet life-altering complication of thyroid and parathyroid surgery. However, the advent of parathyroid cryopreservation, and subsequent autotransplantation of parathyroid tissue, revolutionized the management of this devastating complication. However, cryopreservation of parathyroid tissue is not widely performed due to the rarity of utilization, the potential high costs, and need for specialized expertise. Furthermore, studies have shown that the viability of the parathyroid tissue is diminished after 2 years, raising more debate about need for cryopreservation. In this chapter, we evaluate data justifying and contradicting the practice of parathyroid cryopreservation.

Keywords

Parathyroid · Autotransplantation · Cryopreservation · Hypoparathyroidism · Hypocalcemia

Introduction

Permanent hypoparathyroidism is a devastating complication of parathyroid and thyroid surgery. Although, hypoparathyroidism can be managed medically with oral calcium and vitamin D, it remains a problematic condition for patients who may

S. Samuel · M. A. Guerrero (✉)
Department of Surgery, Banner University Medical Center, University of Arizona, Tucson, AZ, USA
e-mail: ssamuel@email.arizona.edu; mguerrero@surgery.arizona.edu

P. Angelos, R. H. Grogan (eds.), *Difficult Decisions in Endocrine Surgery*, Difficult Decisions in Surgery: An Evidence-Based Approach,
https://doi.org/10.1007/978-3-319-92860-9_22

still experience the deleterious effects of hypocalcemia such as osteoporosis, arrhythmias, tetany and cataracts [1]. Permanent hypoparathyroidism also produces high financial costs resulting from frequent testing of calcium levels, hospital admissions for intravenous treatment, and lifetime calcium supplementation [2]. Adhering to meticulous intra-operative dissection during initial parathyroidectomy or thyroidectomy can significantly reduce the risk of hypoparathyroidism. The use of parathyroid gland autotransplantation (immediate or delayed) in patients with recurrent hyperparathyroidism or multiglandular hyperparathyroidism has also been shown to reduce the risk of permanent hypoparathyroidism [3]. It has been reported that up to 10% of patients undergoing initial parathyroidectomy for multi-glandular parathyroid hyperplasia and 30% of patients undergoing reoperation for persistent or recurrent hyperparathyroidism develop permanent hypoparathyroid-ism [4]. An acceptable risk of surgical hypoparathyroidism after initial surgery is approximately 1–2% [5], but the risk increases to more than 5% with reoperations. Enhanced methods in the preservation of parathyroid tissues have permitted the delayed autotransplantation of parathyroid tissue to help reduce permanent hypo-parathyroidism [5]. In this chapter, we evaluate data justifying and contradicting the practice of parathyroid cryopreservation (Tables 22.1, 22.2, 22.3, 22.4, 22.5, 22.6).

Samuel Wells first described parathyroid cryopreservation in 1976 [6]. The same group further showed that cryopreserved parathyroid tissue maintained functionality after delayed autotransplantation by measuring parathyroid hormone (PTH) [7]. Although cryopreservation of parathyroid tissue with delayed autotransplantation has been widely accepted as a method to prevent permanent hypoparathyroidism, the

Table 22.1 PICO table

Population	Patients undergoing subtotal parathyroidectomy or total with autotransplantation
Intervention	Cryopreservation of parathyroid
Comparator	No cryopreservation
Outcome	Permanent hypoparathyroidism

Table 22.2 Indications for parathyroid cryopreservation

Initial neck operations: Familial primary hyperparathyroidism Secondary hyperparathyroidism Tertiary hyperparathyroidism
Redo neck operations: Persistent hyperparathyroidism Recurrent hyperparathyroidism Parathyroidectomy after thyroidectomy Redo central neck dissection for thyroid cancer

Table 22.3 Billing and reimbursement information for parathyroid cryopreservation [8]

Procedure	CPT code or TMID code	Professional (P) or technical (T) fee, $	Medicare reimbursement, $	Commercial payors reimbursement, $
Parathyroid cryopreservation (operating room portion)	60,669	574 (P)[a]	82	195–401[b]
Parathyroid cryopreservation (laboratory processing and storage portion)	88,399,099	1000 (T)[c]	None	300–500

TMID transaction master charge ID
[a]There is no technical fee for the procedure in the operating room
[b]Some commercial payors bundle this procedure with the main parathyroidectomy procedure (CPT 60500 series) and do not issue separate reimbursement. Those payors who do reimburse usually require that the hospital's billing specialist sends additional information, such as the operative report, before payment
[c]This fee covers processing by the laboratory and indefinite storage time. The same fee is also applied for the process of parathyroid thawing for reimplantation

Table 22.4 Parathyroid tissue cryopreservation, autotransplantation, and cure rates

Study	# of cryopreserved patients	# of autotransplants	No Fxn #, (%)	Partial Fxn #, (%)	Full Fxn #, (%)	Mean F/U (mths)
Caccitolo et al. [3]	112	15	9, (60%)	3, (20%)	3, (20%)	15
Cohen et al. [4]	448	30	8, (31%)	6, (23%)	12, (46%)	24
Wells et al. [7]	6	6	1, (17%)	0	5, (83%)	23
Herrera et al. [10]	NA	12	7, (59%)	3, (25%)	1, (8%)	60
Saxe et al. [11]	NA	12	5, (42%)	1, (8%)	6, (50%)	18
Brennan et al. [12]	NA	7	3, (43%)	1, (14%)	3(43%)	NA
Wagner et al. [14]	25	25	NA	NA	16, (64%)	40
Feldman et al. [15]	NA	26	11, (42%)	4, (15%)	8, (31%)	35
Borot et al. [19]	1376	21	17, (80%)	2, (10%)	2, (10%)	26
Shepet, et al. [21]	442	4	3, (75%)	0	1, (25%)	24

No Fxn No function, *Partial Fxn* Partial Function, Full Fxn Full function, *mean F/U* mean Follow-up, # number, *mths* months

Table 22.5 GRADE recommendation criteria

A: Strongly recommend	The recommendation is based on good evidence that the service or intervention can improve important health outcomes. Evidence includes consistent results from well-designed, well-conducted studies in representative populations that directly assess effects on health outcomes
B: Recommend	The recommendation is based on fair evidence that the service or intervention can improve important health outcomes. The evidence is sufficient to determine effects on health outcomes, but the strength of the evidence is limited by the number, quality, or consistency of the individual studies; generalizability to routine practice; or indirect nature of the evidence on health outcomes
C: Recommend	The recommendation is based on expert opinion
D: Recommend against	The recommendation is based on expert opinion
E: Recommend against	The recommendation is based on fair evidence that the service or intervention does not improve important health outcomes or that harms outweigh benefits
F: Strongly recommend against	The recommendation is based on good evidence that the service or intervention does not improve important health outcomes or that harms outweigh benefits
I: Recommends neither for nor against	Evidence is insufficient to recommend for or against

Adapted from the U.S. Preventive Services Task Force, Agency for Healthcare Research and Quality [22]

Table 22.6 Level of evidence of studies

Level of evidence	Treatment study
I	Randomized controlled trials with adequate statistical power to detect differences
II	Lower quality randomized control trials
III	Case control studies
IV	Case series with no comparison groups
V	Expert opinion

practice is cumbersome and costly and some endocrine surgeons have questioned its routine application. This chapter focuses on the evidence in favor and against parathyroid gland cryopreservation. Specific recommendations will be addressed:

Does cryopreservation affect cellular viability and graft function?
Does the cost of cryopreservation support its use?
Should parathyroid cryopreservation be utilized?

Cryopreservation of Parathyroid Tissue

Cryopreservation allows the storage of parathyroid tissue with preservation of the tissue/cell integrity and function for delayed autotransplantation [6, 7]. Since its description, parathyroid cryopreservation has been utilized mainly in the setting of subtotal or total parathyroidectomy for hereditary primary hyperparathyroidism, and persistent or recurrent hyperparathyroidism [3, 6, 8, 9] (Table 22.2).

The technique of cryopreservation commences by confirming parathyroid tissue by frozen section. The parathyroid gland is then minced into 40 pieces measuring 1 × 1 × 1 mm [5]. These pieces are then immersed in ice-chilled saline in a sterile vial or syringe. The patient's blood or fetal calf serum can be used as the freezing media. However, the typical freezing medium contains Roswell Park Memorial Institute (RPMI) 1640 solution. The Mayo clinic cooling technique involves the placement of the vials in dry ice pre-chilled to approximately −55 °C to −60 °C for an hour to allow cooling by −1 °C per minute [10]. Some authors endorse placing the vials in −60 °C ethyl alcohol bath [11] or a −70 °C bath [4]. After cooling the vials are placed in a liquid nitrogen storage tank for the long term at temperatures ranging from −170 °C [4, 12], −180 °C [6, 13], −190 °C [11], or − 196 °C [14].

In the event that delayed autotransplantation is required, the vials containing the parathyroid tissue are removed from the liquid nitrogen baths and shaken in a bath of warm water at 37 °C [13] or 42 °C [11] until the parathyroid tissue is thawed. The pieces of tissue are then washed three times at 37 °C in RPMI 1640 solution [10, 11] to rinse off the DMSO. Up to 40 pieces of the parathyroid tissue are then implanted using local anesthesia into the non-dominant forearm. The wound is marked with a metal clip in the case of future re-exploration. The success of the autotransplantation is defined as:

1. Complete function: Asymptomatic and eucalcemic patient
2. Partial function: Hypocalcemic patient, but lower required dosage of preoperative medication
3. Non-Function: Hypocalcemic patient and no change in dosage of preoperative medication

Parathyroid Graft Function and Cellular Viability

There exists variability regarding the success of delayed autotransplantation following cryopreservation. In comparison to immediate fresh parathyroid autotransplantation, delayed autotransplantation has been associated with reduced success rates (55% versus 17%, respectively) [10]. Other studies have demonstrated that immediate fresh autotransplantation can achieve functionality rate over 90% [4, 14], whereas the success rate of delayed autotransplantation varies from 18% to 83% [4, 7, 10, 15, 16]. However, other studies show that delayed autotransplantation following cryopreservation is successful [8] and some show no difference in the function of cryopreserved tissue when compared to immediate autotransplantation [6, 16, 17]. One study demonstrated a 100% success in nine patients who required delayed parathyroid autotransplantation [8]. Hypocalcemia was corrected in all nine patients with delayed autotransplantation occurring between 3 and 22 months from their initial operation [8].

It may be argued that in order to maximize the chances for a successful delayed autotransplantation that cryopreservation should be performed in only experienced centers. Several single institution studies have shown relatively high rates of graft functionality of 46% to 83% [4, 10, 14, 18]. A longitudinal study performed over the course of 10 years showed that 16 (64%) of 25 patients were eucalcemic and free of hypoparathyroid symptoms off of medication and that the remaining nine patients who still required calcium supplements required less supplementation in comparison to the preoperative dose [14]. It is plausible that use in a single high volume institution provides standardization of specimen acquisition and storage, thereby resulting in higher autotransplantation success rates. This is exemplified by the fact that one of the highest reported success rate (83%) is from the institution where cryopreservation was first described [18]. Yet, a recent multi-institutional study evaluated cryopreservation and autotransplantation in nine separate centers and found that only 20 patients underwent delayed autotransplantation and 80% were nonfunctional [19]. The authors recommended abandoning the practice of cryopreservation [19].

The etiology for the difference in success rate between immediate and delayed autotransplantation is not fully understood; the tissues are equally viable with no difference in secretory ability, but the reason for the decrease in function when the tissue is autotransplanted is unknown [20]. Wagner et al. conducted an investigation that showed that cryopreservation did not affect the secretory function and regulation of PTH secretion of parathyroid tissue [17]. There was no difference in viability, but investigation under light microscopy showed partial necrosis of the cryopreserved parathyroid tissue, leading to the recommendation of implanting 20–40 parathyroid tissue fragments to attain successful autotransplantation [17]. More recent studies showed a decrease in function and cell viability with lengthened periods of cryopreservation storage time up to and after 22 months [4, 13].

It has been suggested that prolonged cryopreservation results in loss of graft function [13]. In a 13-year prospective analysis, Cohen and colleagues showed that 60% of cryopreserved parathyroid autotransplantations were functional [4]. The authors did note that graft failure was related to length of cryopreservation. The study reported that no grafts function when stored longer than 22 months [4]. Another study found that 71% of parathyroid cells were viable when cryopreservation storage time was less than 24 months, but drastically fell to 1% when storage time exceeded that time point [13]. Other studies have also indicated a progressive diminished cellular viability with length of cryopreservation [6, 16, 17].

Does Cryopreservation Affect Cellular Viability and Graft Function?

Level IV Evidence The majority data show that graft functionality is reduced with cryopreservation and delayed autotransplantation when compared to immediate fresh autotransplantation. Furthermore, studies have shown that cellular viability decreases with prolonged storage time beyond 22 months and may account for the decreased function.

Financial Cost

Along with the lack of consensus regarding the function and viability of cryopreserved parathyroid tissue, there is still concern regarding the costs related to storage of parathyroid tissue required for cryopreservation. The technique of cryopreservation itself and storage is relatively inexpensive (Table 22.3) [8]. However, another issue to consider is whether cryopreservation is utilized sufficiently to account for these costs. For instance, one study reported a cryopreservation rate of only 4% [3]. Therefore, cryopreservation may be theoretically applicable, but practically unfeasible due to the low indications for cryopreservation and low rate of cryopreservation [3].

Another point of contention is whether delayed autotransplantation produces sufficient success to account for costs of the procedure, storage, and disposal (Table 22.3). Some may argue that there is low utilization of cryopreservation and that the time and costs of cryopreservation outweigh the benefits. One study, for example, reported that out of 3080 parathyroid operations only 4% underwent cryopreservation with a success rate of 23% [3]. In 2010, a French multicenter study determined that only 2% of patients underwent delayed autotransplantation of cryopreserved tissue, with a low cure rate of 10% [19]. Based on these results, they recommended that cryopreservation only be performed in large centers for patients with parathyroid hyperplasia and tissues should be discarded when patient no longer displays symptoms of hypoparathyroidism and after 1 year of preservation [19].

Another study determined that cryopreservation was not cost effective with the need for re-implantation being quite low at 1% [21]. The study evaluated 442 patients who underwent parathyroid cryopreservation over a decade and found that only 1 out of the 4 patients that required autotransplantation had a successful outcome [21]. These results parallel those of other studies [3, 19] showing a high rate of cryopreservation with low utilization of cryopreserved parathyroid and low success rates. This had led to some acknowledging the utility of cryopreservation, but deeming it economically unrealistic for all patients with parathyroid disease [9].

An opposing study showed that delayed autotransplantation following cryopreservation is successful [8]. Hypocalcemia was corrected in all nine patients with delayed autotransplantation occurring between 3 and 22 months from their initial operation. The authors determined that storage costs were inexpensive at their institution; specimen preparation and storage fees were reimbursable, and patients were not charged if the specimens were stored beyond 2 years [8]. However, although the study [8] performed cryopreservation in over a third of the patients, less than 2% required delayed parathyroid autotransplantation.

Does the Cost of Parathyroid Cryopreservation Support Its Use?

Level III and IV evidence: Data available suggest that the low utilization of cryopreservation, and low use of delayed parathyroid autotransplantation does not offset the overall cost of parathyroid tissue cryopreservation and autotransplantation.

Conclusion

The advent of parathyroid cryopreservation provided a means to treat the devastating complication of permanent hypoparathyroidism. Theoretically cryopreservation of parathyroid tissue is an essential tool for an endocrine surgeon, yet practically its use has not gained wide application. A clear alternative is to immediately autotransplant parathyroid tissue in the forearm to protect against permanent hypoparathyroidism and to extract the autograft if permanent hypoparathyroidism does not develop. Given the varied data on cryopreservation usage, graft functionality, and clinical success continued usage will likely wane. From the available data, the following recommendations are made.

Recommendations

Routine Use of Cryopreservation

Recommendation (GRADE I): Data show that since the first description, cryopreservation utilization is exceedingly low. Therefore, it is the author's conclusion that the routine practice of cryopreservation in individual centers may have limited clinical utility. Furthermore, tissue stored beyond 22 months should be considered for disposal.

Selective Use of Cryopreservation

Recommendation (GRADE I): Data show that there is no cost benefit for selective cryopreservation in low volume situations. An exception would be at high volume academic centers that are using cryopreservation or in pooled high-volume situations.

Delayed Autograft Transplantation

Recommend against (GRADE E): Based on available data, the authors do not recommend continued practice of delayed autotransplantation since studies have shown low utilization and low success rates. For centers that frequently cryopreserve tissue, it is recommended that delayed autotransplantation not extend beyond 22 months.

References

1. Flechner SM, Berber E, Askar M, Stephany B, Agarwal A, Milas M. Allotransplantation of cryopreserved parathyroid tissue for severe hypocalcemia in a renal transplant recipient. Am J Transplant. 2010;10:2061–5.
2. Larrad Jiménez A, Hernández Hernández JR. Parathyroid transplantation. Endocrinología y Nutrición (English Edition). 2013;60(4):161–3.

3. Caccitolo JA, Farley DR, van Heerden JA, Grant CS, Thompson GB, Sterioff S. The current role of parathyroid cryopreservation and autotransplantation in parathyroid surgery: an institutional experience. Surgery. 1997;122:1062–7.
4. Cohen MS, Dilley WG, Wells SA Jr, et al. Long-term functionality of cryopreserved parathyroid autografts: a 13-year prospective analysis. Surgery. 2005;138:1033–40.
5. Guerrero MA. Cryopreservation of parathyroid glands. Int J Endocrinol. 2010.
6. Wells SA Jr, Ellis GJ, Gunnells JC, et al. Parathyroid autotransplantation in primary parathyroid hyperplasia. N Engl J Med. 1976;295:57–62.
7. Wells SA Jr, Farndon JR, Dale JK, Leight GS, Dilley WG. Long-term evaluation of patients with primary parathyroid hyperplasia managed by total parathyroidectomy and heterotopic autotransplantation. Ann Surg. 1980;192:451–8.
8. Agarwal A, Waghray A, Gupta S, Sharma R, Milas M. Cryopreservation of parathyroid tissue: an illustrated technique using the Cleveland Clinic protocol. J Am Coll Surg. 2013;216(1):e1–9.
9. Schneider R, Ramaswamy A, Slater EP, Bartsch DK, Schlosser K. Cryopreservation of parathyroid tissue after parathyroid surgery for renal hyperparathyroidism: does it really make sense? World J Surg. 2012;36(11):2598–604.
10. Herrera M, Grant C, van Heerden JA, Fitzpatrick LA. Parathyroid autotransplantation. Arch Surg. 1992;127:825–9.
11. Saxe AW, Spiegel AM, Marx SJ, Brenman MF. Deferred parathyroid autografts with cryopreserved tissue after reoperative parathyroid surgery. Arch Surg. 1982;117(5):538–43.
12. Brennan MF, Brown EM, Sears HF, Aurbach GD. Human parathyroid cryopreservation: in vitro testing of function by parathyroid hormone release. Ann Surg. 1978;187(1):87–90.
13. Guerrero MA, Evans DB, Lee JE, et al. Viability of cryopreserved parathyroid tissue: when is continued storage versus disposal indicated? World J Surg. 2008;32:836–9.
14. Wagner PK, Seesko HG, Rothmund M. Replantation of cryopreserved human parathyroid tissue. World J Surg. 1991;15(6):751–5.
15. Feldman AL, Sharaf RN, Skarulis MC, et al. Results of heterotopic parathyroid autotransplantation: a 13-year experience. Surgery. 1999;126:1042–8.
16. Saxe A. Parathyroid transplantation: a review. Surgery. 1984;95:507–26.
17. Wagner PK, Rumpelt HJ, Krause U, Rothmund M. The effect of cryopreservation on hormone secretion in vitro and morphology of human parathyroid tissue. Surgery. 1986;99:257–64.
18. Wells SA Jr, Gunnells JC, Shelburne JD. Transplantation of the parathyroid glands in man: clinical indications and results. Surgery. 1975;78:34–44.
19. Borot S, Lapierre V, Carnaille B, Goudet P, Penfornis A. Results of cryopreserved parathyroid autografts: a retrospective multicenter study. Surgery. 2010;147(4):529–35.
20. Herrera MF, Grant CS, Van Heerden JA, Jacobsen D, Weaver A, Fitzpatrick LA. The effect of cryopreservation on cell viability and hormone secretion in human parathyroid tissue. Surgery. 1992;112:1096–102.
21. Shepet K, Alhefdhi A, Usedom R, Sippel R, Chen H. Parathyroid cryopreservation after parathyroidectomy: a worthwhile practice? Ann Surg Oncol. 2013;20(7):2256–60.
22. U.S. Preventive Services Task Force Ratings. Strength of recommendations and quality of evidence. Guide to clinical preventive services, third edition: periodic updates. Rockville: Agency for Healthcare Research and Quality; 2000–2003.

Should Antibiotic Prophylaxis Be Given Prior to Thyroidectomy or Parathyroidectomy?

23

Jacob Moalem

Abstract

Although thyroid and parathyroid operations are very commonly performed, until recently there has been very little evidence to inform the decision of whether or not preoperative antibiotic prophylaxis should be given. It is interesting to note that while most surgeons would agree that clean operations that do not involve prosthetic implants do not generally require antibiotic prophylaxis, most endocrine surgeons give their patients preoperative antibiotic prophylaxis always or nearly always.

Keywords

Antibiotic prophylaxis · Thyroidectomy · Parathyroidectomy · Wound infection

Wound infections following thyroid or parathyroid operations are rare. Most large studies report a wound infection rate of less than 1%, although it is unknown whether that low infection rate is achieved with or without preoperative antibiotic prophylaxis. Recently, two prospective randomized trials have been reported on this subject [1, 2] (Table 23.1). Both studies, totaling more than 2500 patients did not demonstrate any benefit to antibiotic prophylaxis. Another retrospective study, reviewing more than 1000 patients, reached the same conclusion [3]. On the other hand, there are several reports of severe and occasionally lethal streptococcal infections following thyroid or parathyroid operations [4–8].

J. Moalem
Department of Surgery, University of Rochester Medical Center, Rochester, NY, USA
e-mail: Jacob_Moalem@urmc.rochester.edu

P. Angelos, R. H. Grogan (eds.), *Difficult Decisions in Endocrine Surgery*, Difficult Decisions in Surgery: An Evidence-Based Approach,
https://doi.org/10.1007/978-3-319-92860-9_23

Table 23.1 Summary of comparative studies evaluating the role of preoperative antibiotic prophylaxis in thyroidectomy and parathyroidectomy

Reference	Patients	Intervention	Comparator	Outcome
Urono [2]	(Prospective) patients who underwent thyroidectomy or parathyroidectomy	541—received piperacillin 541 received cefazolin	1082 received no antibiotic prophylaxis	No difference in SSI rate
Avenia [1]	(Prospective) patients who underwent thyroidectomy	250 received Ampicillin/sulbactam	250 received no antibiotic prophylaxis	No difference in SSI
DePalma [3]	(Retrospective) patients who underwent thyroidectomy	1132 patients who received antibiotic prophylaxis	1794 received no antibiotic prophylaxis	No difference in SSI
Lu [19]	(Retrospective) patients who underwent thyroidectomy	1166 patients who received no antibiotic prophylaxis	None	One SSI
Dionigi [23]	(Prospective, nonrandomized)	50 patients who received first generation cephalosporin	191 received no antibiotic prophylaxis	No difference in SSI

SSI skin/soft tissue infection

To date, there are no data to support routine antibiotic prophylaxis prior to thyroid or parathyroid surgery. This decision should be individualized according to surgeon experience, previous results, and patient and operative considerations that may increase the risk for wound infection.

Thyroidectomy and parathyroidectomy together account for the vast majority of endocrine operations done, and are nearly always classified as clean cases. Although the routine use of prophylactic antibiotics is not generally recommended in clean cases, [9] the impact of a superficial or deep wound infection in a cervical incision can be great and the risk attributed to a single dose of antibiotics is low. Therefore, it remains controversial whether prophylactic antibiotics should be used prior to thyroidectomy or parathyroidectomy. Nevertheless, since the introduction of the Surgical Care Improvement Project (SCIP) in 2004, an active decision regarding the administration of preoperative antibiotics must be made in every case, and in cases where no antibiotics are given, justification must be documented in the chart.

As a recent international survey of endocrine surgeons has shown, there is substantial variation in practice patterns relating to the use of preoperative antibiotic prophylaxis prior to thyroid or parathyroid surgery: Nearly two thirds of endocrine surgeons stated that they used preoperative antibiotics almost always (more than 90% of the time) while 26% of endocrine surgeons stated that they used preoperative antibiotics almost never (less than 10%) prior to thyroidectomy or parathyroidectomy. In that study, surgeons who worked in Asia (58%) were more likely than their European (8.8%) or American (29%) counterparts to always or almost always give preoperative antibiotics. Surgeons who worked in community hospitals were more likely to almost always give antibiotics than those who worked in University or Affiliated medical centers [10].

In this chapter, the available evidence that pertains to this important question will be summarized and graded, with the hope that it will help surgeons make more individualized decisions regarding the use or the withholding of preoperative antibiotic prophylaxis prior to thyroid or parathyroid surgery.

Prevalence and Predictors of Wound Infections Following Thyroid or Parathyroid Surgery

A classic prospective study of more than 20,000 surgical wounds at a Minneapolis VA hospital was one of the most important in demonstrating the benefit of preoperative antibiotic prophylaxis in clean and clean- contaminated operations. In that study, the administration of antibiotic prophylaxis was associated with a reduction in wound infection rates from 5.1% to 0.8% in clean cases, and from 10.1% to 1.3% in clean—contaminated wounds [11].

Among large series of unselected patients who underwent thyroidectomy, low but highly variable wound infection rates have been reported. In the largest series of patients who underwent thyroidectomy, including nearly 15,000 patients in Italy, the wound infection rate was 0.3% [12]. A well- designed prospective study of postoperative complications after thyroidectomy for multinodular goiters also revealed an infection rate of 0.3% (1/300) [13].

A recent review of the American College of Surgeons' National Surgical Quality Improvement Program (ACS-NSQIP) user files between 2005 and 2011 again revealed a surgical site infection (SSI) rate of 0.36% (N = 179) among nearly 50,000 patients who underwent thyroidectomy. In that study, ¾ of the infections were classified as SSIs, and the rest were organ space infections or deep incisional infections. While preoperative factors such as obesity, alcohol use, and non-independent status were predictive of postoperative wound infection, these were not nearly as important as intraoperative variables that cannot always be predicted preoperatively. A wound classification of clean—contaminated (the result of intraoperative tracheal or esophageal injury) was by far the most predictive factor for wound infection (Odds ratio = 6.1), followed by prolonged operative time. No information is available regarding the use of antibiotic prophylaxis in the patients who were included in that study [14] (Table 23.2).

Table 23.2 Summary of non comparative studies

Author	Type	Major finding
Elfenbein [14]	#	OR time and wound classification were most predictive of postop SSI. Preop factors less predictive, included obesity, alcohol use, and non-independent status
Moalem [10]	@	Use of preoperative antibiotics varies widely and appears dogmatic (88% of endocrine surgeons use abx almost always (62%) or almost never (26%))
Hardy [6]	@	40% of surgeons had at least one patient with severe postthyroidectomy wound infection; 9% had at least one patient with necrotizing wound infection

= NSQIP review. @ = Survey study

Reasons (and Supportive Data) to Consider Administering Preoperative Antibiotics Routinely Prior to Thyroid or Parathyroid Surgery

Although thyroid and parathyroid operations are nearly always classified as clean cases, infections still occur. A recent survey of members of the British Association of Endocrine Surgeons revealed that 40 of 100 respondents to a survey had at least one patient with a severe wound infection that required intravenous antibiotics or surgical drainage. In addition, nine surgeons had patients with fulminant wound infections, of whom six died [6]. A study from France, where severe infections are reported to government authorities, described three cases of fulminant streptococcal infections, which were rapidly lethal in two patients (death occurred on postoperative days 4 and 12 despite intensive care and debridement), and resulted in a prolonged ICU stay in the third. Those three cases occurred in geographically distinct areas in France, and no causative factor was discovered [5]. In contrast, a report from the Center for Disease Control in the United States described an outbreak of severe necrotizing group-A strep among three patients who underwent thyroid and parathyroid surgery in late 1996 [4]. Two of those patients died from the infection, and the third was discharged after a prolonged ICU stay. All three cases were attributed to subclinical infection among health care workers who were in contact with the patients.

A few other case reports of severe streptococcal infections following thyroid surgery exist [7, 8]. Curiously, such devastating infections tend to affect young, fit adults who appear to have intact immunity and no known risk factors for infection [15].

Superficial wound infections are far more common than the necrotizing wound infections reported above. Among large series of outcome—related studies of thyroidectomy, wound infection is commonly not reported [16]. Nevertheless, some studies have revealed wound infection rates as high as 5.3% among patients who underwent conventional thyroidectomy [17]. In other series of patients who underwent clean surgery, infection rates as high as 16% have been reported among high—risk patients [18].

The cosmetically sensitive location of the scar (and therefore, of a potential wound infection) greatly increases the impact of an otherwise simple SSI, and also limits therapeutic options. Whereas, most superficial wound infections are readily treated with suture removal or incision and drainage, the proximity of the cervical incision to critical structures precludes open packing and regular dressing changes. Moreover, such treatment and healing by secondary intent can be associated with a suboptimal long-term cosmetic result in a highly visible and sensitive area.

Finally, in an era of protocol-driven care pathways, where substantial efforts to standardize care and reduce variability are made, some surgeons may be disincentivized to personalize care and simply order antibiotic prophylaxis routinely, per hospital perioperative policy.

Reasons (and Supportive Data) to Consider NOT Administering Preoperative Antibiotics Routinely Prior to Thyroid or Parathyroid Surgery

To date, no study has demonstrated benefit with the routine administration of prophylactic antibiotics. Three comparative studies have been done to address this question. A retrospective review recently compared 1132 patients who underwent thyroid surgery and received antibiotic prophylaxis to 1794 patients who did not. That study found an overall wound infection rate of 1%, but no difference between the two groups [3]. A recent prospective randomized study compared 1082 patients who underwent thyroid or parathyroid surgery and received antibiotic prophylaxis (evenly split between cefazolin and piperacillin) to 1082 patients who did not receive antibiotics. That study did not demonstrate a difference in SSI, with one SSI (0.09%) in the antibiotic group, and three (0.28%) in the no antibiotic group ($p = 0.371$). Interestingly, preoperative antibiotics were associated with a lower urinary tract infection (UTI) rate (3 vs. 17, $p = 0.002$) in this large cohort of patients. Notably, 84% of the UTI's in that series were in patients who had an indwelling urinary catheter [2].

Finally, a multicenter prospective randomized double blind study was conducted on 500 patients who underwent thyroidectomy. Half received ampicillin/sulbactam as prophylaxis, and half received none. No difference in SSI rate was found, with two infections in the antibiotic group, and only one in the no antibiotic group [1]. In addition, a large retrospective case series of patients who underwent thyroid operations without antibiotic prophylaxis reported a single infection among more than 1000 patients [19, 20]. These findings demonstrate that with meticulous technique, scrupulous maintenance of sterile conditions, and attention to hemostasis very low infection rates can be readily achieved even without antibiotic prophylaxis.

Recently, the overuse of antibiotic prophylaxis has been cited as a possible contributing factor to the development of antibiotic resistance [21, 22]. Additionally, adverse reactions such as renal or hepatic toxicity, allergic reactions, and the development of opportunistic infections are all possible even after a single dose of antibiotics. Taken together, one could easily argue that the societal and individual harm that is caused by routine, unnecessary antibiotic prophylaxis prior to these common and clean operations may be greater than the benefit that they are intended to confer.

Conclusions

Infections following thyroid or parathyroid operations are very uncommon, partly because of the clean nature of these operations, but also because of the very rich blood supply in the neck. To date, only two randomized studies have been done in an effort to determine the necessity of antibiotic prophylaxis prior to these operations. Both studies failed to show a benefit to antibiotic prophylaxis. On the other hand, there are a few case reports describing serious and even lethal wound infections following thyroid and parathyroid operations. It is unclear whether antibiotic prophylaxis would prevent such infections, and in most of the reports is it not mentioned whether the patients received antibiotic prophylaxis [4–7].

Recommendations

There are no data to support the routine administration of preoperative antibiotic prophylaxis prior to thyroid or parathyroid operations. However, because of the paucity of level one data, and the wide range of wound infections reported in the literature, it is recommended that surgeons carefully scrutinize their own outcomes as it relates to wound infections and individualize this decision. Selective use of antibiotic prophylaxis may be appropriate, but to date, no preoperative patient factor (diabetes, obesity, immunocompromised patient) or operative factor (reoperation) has been proven to increase the risk of infection, or to be associated with increased benefit from preoperative antibiotic prophylaxis (grade B recommendation).

References

1. Avenia N, Sanguinetti A, Cirocchi R, Docimo G, Ragusa M, Ruggiero R, et al. Antibiotic prophylaxis in thyroid surgery: a preliminary multicentric Italian experience. Ann Surg Innov Res. 2009;3:10.
2. Uruno T, Masaki C, Suzuki A, Ohkuwa K, Shibuya H, Kitagawa W, et al. Antimicrobial prophylaxis for the prevention of surgical site infection after thyroid and parathyroid surgery: a prospective randomized trial. World J Surg. 2015;39(5):1282–7.
3. De Palma M, Grillo M, Borgia G, Pezzullo L, Lombardi CP, Gentile I. Antibiotic prophylaxis and risk of infections in thyroid surgery: results from a national study (UEC-Italian endocrine surgery units association). Updat Surg. 2013;65(3):213–6.
4. Control CD. Prevention. Nosocomial group a streptococcal infections associated with asymptomatic health-care workers--Maryland and California, 1997. MMWR Morb Mortal Wkly Rep. 1999;48(8):163.
5. Faibis F, Sapir D, Luis D, Laigneau P, Lepoutre A, Pospisil F, et al. Severe group a streptococcus infection after thyroidectomy: report of three cases and review. Surg Infect. 2008;9(5):529–31.
6. Hardy R, Forsythe J. Uncovering a rare but critical complication following thyroid surgery: an audit across the UK and Ireland. Thyroid. 2007;17(1):63–5.
7. Hung JA, Rajeev P. Streptococcal toxic shock syndrome following total thyroidectomy. Ann R Coll Surg Engl. 2013;95(7):457–60.
8. Karlik JB, Duron V, Mermel LA, Mazzaglia P. Severe group a streptococcus surgical site infection after thyroid lobectomy. Surg Infect. 2013;14(2):216–20.
9. Bratzler DW, Dellinger EP, Olsen KM, Perl TM, Auwaerter PG, Bolon MK, et al. Clinical practice guidelines for antimicrobial prophylaxis in surgery. Am J Health Syst Pharm. 2013;70(3):195–283.
10. Moalem J, Ruan DT, Farkas RL, Shen WT, Kebebew E, Duh QY, et al. Patterns of antibiotic prophylaxis use for thyroidectomy and parathyroidectomy: results of an international survey of endocrine surgeons. J Am Coll Surg. 2010;210(6):949–56.
11. Olson M, O'Connor M, Schwartz ML. Surgical wound infections. A 5-year prospective study of 20,193 wounds at the Minneapolis VA medical center. Ann Surg. 1984;199(3):253–9.
12. Rosato L, Avenia N, Bernante P, De Palma M, Gulino G, Nasi PG, et al. Complications of thyroid surgery: analysis of a multicentric study on 14,934 patients operated on in Italy over 5 years. World J Surg. 2004;28(3):271–6.

13. Zambudio AR, Rodríguez J, Riquelme J, Soria T, Canteras M, Parrilla P. Prospective study of postoperative complications after total thyroidectomy for multinodular goiters by surgeons with experience in endocrine surgery. Ann Surg. 2004;240(1):18.
14. Elfenbein DM, Schneider DF, Chen H, Sippel RS. Surgical site infection after thyroidectomy: a rare but significant complication. J Surg Res. 2014;190(1):170–6.
15. Martin PR, Høiby EA. Streptococcal Serogroup: a epidemic in Norway 1987–1988. Scand J Infect Dis. 1990;22(4):421–9.
16. Chadwick D. Fourth National Audit Report, The British Association of Endocrine and Thyroid Surgeons. 2012. Available at http://www.baets.org.uk/wp-content/uploads/2013/05/4th-National-Audit.pdf. Accessed 24 Mar 2015.
17. Dionigi G, Boni L, Rovera F, Rausei S, Dionigi R. Wound morbidity in mini-invasive thyroidectomy. Surg Endosc. 2011;25(1):62–7.
18. Haley RW, Culver DH, Morgan WM, White JW, Emori TG, Hooton TM. Identifying patients at high risk of surgical wound infection: a simple multivariate index of patient susceptibility and wound contamination. Am J Epidemiol. 1985;121(2):206–15.
19. Lu Q, Xie S-Q, Chen S-Y, Chen L-J, Qin Q. Experience of 1166 thyroidectomy without use of prophylactic antibiotic. Biomed Res Int. 2014;2014:1–5.
20. Qin Q, Li H, Wang L-B, Li A-H, Chen L-J, Lu Q. Thyroid surgery without antibiotic prophylaxis: experiences with 1,030 patients from a teaching hospital in China. World J Surg. 2014;38(4):878–81.
21. Porco TC, Gao D, Scott JC, Shim E, Enanoria WT, Galvani AP, et al. When does overuse of antibiotics become a tragedy of the commons? PLoS One. 2012;7(12):e46505.
22. Davey P, Brown E, Charani E, Fenelon L, Gould IM, Holmes A, et al. Interventions to improve antibiotic prescribing practices for hospital inpatients. Cochrane Libr. 2013.
23. Dionigi G, Rovera F, Boni L, Castano P, Dionigi R. Surgical site infections after thyroidectomy. Surg Infect. 2006;7(Supplement 2):s-117–s-20.

The Value of Intraoperative Parathyroid Hormone Monitoring in Primary Hyperparathyroidism Cases That Are Localized with Two Imaging Studies

24

Jennifer H. Kuo and Wen T. Shen

Abstract

Minimally invasive parathyroidectomy has become a preferred approach for primary hyperparathyroidism in patients with a single parathyroid adenoma. Preoperative localization studies and intraoperative parathyroid hormone (ioPTH) are important adjuncts, with surgeons often relying on ioPTH to confirm cure. The utility of ioPTH in patients with two concordant preoperative localization studies that accurately predict single parathyroid adenomas, remains controversial. This chapter explores the evidence for the use of ioPTH is this setting.

Keywords

Minimally invasive parathyroidectomy · Concordant preoperative studies · IOPTH

J. H. Kuo
Division of GI/Endocrine Surgery, Columbia University, New York, NY, USA
e-mail: jhk2029@cumc.columbia.edu

W. T. Shen (✉)
Department of Surgery, University of California, San Francisco/Mt. Zion Medical Center, San Francisco, CA, USA
e-mail: wen.shen@ucsfmedctr.org

P. Angelos, R. H. Grogan (eds.), *Difficult Decisions in Endocrine Surgery*, Difficult Decisions in Surgery: An Evidence-Based Approach,
https://doi.org/10.1007/978-3-319-92860-9_24

Study Design

We performed a comprehensive PubMed database search of the use of intraoperative parathyroid hormone monitoring in minimally invasive parathyroidectomy. Our search returned 148 articles. The pertinent articles are summarized in this chapter.

Discussion

Our literature search reveals that there is minimal supporting evidence to provide definitive recommendations. Change in surgical management guided by ioPTH use occurs 0.03–10% of the time and there is modest evidence to suggest that the use of ioPTH does not statistically increase the success of biochemical cure with a minimal difference in cure rates (normal calcium and PTH levels at 6 months, 90–99% without ioPTH, 97–99% with ioPTH). There is insufficient evidence to discern a difference in recurrence, length of operation, or length of hospitalization. The marginal added benefit of ioPTH in patients with concordant preoperative imaging studies needs to be weighed against the added cost and increased operating time. As surgeons become more familiar with interpreting preoperative imaging studies and performing their own ultrasounds, they may move towards utilizing intraoperative parathyroid hormone measurement on a more selective basis (Table 24.1).

Introduction

Primary hyperparathyroidism is a common endocrine disorder that is becoming more prevalent in the United States, with 100,000 new cases diagnosed each year [1, 2]. It is classically characterized and diagnosed by high levels of both serum calcium and intact parathyroid hormone (ioPTH), in the setting of a normal vitamin D 25-OH level. Both sporadic and familial forms of the disease exist, with the vast majority of patients having sporadic disease. Most patients with sporadic disease have a single parathyroid adenoma, but involvement of more than one gland, either in the form of multiple adenomas or four-gland hyperplasia, occurs 15–20% of the time.

Table 24.1 PICO table

Population	Patients with sporadic primary hyperparathyroidism with two concordant preoperative localizing studies
Intervention	No intraoperative parathyroid hormone monitoring
Comparator	Intraoperative parathyroid hormone monitoring
Outcome	• Recurrence • Length of operation • Cost

The only curative treatment for primary hyperparathyroidism is surgery and removal of abnormal, overactive parathyroid gland(s). For patients with symptomatic disease and asymptomatic patients who meet criteria for surgery [3], parathyroidectomy is an effective therapy that cures the disease, decreases the risk of kidney stones, improves bone mineral density, and may decrease fracture risk and modestly improve some quality of life measurements.

The goal of parathyroidectomy in primary hyperparathyroidism is biochemical cure of the disease with normalization of both serum calcium and iPTH 6 months after surgery. Traditionally, the standard surgical approach was a bilateral neck exploration, usually under general anesthesia [4]. Bilateral exploration relies on visual and weight-based estimations of gland size to distinguish single adenoma from multiglandular disease. Over the last two decades, the preferred surgical approach for primary hyperparathyroidism has become minimally invasive parathyroidectomy, which targets a single hyperfunctioning gland with a smaller incision. This approach has been shown to be as successful as traditional bilateral exploration [5, 6], and is associated with decreased operative time and less morbidity [7]. The success of minimally invasive parathyroidectomy was made possible by advancements in preoperative localization studies and the introduction of intraoperative parathyroid hormone monitoring.

Concordant Preoperative Imaging

Preoperative localization studies permit the surgeon to limit the operative field to the region where a single radiologic focus is identified. Surgeons often use agreement (or concordance) of two preoperative imaging studies to guide focused exploration in minimally invasive parathyroidectomy. Concordance or agreement of ultrasonography (Fig. 24.1) and one other imaging study, most commonly nuclear medicine technetium-99m-sestamibi scans (MIBI, Fig. 24.2), used for the preoperative

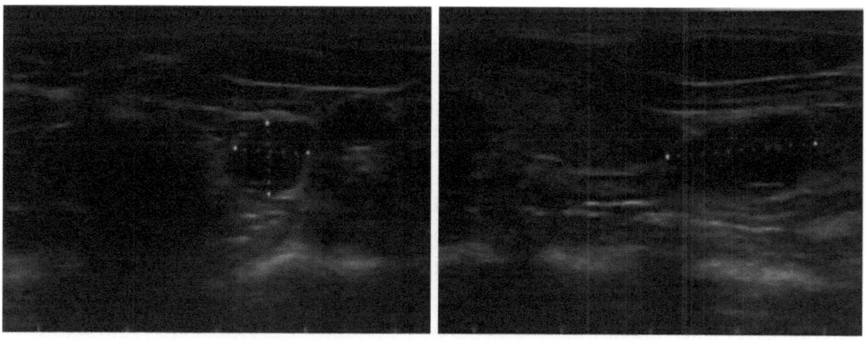

Fig. 24.1 Ultrasound imaging of a left lower parathyroid adenoma

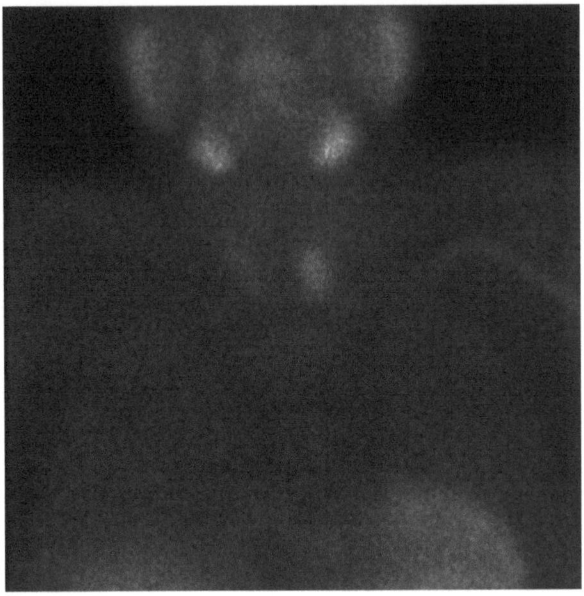

Fig. 24.2 Sestamibi scan of a left upper parathyroid adenoma in the tracheoesophageal groove

localization of hyperfunctioning parathyroid glands, successfully predicts the location of a single hyperfunctioning parathyroid gland in 93–97% of patients with single-gland disease [6, 8, 9].

Intraoperative Parathyroid Hormone Monitoring

Intraoperative parathyroid hormone monitoring (ioPTH) takes advantage of the short half-life (3–5 min) of PTH and utilizes a rapid immunochemiluminescence assay technique that allows measurements while the patient is still in the operating room [10–12]. The assay can be completed with a turnaround time of 8–20 min. Accuracy of ioPTH is dependent upon the surgeon's knowledge and familiarity with PTH dynamics. Two general protocols for ioPTH are widely accepted and produce reliable results. The first is widely known as the "Miami Criterion" requiring a >50% drop in PTH value. This method requires four intraoperative PTH samples: at the time of incision, before excision of the gland, and 5 and 10 min after excision of the gland. A drop in PTH values of >50% from the highest level is used as criterion to conclude surgery. If the PTH value does not drop appropriately by 10 min after gland excision, a repeat PTH level can be drawn at 20 min. In most patients, the Miami criterion is met with this additional measurement [13, 14]. If the criterion is not met, further exploration of the other glands is mandated and additional glands are removed (with repeat measurements of PTH) until the criterion is fulfilled. Use of the Miami criterion further increases the success rate of minimally invasive parathyroidectomy by 1–3% [6, 15] and can also predict normal postoperative calcium levels for at least 6 months [16]. Other surgeons use a modified Miami criterion that requires a >50% percent drop from the highest level and a return of PTH values to the normal range as the criteria to conclude surgery. The use of both of these criteria can predict postoperative normal or low calcium levels with an excellent accuracy of 97% [17].

Although the merits of ioPTH are clear, false-positive and false-negative results can occur. Although rare [18, 19], false-positive results where there is a drop in PTH followed by persistent postoperative hyperparathyroidism, suggests the possibility for a multiple endocrine neoplasia (MEN) syndrome, parathyroid carcinoma, or other familial causes of hyperparathyroidism. More commonly, false-negative PTH results can occur at a rate of 1.2–9.8% [15] and have been associated with (1) PTH levels drawn from an ipsilateral internal jugular vein to a single adenoma where it can take longer for the PTH level to drop, (2) PTH levels that continue to rise after the pre-excision level is drawn or (3) or slower PTH kinetics that require a longer time to drop to normal range when using the modified Miami criterion. False-negative rates can lead to an increase in anesthesia time and continuation of unnecessary surgical exploration, potentially increasing surgical complications and costs [15]. Therefore, the use of IOPTH as a guide to determine the necessary extent of parathyroid exploration remains controversial, especially in the cohort of patients with concordant preoperative imaging that accurately predicts single gland disease in 93–97% of patients.

Search Strategy

We performed a comprehensive review of the literature related to the use of intraoperative parathyroid hormone monitoring in minimally invasive parathyroidectomy. A literature search was conducted in the PubMed database using the key words: primary hyperparathyroidism, parathyroidectomy, parathyroid surgery, preoperative imaging, and intraoperative parathyroid hormone monitoring. Searches were limited to the English language, human subjects, and literature published in the last 10 years. Our search returned 148 articles. Studies evaluating secondary, tertiary, familial, malignant, or non-classical primary hyperparathyroidism, reoperative surgery, bilateral neck exploration, single preoperative localization study, and/or discordant or missing concordant preoperative localization studies were excluded. Table 24.2 provides a summary of studies pertinent to our discussion.

Discussion

Although it is generally agreed that surgery is the fastest, most durable, and most cost-effective treatment for primary hyperparathyroidism, and that minimally invasive parathyroidectomy provides equivalent rates of cure as the more traditional bilateral neck exploration in the setting of appropriate adjunct studies, there is still little consensus as to what those adjunct studies should be. Few would dispute the utility of intraoperative parathyroid hormone monitoring in patients with multiglandular disease, reoperative cases, or in cases with discordant preoperative localization. However, regarding the utility of intraoperative parathyroid hormone in cases

Table 24.2 Summary table of studies evaluating the role of ioPTH in primary hyperparathyroidism patients with two concordant preoperative studies

Study/Year	Population	Study type	Number of patients	Use of IOPTH	Conversion to bilateral exploration	Length of operation	Length of hospitalization	% Cure at 6 months	Recurrence	Quality of evidence
Chen et al. (2005)	1HPT with concordant localization	(a) Retrospective (no ioPTH) and (b) prospective (ioPTH)	345	54.5% (188/345)	(a) Na (b) 10.6%	Na	(a) 2.0 ± 0.3 days (b) 0.3 ± 0 days	(a) 90% (b) 99%	(a) Na (b) 1% (2/188)	Moderate
Cho et al. (2011)	1HPT with concordant localization	Prospective cohort study	119	No	10.9% (13 of 119)	Na		97%	Na	Moderate
Elfenbein et al. (2014)	1HPT with concordant localization	Retrospective	1421	Yes	Na	Na	Na	98%	Na	Moderate
Gawande et al. (2006)	1HPT with concordant localization	Retrospective	319	Yes	1% (3/319)	Na	Na	99%	Na	Moderate
Haciyanli et al (2009)	1HPT with concordant localization	Prospective	30	No	Na	Na	Na	96.7%	Na	Low
Mihai et al. (2006)	1HPT with concordant localization	Retrospective	150	No	0.03%	Na	Na	99.3%	0%	Moderate
Zawawi et al. (2013)	1HPT with concordant localization	Retrospective and prospective	186	Yes	Na	+30.9 min	Na	Na (96.7% correlated with hypercellular tissue on frozen section without ioPTH)	Na	Moderate

of primary hyperparathyroidism and two concordant preoperative imaging studies, there remains controversy as to whether or not the marginal benefit of ioPTH monitoring is enough to warrant its use.

Our literature search conducted to specifically address this question reveals that there is minimal supporting evidence to provide definitive recommendations. Although there are no randomized controlled trials directly comparing the use of ioPTH in 1HPT patients with concordant studies, change in surgical management guided by ioPTH use occurred 0.03–10% [20–23] of the time and the difference in cure rates (normal calcium and PTH levels at 6 months) is minimal (90–99% without ioPTH, 97–99% with ioPTH). This incremental difference in cure rates is not statistically significant. Only two studies were able to provide information on recurrence [20, 23]. In addition, very little information could be found regarding the actual difference in length of operation [24] and length of hospitalization [20]. Thus, there is modest evidence to suggest that the use of ioPTH does not statistically increase the success of biochemical cure for minimally invasive parathyroidectomy in patients with primary hyperparathyroidism and two concordant preoperative localization studies. In addition, there is insufficient evidence to determine whether the use of ioPTH has any discernible effect on other clinical outcomes such as length of operation time, length of hospital stay, and recurrence rates.

Surgeon-Performed Ultrasound

Concordance of preoperative localization studies most often refers to an ultrasound and a MIBI scan. Little distinction has been made between a radiology-performed ultrasound (most often performed by radiological technicians and then read by a radiologist) and a surgeon-performed ultrasound (SUS). It has been postulated that an ultrasound performed by a dedicated parathyroid sonographer with a better understanding of the embryological origins of ectopic glands, has greater accuracy in detecting parathyroid adenomas. As a single test, SUS has been shown to be as accurate as MIBI with a sensitivity of 77–87% [25, 26]. When used in conjunction with MIBI, concordance of the two studies can be found 82.5% of the time [27] and provides additional information about localization 14% of the time [28]. SUS has proven most helpful in localization of parathyroid glands when MIBI scans have been negative [26, 28]. In addition, surgeon-performed ultrasound has the added benefit of evaluating concomitant thyroid pathology that can occur in 33–51% of patients [29, 30]. In our own series, we found that concordance of a MIBI scan with a surgeon-performed ultrasound (SUS) was more accurate than concordance with a radiology-performed ultrasound at predicting single glandular disease (93.7% vs. 89.1%), but concordance of MIBI with both a radiology-performed ultrasound and SUS was most accurate, at 94.8%. The addition of ioPTH was beneficial in patients with MIBI concordance with a radiology-performed ultrasound (+8.0%, $p < 0.0001$), but did not make a significant difference in patients with concordance of a SUS and MIBI, or concordance of a radiology performed ultrasound, SUS, and MIBI (unpublished results).

Cost-Effectiveness of Iopth Use in Primary Hyperparathyroidism

The argument against the use of intraoperative parathyroid hormone monitoring fundamentally hinges on the cost-effectiveness of the test; that is, does the added cost of ioPTH monitoring justify its incremental effectiveness? Morris et al. evaluated [15] the cost of ioPTH using a base-case of a 60 year-old woman with a biochemical diagnosis of primary hyperparathyroidism who met the NIH 2002 consensus guidelines for parathyroidectomy. They found that ioPTH improved the success rate of their base-case scenario from 96.3 to 98.8%, and the IOPTH strategy increases cost by 3.8%. IoPTH was the most cost-saving strategy when assay costs were less than $110 or the cost of the operation was greater than $12,000. Although this study did not explicitly address the cost of ioPTH in patients with two concordant preoperative imaging studies, it is still pertinent to the patient population with two concordant studies as the success rate of parathyroidectomy without ioPTH was set at 96.3%, similar to the overall success rates of parathyroidectomies in our cohort. The results of this study suggest that there is definitely an incremental cost accrued with the use of ioPTH, even though the study did not directly address the effectiveness of the adjunct test.

Recommendation

Our review of the literature on parathyroid surgery over the last decade demonstrates that intraoperative parathyroid hormone monitoring may not be required in patients with sporadic primary hyperparathyroidism and concordant preoperative localization studies. ioPTH appears to provide modest incremental value to surgical outcomes, and comes at added cost and increased operating time. As surgeons become more familiar with interpreting preoperative imaging studies and performing their own ultrasound in the clinic and operating room, they may move towards utilizing intraoperative parathyroid hormone measurement on a more selective basis. Nonetheless, many surgeons (including the authors) will likely continue to use ioPTH as a "fail-safe" measure intended to maximize operative success (and also provide reassurance to both surgeon and patient that the operation is indeed over).

References

1. Yeh MW, Ituarte PH, Zhou HC, Nishimoto S, Liu IL, Harari A, et al. Incidence and prevalence of primary hyperparathyroidism in a racially mixed population. J Clin Endocrinol Metab. 2013;98(3):1122–9. https://doi.org/10.1210/jc.2012-4022. PMID: 23418315; PMCID: PMC3590475.
2. Press DM, Siperstein AE, Berber E, Shin JJ, Metzger R, Monteiro R, et al. The prevalence of undiagnosed and unrecognized primary hyperparathyroidism: a population-based analysis from the electronic medical record. Surgery. 2013;154(6):1232–7. discussion 7-8. PMID: 24383100.

3. Bilezikian JP, Khan AA, Potts JT Jr. Third International Workshop on the Management of Asymptomatic Primary H. Guidelines for the management of asymptomatic primary hyperparathyroidism: summary statement from the third international workshop. J Clin Endocrinol Metab. 2009;94(2):335–9. https://doi.org/10.1210/jc.2008-1763. PMID: 19193908; PMCID: PMC3214274.
4. Silverberg SJ, Bilezikian JP. Asymptomatic primary hyperparathyroidism: a medical perspective. Surg Clin North Am. 2004;84(3):787–801. https://doi.org/10.1016/j.suc.2004.03.002. PMID: 15145235.
5. Irvin GL 3rd, Prudhomme DL, Deriso GT, Sfakianakis G, Chandarlapaty SK. A new approach to parathyroidectomy. Ann Surg. 1994;219(5):574–9. discussion 9-81. PMID: 8185406; PMCID: PMC1243192.
6. Irvin GL 3rd, Solorzano CC, Carneiro DM. Quick intraoperative parathyroid hormone assay: surgical adjunct to allow limited parathyroidectomy, improve success rate, and predict outcome. World J Surg. 2004;28(12):1287–92. https://doi.org/10.1007/s00268-004-7708-6. PMID: 15517474.
7. Norman J, Chheda H, Farrell C. Minimally invasive parathyroidectomy for primary hyperparathyroidism: decreasing operative time and potential complications while improving cosmetic results. Am Surg. 1998;64(5):391–5. discussion 5-6. PMID: 9585770.
8. Smith N, Magnuson JS, Vidrine DM, Kulbersh B, Peters GE. Minimally invasive parathyroidectomy: use of intraoperative parathyroid hormone assays after 2 preoperative localization studies. Arch Otolaryngol Head Neck Surg. 2009;135(11):1108–11. https://doi.org/10.1001/archoto.2009.160. PMID: 19917923.
9. Lew JI, Solorzano CC, Montano RE, Carneiro-Pla DM, Irvin GL 3rd. Role of intraoperative parathormone monitoring during parathyroidectomy in patients with discordant localization studies. Surgery. 2008;144(2):299–306. https://doi.org/10.1016/j.surg.2008.03.039. PMID: 18656639.
10. Carneiro DM, Irvin GL 3rd. Late parathyroid function after successful parathyroidectomy guided by intraoperative hormone assay (QPTH) compared with the standard bilateral neck exploration. Surgery. 2000;128(6):925–9. https://doi.org/10.1067/msy.2000.109964. discussion 35-6. PMID: 11114625.
11. Sokoll LJ, Drew H, Udelsman R. Intraoperative parathyroid hormone analysis: a study of 200 consecutive cases. Clin Chem. 2000;46(10):1662–8. PMID: 11017947.
12. Delbridge LW, Dolan SJ, Hop TT, Robinson BG, Wilkinson MR, Reeve TS. Minimally invasive parathyroidectomy: 50 consecutive cases. Med J Aust. 2000;172(9):418–22. PMID: 10870533.
13. Carneiro DM, Solorzano CC, Nader MC, Ramirez M, Irvin GL 3rd. Comparison of intraoperative iPTH assay (QPTH) criteria in guiding parathyroidectomy: which criterion is the most accurate? Surgery. 2003;134(6):973–9. https://doi.org/10.1016/j.surg.2003.06.001. discussion 9-81. PMID: 14668730.
14. Di Stasio E, Carrozza C, Pio Lombardi C, Raffaelli M, Traini E, Bellantone R, et al. Parathyroidectomy monitored by intra-operative PTH: the relevance of the 20 min end-point. Clin Biochem. 2007;40(9–10):595–603. https://doi.org/10.1016/j.clinbiochem.2006.12.007. PMID: 17349989.
15. Morris LF, Zanocco K, Ituarte PH, Ro K, Duh QY, Sturgeon C, et al. The value of intraoperative parathyroid hormone monitoring in localized primary hyperparathyroidism: a cost analysis. Ann Surg Oncol. 2010;17(3):679–85. https://doi.org/10.1245/s10434-009-0773-1. Epub 2009/11/04. PMID: 19885701; PMCID: PMC2820694.
16. Irvin GL 3rd, Dembrow VD, Prudhomme DL. Clinical usefulness of an intraoperative "quick parathyroid hormone" assay. Surgery. 1993;114(6):1019–22. discussion 22-3. PMID: 8256205.
17. Richards ML, Thompson GB, Farley DR, Grant CS. An optimal algorithm for intraoperative parathyroid hormone monitoring. Arch Surg. 2011;146(3):280–5. https://doi.org/10.1001/archsurg.2011.5. PMID: 21422358.
18. Schneider DF, Mazeh H, Sippel RS, Chen H. Is minimally invasive parathyroidectomy associated with greater recurrence compared to bilateral exploration? Analysis of more than 1,000

cases. Surgery. 2012;152(6):1008–15. https://doi.org/10.1016/j.surg.2012.08.022. PMID: 23063313; PMCID: PMC3501613.

19. Greene AB, Butler RS, McIntyre S, Barbosa GF, Mitchell J, Berber E, et al. National trends in parathyroid surgery from 1998 to 2008: a decade of change. J Am Coll Surg. 2009;209(3):332–43. https://doi.org/10.1016/j.jamcollsurg.2009.05.029. PMID: 19717037.
20. Chen H, Pruhs Z, Starling JR, Mack E. Intraoperative parathyroid hormone testing improves cure rates in patients undergoing minimally invasive parathyroidectomy. Surgery. 2005;138(4):583–7.; discussion 7-90. Epub 2005/11/05. PMID: 16269285. https://doi.org/10.1016/j.surg.2005.06.046.
21. Gawande AA, Monchik JM, Abbruzzese TA, Iannuccilli JD, Ibrahim SI, Moore FD Jr. Reassessment of parathyroid hormone monitoring during parathyroidectomy for primary hyperparathyroidism after 2 preoperative localization studies. Arch Surg. 2006;141(4):381–4. https://doi.org/10.1001/archsurg.141.4.381. discussion 4. Epub 2006/04/19. PMID: 16618896.
22. Cho NL, Gawande AA, Sheu EG, Moore FD Jr, Ruan DT. Critical role of identification of the second gland during unilateral parathyroid surgery: a prospective review of 119 patients with concordant localization. Arch Surg. 2011;146(5):512–6. https://doi.org/10.1001/archsurg.2011.91. Epub 2011/05/18. PMID: 21576603.
23. Mihai R, Palazzo FF, Gleeson FV, Sadler GP. Minimally invasive parathyroidectomy without intraoperative parathyroid hormone monitoring in patients with primary hyperparathyroidism. Br J Surg. 2007;94(1):42–7. Epub 2006/11/04. PMID: 17083106. https://doi.org/10.1002/bjs.5574.
24. Zawawi F, Mlynarek AM, Cantor A, Varshney R, Black MJ, Hier MP, et al. Intraoperative parathyroid hormone level in parathyroidectomy: which patients benefit from it? J Otolaryngol Head Neck Surg. 2013;42:56. https://doi.org/10.1186/1916-0216-42-56. Epub 2013/12/20. PMID: 24350891; PMCID: PMC3878236.
25. Deutmeyer C, Weingarten M, Doyle M, Carneiro-Pla D. Case series of targeted parathyroidectomy with surgeon-performed ultrasonography as the only preoperative imaging study. Surgery. 2011;150(6):1153–60. Epub 2011/12/06. PMID: 22136835. https://doi.org/10.1016/j.surg.2011.09.041.
26. Solorzano CC, Lee TM, Ramirez MC, Carneiro DM, Irvin GL. Surgeon-performed ultrasound improves localization of abnormal parathyroid glands. Am Surg. 2005;71(7):557–62. discussion 62-3. Epub 2005/08/11. PMID: 16089118.
27. Aliyev S, Agcaoglu O, Aksoy E, Birsen O, Milas M, Mitchell J, et al. An analysis of whether surgeon-performed neck ultrasound can be used as the main localizing study in primary hyperparathyroidism. Surgery. 2014;156(5):1127–31. Epub 2014/12/03. PMID: 25444313. https://doi.org/10.1016/j.surg.2014.05.009.
28. Adler JT, Chen H, Schaefer S, Sippel RS. What is the added benefit of cervical ultrasound to (9)(9)mTc-sestamibi scanning in primary hyperparathyroidism? Ann Surg Oncol. 2011;18(10):2907–11. Epub 2011/04/22. PMID: 21509629. https://doi.org/10.1245/s10434-011-1724-1.
29. Alkhalili E, Tasci Y, Aksoy E, Aliyev S, Soundararajan S, Taskin E, et al. The utility of neck ultrasound and Sestamibi scans in patients with secondary and tertiary hyperparathyroidism. World J Surg. 2014;39(3):701–5. Epub 2014/11/21. PMID: 25409841. https://doi.org/10.1007/s00268-014-2878-3.
30. Morita SY, Somervell H, Umbricht CB, Dackiw AP, Zeiger MA. Evaluation for concomitant thyroid nodules and primary hyperparathyroidism in patients undergoing parathyroidectomy or thyroidectomy. Surgery. 2008;144(6):862–6.; discussion 6-8. Epub 2008/12/02. PMID: 19040989. https://doi.org/10.1016/j.surg.2008.07.029.

Transperitoneal Versus Retroperitoneal Laparoscopic Adrenalectomy

25

Amudhan Pugalenthi and Eren Berber

Abstract

Over the last two decades, laparoscopic adrenalectomy (LA) has become the gold standard for the removal of benign adrenal tumors. There are two approaches that are popular. Gagner et al. demonstrated the laparoscopic transperitoneal approach in 1992. A year later, Mercan described the posterior retroperitoneal approach. Laparoscopic transperitoneal adrenalectomy (LTA) was the approach initially adopted by surgeons because of a familiar anatomy, but recently the posterior retroperitoneal adrenalectomy (PRA) has gained widespread acceptance because of avoidance of intra-abdominal organs during resection. Although proponents of each approach claim superiority of one method over other, there is no conclusive data available in the literature that demonstrates the superiority of one over the other. In this article, we will compare the outcomes from published data on the retroperitoneal and transperitoneal approach for adrenalectomy with evidence using the GRADE approach.

Keywords

Laparoscopy · Transperitoneal · Posterior · Retroperitoneal · Adrenalectomy

A. Pugalenthi · E. Berber (✉)
Department of Endocrine Surgery, Cleveland Clinic, Cleveland, OH, USA
e-mail: berbere@ccf.org

P. Angelos, R. H. Grogan (eds.), *Difficult Decisions in Endocrine Surgery*, Difficult Decisions in Surgery: An Evidence-Based Approach,
https://doi.org/10.1007/978-3-319-92860-9_25

Introduction

Laparoscopic adrenalectomy (LA) is the current "gold standard" for removal of benign adrenal tumors. Gagner et al. performed the first transperitoneal adrenalectomy in 1992 [1]. A year later, Mercan described the posterior retroperitoneal approach [2]. Laparoscopic transperitoneal adrenalectomy (LTA) was the approach initially adopted by surgeons because of a familiar anatomy, but recently the posterior retroperitoneal adrenalectomy (PRA) has gained widespread acceptance because of avoidance of intra-abdominal organs during resection. Although proponents of each approach claim superiority of one method over other, there is no conclusive data available in the literature that demonstrates the superiority of one over the other [3]. Two of the three published meta-analyses comparing the two approaches (PRA vs. LTA) concluded equivalent outcomes [3, 4], while the third one [5] claimed that the posterior approach had a superior short-term outcome. In this article, we will compare the outcomes from published data on the retroperitoneal and transperitoneal approach for adrenalectomy with evidence using the GRADE approach (http://www.gradeworkinggroup.org).

Search Strategy

We conducted a PubMed search for the following key words: "Laparoscopic", "Adrenalectomy", "Posterior approach" and "Transperitoneal". The search strategy is based on *PICO* elements as shown in Table 25.1.

The search was limited to English language and human studies. All the articles were reviewed; the best studies for this review were selected based their relevance with review of their significant references. Outcomes assessed include: complication rate, conversion rate, and length of hospital stay, operative time and tumor size.

Posterior Retroperitoneal Adrenalectomy

Mercan et al. published his initial series of 11 patients who underwent posterior adrenalectomy with no complications and no conversions to open procedure. Encouraged by this several surgeons adopted this approach and studies have been published that show benefit of this approach (Table 25.2). Although transperitoneal approach is the widely preferred approach for adrenalectomy, the posterior approach has its own advantages. The posterior approach gives a direct access to the adrenal

Table 25.1 PICO table

*P*opulation	Patients undergoing adrenalectomy
*I*ntervention	Retroperitoneal
*C*omparator	Transperitoneal
*O*utcomes	Complications, length of operation, postoperative morbidity

Table 25.2 Selected studies of Posterior Retroperitoneal Adrenalectomy (PRA)

Author, Year Country	*n*	Tumor size[a] (cm)	OR time (min)	LOS[a] (days)	Complications (%)	Conversion (%)	Quality of evidence
Mercan, 1995 [2] Turkey	11	3.6	150	3	0	0	High
Siperstein, 2000 [20] USA	33	3.2	176	1.4	0	0	High
Salomon, 2001 [21] France	115	3.1	118	4	12	0.8	High
Walz, 2006 [6] Germany	560	2.9	67	NA	16	1.7	High
Perrier, 2008 [22] USA	68	3.4	121	3	16	9	High
Cabalag, 2013 [23] Australia	50	3.4	70	1	8	0	Moderate

n number of adrenalectomies, *OR* operative, *LOS* length of stay, *NA* not available
[a]Median

gland thus minimizing the need for additional dissection as in the transabdominal approach. On the right side, it avoids the mobilization of the liver and on the left side it avoids mobilizing the spleen and splenic flexure of the colon that may be required in a transperitoneal approach. This is especially beneficial in patients with prior abdominal surgeries and adhesions. For bilateral tumors there is no need for repositioning. The disadvantage though is the limited space that can be created in the retroperitoneum. The upper limit of lesion size is 6–7 cm in various publications. The median tumor size ranges from 2.9 to 3.6 cm in the studies shown in Table 25.2. Conversion rate is less than 2%. Walz et al. [6] popularized this technique by reporting a large patient series with low morbidity. The mortality was zero, the major complication rate was 1.3%, and minor complication rate was 14.4%. The mean operating time of 560 procedures was (67 ± 40 min). This and other studies have demonstrated that in appropriately selected patients the posterior approach is safe and effective (Table 25.2).

Lateral Transperitoneal Adrenalectomy

After Gagner demonstrated the lateral transperitoneal approach for LA in 1991 [1], adrenalectomy has evolved from an open procedure performed by a chevron or thoracoabdominal incision to one that the can be performed via a minimally invasive approach. Many surgeons prefer the LTA because of the familiar operative field with the largest working space. Several studies have been published since then prove LTA to be safe and effective. The surgery can be performed at optimal insufflation pressures (12–15 mm of Hg) with adequate visualization. The reported rates of complication vary from 0.3 to 12%, but majority of them being minor complications. The length of stay is less than 5 days, with most studies reporting 1–2 days

Table 25.3 Selected studies of Lateral Transperitoneal Adrenalectomy (LTA)

Author, Year Country	*n*	Tumor size[a] (cm)	OR time (min)	LOS[a] (days)	Complications (%)	Conversion (%)	Quality of evidence
Gagner, 1997 [1] USA	100	<5	123	2.4	12	3	High
Pillinger, 2002 [24] Australia	59	7–11	175	4	8	5	High
Kalady, 2004 [25] USA	74	5.2	171	3.4	11	11	Moderate
Nguyen, 2011 [26] USA	154	3.6	156	3.4	0.2	0.2	High
Hirano, 2014 [27] Japan	76	2.7	205	NA	0.3	7	Low
Paganini, 2014 [17] Italy	64	4.5	92	4.8	6	3	Low

n number of adrenalectomies, *OR* operative, *LOS* length of stay, *NA* not available
[a]Median

(Tables 25.3 and 25.4). The disadvantage of the lateral approach however is that it requires repositioning for bilateral tumor. It is relatively difficult in patients who had previous abdominal surgeries due to intraoperative adhesions.

Posterior Approach vs. Lateral Approach–The Evidence

There is no general consensus regarding the optimal approach in the resection of benign adrenal tumors: RPA vs. LTA. Surgeons therefore base their practice upon local expertise and preference. The majority of studies comparing these two approaches are retrospective studies. Till date four prospective randomized studies [7–10] and three metaanalyses [3–5] have compared the two approaches. Although the indications for LA are well established, but for a given patient which approach is better has not been resolved. We will analyze the outcomes from selected studies comparing the two approaches.

Complications

The overall complication rate for PRA ranges from 0 to 18%. Barczynski et al. reported in their randomized study, a rate of 18%. All of them were either grade 1 or grade 2. In the LTA group the complications ranged from 2.6 to 31% (Table 25.4). Our group reported no complications in the PRA group but three mortalities as a result of cardiac and pulmonary complications in their LTA group. This was related to the fact that the patients with smaller tumors were approached by the posterior technique, whereas more complex cases were operated by lateral transabdominal approach. The patients who underwent PRA group are reported to have lesser

Table 25.4 Selected studies comparing Lateral Transperitoneal adrenalectomy (LTA) vs. Posterior Retroperitoneal adrenalectomy (PRA)

Author, Year Country	Approach	*n*	Tumor size[a] (cm)	OR time (min)	LOS[a] (days)	Complications (%)	Conversions (%)	Quality of evidence
Fernandez, 1996[b] [7] Spain	PRA	11	NA	105	2.7	0	0	High
	LTA	10	NA	88	3	20	0	
Naya, 2002 [28] Japan	PRA	22	NA	221	9.5	14	14	Very low
	LTA	28	NA	201	9.0	7	14	
Rubinstein, 2005[b] [8] USA	PRA	32	2.6	126	1	3.2	3	High
	LTA	25	2.7	130	1	8	4	
Gockel, 2005 [15] Germany	PRA	135	3.5	120	5	8.3	3	High
	LTA	132	3.5	85	6.5	3	1.5	
Lombardi, 2008 [16] Italy	PRA	38	3.6	114	5.6	5	NA	Low
	LTA	38	3.7	135	6.2	2.6	NA	
Berber, 2009 [11] USA	PRA	90	2.8	138	1–2	0	2	High
	LTA	69	4.4	157	1–2	4	3	
Mohammadi-Fallah, 2013[b] [9] Iran	PRA	13	2.6	127	3	8	8	Low
	LTA	11	2.9	129	3.7	8	0	
Barczynski, 2014[b] [10] Poland	PRA	33	3.9	50	2.9	18	0	Very high
	LTA	32	4.0	77	4.4	31	0	
Epelboym, 2014 [29] USA	PRA	81	NA	80	1	4	0	Low
	LTA	130	NA	130	2	7	3	

n number of adrenalectomies, *OR* operative, *LOS* length of stay, *NA* not available
[a]Median
[b]Prospective randomized study

overall complication rate than those undergoing LTA in most of the studies (Table 25.4). Among the four randomized studies, one study reported a similar [9], and three studies reported lower complication rate for PRA group compared to LTA [7, 8, 10]. In a recent metaanalyses by Constantinides et al. no difference was found in the complication rate between the two approaches. In the largest series of 560 adrenalectomies by the posterior approach Walz et al. reported 7 (1.2%) major and 83 (12%) minor complications.

Operative Time

Majority of the studies listed in Table 25.4 do not show much difference in terms of operative time between the two approaches (PRA vs. LTA). The median operative times for PRA ranged from 50 to 221 min and for LTA from 77 to 201 min. Although it is likely that preoperative factors may have resulted in selection bias for a particular approach, three out of the four randomized studies did not show a significant difference in operative time between the two approaches [8–10]. In a recent randomized control trial (RCT), Barczynski et al. reported that on multivariable analysis, body mass index >30 and lateral approach predicted prolonged operative time of >90 min [10]. It has also been shown that there is a relative continuation of learning curve even after 500 cases [6].

Conversion

Conversion rate from LA to open procedure ranges from 0 to 8% for the posterior approach and 0–4% for lateral approach (Table 25.4). Only one study by Naya et al. reported high conversion rates of 14% for both approaches. Among the four RCTs three reported zero conversions in the LTA group and two reported zero conversions in the PRA group. At our institution, our conversion rate for PRA is 2% and for LTA is 3% [11]. Most common reasons for conversion from the posterior approach to open are bleeding, failure to make progress, difficulty to create or maintain pneumoperitoneum. Most common reasons for conversion to open from LTA are bleeding, failure to make progress, injury to pancreas or spleen [3]. Walz et al. reported 11 conversions out of the total 560 posterior adrenalectomies. Of these, two were converted to a lateral laparoscopic approach and nine were converted to an open procedure. In the same report no conversions to open occurred after the 33rd PRA [12]. Based on conversion rates, it is believed that the learning curve for the operative techniques for both LTA and PRA is between 30 and 40 cases [13, 14].

Tumor Size

Three of the four randomized studies did not find any statistically significant difference in tumor size between the PRA and the LTA group [8–10], the fourth study by Fernandez-Cruz however did not report a tumor size [7]. In the literature, the median tumor size for PRA ranges from 2.6 to 3.9 cm and for LTA between 2.7 and 4.4 cm (Table 25.4). Walz et al. reported that they routinely selected tumors up to 7 cm without suspicion of malignancy for the posterior approach [6]. In our experience, benign tumors <6 cm are considered for the posterior approach if the body habitus of the patient is appropriate [11]. Nigri et al. and Chen et al. reported no significant difference in tumor size between the two approaches in their meta-analyses [4, 5]. Although the studies did not show a difference in tumor size for the two surgical approaches, in our experience, those patients with smaller tumors are preferentially channeled to PRA.

Length of Stay

Patients who undergo PRA were shown to have shorter length of stay (LOS) compared to patients who had LTA in most studies [7, 9, 10, 15–17]. However the LOS was similar in two studies [8, 11]. In all the four randomized studies the median length of stay in the PRA group was ≤3 days and after LTA was <4.5 days (Table 25.4). It has been speculated that the shorter length after PRA might be related to lesser postoperative pain in the posterior approach allowing earlier discharge of the patients from hospital [18]. Walz et al. reported that half their patients ($n = 142$) did not require any postoperative analgesia, and only five required analgesia for more than 24 h [12]. Chen et al. and Constantinides et al. reported in their metaanalyses, shorter LOS in patients who underwent PRA than LTA [3, 5]. On the other hand Nigri et al. metaanalyses showed there was no significant difference in the LOS stay between LTA and PRA [4].

Conclusion

For the past two decades numerous authors have reported their experience from different parts of the world regarding laparoscopic adrenalectomy. Overall, the literature shows a low morbidity for both PRA and LTA in experienced hands. Although the patient selection criteria for a given approach have not been strictly defined, except for tumor size, there is a suggestion in most studies that the postoperative pain, morbidity and length of stay may be less after PRA compared to LTA. There are definite advantages of PRA in patients with bilateral tumors, and abdominal adhesions. Nevertheless, it should be borne in mind that the posterior technique requires special training to operate in a smaller and less familiar space.

A Personal View of Laparoscopic Adrenalectomy

The authors believe that a comprehensive adrenal tumor program should offer both options to the patients. Due to the ease of access and avoidance of intra-peritoneal manipulation, we preferentially consider the PR approach in any patient presenting with tumors less than 6 cm. Nevertheless, for a patient to qualify a patient for the

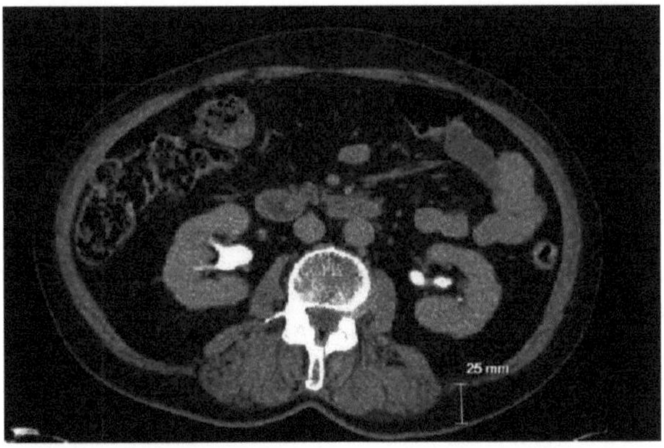

Fig. 25.1 Gerota's fascia-to-skin distance- The line shows the distance between skin and Gerota's fascia at a level, 1 cm below the 12th rib, which is favourable for the posterior approach

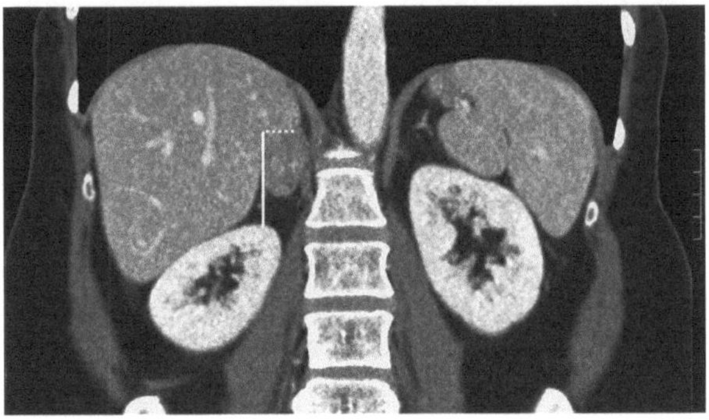

Fig. 25.2 The tumor-kidney relationship is favourable for a posterior approach as shown by the vertical (solid) line. The adrenal tumor is located well above the superior pole of the kidney

posterior approach, we look at additional topographical parameters, such as the thickness of the soft tissues below the 12th rib (where the first trocar is inserted), and the relationship between the 12th rib and the renal hilum (the best candidates are those in whom the 12th rib is -rostral to the renal hilum) (Fig. 25.1). Those tumors that are superior to the upper pole of the kidney are also better candidates for the posterior approach (Fig. 25.2). By adhering to these principles and selecting a technique tailored to the tumor and topographic features in a given patient, we were able to achieve a low morbidity and conversion rate in our series [19]. Laparoscopic ultrasound was crucial in our experience to maintain the safety of both approaches by recognizing the critical structures early during the dissection. We feel that LTA and PRA are complementary and not competitive to each other and also that they enhance the training of the future endocrine surgeons.

References

1. Gagner M, Lacroix A, Bolte E. Laparoscopic adrenalectomy in Cushing's syndrome and pheochromocytoma. N Engl J Med. 1992;327(14):1033.
2. Mercan S, Seven R, Ozarmagan S, Tezelman S. Endoscopic retroperitoneal adrenalectomy. Surgery. 1995;118(6):1071–5. discussion 5-6.

3. Constantinides VA, Christakis I, Touska P, Palazzo FF. Systematic review and meta-analysis of retroperitoneoscopic versus laparoscopic adrenalectomy. Br J Surg. 2012;99(12):1639–48.
4. Nigri G, Rosman AS, Petrucciani N, Fancellu A, Pisano M, Zorcolo L, et al. Meta-analysis of trials comparing laparoscopic transperitoneal and retroperitoneal adrenalectomy. Surgery. 2013;153(1):111–9.
5. Chen W, Li F, Chen D, Zhu Y, He C, Du Y, et al. Retroperitoneal versus transperitoneal laparoscopic adrenalectomy in adrenal tumor: a meta-analysis. Surg Laparosc Endosc Percutan Tech. 2013;23(2):121–7.
6. Walz MK, Alesina PF, Wenger FA, Deligiannis A, Szuczik E, Petersenn S, et al. Posterior retroperitoneoscopic adrenalectomy--results of 560 procedures in 520 patients. Surgery. 2006;140(6):943–8. discussion 8-50.
7. Fernandez-Cruz L, Saenz A, Benarroch G, Astudillo E, Taura P, Sabater L. Laparoscopic unilateral and bilateral adrenalectomy for Cushing's syndrome. Transperitoneal and retroperitoneal approaches. Ann Surg. 1996;224(6):727–34. discussion 34-6.
8. Rubinstein M, Gill IS, Aron M, Kilciler M, Meraney AM, Finelli A, et al. Prospective, randomized comparison of transperitoneal versus retroperitoneal laparoscopic adrenalectomy. J Urol. 2005;174(2):442–5. discussion 5.
9. Mohammadi-Fallah MR, Mehdizadeh A, Badalzadeh A, Izadseresht B, Dadkhah N, Barbod A, et al. Comparison of transperitoneal versus retroperitoneal laparoscopic adrenalectomy in a prospective randomized study. J Laparoendosc Adv Surg Tech Part A. 2013;23(4):362–6.
10. Barczynski M, Konturek A, Nowak W. Randomized clinical trial of posterior retroperitoneoscopic adrenalectomy versus lateral transperitoneal laparoscopic adrenalectomy with a 5-year follow-up. Ann Surg. 2014;260(5):740–7. discussion 7-8.
11. Berber E, Tellioglu G, Harvey A, Mitchell J, Milas M, Siperstein A. Comparison of laparoscopic transabdominal lateral versus posterior retroperitoneal adrenalectomy. Surgery. 2009;146(4):621–5. discussion 5-6.
12. Walz MK, Peitgen K, Walz MV, Hoermann R, Saller B, Giebler RM, et al. Posterior retroperitoneoscopic adrenalectomy: lessons learned within five years. World J Surg. 2001;25(6):728–34.
13. Guerrieri M, Campagnacci R, De Sanctis A, Baldarelli M, Coletta M, Perretta S. The learning curve in laparoscopic adrenalectomy. J Endocrinol Investig. 2008;31(6):531–6.
14. Schreinemakers JM, Kiela GJ, Valk GD, Vriens MR, Rinkes IH. Retroperitoneal endoscopic adrenalectomy is safe and effective. Br J Surg. 2010;97(11):1667–72.
15. Gockel I, Kneist W, Heintz A, Beyer J, Junginger T. Endoscopic adrenalectomy: an analysis of the transperitoneal and retroperitoneal approaches and results of a prospective follow-up study. Surg Endosc. 2005;19(4):569–73.
16. Lombardi CP, Raffaelli M, De Crea C, Sollazzi L, Perilli V, Cazzato MT, et al. Endoscopic adrenalectomy: is there an optimal operative approach? Results of a single-center case-control study. Surgery. 2008;144(6):1008–14. discussion 14-5.
17. Paganini AM, Balla A, Guerrieri M, Lezoche G, Campagnacci R, D'Ambrosio G, et al. Laparoscopic transperitoneal anterior adrenalectomy in pheochromocytoma: experience in 62 patients. Surg Endosc. 2014;28(9):2683–9.
18. Kiriakopoulos A, Economopoulos KP, Poulios E, Linos D. Impact of posterior retroperitoneoscopic adrenalectomy in a tertiary care center: a paradigm shift. Surg Endosc. 2011;25(11):3584–9.
19. Agcaoglu O, Aliyev S, Karabulut K, Siperstein A, Berber E. Robotic vs laparoscopic posterior retroperitoneal adrenalectomy. Arch Surg. 2012;147(3):272–5.
20. Siperstein AE, Berber E, Engle KL, Duh QY, Clark OH. Laparoscopic posterior adrenalectomy: technical considerations. Arch Surg. 2000;135(8):967–71.
21. Salomon L, Soulie M, Mouly P, Saint F, Cicco A, Olsson E, et al. Experience with retroperitoneal laparoscopic adrenalectomy in 115 procedures. J Urol. 2001;166(1):38–41.
22. Perrier ND, Kennamer DL, Bao R, Jimenez C, Grubbs EG, Lee JE, et al. Posterior retroperitoneoscopic adrenalectomy: preferred technique for removal of benign tumors and isolated metastases. Ann Surg. 2008;248(4):666–74.
23. Cabalag MS, Mann GB, Gorelik A, Miller JA. Posterior retroperitoneoscopic adrenalectomy: outcomes and lessons learned from initial 50 cases. ANZ J Surg. 2014;85(6):478–82.

24. Pillinger SH, Bambach CP, Sidhu S. Laparoscopic adrenalectomy: a 6-year experience of 59 cases. ANZ J Surg. 2002;72(7):467–70.
25. Kalady MF, McKinlay R, Olson JA Jr, Pinheiro J, Lagoo S, Park A, et al. Laparoscopic adrenalectomy for pheochromocytoma. A comparison to aldosteronoma and incidentaloma. Surg Endosc. 2004;18(4):621–5.
26. Nguyen PH, Keller JE, Novitsky YW, Heniford BT, Kercher KW. Laparoscopic approach to adrenalectomy: review of perioperative outcomes in a single center. Am Surg. 2011;77(5):592–6.
27. Hirano D, Hasegawa R, Igarashi T, Satoh K, Mochida J, Takahashi S, et al. Laparoscopic adrenalectomy for adrenal tumors: a 21-year single-institution experience. Asian J Surg. 2014;38(2):79–84.
28. Naya Y, Nagata M, Ichikawa T, Amakasu M, Omura M, Nishikawa T, et al. Laparoscopic adrenalectomy: comparison of transperitoneal and retroperitoneal approaches. BJU Int. 2002;90(3):199–204.
29. Epelboym I, Digesu CS, Johnston MG, Chabot JA, Inabnet WB, Allendorf JD, et al. Expanding the indications for laparoscopic retroperitoneal adrenalectomy: experience with 81 resections. J Surg Res. 2014;187(2):496–501.

Bilateral Adrenalectomy Versus Medical Management for Cushing's Syndrome with Bilateral Adrenal Hyperplasia

26

Colleen Majewski

Abstract

Cushing's syndrome due to bilateral adrenal hyperplasia is a rare disease with a high morbidity and mortality rate. The hypercortisolism found in Cushing's syndrome leads to obesity and its associated diseases, higher risk of infections, and conditions associated with collagen breakdown. Surgical resection of the source of cortisol is curative but results in a patient with permanent adrenal insufficiency and the need for life-long medications. Bilateral adrenalectomy has been the standard treatment, but a unilateral adrenalectomy has provided good outcomes and reduces the chance of life-long hypoadrenalism. Laparscopic and synchronous removal of the adrenal glands has offered a cure with less complications and morbidity. Medical therapies decrease cortisol production by inhibiting ACTH, inhibiting cortisol, or blocking the action of cortisol at the level of the glucocorticoid receptor. Combination medical therapy can offer faster improvement in cortisol levels. The following chapter reviews the benefits and risks of surgical versus medical therapy in patients with Cushing's syndrome due to bilateral adrenal hyperplasia.

Keywords

Cushing's syndrome · Hypercortisolism · Adrenalectomy · Bilateral adrenal hyperplasia · Medical therapy

C. Majewski
Division of Endocrinology, Department of Medicine, Northwestern University, Chicago, IL, USA
e-mail: Colleen.Majewski@nm.org

P. Angelos, R. H. Grogan (eds.), *Difficult Decisions in Endocrine Surgery*, Difficult Decisions in Surgery: An Evidence-Based Approach,
https://doi.org/10.1007/978-3-319-92860-9_26

Introduction

Cushing's syndrome is a rare yet serious medical condition that is both challenging to diagnose and treat. Cushing's syndrome refers to adrenocortical hyperfunction leading to elevated levels of cortisol. The elevated cortisol level leads to atrophy of both the pituitary corticotrophs and the normal adrenal cells of the zona fasciculata and reticularis. Primary adrenocortical dysfunction is due to an adrenocortical tumor, micronodular dysplasia, or ACTH-independent macronodular hyperplasia. The most common cause of ACTH-independent Cushing's syndrome is a unilateral adrenal adenoma. Adrenal adenomas or carcinomas account for 18–20% of all causes of ACTH-independent Cushing's syndrome. Primary pigmented nodular adrenocortical disease (PPNAD) accounts for less than 1% of all cases of Cushing's syndrome. The familial form of PPNAD is referred to as Carney syndrome or Carney complex, which is an autosomal dominant syndrome. Patients with Carney complex have skin findings of pigmented lentigines and blue nevi, and they also have multiple endocrine and nonendocrine neoplasms [1]. Bilateral macronodular adrenal hyperplasia (BMAH) also accounts for less than 1% of cases of Cushing's syndrome [2]. In BMAH the adrenal glands contain multiple nonpigmented nodules greater than 5 mm in diameter. The adrenal nodules in BMAH appear to involve receptors that respond to gastric inhibitory polypeptide, vasopressin, beta-adrenergic agents, serotonin, luteinizing hormone and chorionic gonadotropin [3]. There is evidence of a genetic basis of BMAH as mutations in ARMC5, a putative suppressor gene, has been found in many familial cases [4].

Cortisol is produced efficiently in adenomas that cause Cushing's syndrome [5]. In adrenal carcinomas, however the cortisol production and steroidogenesis is inefficient, resulting in higher levels of cortisol precursors such as 17-ketosteroid and DHEA-S [6] (Fig. 26.1). There is also evidence of production of aldosterone and androgen precursors in patients with adrenal carcinomas [6].

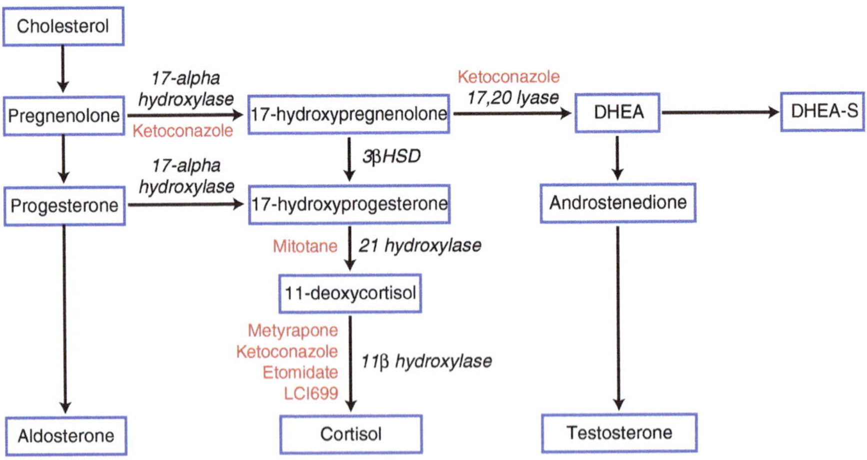

Fig. 26.1 Site of action of steroidogenesis blocking agents used in Cushing's syndrome

The clinical effects of hypercortisolism include obesity, hypertension, diabetes mellitus, depression, muscle weakness, oligomenorrhea, and increased risk of infection [7]. It is essential to treat patients with Cushing's syndrome given the increase in morbidity and mortality associated with this condition. Surgery, which involves removing the cortisol-producing tumor can be curative, but is still associated with risks. Medical therapies to lower cortisol levels or decrease its effects are available and newer agents are being developed and studied. There are risks with both the medical and surgical management of Cushing's syndrome due to bilateral adrenal hyperplasia.

Surgical Management

For most surgeries to treat Cushing's syndrome, imaging is an important tool that helps guide surgical management. Computed tomography (CT) is an excellent imaging technique to view the adrenal glands and to view pathology within the adrenal glands. Magnetic resonance imaging (MRI) is another modality that can be used to clearly image the adrenal glands [8]. CT and MRI are accurate in identifying features that are consistent with an adrenal adenoma, carcinoma, and hyperplasia. Rockall et al. compared the CT and MRI findings of patients with Cushing's syndrome to the pathology of the surgically removed adrenal glands [9]. They found that benign functioning adrenal nodules could not be distinguished from benign non-functioning adrenal nodules based on CT and MRI imaging findings [9]. Further studies have corroborated the inability of traditional imaging such as MRI or CT in determining functionality of adrenal masses or adrenal hyperplasia [10, 11].

Imaging studies using NP-59 ([6-β^{131}I]iodomethyl-19-norcholesterol) have been limited by its availability [10, 11]. NP-59 was introduced in the 1970s to assess adrenal cortical function [12]. However, it has not been commonly used in the United States because it was never approved by the US Food and Drug Administration and only a few centers in the US had approved protocols for the use of NP-59 [12]. This substance is currently unavailable in the US. Thus, further studies are often required to confirm functionality of adrenal pathology, particularly when bilateral pathology is seen.

If imaging demonstrates bilateral adrenal pathology in Cushing's syndrome adrenal vein sampling (AVS) has been demonstrated to help lateralize the source of cortisol hypersecretion. Traditionally the use of adrenal vein sampling has been used successfully to determine laterality of aldosterone-producing adenomas. Adrenal vein sampling in patients with primary hyperaldosteronism has shown repeatedly that the left adrenal vein is difficult to accurately catheterize [13]. In 85% of patients, the concentration of cortisol is higher in the right adrenal vein compared to the left adrenal vein, and a cortisol-corrected aldosterone level is used to determine laterality [13]. Thus, cortisol is the baseline hormone used to verify successful catheterization of the adrenal veins. Also, cortisol is the reference hormone used during AVS in a patient with primary hyperaldosteronism. Since cortisol is the hormone of interest in Cushing's syndrome, it cannot be used as the baseline or reference hormone.

Young et al. has used adrenal vein sampling to help lateralize the source of elevated cortisol production [14]. They evaluated ten patients with bilateral adrenal masses and ACTH-independent Cushing's syndrome or subclinical Cushing's syndrome. After 2 days of dexamethasone, every subject underwent adrenal vein sampling with measurement of adrenal vein and peripheral vein cortisol and epinephrine. Oral dexamethasone was used prior to the procedure to reduce endogenous ACTH secretion from interfering with the interpretation of adrenal gland cortisol secretion [14]. The catheterization of the adrenal veins was considered successful if the concentration of epinephrine in the adrenal vein exceeded the peripheral vein concentration by more than 100 pg/mL. They found an adrenal vein to peripheral vein cortisol gradient of greater than 6.5 was consistent with a cortisol-secreting adenoma. All patients underwent a unilateral or bilateral adrenalectomy based on these results. Eight of the ten patients had a bilateral source of elevated cortisol, five patients with bilateral adrenal hyperplasia and three patients with bilateral cortisol-secreting adenomas. The other two patients had ACTH-independent macronodular adrenal hyperplasia (AIMAH). An adrenal vein to peripheral vein cortisol gradient of less than 3.3 was deemed not clinically important based on long-term postoperative follow-up. The cortisol gradient of one adrenal gland compared to the opposite adrenal gland also revealed predictive power in this study. The authors found a cortisol lateralization ratio of 2.3 or greater was consistent with cortisol hypersecretion from one adrenal gland, whereas a ratio of less than two in patients with bilateral cortisol hypersecretion. The surgical approach was laparoscopic in all but two patients. The patients were followed for 36 months and hypercortisolism did not recur [14].

Another study has used aldosterone as the reference hormone in helping to lateralize a source of elevated cortisol [15]. However, this may not be as accurate because aldosterone secretion during the AVS cannot be stimulated by cosyntropin infusion as can be done with cortisol [13].

Once it is determined to go forward with a bilateral adrenalectomy, there are different surgical approaches that have been studied when removing both adrenal glands. Raffaelli et al. compared three different surgical techniques for a synchronous endoscopic bilateral adrenalectomy: transabdominal laparoscopic, simultaneous posterior retroperitoneoscopic, and robot-assisted [16]. Of the 29 patients included in the study, 5 underwent the transabdominal laparoscopic, 11 underwent the simultaneous posterior retroperitoneoscopic, and 11 patients underwent the robot-assisted technique. The operating time was significantly shorter for the simultaneous posterior retroperitoneoscopic compared to the other two approaches. There were no significant differences in the complications among the three different approaches [16].

Aggarwal et al. reviewed 19 cases of patients with Cushing's syndrome that underwent a laparoscopic bilateral transperitoneal adrenalectomy. The operation was synchronous in 15 patients and staged in the other 4 patients. All of the surgeries were completed laparoscopically with no conversions to an open procedure and there were no major intraoperative complications [17].

Another center analyzed all laparoscopic lateral transabdominal adrenalectomies done for all adrenal lesions performed over a 10 year period from April 2000 to March 2010. Seventy-two of the 215 surgeries were done for patients with Cushing's syndrome. The other procedures were for Conn's syndrome ($n = 90$), pheochromocytoma ($n = 30$), metastatic disease ($n = 8$), incidentalomas ($n = 10$), and other adrenal pathology ($n = 5$). Patients with Cushing's disease that underwent a bilateral adrenalectomy had the highest complication rate. The authors concluded that the higher complication rate in this group was related to the comorbidities often seen in patients with hypercortisolism, such as obesity with large amounts of retroperitoneal fat leading to difficulty localizing the adrenal gland and coagulopathies leading to higher bleeding rates [18].

A series of 50 patients with Cushing's syndrome that underwent bilateral adrenalectomy at two German centers was reported by Osswald, et al. Of the 50 patients followed, 34 had pituitary Cushing's disease, 9 had ectopic Cushing's syndrome, and 9 had ACTH-independent bilateral adrenal hyperplasia. The patients were followed for a median of 11 years and all patients were in remission after surgery. Most of the Cushing's related comorbidities such as hypertension, diabetes mellitus, muscle weakness and physical stigmata improved significantly after surgery. Psychiatric illness attributed to hypercortisolism did not change. Sixty-three percent of the patients had at least one episode of adrenal crisis requiring IV glucocorticoids. After 25 years, 95% of the patients with Cushing's disease were still living [19].

A meta-analysis of 37 studies that investigated the outcome of patients with Cushing's syndrome that were treated with bilateral adrenalectomy concluded this procedure as a relatively safe and effective treatment option. Of the 1320 patients included in the meta-analysis, 82% had Cushing's disease, 13% had ectopic Cushing's syndrome, and 5% had primary adrenal hyperplasia. Surgical mortality after bilateral adrenalectomy was 3% and surgical morbidity was 18%. Less than 2% of all patients had a recurrence of hypercortisolism. However, 46% of the patients died within the first year after surgery. The symptoms of hypertension, obesity and depression improved in the majority of patients. There were 9.3 adrenal crises per 100 patient years [20].

Some surgeons have attempted to remove one adrenal gland even in cases of likely bilateral cortisol hypersecretion. Xu et al. evaluated the role of a unilateral adrenalectomy in Cushing's syndrome [21]. They followed 27 patients with ACTH-independent Cushing's syndrome caused by bilateral adrenocortical hyperplasia that were treated with a unilateral adrenalectomy, 14 patients with AIMAH and 13 patients with PPNAD. Twenty-five patients were cured by unilateral adrenalectomy after a median followup of 69 months (AIMAH) and 47 months (PPNAD). One patient with AIMAH and one patient with PPNAD went on to have removal of the contralateral adrenal gland [21].

Another series retrospectively evaluated 16 patients with bilateral macronodular adrenal hyperplasia (BMAH) [22]. Twelve of the 16 patients underwent unilateral adrenalectomy and were followed over time to assess for recurrence. Three of the 12 patients had long-term remission over an average of 106 months of follow up. Recurrence occurred in the other eight patients after a range of 12–180 months [22]. An additional center reported on 23 patients with ACTH-independent macronodular adrenocortical hyperplasia. Fifteen of the 23 patients underwent a unilateral adrenalectomy. Of these 15 patients, 3 went on to have the contralateral adrenal gland removed due to recurrence after 2–8 years of followup [23]. Given the morbidity and mortality related to surgery and post-operative complications in a patient with hypercortisolism, consideration for unilateral adrenalectomy should be made.

The most common concern after a unilateral or bilateral adrenalectomy is the need for adrenal hormone replacement. Even in patients with a unilateral source of cortisol hypersecretion, the suppressed pituitary corticotrophs need time to recover their ability to secrete ACTH and patients need to be treated with cortisol replacement for a period of time. The recovery of patients with adrenal Cushing's syndrome is typically slower than in the patient with pituitary Cushing's disease or the patient with ectopic Cushing's syndrome [24]. Ninety-one patients with either Cushing's disease, unilateral adrenal Cushing's syndrome, or ectopic Cushing's syndrome were followed for 5 years after curative therapy. The probability of recovering adrenal function was 82% in ectopic Cushing's syndrome, 58% in pituitary Cushing's disease, and 38% in unilateral adrenal Cushing's syndrome [24]. This slow recovery and possibility of no recovery even in a patient with a unilateral adrenalectomy should be considered when deciding whether to treat patients medically or surgically. It is imperative to educate patients on the importance of taking cortisol and aldosterone replacement medications life-long after a bilateral adrenalectomy. Patients must be instructed on how to manage the dose of cortisol replacement during times of illness or stress. All patients with a history of a bilateral adrenalectomy should have immediate access to intramuscular hydrocortisone or dexamethasone in case of emergency.

The patient's improvement in quality of life after a bilateral adrenalectomy is also important to assess. A group of 28 patients that underwent laparoscopic bilateral adrenalectomy for Cushing's syndrome were given a disease-specific questionnaire covering all clinically relevant symptoms associated with Cushing's syndrome. This group of 28 patients was compared to a group of 60 patients that underwent a thyroidectomy, and findings were matched for age, gender, and time of surgery. Ninety-two percent of the patients that underwent a laparoscopic bilateral adrenalectomy reported a significant improvement in their Cushingoid features and 84% reported a significant improvement in their emotional-behavioral symptoms. All of the patients reported an improvement in their overall quality of life [25].

Medical Management

Hypercortisolism due to bilateral adrenal hyperplasia is primarily treated surgically. However, surgery may not lead to a complete cure, and given the risks of surgery and potential comorbidities of the patient, surgery may not be the best option. Medical treatment of Cushing's syndrome includes medications directed against the different components of the hypothalamic-pituitary-adrenal axis. Medications such as dopamine agonists and somatostatin analogs are directed against the pituitary gland to decrease ACTH secretion. Other therapies act at the level of the adrenal gland and inhibit enzyme pathways leading to cortisol synthesis. Finally there are drugs that act to block the actions of cortisol at the level of the glucocorticoid receptor (Fig. 26.2).

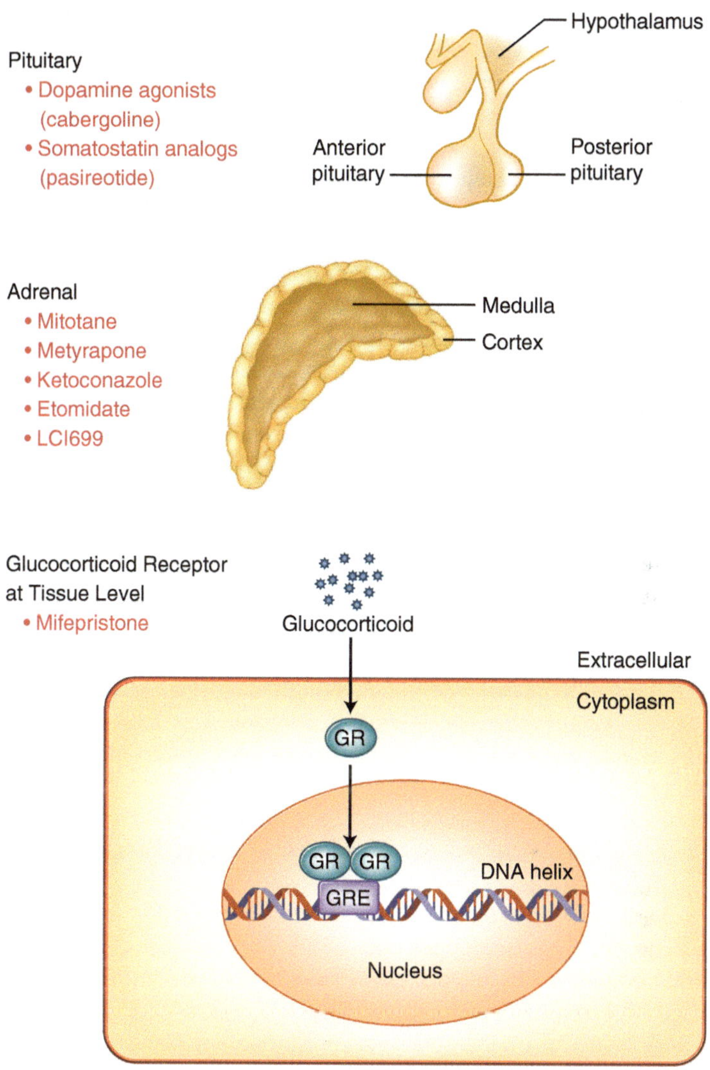

Fig. 26.2 Site of action of medications used to treat Cushing's syndrome

The first medical treatment used for hypercortisolism was cyproheptadine which is an anti-serotonin agent [26]. More effective treatments have emerged and this agent is no longer used to treat Cushing's syndrome.

Mitotane acts at the level of the adrenal gland by inhibiting 11β hydroxylase and cholesterol side chain cleavage. This agent has been used for the treatment of adrenal cancer, and at lower doses of 2–4 g per day it has been used in Cushing's syndrome. Baudry et al. reviewed 76 patients with Cushing's disease at one center that were treated with mitotane [27]. The levels of 24 h urinary free cortisol were measured and remission was defined as normalization of the urine cortisol. Seventy-two percent of the patients achieved remission after a median of 6.7 months, and 71% of those that went into remission subsequently developed a recurrence after a median of 13.2 months [27]. The drug was discontinued in 29% of patients due to intolerance [27]. Mitotane is a potent inducer of CYP3A4, contributing to its many drug interactions and limitations in use [28].

Metyrapone also acts at the level of the adrenal gland blocking the conversion of 11-deoxycortisol to cortisol. It blocks the 11-hydoxylase enzyme, leading to a decrease in cortisol production. In a recent series by Valassi et al., 23 patients were treated with metyrapone preoperatively for an average of 4 months [29]. Cortisol levels normalized in 6 of the 23 patients, and cortisol levels improved in 7 other patients. Common side effects of metyrapone include hirsutism and hypertension. A prior series by Verhelst et al. described an increase in ACTH levels due to the lack of negative feedback from cortisol [30]. The increase in ACTH levels eventually overcame the effects of metyrapone, leading to elevated cortisol levels. The increase in ACTH levels also led to elevated levels of androgens and 11-deoxycortisol, the clinical effects of which were hirsutism and hypertension [30]. The elevated levels of 11-deoxycortisol that occur with use of metyrapone can falsely elevate the cortisol levels if they are measured using a standard immunoassay. Given this finding, it is recommended that cortisol be measured using liquid chromatography with tandem mass spectrometry [31].

Ketoconazole, the imidazole antifungal, is another agent that acts at the level of the adrenal gland to reduce cortisol production. It can decrease cortisol production at doses of 400–1200 mg per day [32]. Ketoconazole was shown in the 1980s to significantly reduce cortisol levels by inhibition of cytochrome P450 enzymes [33]. It has further been demonstrated to inhibit side chain cleavage, 17-hydroxylase, 17,20 lyase, 11β-hydroxylase, and aldosterone synthase [34]. The side effects of ketoconazole include hepatotoxicity, gastrointestinal complaints, and hypogonadism in men. Castinetti, et al. compiled retrospective data from 200 patients with Cushing's disease treated with ketoconazole followed for 9–65 months. When treatment with ketoconazole was stopped due to cure or intolerance of the drug, 50% of patients had normal urinary free cortisol (UFC), 25% of patients had at least a 50% decrease in UFC, and 25% had no change in UFC [32]. Mild increases in liver enzymes (less than 5 times the upper limit of normal) were observed in 13.5% of patients, and severe increases in liver enzymes (more than 5 times the upper limit of normal) were observed in 2.5% of patients. The increase in liver enzymes occurred within 4 weeks of starting ketoconazole or a dose increase. All increases in liver enzymes returned to normal when the drug was stopped. Forty-one percent of patients stopped the treatment due to inability to tolerate the drug [32]. Ketoconazole is an inhibitor of CYP3A4 and thus can affect the metabolism and dosing of other drugs that use this system, such as amiodarone, carbamazepine, amitriptyline, SSRIs, benzodiazepines, calcium channel blockers, statins, and cochicine [35]. Despite the frequent use of ketoconazole for hypercortisolism, it is not available for use in many countries. The US FDA has never approved the use of ketoconazole for treatment of Cushing's syndrome. In 2013, the US FDA issued a "black box warning" regarding liver toxicity with use of ketoconazole.

Another imidazole antifungal that has been used to decrease cortisol levels is etomidate. This drug also inhibits 11β-hydroxylase, aldosterone synthase, and side chain cleavage [36]. Etomidate was found to cause adrenal insufficiency during use as an anesthetic. It can be given intravenously to rapidly decrease cortisol levels. It has primarily been used short-term to lower cortisol levels before surgery. Due to its rapid action it has been used along with hydrocortisone to help normalize cortisol levels [36].

There are case reports using trilostane for the treatment of AIMAH. Trilostane inhibits the synthesis of cortisol by competitive and reversible blocking of 3β-hydroxysteroid dehydrogenase. Obata et al. reports on a case of a patient with Cushing's syndrome due to AIMAH treated with trilostane successfully for 7 years [37].

LCI699 is a new agent that is currently being investigated for use in Cushing's disease. It is a potent inhibitor of aldosterone synthase and 11β-hydroxylase [38]. Twelve patients with Cushing's disease were treated with LCI699. By day 70 of treatment, all 12 patients achieved a 50% or greater reduction in levels of urinary free cortisol compared to baseline [38]. The mean levels of 11-deoxycortisol, 11-deoxycorticosterone, and ACTH levels increased during treatment with LCI699, but these levels declined after treatment discontinuation [38]. Mean systolic blood pressure decreased by 10 mmHg and mean diastolic blood pressure decreased by 6 mmHg from baseline [38]. The most common adverse effects were fatigue, nausea, and headache. No serious adverse events were reported [38].

Mifepristone is a glucocorticoid receptor antagonist and it has a tenfold higher affinity for the glucocorticoid receptor than cortisol [38]. In the SEISMIC trial, 43 patients with Cushing's disease, 4 with ectopic ACTH syndrome and 3 with adrenal cancer were treated with mifepristone. The cortisol levels were not used as an endpoint due to the rise in ACTH and cortisol levels during treatment with this glucocorticoid receptor blocker. There were significant improvements in weight and quality of life. Sixty percent of these subjects had more than a 25% reduction in glucose area under the curve (AUC) during oral glucose tolerance test [39]. There was not a consistent improvement in blood pressure due to the high cortisol levels overwhelming the enzyme type 2 11-β-hydroxysteroid dehydrogenase, which converts cortisol to cortisone. At high levels cortisol can activate the mineralocorticoid receptor resulting in the clinical effects of salt retention and hypertension. Coadministration with a mineralocorticoid receptor block such as spironolactone and eplerenone can ameloriate the hypertensive effects of mifepristone [40]. The most common adverse events reported were fatigue, nausea, headache, low potassium, arthraligia, vomiting, edema, and endometrial thickening in women [39]. The endometrial thickening is related to progesterone receptor blocking actions of mifepristone. Before beginning treatment, it is recommended to check potassium and consider starting spironolactone or eplerenone if needed [39]. Start at a dose of 300 mg daily and increase to a maximum dose of 1200 mg daily [41]. Monitoring of the success of treatment can be challenging with mifepristone given the expected rise in ACTH and cortisol levels, leaving no biochemical parameters to monitor, and contributing to the risk of overdose. If an overdose leading to adrenal insufficiency is expected, treatment with high doses of dexamethasone is recommended to overcome the glucocorticoid receptor blockade [40]. Post hoc analysis of the SEISMIC trial confirmed that mifepristone had a progressive clinical benefit with a higher proportion of responders at the study end [42]. Mifepristone is approved by the US FDA for use in the treatment of hyperglycemia associated with Cushing's syndrome [39].

The dopamine agonist cabergoline has been used to treat Cushing's syndrome at the level of the pituitary gland. D2 dopamine receptors have been found in corticotroph adenomas [43]. Pivonello found 80% of corticotroph adenomas expressed dopamine receptors. All of the adenomas with dopamine expression respond to the use of cabergoline with a 50% or more reduction in ACTH levels [43]. Use of cabergoline is a more appropriate therapy in pituitary Cushing's disease and does not have a known role in the treatment of hypercortisolism due to bilateral adrenal hyperplasia.

Another agent that can improve hypercortisolism at the level of the pituitary gland is pasireotide. Corticotroph adenomas express somatostatin receptors, particularly subtypes 1, 2, 3 and 5 [44]. Pasireotide is particularly potent agonist of the somatostatin receptor subtype 5 [44]. Colao et al. randomly assigned 162 patients with Cushing's disease to pasireotide 600 mcg or pasireotide 900 mcg twice daily for 12 months [45]. Fifteen percent of the 600 mcg group and 26% of the 900 mcg group had a normalization of 24 h urine free cortisol levels [45]. Interestingly, despite the improvement in cortisol levels, there was an increase in hyperglycemia-related adverse events in 118 of the 162 patients [45]. The hyperglycemia seen with pasiretotide appears to be related to a decrease in insulin secretion and a decrease in incretin hormone response [46]. Given this side effect of hyperglycemia, another study investigated the use of the glucagon-like peptide 1 analog (GLP-1) liraglutide and the DPP-IV inhibitor vildagliptin in patients treated with pasireotide [47]. Ninety healthy male volunteers were randomized to pasireotide alone or in combination with metformin, nateglinide, vildagliptin, or liraglutide. The pasireotide-induced hyperglycemia was reduced by all agents, but viladagliptin and liraglutide were associated with the biggest improvement in hyperglycemia [47].

Combination medical therapies for Cushing's syndrome have been studied as well, but not extensively given the rarity of the condition. The combination of three adrenal steroidogenesis inhibitors mitotane, metyrapone, and ketoconazole was investigated by Kamenicky et al. [48]. Given mitotane's slower onset of action, the authors investigated the combination of mitotane with metyrapone and ketoconazole in 11 patients with severe Cushing's disease. All of the patients had a significant reduction in levels of 24 h urinary free cortisol within 24–48 h of the start of treatment [48]. In 7 of the 11 patients, metyrapone and ketoconazole were discontinued after 3.5 months and the 24 h urinary free cortisol remained controlled. The most common adverse effects of the combination therapy were gastrointestinal discomfort, a rise in total cholesterol levels, and a rise in gamma-glutamyl transferase [48].

Discussion

Most patients with Cushing's syndrome have ACTH-dependent disease [49–51]. In this chapter, we review the management of patients with ACTH-independent Cushing's syndrome with bilateral adrenal hyperplasia. The majority of patients with

ACTH-independent hypercortisolism have an obvious unilateral source on imaging [52]. The small subset of patients with ACTH-independent Cushing's syndrome with bilateral adrenal sources found on imaging are a challenge to manage. A functioning versus non-functioning adrenal mass cannot be determined based on imaging. However, the use of adrenal vein sampling as described by Young, et al. can provide guidance for surgical management [14]. Most patients are cured with bilateral adrenalectomy. However, given the need for long-term adrenal replacement and risk of adrenal crisis, some surgeons have performed unilateral adrenalectomy with successful results. For those patients that are not good surgical candidates or have a recurrence after surgery, there are several medical therapies that are available. The therapies that have demonstrated some success in Cushing's syndrome due to bilateral adrenal hyperplasia act by inhibiting cortisol synthesis or blocking the glucocorticoid receptor. Combination therapy should be considered in order to quickly reduce levels of cortisol. Overall, patients with Cushing's syndrome due to bilateral adrenal hyperplasia have a high morbidity and mortality rate without treatment. Both surgical and medical therapies should be considered for this patient population.

References

1. Stratakis CA, Kirschner LS, Carney JA. Clinical and molecular features of the Carney complex: diagnostic criteria and recommendations for patient evaluation. J Clin Endocrinol Metab. 2001;86(9):4041–6.
2. Lacroix A, Ndiaye N, Tremblay J, Hamet P. Ectopic and abnormal hormone receptors in adrenal Cushing's syndrome. Endocr Rev. 2001;22(1):75–110.
3. Lacroix A, Bourdeau I, Lampron A, Mazzuco TL, Tremblay J, Hamet P. Aberrant G-protein coupled receptor expression in relation to adrenocortical overfunction. Clin Endocrinol. 2010;73(1):1–15.
4. Ravikumar A, Levine AC. Genetic basis of bilateral macronodular hyperplasia. Endocr Pract. 2015;21(4):390–4.
5. Beuschlein F, Schulze E, Mora P, Gensheimer HP, Maser-Gluth C, Allolio B, et al. Steroid 21-hydroxylase mutations and 21-hydroxylase messenger ribonucleic acid expression in human adrenocortical tumors. J Clin Endocrinol Metab. 1998;83(7):2585–8.
6. Arlt W, Biehl M, Taylor AE, Hahner S, Libe R, Hughes BA, et al. Urine steroid metabolomics as a biomarker tool for detecting malignancy in adrenal tumors. J Clin Endocrinol Metab. 2011;96(12):3775–84.
7. Howlett TA, Rees LH, Besser GM. Cushing's syndrome. Clin Endocrinol Metab. 1985;14(4):911–45.
8. Lumachi F, Marchesi P, Miotto D, Motta R. CT and MR imaging of the adrenal glands in cortisol-secreting tumors. Anticancer Res. 2011;31(9):2923–6.
9. Rockall AG, Babar SA, Sohaib SA, Isidori AM, Diaz-Cano S, Monson JP, et al. CT and MR imaging of the adrenal glands in ACTH-independent cushing syndrome. Radiographics. 2004;24(2):435–52.
10. Lumachi F, Zucchetta P, Marzola MC, Bui F, Casarrubea G, Angelini F, et al. Usefulness of CT scan, MRI and radiocholesterol scintigraphy for adrenal imaging in Cushing's syndrome. Nucl Med Commun. 2002;23(5):469–73.
11. Yu KC, Fraker DL, Ziessman HA. Atlas of iodocholesterol scintigraphy (NP-59) in Cushing's syndrome with CT and MR correlation. Clin Nucl Med. 1996;21(2):136–41.
12. Sarkar SD, Cohen EL, Beierwaltes WH, Ice RD, Cooper R, Gold EN. A new and superior adrenal imaging agent, 131I-6beta-iodomethyl-19-nor-cholesterol (NP-59): evaluation in humans. J Clin Endocrinol Metab. 1977;45(2):353–62.

13. Young WF, Stanson AW, Thompson GB, Grant CS, Farley DR, van Heerden JA. Role for adrenal venous sampling in primary aldosteronism. Surgery. 2004;136(6):1227–35.
14. Young WF Jr, du Plessis H, Thompson GB, Grant CS, Farley DR, Richards ML, et al. The clinical conundrum of corticotropin-independent autonomous cortisol secretion in patients with bilateral adrenal masses. World J Surg. 2008;32(5):856–62.
15. Domino JP, Chionh SB, Lomanto D, Katara AN, Rauff A, Cheah WK. Laparoscopic partial adrenalectomy for bilateral cortisol-secreting adenomas. Asian J Surg. 2007;30(2):154–7.
16. Raffaelli M, Brunaud L, De Crea C, Hoche G, Oragano L, Bresler L, et al. Synchronous bilateral adrenalectomy for Cushing's syndrome: laparoscopic versus posterior retroperitoneoscopic versus robotic approach. World J Surg. 2014;38(3):709–15.
17. Aggarwal S, Yadav K, Sharma AP, Sethi V. Laparoscopic bilateral transperitoneal adrenalectomy for Cushing syndrome: surgical challenges and lessons learnt. Surg Laparosc Endosc Percutan Tech. 2013;23(3):324–8.
18. Sommerey S, Foroghi Y, Chiapponi C, Baumbach SF, Hallfeldt KK, Ladurner R, et al. Laparoscopic adrenalectomy--10-year experience at a teaching hospital. Langenbecks Arch Surg. 2015;400(3):341–7.
19. Osswald A, Plomer E, Dimopoulou C, Milian M, Blaser R, Ritzel K, et al. Favorable long-term outcomes of bilateral adrenalectomy in Cushing's disease. Eur J Endocrinol. 2014;171(2):209–15.
20. Ritzel K, Beuschlein F, Mickisch A, Osswald A, Schneider HJ, Schopohl J, et al. Clinical review: outcome of bilateral adrenalectomy in Cushing's syndrome: a systematic review. J Clin Endocrinol Metab. 2013;98(10):3939–48.
21. Xu Y, Rui W, Qi Y, Zhang C, Zhao J, Wang X, et al. The role of unilateral adrenalectomy in corticotropin-independent bilateral adrenocortical hyperplasias. World J Surg. 2013;37(7):1626–32.
22. Albiger NM, Ceccato F, Zilio M, Barbot M, Occhi G, Rizzati S, et al. An analysis of different therapeutic options in patients with Cushing's syndrome due to bilateral macronodular adrenal hyperplasia: a single-centre experience. Clin Endocrinol. 2015;82(6):808–15.
23. Li J, Yang CH. Diagnosis and treatment of adrenocorticotrophic hormone-independent macronodular adrenocortical hyperplasia: a report of 23 cases in a single center. Exp Ther Med. 2015;9(2):507–12.
24. Berr CM, Di Dalmazi G, Osswald A, Ritzel K, Bidlingmaier M, Geyer LL, et al. Time to recovery of adrenal function after curative surgery for Cushing's syndrome depends on etiology. J Clin Endocrinol Metab. 2015;100(4):1300–8.
25. Neychev V, Steinberg SM, Yang L, Mehta A, Nilubol N, Keil MF, et al. Long-term outcome of bilateral laparoscopic adrenalectomy measured by disease-specific questionnaire in a unique group of patients with Cushing's syndrome. Ann Surg Oncol. 2015;22(Suppl 3): S699–706.
26. Krieger DT, Amorosa L, Linick F. Cyproheptadine-induced remission of Cushing's disease. N Engl J Med. 1975;293(18):893–6.
27. Baudry C, Coste J, Bou Khalil R, Silvera S, Guignat L, Guibourdenche J, et al. Efficiency and tolerance of mitotane in Cushing's disease in 76 patients from a single center. Eur J Endocrinol. 2012;167(4):473–81.
28. van Erp NP, Guchelaar HJ, Ploeger BA, Romijn JA, Hartigh J, Gelderblom H. Mitotane has a strong and a durable inducing effect on CYP3A4 activity. Eur J Endocrinol. 2011; 164(4):621–6.
29. Valassi E, Crespo I, Gich I, Rodriguez J, Webb SM. A reappraisal of the medical therapy with steroidogenesis inhibitors in Cushing's syndrome. Clin Endocrinol. 2012;77(5):735–42.
30. Verhelst JA, Trainer PJ, Howlett TA, Perry L, Rees LH, Grossman AB, et al. Short and long-term responses to metyrapone in the medical management of 91 patients with Cushing's syndrome. Clin Endocrinol. 1991;35(2):169–78.
31. Monaghan PJ, Owen LJ, Trainer PJ, Brabant G, Keevil BG, Darby D. Comparison of serum cortisol measurement by immunoassay and liquid chromatography-tandem mass spectrometry in patients receiving the 11beta-hydroxylase inhibitor metyrapone. Ann Clin Biochem. 2011;48(Pt 5):441–6.

32. Castinetti F, Guignat L, Giraud P, Muller M, Kamenicky P, Drui D, et al. Ketoconazole in Cushing's disease: is it worth a try? J Clin Endocrinol Metab. 2014;99(5):1623–30.
33. Dandona P, Mohiuddin J, Prentice HG. Ketoconazole and adrenocortical secretion. Lancet. 1985;1(8422):227.
34. Feelders RA, Hofland LJ. Medical treatment of Cushing's disease. J Clin Endocrinol Metab. 2013;98(2):425–38.
35. Molitch ME. Current approaches to the pharmacological management of Cushing's disease. Mol Cell Endocrinol. 2015;408:185–9.
36. Preda VA, Sen J, Karavitaki N, Grossman AB. Etomidate in the management of hypercortisolaemia in Cushing's syndrome: a review. Eur J Endocrinol. 2012;167(2):137–43.
37. Obata Y, Yamada Y, Baden MY, Hosokawa Y, Saisho K, Tamba S, et al. Long-term efficacy of trilostane for Cushing's syndrome due to adrenocorticotropin-independent bilateral macronodular adrenocortical hyperplasia. Intern Med. 2011;50(21):2621–5.
38. Bertagna X, Pivonello R, Fleseriu M, Zhang Y, Robinson P, Taylor A, et al. LCI699, a potent 11beta-hydroxylase inhibitor, normalizes urinary cortisol in patients with Cushing's disease: results from a multicenter, proof-of-concept study. J Clin Endocrinol Metab. 2014;99(4):1375–83.
39. Fleseriu M, Biller BM, Findling JW, Molitch ME, Schteingart DE, Gross C, et al. Mifepristone, a glucocorticoid receptor antagonist, produces clinical and metabolic benefits in patients with Cushing's syndrome. J Clin Endocrinol Metab. 2012;97(6):2039–49.
40. Fleseriu M, Molitch ME, Gross C, Schteingart DE, Vaughan TB 3rd, Biller BM. A new therapeutic approach in the medical treatment of Cushing's syndrome: glucocorticoid receptor blockade with mifepristone. Endocr Pract. 2013;19(2):313–26.
41. Fleseriu M. Medical treatment of Cushing disease: new targets, new hope. Endocrinol Metab Clin N Am. 2015;44(1):51–70.
42. Katznelson L, Loriaux DL, Feldman D, Braunstein GD, Schteingart DE, Gross C. Global clinical response in Cushing's syndrome patients treated with mifepristone. Clin Endocrinol. 2014;80(4):562–9.
43. Pivonello R, Ferone D, de Herder WW, Kros JM, De Caro ML, Arvigo M, et al. Dopamine receptor expression and function in corticotroph pituitary tumors. J Clin Endocrinol Metab. 2004;89(5):2452–62.
44. Hofland LJ, Lamberts SW. The pathophysiological consequences of somatostatin receptor internalization and resistance. Endocr Rev. 2003;24(1):28–47.
45. Colao A, Petersenn S, Newell-Price J, Findling JW, Gu F, Maldonado M, et al. A 12-month phase 3 study of pasireotide in Cushing's disease. N Engl J Med. 2012;366(10):914–24.
46. Henry RR, Ciaraldi TP, Armstrong D, Burke P, Ligueros-Saylan M, Mudaliar S. Hyperglycemia associated with pasireotide: results from a mechanistic study in healthy volunteers. J Clin Endocrinol Metab. 2013;98(8):3446–53.
47. Breitschaft A, Hu K, Hermosillo Resendiz K, Darstein C, Golor G. Management of hyperglycemia associated with pasireotide (SOM230): healthy volunteer study. Diabetes Res Clin Pract. 2014;103(3):458–65.
48. Kamenicky P, Droumaguet C, Salenave S, Blanchard A, Jublanc C, Gautier JF, et al. Mitotane, metyrapone, and ketoconazole combination therapy as an alternative to rescue adrenalectomy for severe ACTH-dependent Cushing's syndrome. J Clin Endocrinol Metab. 2011;96(9):2796–804.
49. Newell-Price J, Bertagna X, Grossman AB, Nieman LK. Cushing's syndrome. Lancet. 2006;367(9522):1605–17.
50. Arnaldi G, Angeli A, Atkinson AB, Bertagna X, Cavagnini F, Chrousos GP, et al. Diagnosis and complications of Cushing's syndrome: a consensus statement. J Clin Endocrinol Metab. 2003;88(12):5593–602.
51. Raff H, Findling JW. A physiologic approach to diagnosis of the Cushing syndrome. Ann Intern Med. 2003;138(12):980–91.
52. Lacroix A, Bourdeau I. Bilateral adrenal Cushing's syndrome: macronodular adrenal hyperplasia and primary pigmented nodular adrenocortical disease. Endocrinol Metab Clin N Am. 2005;34(2):441–58. x.

Routine Screening for Primary Hyperaldosteronism in Hypertensive Patients: Yes or No?

27

Konstantinos P. Economopoulos and Carrie C. Lubitz

Abstract

Primary hyperaldosteronism is the most common cause of secondary hypertension and endocrine-related hypertension and is characterized by autonomous, inappropriately elevated serum aldosterone, arising from either an aldosterone producing adenoma or bilateral adrenal hyperplasia. In comparison to matched patients with primary (essential) hypertension, patients with both subtypes of primary hyperaldosteronism have increased odds of stroke, non-fatal heart attack and atrial fibrillation. Moreover, patients with primary hyperaldosteronism have worse psychosocial and quality of life scores when compared to patients with primary hypertension. Although treatment guidelines for primary hyperaldosteronism vary, diagnosis is usually focused on identifying serum hyperaldosteronism and subsequently by differentiating between unilateral and bilateral disease with imaging (CT or MRI) and/or adrenal-venous sampling. Most patients with aldosterone producing adenoma can be managed successfully with laparoscopic adrenalectomy, not only by curing their hypertension, but also by reversing cardiovascular and renal complications. Moreover, primary hyperaldosteronism patients diagnosed with bilateral-adrenal hyperplasia can likewise have improvement in hypertension and downstream cardiovascular outcomes with appropriate mineralocorticoid-receptor antagonist treatment.

Keywords

Primary hyperaldosteronism · Secondary hypertension · Screening · Adrenal venous sampling · Adrenalectomy · Mineralocorticoid receptor antagonists

K. P. Economopoulos
Department of Surgery, Duke University, Durham, NC, USA

C. C. Lubitz (✉)
Department of Surgery, Massachusetts General Hospital, Boston, MA, USA

Institute for Technology Assessment, Boston, MA, USA
e-mail: CLUBITZ@mgh.harvard.edu

P. Angelos, R. H. Grogan (eds.), *Difficult Decisions in Endocrine Surgery*, Difficult Decisions in Surgery: An Evidence-Based Approach, https://doi.org/10.1007/978-3-319-92860-9_27

What Is the Public Health Impact of Hypertension?

Hypertension (HTN; see table 1 for most commonly used abbreviations) is the leading cause of heart disease, stroke and death and costs the U.S. over 46 billion annually [1]. Seventy-six million Americans and one billion people worldwide suffer from the disease [2]. The primary goals of treatment of HTN, as these are listed by the Joint National Committee on prevention, evaluation, and treatment of high blood pressure are: (1) Targeting modifiable lifestyle risk factors, (2) Treating end-organ damage, and (3) Identifying the cause of the disease.

Resistant hypertension (RH), defined as failure to meet goal BP with a three-drug antihypertensive regimen, including a diuretic, in a compliant patient, is estimated between 12 and 30% of the hypertensive population [3–5]. Morbidity and death are even greater with RH. As outlined by expert and commonly practices, a work-up for secondary causes of hypertension is postponed until standard treatment for primary hypertension has failed [3, 6–8]. The clinical approach to these patients is a matter of debate and on-going research. We argue that earlier approaches to subtype differentiation and treatment of potentially curable causes of hypertension are of paramount public health concern.

Why Should We Screen for Primary Hyperaldosteronism?

Primary hyperaldosteronism (PA) is the most common cause of secondary HTN and is characterized by autonomous, inappropriately elevated serum aldosterone, arising from either an aldosterone-producing adenoma (APA) or bilateral adrenal hyperplasia (BAH) [9–14]. Recent reports indicate a higher prevalence of PA than previously thought. This may be attributable to improvements in our diagnostic armamentarium (e.g. increased use of screening with aldosterone-renin ratio) and increased use and quality of abdominal imaging. Best estimates of the prevalence of PA in hypertensive population are approximately 10% [15]; the prevalence of PA in the resistant hypertensive population is more than two times higher, almost 23% [3, 16–18]. Most patients with aldosterone producing adenoma (APA) can be managed successfully with laparoscopic adrenalectomy. Depending on the definition of "cure", 33–77% are cured or benefited by surgery [19–23]. It has been shown that treatment of aldosterone excess results in vascular remodeling, reversal of ventricular hypertrophy and reverses cardiovascular and renal complications [21, 24].

Given 1/8 of the hypertensive population has resistant hypertension, approximately 1/5 of patients with resistant hypertension have PA, and half of patients with PA have unilateral disease, we estimate over a million hypertensive patients in the U.S. could be potentially cured with surgery [13, 25, 26]. Not only could we potentially cure those patients with unilateral disease with screening, we can also identify those patients with bilateral adrenal hyperplasia likely to benefit from disease-targeted mineralocorticoid-receptor antagonists. Disease-specific therapy—either medical or surgical is more effective [26–33]. In comparison to primary hypertensive patients matched for blood pressure, patients with PA have four times increased odds of stroke, seven times increased odds of non-fatal myocardial infarction, and 12 times increased odds of atrial fibrillation [14]. Moreover, it has been consistently shown length of time with hypertension is correlated with failure of cure following surgery for APA [22, 23].

Are Clinical Signs and Symptoms of Primary Hyperaldosteronism Helpful?

Patients with PA are difficult to distinguish from patients with primary hypertension. Frequently, HTN is the only clinical sign of PA, making its diagnosis extremely challenging. Because of this, PA is frequently over-looked and under-diagnosed. PA is characterized by inappropriately elevated plasma aldosterone, non-suppressible with sodium, which causes serum hypernatremia, hypokalemia, metabolic alkalosis, and suppression of renin [10]. Given that many patients with all forms of hypertension are on a number of anti-hypertensive medications that can affect the renin-angiotensin system, minor electrolyte abnormalities often go unnoticed. In rare instances, patients can present with muscle weakness, muscle cramping, myalgia and tremor which are the signs and symptoms of hypokalemia. While hypokalemia is commonly referenced as a distinguishing feature of patients with PA, it is present in <40% of patients with the disease [34]. Even more rarely, patients may be diagnosed during biochemical and/or hormonal evaluation of an adrenal incidentaloma with early-onset HTN or stroke [35]. Age nor gender is helpful in distinguishing PA within the hypertensive population with a mean age of diagnosis of PA of 52 years old and close to equivalent rate between men and women [36]. Moreover, there is no increased race or ethnicity-specific incidence of PA [36]. In sum, a high index of suspicion and systematic screening for patients with PA are the only clear way to identify potentially curable disease.

Who Should We Screen for Primary Hyperaldosteronism and How?

There is no consensus among experts on who should be screened for PA and currently there are no guidelines recommending the screening of all primary hypertensive patients for PA [11, 12, 36, 37]. However, it is agreed in the field that patients who fail to have their blood pressure corrected following concurrent administration of three antihypertensive medications with one diuretic (i.e. resistant hypertension), should be screened for secondary causes of hypertension [3, 7, 8]. Other possible entities causing secondary hypertension and their biochemical profiles should be considered while screening these patients (Table 27.1).

Serum potassium levels were historically used to be the only screening tool for the diagnosis of PA. However, hypokalemia is currently known to occur in less than 38% of the PA population, rendering it an inappropriate screening test for PA [15]. While hypokalemia is not a sensitive screening test, in a patient with

Table 27.1 Biochemical profiles of different causes of secondary hypertension

Disease	Potassium	Aldosterone	Renin
Aldosterone-producing adenoma	50%↓↓	↑↑	↓
Bilateral adrenal hyperplasia	17%↓	↑↑	↓
Loop-diuretic therapy	↓	↓	↑
Renal artery stenosis	↓	↑	↑
Congenital adrenal hyperplasia	↓	↓	↓
Cushing's syndrome	↓	↓	↓
Familial hyperaldosteronism			
Type I or GRA	Normal	↑↑	↓
Type II	↓	↑	↓
Type III	↓	↑	↓

difficult-to-control hypertension, hypokalemia is predictive of PA and other secondary etiologies of hypertension. Patients with hypertension and hypokalemia should be screened for iatrogenic causes (e.g. loop-diuretic therapy, exogenous steroids), anatomic abnormalities (e.g. renal artery stenosis), as well as other congenital and acquired pathologies (APA, BAH, congenital adrenal hyperplasia, familial hyperaldosteronism, ectopic ACTH production and Cushing's disease). Patients with an incidentaloma found on abdominal imaging should undergo a hormonal and biochemical diagnostic work-up.

Aldosterone-to-renin ratio (ARR) has been proposed as the gold standard initial diagnostic tool for PA in hypertensive patients by most endocrine and cardiovascular societies. However, published guidelines on threshold ratios (conventional threshold ARR ≥ 20) and subsequent steps in management substantially differ among different societies (Table 27.2) [3, 7, 8, 38]. Given the obscure clinical picture of PA and the disagreement in the optimal diagnostic method, some experts recommend use of a combination of tests. The American Heart Association and American Association of Clinical Endocrinologists (AACE)/American Association of Endocrine Surgeons (AAES) guidelines use an absolute serum aldosterone level ≥ 15 ng/dL in addition to an ARR ≥ 20 for diagnosis of PA. An ARR > 30 and a serum aldosterone >20 ng/dL was shown to have both sensitivity and specificity >90% in diagnosing APA [39]. Rossi et al. developed a model with superior diagnostic accuracy using a combination of plasma renin activity, potassium, and either serum aldosterone or captopril-suppressed aldosterone [40]. The threshold value utilized by a clinician may also vary depending on the lateralization strategy at that institution. Knowledge and application of testing characteristics (i.e. using a higher threshold increased false-negatives) is essential to guide clinical decision making.

Although ARR is the best screening test we have for the diagnosis and differentiation of PA, its accuracy depends on many factors, such as age, posture, time of day, medications, serum electrolyte levels and cause of hypertension [8]. It is essential that the clinician is aware of how the aforementioned factors affect the ARR results (Table 27.3). Confirmatory testing is recommended with either administration of oral or intravenous saline, captopril, or fludrocortisone as the specificity of

Table 27.2 Consensus guideline recommendations for PA screening

Guidelines	Criterion for screening	Suggested ARR threshold	Confirmatory test	Imaging	AVS
AACE/AAES Guidelines for the Management of Adrenal Incidentalomas [35]	Incidental adrenal nodules + HTN, new HTN, HTN + hypokalemia, resistant HTN	ARR ≥ 20 + plasma aldosterone ≥ 15 ng/dL	Oral salt loading or saline infusion testing	CT	Yes, in all except age < 40 + unilateral 1 cm nodule on CT (directly to surgery)
American Heart Association Guidelines for Resistant Hypertension [3]	Resistant hypertension	ARR 20–30 (using minimum renin 0.5 ng/mL/h) ± plasma aldo ≥ 15 ng/dL	–	–	–
Endocrine Society clinical practice guidelines [8]	JNC 7 [7] stage 2, resistant HTN, hypokalemia, incidentalomas, family history	ARR 20–40	Oral sodium, saline infusion, captopril, or fludrocortisone suppression testing	CT	Yes, in all surgical candidates
ESH/SSC Guidelines for the management of arterial hypertension	Incidental adrenal nodules + HTN, new HTN, HTN + hypokalemia, resistant HTN	ARR ≥ 20 + plasma aldosterone ≥ 15 ng/dL	Oral salt loading or saline infusion testing	CT	Yes, in all except age < 40 + unilateral 1 cm nodule on CT

AACE American Association of Clinical Endocrinologists, *AAES* American Association of Endocrine Surgeons, *ARR* plasma renin to aldosterone ratio, *ESH* European Society of Hypertension, *ESC* European Society of Cardiology

Table 27.3 Factors that affect the aldosterone-renin ratio (ARR)

Factor	Effect on ARR
Increased age	FP
Hypokalemia	FN
Hypernatremia	FP
Pregnancy	FN
Renal failure	FP
Resistant hypertension	FN
Drugs	
Diuretics	FN
ACE inhibitors	FN
ARBs	FN
β-blockers	FP
CCB	FN

FP false-positive (FP), decreased specificity, *FN* false-negative, decreased sensitivity

screening tests are low. Oral load of 5 g sodium diet for 3 days is followed by a 24 h urinary aldosterone level; when urinary aldosterone is greater than 12 μg the diagnosis of PA is confirmed. Also, intravenous load of 2 L saline infused over 4 h is followed by quantification of serum aldosterone; serum aldosterone >10 ng/dL confirms PA. However, confirmatory suppression testing could be potentially dangerous, especially for patients with exacerbation of congestive heart failure [37, 41]. For the most accurate measurements of confirmatory testing: (1) hypokalemia should be corrected, (2) hypertension should be controlled and (3) patients should not be under treatment with a mineralocorticoid receptor antagonist, such as spironolactone or eplerenone, for 6 weeks prior to testing. On the contrary, screening with ARR has been shown to still be useful without withdrawing anti-hypertensive medications and should be utilized in cases where discontinuation of medications may be harmful [8, 17, 36].

How Do We Identify Appropriate Patients for Adrenalectomy?

The next step after confirming a serological diagnosis of PA is to identify if this is due to unilateral (APA or unilateral hyperplasia) or bilateral adrenal disease (BAH). The great majority of patients with unilateral disease treated with adrenalectomy have improvement if not cure from their hypertension [42]. Given that most aldosteronomas are benign and fewer than two centimeters, nearly all tumors can be removed laparoscopically. Although it has been noted that APA patients have higher systolic blood pressure, lower serum potassium and higher aldosterone levels compared to BAH patients on average, there is no single diagnostic test to successfully differentiate the two pathologic entities [43–45]. This is mainly because APA, BAH and primary hypertension could all present with systolic blood pressure and spontaneous hypokalemia while on numerous antihypertensive medications and varying clinical settings in which the blood pressure is assessed [18]. Prior to pursuing lateralization, a thorough discussion with the patient about the risks and benefits of surgery as well as the benefits and potential side effects of medical therapy (i.e. mineralocorticoid receptor antagonists) is needed.

Identifying the right candidates for adrenalectomy remains challenging. Frequently, the first step in assessing unilateral versus bilateral aldosterone-excess is by non-invasive imaging techniques (traditionally with CT scan). The major drawback of CT scan is that it does not provide us with any information regarding the functionality of the adrenal tumors. Also, aldosteronomas are frequently small tumors, thus increasing the false-negative rates and decreasing the sensitivity of CT scan. Rossi et al. reported on 1125 PA patients and found that 17% of them had tumors <1 cm, while 45% had tumors <2 cm [18]. In addition, non-functional adenomas increase with age, leading to high-false positive rates and decreased specificity of CT scan in the elderly. Magill et al. reported an accuracy rate of CT of 37% when is directly compared to adrenal venous sampling (AVS) [45]. Young et al. performed a direct comparison of AVS and CT scan lateralization results on 194 PA patients. In their study, 41% of patients who had negative CT scans had positive AVS results, CT identified the wrong adrenal gland in 21% of the patients and AVS falsely diagnosed four patients with bilateral adrenal hyperplasia [46]. However, CT scan is particularly helpful in assessing for large adrenal tumors, with tumors larger than 4 cm raising the suspicion for aldosterone-secreting adrenocortical carcinoma. Due to the aforementioned weaknesses of CT, we believe that AVS should be performed in all patients willing to undergo surgery (Fig. 27.1). Because incidental non-functional adrenal nodules in patients younger than 40 years old are rare, the AACE/AAES experts recommend proceeding with adrenalectomy without AVS when CT scan shows a unilateral microadenoma (with clear ARR elevation) [35].

Adrenal venous sampling is a costly and difficult procedure that is not available in all hospitals and clinics, but it remains one of the best diagnostic tools for

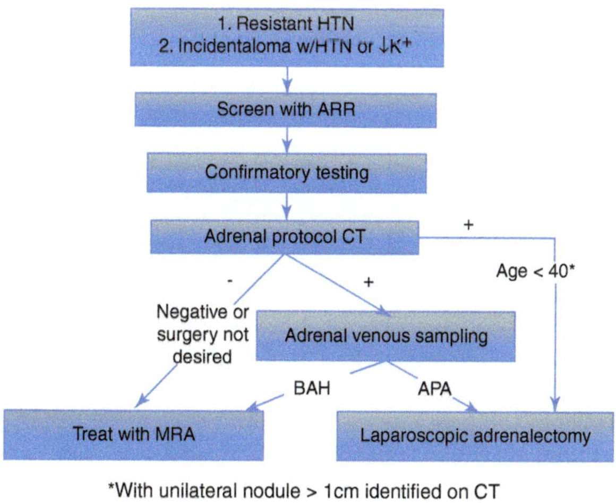

Fig. 27.1 Algorithm for diagnosis and treatment of surgically-correctable primary aldosteronism

lateralization of PA patients to date. It requires cannulation of both adrenal veins and inferior vena cava (IVC) and comparison of aldosterone and cortisol levels in these specific regions of venous circulation. ACTH stimulation is used to amplify potential laterality by reducing stress-induced fluctuations during cannulation and sampling, assisting in differentiating IVC versus right adrenal vein cannulation (adrenal to IVC cortisol ratio greater than 5 indicates proper placement in the right adrenal vein) and maximizing aldosterone secretion [46, 47]. Cortisol measurements are used to normalize aldosterone levels and cortisol-adjusted aldosterone lateralization ratio greater than 4 is indicative for adrenalectomy with a sensitivity ranging from 78 to 98% [45, 46, 48].

Successful catheterization of both adrenal veins ranges from 95% to 97% in experienced centers [43, 46]. However, in low volume centers with minimal experience with the procedure this rate could drop as low as 10% [49]. Complications due to AVS and adrenal vein rupture are seen in less than 3% and 1%, respectively, in high-volume centers [43, 46].

The main limitation of AVS is the variation in indication, technique and diagnostic cut-off values proposed by different research groups [43, 45, 46, 50]. Limited access to the procedure, technical difficulty, high cost and potential complications (such as hematoma, adrenal infarction and aortic dissection) are cited as arguments against using AVS regularly [51]. Successful categorization of PA patients in APA and BAH subtypes ranges from 63% to 97% in the literature [45, 52, 53].

Given the inaccuracies of CT and relatively low morbidity of AVS, we recommend AVS when available. Whether or not utilizing AVS in every case is a cost-effective approach has not been evaluated to date.

Routine Screening for Primary Hyperaldosteronism in Hypertensive Patients?

Yes. PA is a prevalent and under-diagnosed disease. While the screening tests for PA and lateralization strategies are imperfect, the benefits of definitive treatment are clear. Prevalence estimates have recently increased, mainly due to successful screening. The more we are looking, the more we are finding. Hypertension is epidemic and PA is the main etiology in at least 10% of this population. Given that approximately half of those patients (i.e. 5% of the hypertensive population) have unilateral disease, we have the potential to help a large group of patients by screening and targeted treatment of patients with PA, especially in the subgroup of patients with high-risk RH. Furthermore, AVS and laparoscopic adrenalectomy are safe procedures and length of stay following surgery and loss of productivity are minimal.

The financial impact of a screening strategy has been less well studied and is forthcoming. Reimel et al. found surgical treatment to be cost-effective compared to medical therapy alone in PA patients [54]. Our group presented our finding that screening all patients with resistant hypertension for PA is cost-effective at accepted willingness to pay thresholds (American Association of Endocrine Surgeons, Boston MA, 2013). It is less clear if screening the primary hypertensive population at large to identify and treat PA patients is cost-effective and is a key focus of on-going work.

In summary, we believe that the health benefits of targeted intervention for the significant portion of PA patients within the primary hypertensive population warrant early screening, especially in those patients with poorly controlled hypertension, those with concomitant hypokalemia, or known adrenal nodules.

References

1. Mozaffarian D, Benjamin EJ, Go AS, Arnett DK, Blaha MJ, Cushman M, et al. Heart disease and stroke statistics--2015 update: a report from the American Heart Association. Circulation. 2015;131(4):e29–322.
2. Rodriguez F, Foody J. Primary prevention of cardiovascular disease. In: Stergiopoulos K, Brown DL, editors. Evidence-based cardiology consult. London: Springer; 2014. p. 149–58.
3. Calhoun DA, Jones D, Textor S, Goff DC, Murphy TP, Toto RD, et al. Resistant hypertension: diagnosis, evaluation, and treatment: a scientific statement from the American Heart Association professional education Committee of the Council for high blood pressure research. Circulation. 2008;117(25):e510–26.
4. Egan BM, Zhao Y, Axon RN, Brzezinski WA, Ferdinand KC. Uncontrolled and apparent treatment resistant hypertension in the United States, 1988 to 2008. Circulation. 2011;124(9):1046–58.
5. Persell SD. Prevalence of resistant hypertension in the United States, 2003–2008. Hypertension. 2011;57(6):1076–80.
6. James PA, Oparil S, Carter BL, Cushman WC, Dennison-Himmelfarb C, Handler J, et al. 2014 evidence-based guideline for the management of high blood pressure in adults: report from the panel members appointed to the eighth joint National Committee (JNC 8). JAMA. 2014;311(5):507–20.
7. Green L. JNC 7 express: new thinking in hypertension treatment. Am Fam Physician. 2003;68(2):228, 30.
8. Funder JW, Carey RM, Fardella C, Gomez-Sanchez CE, Mantero F, Stowasser M, et al. Case detection, diagnosis, and treatment of patients with primary aldosteronism: an endocrine society clinical practice guideline. J Clin Endocrinol Metab. 2008;93(9):3266–81.
9. Fagugli RM, Taglioni C. Changes in the perceived epidemiology of primary hyperaldosteronism. Int J Hypertens. 2011;2011:162804.
10. Fardella CE, Mosso L, Gomez-Sanchez C, Cortes P, Soto J, Gomez L, et al. Primary hyperaldosteronism in essential hypertensives: prevalence, biochemical profile, and molecular biology. J Clin Endocrinol Metab. 2000;85(5):1863–7.
11. Gordon RD, Stowasser M. Primary aldosteronism: the case for screening. Nat Clin Pract Nephrol. 2007;3(11):582–3.
12. Lim PO, Rodgers P, Cardale K, Watson AD, MacDonald TM. Potentially high prevalence of primary aldosteronism in a primary-care population. Lancet. 1999;353(9146):40.
13. Strauch B, Zelinka T, Hampf M, Bernhardt R, Widimsky J Jr. Prevalence of primary hyperaldosteronism in moderate to severe hypertension in the Central Europe region. J Hum Hypertens. 2003;17(5):349–52.
14. Milliez P, Girerd X, Plouin PF, Blacher J, Safar ME, Mourad JJ. Evidence for an increased rate of cardiovascular events in patients with primary aldosteronism. J Am Coll Cardiol. 2005;45(8):1243–8.
15. Mulatero P, Stowasser M, Loh KC, Fardella CE, Gordon RD, Mosso L, et al. Increased diagnosis of primary aldosteronism, including surgically correctable forms, in centers from five continents. J Clin Endocrinol Metab. 2004;89(3):1045–50.
16. Eide IK, Torjesen PA, Drolsum A, Babovic A, Lilledahl NP. Low-renin status in therapy-resistant hypertension: a clue to efficient treatment. J Hypertens. 2004;22(11):2217–26.
17. Gallay BJ, Ahmad S, Xu L, Toivola B, Davidson RC. Screening for primary aldosteronism without discontinuing hypertensive medications: plasma aldosterone-renin ratio. Am J Kidney Dis. 2001;37(4):699–705.

18. Rossi GP, Bernini G, Caliumi C, Desideri G, Fabris B, Ferri C, et al. A prospective study of the prevalence of primary aldosteronism in 1,125 hypertensive patients. J Am Coll Cardiol. 2006;48(11):2293–300.
19. Rutherford JC, Stowasser M, Tunny TJ, Klemm SA, Gordon RD. Laparoscopic adrenalectomy. World J Surg. 1996;20(7):758–60. discussion 61.
20. Lo CY, Tam PC, Kung AW, Lam KS, Wong J. Primary aldosteronism. Results of surgical treatment. Ann Surg. 1996;224(2):125–30.
21. Rossi GP, Cesari M, Cuspidi C, Maiolino G, Cicala MV, Bisogni V, et al. Long-term control of arterial hypertension and regression of left ventricular hypertrophy with treatment of primary aldosteronism. Hypertension. 2013;62(1):62–9.
22. Letavernier E, Peyrard S, Amar L, Zinzindohoue F, Fiquet B, Plouin PF. Blood pressure outcome of adrenalectomy in patients with primary hyperaldosteronism with or without unilateral adenoma. J Hypertens. 2008;26(9):1816–23.
23. van der Linden P, Steichen O, Zinzindohoue F, Plouin PF. Blood pressure and medication changes following adrenalectomy for unilateral primary aldosteronism: a follow-up study. J Hypertens. 2012;30(4):761–9.
24. Rossi GP, Bolognesi M, Rizzoni D, Seccia TM, Piva A, Porteri E, et al. Vascular remodeling and duration of hypertension predict outcome of adrenalectomy in primary aldosteronism patients. Hypertension. 2008;51(5):1366–71.
25. Calhoun DA. Hyperaldosteronism as a common cause of resistant hypertension. Annu Rev Med. 2013;64:233–47.
26. Judd E, Calhoun DA. Apparent and true resistant hypertension: definition, prevalence and outcomes. J Hum Hypertens. 2014;28(8):463–8.
27. Ahmed AH, Gordon RD, Sukor N, Pimenta E, Stowasser M. Quality of life in patients with bilateral primary aldosteronism before and during treatment with spironolactone and/or amiloride, including a comparison with our previously published results in those with unilateral disease treated surgically. J Clin Endocrinol Metab. 2011;96(9):2904–11.
28. Vaclavik J, Sedlak R, Plachy M, Navratil K, Plasek J, Jarkovsky J, et al. Addition of spironolactone in patients with resistant arterial hypertension (ASPIRANT): a randomized, double-blind, placebo-controlled trial. Hypertension. 2011;57(6):1069–75.
29. Gaddam K, Corros C, Pimenta E, Ahmed M, Denney T, Aban I, et al. Rapid reversal of left ventricular hypertrophy and intracardiac volume overload in patients with resistant hypertension and hyperaldosteronism: a prospective clinical study. Hypertension. 2010;55(5):1137–42.
30. Waldmann J, Maurer L, Holler J, Kann PH, Ramaswamy A, Bartsch DK, et al. Outcome of surgery for primary hyperaldosteronism. World J Surg. 2011;35(11):2422–7.
31. Pang TC, Bambach C, Monaghan JC, Sidhu SB, Bune A, Delbridge LW, et al. Outcomes of laparoscopic adrenalectomy for hyperaldosteronism. ANZ J Surg. 2007;77(9):768–73.
32. Catena C, Colussi G, Lapenna R, Nadalini E, Chiuch A, Gianfagna P, et al. Long-term cardiac effects of adrenalectomy or mineralocorticoid antagonists in patients with primary aldosteronism. Hypertension. 2007;50(5):911–8.
33. Rossi GP, Pitter G, Bernante P, Motta R, Feltrin G, Miotto D. Adrenal vein sampling for primary aldosteronism: the assessment of selectivity and lateralization of aldosterone excess baseline and after adrenocorticotropic hormone (ACTH) stimulation. J Hypertens. 2008;26(5):989–97.
34. Young WF Jr. Minireview: primary aldosteronism--changing concepts in diagnosis and treatment. Endocrinology. 2003;144(6):2208–13.
35. Zeiger MA, Thompson GB, Duh QY, Hamrahian AH, Angelos P, Elaraj D, et al. The American Association of Clinical Endocrinologists and American Association of Endocrine Surgeons medical guidelines for the management of adrenal incidentalomas. Endocr Pract. 2009;15(Suppl 1):1–20.
36. Schwartz GL, Chapman AB, Boerwinkle E, Kisabeth RM, Turner ST. Screening for primary aldosteronism: implications of an increased plasma aldosterone/renin ratio. Clin Chem. 2002;48(11):1919–23.
37. Mulatero P, Dluhy RG, Giacchetti G, Boscaro M, Veglio F, Stewart PM. Diagnosis of primary aldosteronism: from screening to subtype differentiation. Trends Endocrinol Metab. 2005;16(3):114–9.

38. Mancia G, Fagard R, Narkiewicz K, Redon J, Zanchetti A, Bohm M, et al. 2013 ESH/ESC Guidelines for the management of arterial hypertension: the Task Force for the management of arterial hypertension of the European Society of Hypertension (ESH) and of the European Society of Cardiology (ESC). J Hypertens. 2013;31(7):1281–357.
39. Weinberger MH, Fineberg NS. The diagnosis of primary aldosteronism and separation of two major subtypes. Arch Intern Med. 1993;153(18):2125–9.
40. Rossi GP, Rossi E, Pavan E, Rosati N, Zecchel R, Semplicini A, et al. Screening for primary aldosteronism with a logistic multivariate discriminant analysis. Clin Endocrinol (Oxf). 1998;49(6):713–23.
41. Mulatero P, Milan A, Fallo F, Regolisti G, Pizzolo F, Fardella C, et al. Comparison of confirmatory tests for the diagnosis of primary aldosteronism. J Clin Endocrinol Metab. 2006;91(7):2618–23.
42. Stowasser M, Gordon RD. Primary aldosteronism--careful investigation is essential and rewarding. Mol Cell Endocrinol. 2004;217(1–2):33–9.
43. Rossi GP, Sacchetto A, Chiesura-Corona M, De Toni R, Gallina M, Feltrin GP, et al. Identification of the etiology of primary aldosteronism with adrenal vein sampling in patients with equivocal computed tomography and magnetic resonance findings: results in 104 consecutive cases. J Clin Endocrinol Metab. 2001;86(3):1083–90.
44. Blumenfeld JD, Sealey JE, Schlussel Y, Vaughan ED Jr, Sos TA, Atlas SA, et al. Diagnosis and treatment of primary hyperaldosteronism. Ann Intern Med. 1994;121(11):877–85.
45. Magill SB, Raff H, Shaker JL, Brickner RC, Knechtges TE, Kehoe ME, et al. Comparison of adrenal vein sampling and computed tomography in the differentiation of primary aldosteronism. J Clin Endocrinol Metab. 2001;86(3):1066–71.
46. Young WF, Stanson AW, Thompson GB, Grant CS, Farley DR, van Heerden JA. Role for adrenal venous sampling in primary aldosteronism. Surgery. 2004;136(6):1227–35.
47. Doppman JL, Gill JR Jr. Hyperaldosteronism: sampling the adrenal veins. Radiology. 1996;198(2):309–12.
48. Satoh F, Abe T, Tanemoto M, Nakamura M, Abe M, Uruno A, et al. Localization of aldosterone-producing adrenocortical adenomas: significance of adrenal venous sampling. Hypertens Res. 2007;30(11):1083–95.
49. Vonend O, Ockenfels N, Gao X, Allolio B, Lang K, Mai K, et al. Adrenal venous sampling: evaluation of the German Conn's registry. Hypertension. 2011;57(5):990–5.
50. Nishikawa T, Omura M. Clinical characteristics of primary aldosteronism: its prevalence and comparative studies on various causes of primary aldosteronism in Yokohama Rosai Hospital. Biomed Pharmacother. 2000;54(Suppl 1):83s–5s.
51. Stewart PM, Allolio B. Adrenal vein sampling for Primary Aldosteronism: time for a reality check. Clin Endocrinol (Oxf). 2009;72(2):146–8.
52. Young WF Jr, Stanson AW, Grant CS, Thompson GB, van Heerden JA. Primary aldosteronism: adrenal venous sampling. Surgery. 1996;120(6):913–9. discussion 9–20.
53. Sheaves R, Goldin J, Reznek RH, Chew SL, Dacie JE, Lowe DG, et al. Relative value of computed tomography scanning and venous sampling in establishing the cause of primary hyperaldosteronism. Eur J Endocrinol. 1996;134(3):308–13.
54. Reimel B, Zanocco K, Russo MJ, Zarnegar R, Clark OH, Allendorf JD, et al. The management of aldosterone-producing adrenal adenomas--does adrenalectomy increase costs? Surgery. 2010;148(6):1178–85. discussion 85.

Routine Glucose Monitoring in Postoperative Pheochromocytoma Patients: Yes or No?

28

Neha Goel and James A. Lee

Abstract

Pheochromocytomas are rare neuroendocrine tumors characterized by the release of catecholamines. In the preoperative setting, the release of these catecholamines can lead to hyperglycemia by promoting liver glycogenolysis and gluconeogenesis, inhibiting pancreatic insulin secretion, and enhancing peripheral insulin resistance. Postoperatively, there is often a period of rebound hypoglycemia that can be dangerously prolonged given the preoperative depletion of glycogen stores secondary to high catecholamine levels. This complication of postoperative hypoglycemia can be extremely detrimental given that it often goes unrecognized secondary to the masking effects of anesthesia. The change in mental status associated with hypoglycemia may be incorrectly attributed to residual anesthesia. Alpha and beta-blockade further blunt the body's natural response to hypoglycemia which is usually tachycardia, palpitations, and sweating. Prolonged, unrecognized hypoglycemia can lead to severe neurologic consequences such as seizures, unconsciousness, or even irreversible brain damage. This complication must therefore be preemptively anticipated and acutely managed. A thorough literature search over the years provides data in favor of routine postoperative glucose monitoring after pheochromocytoma resection. Given the high stakes involved with missing this relatively common diagnosis seen in 4–15% of pheochromocytoma patients undergoing resection, a GRADE 1C

N. Goel (✉)
Department of Surgery, New York Presbyterian-Columbia University Medical Center, New York, NY, USA
e-mail: ng2362@cumc.columbia.edu

J. A. Lee
Department of Surgery, Columbia University Medical Center, New York, NY, USA
e-mail: jal74@cumc.columbia.edu

P. Angelos, R. H. Grogan (eds.), *Difficult Decisions in Endocrine Surgery*, Difficult Decisions in Surgery: An Evidence-Based Approach,
https://doi.org/10.1007/978-3-319-92860-9_28

recommendation for routine monitoring in all postoperative pheochromocytoma patients for the first 5 h has been deemed appropriate.

Keywords
Pheochromocytoma resection · Postoperative hypoglycemia · Unrecognized hypoglycemia · Routine postoperative glucose monitoring in all patients · Elevated preoperative urine metanephrine levels · Alpha and beta blockade · Neurologic complications

Background

Pheochromocytomas are rare neuroendocrine tumors characterized by the release of catecholamines. These neoplasms arise from chromaffin cells of the adrenal medulla and present with signs and symptoms consistent with catecholamine excess. Classical symptoms include palpitations, paroxysmal hypertension, tachycardia, headaches, and diaphoresis [1]. Patients may also have acute attacks of pallor, nausea, and panic attacks lasting several minutes [2]. More elusive symptoms of weight loss and fatigue have also been seen with pheochromoctyomas [3]. In extreme cases patients may have florid heart failure, or takotsubo cardiomyopathy, secondary to a catecholamine surge [3]. More subtle signs may include new onset diabetes as a result of glycogenolysis and insulin inhibition due to catecholamine release [4]. Given the complex nature of this tumor, meticulous perioperative management is extremely important. Table 28.1 summarizes the studies using the Population, Intervention, Comparator, and Outcomes (PICO) format.

Preoperative Hemodynamic Changes and Management

Preoperative management of the patient consists of catecholamine blockade, specifically using alpha-adrenergic blockers for hypertension and beta-blockers for tachycardia. The most commonly used alpha-blocker is phenoxybenzamine secondary to its irreversible and non-selective nature. The drug is titrated as needed and patients usually achieve their goal dose within 10–14 days. Clinical signs of the optimal dose are a stuffy nose and slight dizziness due to postural hypotension [5]. Another alternative to phenoxybenzamine is doxazosin, a selective and reversible alpha-blocker. However, unlike phenoxybenzamine, strong catecholamine bursts can displace doxazosin from its receptor binding site and reduce its efficacy [6]. On

Table 28.1 PICO table

*P*opulation	Postoperative pheochromocytoma patients
*I*ntervention	Routine glucose monitoring
*C*omparator	Selective glucose monitoring
*O*utcomes	Complications, ICU admission

the other hand, some believe that reduced postoperative hypotension may be a benefit of doxazosin [7–9]. During alpha blockade, it is imperative to also replete the intravascular volume as the alpha-mediated vasoconstriction is released. Calcium channel blockers are also occasionally used to control refractory hypertension [10].

Patients with preoperative tachycardia can be managed with a cardioselective beta1-blocker such as metoprolol, bisoprolol, or atenolol [9]. Intraoperative tachycardia is usually controlled using a short acting beta1- blocker such as esmolol [11]. Unlike the other selective beta1-blockers, labetolol, a combined alpha1 and beta-blocker has mixed reviews in terms of its use [12]. Reports of orthostatic hypotension and hypertensive crisis have been observed [13–15].

Preoperative Hyperglycemia

In addition to the aforementioned hemodynamic changes caused by pheochromocytomas, endocrine changes are also well documented. La Batide-Alanore et al. reports the rate of diabetes of 68 of 191 (35.6%) patients with pheochromocytoma. Pheochromocytoma patients with or without diabetes did not differ in body mass index, plasma noradrenaline concentration, metanephrine excretion, or tumor characteristics. Age, duration of hypertension, and plasma epinephrine concentration were significantly and independently associated with diabetes in patients with pheochromocytoma. Specifically, pheochromocytoma patients with diabetes were younger, more likely female, and had a lower body mass index than those with essential hypertension ($P < 0.01$). After adjustment for these three variables, the odds ratio for pheochromocytoma in hypertensive patients with diabetes was 5.5 (95% confidence interval, 3.5–8.7). For patients younger than 51 years old with a body mass index <25 kg/m^2, the odds ratio was 18.9 (95% confidence interval, 5.9–58.8) [4]. The use of preoperative alpha or beta blockade has not proven very effective in controlling preoperative glucose levels [16]. In fact, alpha and beta blockade may inhibit the symptoms of hypoglycemia such as palpitations, diaphoresis, and tremors, leading to a precarious situation.

Overall, diabetes is present in one of three patients with pheochromocytoma. In young patients with hypertension and normal body weight, the presence of diabetes should be used to further investigate the presence of a pheochromocytoma. In severe cases, patients may initially present with diabetic ketoacidosis [4].

The hyperglycemia seen with pheochromocytomas can be attributed to an imbalance in glucose homeostasis. Normal glucose levels are maintained by a system of checks and balances involving the liver, the pancreas, and the adrenal gland, all of which are under control of the autonomic nervous system [17]. Over the years, much research has been conducted on the effect of catecholamines and glucose control.

Both the liver and pancreas are innervated by the autonomic nervous system. Catecholamine release secondary to the pheochromocytoma promotes liver glycogenolysis and gluconeogenesis. Epinephrine is the predominant driver of this phenomenon in the liver through beta-adrenergic stimulation [17, 18]. Additionally, hepatic glucoreceptors have been hypothesized to be coupled with capsaicin-sensitive afferent nerves to convey blood glucose levels to the central nervous system [17].

The autonomic nervous system controls pancreatic islet cell insulin secretion, and in turn has a major effect in glucose homeostasis. Catecholamines inhibit pancreatic insulin secretion through agonist effects on alpha2-adrenergic receptors [19]. This has been replicated in human study patients where the administration of norepinephrine inhibits insulin release from pancreatic beta cells [20]. Furthermore, the administration of phentolamine, an alpha-receptor blocker, counteracts the inhibitive effect of catecholamines on insulin secretion [19]. Ostenson et al. also reported that alpha2-receptor agonists inhibit insulin release. Besides the well documented adrenergic and cholinergic effects on pancreatic islet cells, the role of neuropeptides is also being researched [21]. Vasoactive intestinal polypeptide, pituitary adenlyate cyclase activating polypeptide, and gastrin releasing peptide are neuropeptides regulated by the parasympathetic nervous system, whereas galanin and neuropeptide Y are part of the sympathetic nervous system [22]. Insulin secretion is stimulated by neuropeptides that are part of the parasympathetic nerves and is inhibited by those which are part of the sympathetic nervous system.

Unlike the liver and the pancreatic islet cells, the adrenal medulla receives its main nerve supply from the greater and lesser splanchnic nerves. Catecholamine secretion by the adrenal medulla is regulated by adrenoceptors, dihydropyridine-sensitive $Ca2+$ channels, and capsaicin-sensitive sensory nerves. In response to stress, the sympathoadrenal system is activated and releases adrenal catecholamines and pancreatic glucagon, both leading to hyperglycemia [17].

Catecholamines also play an important role in enhancing peripheral insulin resistance. Administration of epinephrine increases peripheral insulin resistance through beta-adrenergic receptors [23]. This has been demonstrated in the pheochromocytoma population by Wiesner et al. who were able to show a reversal of insulin resistance after tumor resection [24]. In extreme situations, this reversal may actually contribute to acute postoperative hypoglycemia.

Postoperative Hypoglycemia

Hypoglycemia following pheochromocytoma resection is an insidious complication that contradicts the hyperglycemia usually seen in postoperative patients secondary to the body's normal response to the stress of surgery. The hypoglycemia following tumor resection can be attributed to the preoperative suppression of endogenous insulin secretion and a reactive postoperative rebound hyperinsulinemia. This reactive rise in insulin results from the sudden decrease in catecholamines and reduction of alpha-receptor stimulation, which preoperatively had inhibitive effects on the pancreatic insulin secreting islet cells [16]. Additionally, once the tumor is resected, the beta cells of the pancreas become rapidly sensitive to the preoperative hyperglycemia and respond with a reactive hyperinsulinemia. Improved peripheral insulin sensitivity with increased glucose use by skeletal muscle further contributes to hypoglycemia [24].

The body's normal compensatory response to hypoglycemia is the release of glucagon, epinephrine, and cortisol to stimulate the sympathetic nervous system to increase blood glucose levels via gluconeogenesis, glycogenolysis, and inhibition of insulin secretion. However, hypoglycemia usually persists in the acute postoperative period since liver glycogen stores are depleted preoperatively by the pheochromocytoma. The use of beta blockers also diminishes sympathetic tone secondary to the stress of surgery and impairs gluconeogenesis and glycogenolysis, further inhibiting recovery from postoperative hypoglycemia [25]. The effect of beta blockers combined with alpha blockers, which increase insulin secretion, exacerbates postoperative hypoglycemia.

Postoperative hypoglycemia can be extremely detrimental given that it often goes unrecognized secondary to the masking effects of anesthesia. The change in mental status associated with hypoglycemia may be attributed to residual anesthesia [26]. Alpha and beta-blockade further blunt the body's natural response to hypoglycemia which is usually tachycardia, palpitations, and sweating. Prolonged, unrecognized hypoglycemia can lead to severe neurologic consequences such as seizures, unconsciousness, or even irreversible brain damage.

Meeke et al. describe a case of a 45 year old female whose symptoms of postoperative drowsiness and mild hypotension were initially thought to be due to the effects of 3.5 h of general anesthesia using enflurane, nitrous oxide, droperidol, and fentanyl. It turned out that hypoglycemia was the cause of this patient's drowsiness. This case report urges physicians to consider hypoglycemia when confronted with a postoperative pheochromocytoma resection patient who fails to fully awaken from anesthesia or in severe cases develops a postoperative coma up to 2 h after surgery [26].

Another case report by Kato et al. describes a 39 year old male with severe hypoglycemia following resection of a right 7.5 × 5 × 7 cm pheochromocytoma. This patient received doxazosin and propranolol for 43 days prior to the adrenalectomy. After 2 h in the intensive care unit, the patient became drowsy and diaphoretic. The patient was found to be hypoglycemic (38 mg/dl) and hyperinsulinemic (63.67 μU/ml, normal being 8.4–8.8 μU/ml). The study concluded with a recommendation for close monitoring of blood glucose for at least 6 h after pheochromocytoma resection [27].

Preoperative Factors Associated with or Predictive of Postoperative Hypoglycemia

Given that hypoglycemia after pheochromocytoma resection can have serious consequences, it behooves one to identify preoperative risk factors that are associated or predictive of postoperative hypoglycemia. A literature review reveals multiple possible factors associated with an increased risk of postoperative hypoglycemia such as greater preoperative urine catecholamine excretion, larger tumor size, longer operative time, and pre-existing diabetes mellitus [16, 28, 29]. Plouin et al. reported a postoperative hypoglycemia rate requiring hypertonic glucose at 15%. This number is supported by Akiba et al. who reported a rate of 13.3% (6 of 45) for severe postoperative hypoglycemia defined as less blood glucose levels less than

50 mg/dL [16]. This group looked at an 8-year-period from 1981 to 1989 where 6 out of 45 pheochromocytoma patients developed severe hypoglycemia (12–50 mg/dl) 2–4.5 h after tumor resection, with an average of 3 h. In order to study the pathophysiology behind postoperative hypoglycemia, levels of plasma immunoreactive insulin (IRI) and glucose were measured at surgery in ten patients with pheochromocytoma, from the beginning of the operation to 5 h after tumor resection. Two of these ten patients developed postoperative hypoglycemia. The highest plasma IRI levels were observed in the two patients with post-resection hypoglycemia and the levels were 174 and 2081 μU/ml. IRI levels in the eight patients without hypoglycemia ranged from 13–222 μU/ml (mean, 77) and were only 14–33 μU/ml (mean, 22) in the five control patients made up of patients with primary aldosteronism and Cushing's syndrome [16].

Akiba et al. also concluded that patients with higher levels of preoperative urine epinephrine and those with either diabetes mellitus or impaired glucose tolerance, identified preoperatively by the World Health Organization criteria, were at a higher risk for postoperative hypoglycemia. These observations suggest that excessive rebound secretion of insulin after removal of a pheochromocytoma occurs because preoperative endogenous insulin secretion is suppressed by the elevated plasma catecholamine level. They also found that intraoperative infusion of glucose and/or postoperative infusion of epinephrine and norepinephrine did not necessarily prevent hypoglycemia. They conclude by recommending glucose monitoring for at least 5 h after tumor resection, however they do not comment on the frequency of glucose checks. They also concluded that patients with high preoperative urine catecholamime levels or impaired glucose intolerance are at high risk. Additionally, based on the findings of a single patient with elevated intraoperative plasma catecholamine levels, they suggest that patients with an extreme increase in intraoperative plasma catecholamines can also be at high risk of postoperative hypoglycemia [16].

Chen et al. conducted a retrospective chart review of patients who underwent pheochromocytoma resection between 1993 and 2013 at two large academic medical centers to elucidate the incidence of postoperative hypoglycemia and to identify predisposing risk factors. The primary endpoint was postoperative hypoglycemia defined as blood glucose less than 55 mg/dl. A total of 213 patients were identified. Nine patients (4.2%) experienced postoperative hypoglycemia, and eight of these patients presented within the first 24 h. The average lowest postoperative glucose in these patients was 41 mg/dl (range 20–53), which occurred between 0.4 and 142 h postoperatively. In the majority of patients (5 of 9), the first episode of hypoglycemia occurred in the first four postoperative hours. In three patients, the first episode was within 24 h. Two of these patients also experienced a second episode of hypoglycemia up to 42 h postoperatively. One patient even had hypoglycemia after 162 h. This patient, however, had undergone a bilateral adrenalectomy complicated by critical illness and the need for total parenteral nutrition [29].

In comparing the patients with and without postoperative hypoglycemia, Chen et al. found no difference in patient demographics, history of diabetes mellitus, preoperative baseline glucose levels, type of preoperative adrenergic receptor blockade received, or operative approach. However, patients with postoperative hypoglycemia had higher preoperative 24-h urinary metanephrine levels (4726 vs. 2461 μg/24 h, $P = 0.05$), longer operative times (270 vs. 142 min, $P < 0.01$), and larger tumors (7.6 vs. 4.6 cm, $P = 0.02$). These patients required frequent intensive care level monitoring (88.9% vs. 34.5%, $P < 0.01$) but there was no statistically significant difference in length of hospital stay (5 vs. 3 days, $P = 0.10$) [29].

Multivariate analysis revealed that the only independent predictors of postoperative hypoglycemia are increased preoperative 24-h urine epinephrine levels ($P = 0.03$) and longer operating time ($P < 0.01$) [29]. This finding of a longer operative time associated with postoperative hypoglycemia is supported by Chernow et al. who concluded that the magnitude of the stress response is proportional to the extent of operation and that postoperatively there may be a component of relative hypoadrenalism contributing to hypoglycemia [30]. Chen et al., much like other studies, does not comment on a recommended frequency or duration for glucose monitoring.

Along with elevated preoperative urine metanephrines and longer operative times, epinephrine-predominant pheochromocytomas may also predispose patients to developing postoperative hypoglycemia. In animal studies prolonged stimulation of adrenergic receptors by epinephrine results in tachyphylaxis and desensitization of these receptors. Additionally, chronic epinephrine exposure and stimulation decreases hepatic glycogen storage levels thereby limiting the body's ability to respond to hypoglycemic episodes [30–32].

The role of diabetes in the development of postoperative hypoglycemia remains unclear. It has been hypothesized that patients with pre-existing type 2 diabetes or glucose intolerance may be at decreased risk because the persistent hyperinsulinemia depletes pancreatic stores and prevents the rebound hyperinsulinemia seen after pheochromocytoma resection [33]. Akiba et al. showed that preoperative diabetes or glucose intolerance was a risk factor, however, Chen et al. and Plouin et al. showed differing results [16, 28, 29].

Plouin et al. looked at a total 165 patients, 25 of which had episodes of postoperative hypoglycemia requiring intravenous hypertonic glucose fluids. In their study, there was no significant difference in the proportion of patients with preoperative hyperglycemia [8 of 25 (32.0%) vs. 43 of 131 (32.8%)], malignant pheochromocytoma [3 of 25 (12.0%) vs. 31 of 131 (23.7%)], or in preoperative plasma catecholamine concentrations between cases with and without hypoglycemia [28].

It is also important to keep in mind that if both hypotension and hypoglycemia occur in a patient after bilateral partial or complete adrenalectomy, suspicions about hypocortisolism and Addisonian crisis should be raised [34]. In these situations, plasma and urinary cortisol and plasma adrenocorticotropic hormone (ACTH) levels should be measured [34]. If the diagnosis of hypocortisolism or Addisonian crisis is made, steroids should be administered immediately [35].

Overall, the only factor associated with postoperative hypoglycemia that has been supported by more than one study is elevated preoperative urine metanephrine levels [16, 29]. Chen et al. also found an association with increased operative times and larger tumors. Some studies have found preoperative diabetes or glucose intolerance to lead to postoperative hypoglycemia, however this has been refuted by more contemporary studies [16, 28, 29].

Recommendations

In conclusion, postoperative hypoglycemia is seen in 4–15% of patients undergoing pheochromocytoma resection [16, 28, 29]. If this complication is not anticipated, it can be missed with detrimental neurologic consequences [16, 28, 29]. A thorough literature search over the years provides data in favor of routine postoperative monitoring of glucose levels after pheochromocytoma resection, however the exact duration and frequency of glucose checks remains up for debate. Studies have recommended close postoperative glucose monitoring anywhere from 2 to 24 h [29, 36]. Based on the studies reviewed, most postoperative hypoglycemic events occurred within the first five postoperative hours, thus routine monitoring equivalent to what an intensive care unit would provide at a given institution for hyperglycemia monitoring, usually at 1 h intervals, should be conducted during the postoperative period [16, 29, 37]. Ongoing routine monitoring should continue if any episodes of hypoglycemia are found and should be continued until glucose levels normalize. It is important to remember that the effects of anesthesia can mask postoperative symptoms of hypoglycemia, thus patients who are still emerging from anesthesia should have routine monitoring outside the recommended 5 h period. Similarly, those patients who remain in critical condition postoperatively and require intubation or are unable to manifest signs and symptoms of hypoglycemia due to alpha or beta-blockade should have routine monitoring of their blood glucose levels. Hemodynamically unstable patients should also have prolonged routine glucose monitoring.

It is also important to note that Chen et al. showed postoperative hypoglycemia to be associated with higher preoperative urine metanephrine levels and those who had undergone longer operations for larger tumors [29]. Thus it may be wise to place these patients with known risk factors for postoperative hypoglycemia in the intensive care unit. Chen et al. also showed that patients with complicated postoperative courses or those requiring bilateral adrenalectomy presented with postoperative hypoglycemia up to 162 h after surgery [29]. These patients should also undergo routine monitoring until they are deemed stable to come out of the intensive care unit on an individual to individual basis.

Patients found to be hypoglycemic should be administered intravenous dextrose solutions immediately. Some studies even recommend routine administration of dextrose containing intravenous fluids with the assumption that by the time hypoglycemia is detected it may be severe and refractory to large amounts of glucose administration. For example, Yanaru et al. describes a case of a 54 year old female who presented with a glucose level of 30 mg/dl 4 h after tumor resection. Despite intravenous administration of glucose at a rate of 15 g/h. with intermittent boluses of 5 g of glucose, it took about 2 h to obtain glucose levels above 100 mg/dl. They recommend that all patients who undergo pheochromocytoma resection have regular postoperative glucose monitoring and receive dextrose-containing fluids routinely. They also had a low threshold for checking serum glucose levels in patients who had excessive drowsiness or hyperadrenergic symptoms postoperatively, and often sent these patients to the intensive care unit [37].

Additional challenges of the immediate postoperative period are blood pressure instability and heart rate control, necessitating close patient monitoring for at least 24–48 h [36]. Since patients are being closely monitored for hemodynamic instability for prolonged periods of time, it only makes sense to routinely monitor patients for hypoglycemia, at least for the first five critical postoperative hours where studies have shown most patients present with this complication.

Despite the well-documented complication of postoperative hypoglycemia after pheochromocytoma resection, all of these studies have limitations associated with either being case studies, case reports, retrospective reviews, or prospective studies with small patient samples. As a result, all of the current available research on postoperative hypoglycemia falls under the GRADE format study design category of observational studies, which places the initial quality of evidence rating as low. Further review of the quality of evidence reveals that it should not be downgraded since there are no serious doubts about the indirectness of evidence, no serious imprecisions, and an unlikely probability of publication bias. The recommendation however can be upgraded because it is likely that there are plausible biases from the observational studies. In particular, the relatively rare nature of this complication often inherently leads to biased results which may actually underestimate the benefit of routine monitoring of hypoglycemia. Thus, the actual treatment effect is likely to be larger than what the data suggests. An overall GRADE of 1C is therefore recommended in favor of routine postoperative glucose monitoring after pheochromocytoma resection. This grade corresponds to a strong recommendation from low quality evidence and clinically fits the GRADE 1C risk/benefit category since the benefits of identifying and treating early hypoglycemia appear to outweigh the risks of severe neurologic consequences if episodes of hypoglycemia are missed. Additionally, this benefit appears to override the burden of routine monitoring [38, 39].

Overall, since no current consensus guidelines exist on routine postoperative glucose monitoring after pheochromocytoma resection, we propose the following guidelines with a GRADE 1C recommendation:

- All postoperative pheochromocytoma patients should have routine glucose monitoring for at least 5 h.
- Patients with preoperative risk factors for hypoglycemia such as elevated urine metanephrine levels or large tumors with an anticipated prolonged operative time should be considered for monitoring in the intensive care unit or monitored setting with a similar level of acuity [29].
- Patients who remain intubated, are hemodynamically unstable, or have delayed emergence from anesthesia should go to the intensive care unit for prolonged routine glucose monitoring on a case by case basis or until institution-dependent discharge criteria from the intensive care unit are met.

To increase the strength of the recommendation, a large multisite prospective randomized control study would prove useful to identify additional factors predictive of this complication and how to preemptively avoid this complication.

Intraoperative or postoperative real-time monitoring of serum insulin, glucagon, and glucose levels may help to anticipate and treat postoperative hypoglycemia before complications arise [29].

References

1. Manger WM, Gifford RW. Clinical and experimental pheochromocytoma. Hoboken: Blackwell Science; 1996.
2. Därr R, Lenders JW, Hofbauer LC, Naumann B, Bornstein SR, Eisenhofer G. Pheochromocytoma - update on disease management. Ther Adv Endocrinol Metab. 2012;3(1):11–26.
3. Prejbisz A, Lenders JW, Eisenhofer G, Januszewicz A. Cardiovascular manifestations of phaeochromocytoma. J Hypertens. 2011;29:2049–60.
4. La Batide-Alanore A, Chatellier G, Plouin PF. Diabetes as a marker of pheochromocytoma in hypertensive patients. J Hypertens. 2003;21:1703–7.
5. Witteles RM, Kaplan EL, Roizen MF. Safe and cost-effective preoperative preparation of patients with pheochromocytoma. Anesth Analg. 2000;91:302–4.
6. Bravo EL, Tagle R. Pheochromocytoma: state-of-the-art and future prospects. Endocr Rev. 2003;24:539–53.
7. Kinney MA, Narr BJ, Warner MA. Perioperative management of pheochromocytoma. J Cardiothorac Vasc Anesth. 2002;16:359–69.
8. Kocak S, Aydintug S, Canakci N. Alpha blockade in preoperative preparation of patients with pheochromocytomas. Int Surg. 2002;87:191–4.
9. Prys-Roberts C, Farndon JR. Efficacy and safety of doxazosin for perioperative management of patients with pheochromocytoma. World J Surg. 2002;26:1037–42.
10. Tokioka H, Takahashi T, Kosogabe Y, Ohta Y, Kosaka F. Use of diltiazem to control circulatory fluctuations during resection of a phaeochromocytoma. Br J Anaesth. 1988;60:582–7.
11. Gray RJ. Managing critically ill patients with esmolol. An ultra short-acting Beta-adrenergic blocker. Chest. 1988;93:398–403.
12. Reach G, Thibonnier M, Chevillard C, Corvol P, Milliez P. Effect of labetalol on blood pressure and plasma catecholamine concentrations in patients with phaeochromocytoma. Br Med J. 1980;280:1300–1.
13. Van Stratum M, Levarlet M, Lambilliotte JP, Lignian H, De Rood M. Use of labetalol during anesthesia for pheochromocytoma removal. Acta Anaesthesiol Belg. 1983;34:233–40.
14. Yabe R, Suenaga K, Niimura S, Itoh N, Tani M, Kunii N, et al. Treatment of pheochromocytoma with dilevalol. J Med. 1987;18:147–52.
15. Briggs RS, Birtwell AJ, Pohl JE. Hypertensive response to labetalol in phaeochromocytoma. Lancet. 1978;1:1045–6.
16. Akiba M, Kodama T, Ito Y, Obara T, Fujimoto Y. Hypoglycemia induced by excessive rebound secretion of insulin after removal of pheochromocytoma. World J Surg. 1990;14:317–24.
17. Yamaguchi N. Sympathoadrenal system in neuroendocrine control of glucose: mechanisms involved in the liver, pancreas, and adrenal gland under hemorrhagic and hypoglycemic stress. Can J Physiol Pharmacol. 1992;70:167–206.
18. Steiner KE, Stevenson RW, Green DR, Cherrington AD. Mechanism of epinephrine's glycogenolytic effect in isolated canine hepatocytes. Metab Clin Exp. 1985;34:1020–3.
19. Ahrén B, Veith RC, Taborsky GJ. Sympathetic nerve stimulation versus pancreatic norepinephrine infusion in the dog: 1. Effects on basal release of insulin and glucagon. Endocrinology. 1987;21:323–31.
20. Porte D, Williams RH. Inhibition of insulin release by norepinephrine in man. Science. 1966;152:1248–50.

21. Ostenson CG, Cattaneo AG, Doxey JC, Efendic S. Alpha-adrenoceptors and insulin release from pancreatic islets of normal and diabetic rats. Am J Phys. 1989;257:439–43.
22. Ahrén B. Autonomic regulation of islet hormone secretion—implications for health and disease. Diabetologia. 2000;43:393–410.
23. Deibert DC, DeFronzo RA. Epinephrine-induced insulin resistance in man. J Clin Investig. 1980;65:717–21.
24. Wiesner TD, Blüher M, Windgassen M, Paschke R. Improvement of insulin sensitivity after adrenalectomy in patients with pheochromocytoma. J Clin Endocrinol Metab. 2003;88:3632–6.
25. Martin R, St. Pierre B, Moliner OR. Phaeochromocytoma and postoperative hypoglycaemia. Can Anaesth Soc J. 1979;26(4):260–2.
26. Meeke RI, O'Keefe JD, Gaffney JD. Phaeochromocytoma removal and postoperative hypoglycaemia. Anaesthesia. 1985;40(11):1093–6.
27. Kato Y, Saga Y, Hou K, Yamaguchi S, Hashimoto H, Kaneko S, Yachiku S. Postoperative hypoglycemia after resection of pheochromocytoma: a case report. Hinyokika Kiyo. 2004;50(7):479–83.
28. Plouin PF, Duclos JM, Soppelsa F, Boublil G, Chatellier G. Factors associated with perioperative morbidity and mortality in patients with pheochromocytoma: analysis of 165 operations at a single center. J Clin Endocrinol Metab. 2001;86:1480–6.
29. Chen Y, Hodin RA, Pandolfi C, Ruan DT, McKenzie TJ. Hypoglycemia after resection of pheochromocytoma. Surgery. 2014;156(6):1404–8.
30. Chernow B, Alexander HR, Smallridge RC, et al. Hormonal responses to graded surgical stress. Arch Intern Med. 1987;147:1273–8.
31. Tsujimoto G, Honda K, Hoffman BB, Hashimoto K. Desensitization of postjunctional alpha 1- and alpha 2-adrenergic receptor-mediated vasopressor responses in rat harboring pheochromocytoma. Circ Res. 1987;61:86–98.
32. Tsujimoto G, Manger WM, Hoffman BB. Desensitization of beta-adrenergic receptors by pheochromocytoma. Endocrinology. 1984;114:1272–8.
33. Cremer GM, Molnar GD, Taylor WF, et al. Studies of diabetic instability. II. Tests of insulinogenic reserve with infusions of arginine, glucagon, epinephrine, and saline. Metab Clin Exp. 1971;20:1083–98.
34. Costello GT, Moorthy SS, Vane DW, Dierdorf SF. Hypoglycemia following bilateral adrenalectomy for pheochromocytoma. Crit Care Med. 1988;16:562–3.
35. Pacak K, Eisenhofer G, Lenders JWM. Pheochromocytoma: diagnosis, localization, and treatment. Birmingham: Blackwell Pub; 2007.
36. Mannelli M. Management and treatment of pheochromocytomas and paragangliomas. Ann N Y Acad Sci. 2006;1073:405–16.
37. Yanaru T, Sugi Y, Higa K, Katori K, Shono S, Nitahara K. Postoperative profound hypoglycemia after resection of adrenaline-predominant pheochromocytoma. Masui. 2007;56(12):1419–21.
38. Guyatt GH, Oxman AD, Kunz R, Falck-Ytter Y, Vist GE, Liberati A, Schünemann HJ, GRADE Working Group. Going from evidence to recommendations. BMJ. 2008;336(7652):1049–51.
39. Guyatt GH, Oxman AD, Vist G, Kunz R, Brozek J, Alonso-Coello P, Montori V, Akl EA, Djulbegovic B, Falck-Ytter Y, Norris SL, Williams JW Jr, Atkins D, Meerpohl J, Schünemann HJ. GRADE guidelines: 4. Rating the quality of evidence-study limitations (risk of bias). J Clin Epidemiol. 2011;64(4):407–15.

Surgical Versus Nonsurgical Management of Malignant Pheochromocytoma

29

Mark S. Cohen and Travis M. Cotton

Abstract

Malignant pheochromocytomas and paragangliomas are rare. Resection of the primary tumor and metastatic lesions, when feasible, is recommended. Goals of resection include improvement of clinical symptoms, reduction of catecholamine excess, local disease control, improved efficacy of subsequent non-operative therapies, and the possibility of improved survival. A R0 or R1 resection clearly provides more robust biochemical improvement when compared to a R2 resection or 'surgical debulking.' Additional non-surgical therapies can be used in conjunction with surgery or as the primary treatment modality in some cases. Non-surgical local therapies include external beam radiation, percutaneous tumor ablation, and directed transarterial chemoembolization. In addition, systemic therapies include radioactive iodine meta-iodobenzylguanidine (^{131}I-MIBG), cytotoxic chemotherapy, and molecular targeted therapy. Care should be taken to provide patients with the appropriate pharmacologic adrenergic blockade prior to the initiation of most therapies. Patients benefit from a multidisciplinary approach at a center familiar with managing malignant pheochromocytoma patients.

Keywords

Malignant pheochromocytoma · Metastatic pheochromocytoma · Pheochromocytoma · ^{131}I-MIBG · External beam radiation therapy · Percutaneous

M. S. Cohen
Department of Surgery, Division of Endocrine Surgery, Taubman Center, Ann Arbor, MI, USA

T. M. Cotton (✉)
Department of Endocrine Surgery, Warren Alpert Medical School of Brown University, Providence, RI, USA

P. Angelos, R. H. Grogan (eds.), *Difficult Decisions in Endocrine Surgery*, Difficult Decisions in Surgery: An Evidence-Based Approach,
https://doi.org/10.1007/978-3-319-92860-9_29

tumor ablation · Transarterial chemoembolization · Cytotoxic chemotherapy · Targeted molecular therapy

Introduction

Translated from the Greek as "dark colored tumor cells," pheochromocytomas were first described in 1886 by Frankel and are functional neuroendocrine tumors that arise from chromaffin cells of the adrenal medulla which secrete catecholamines [1]. While quite rare in the general population, with an incidence of approximately 0.005%, there is evidence to suggest an incidence as high as 0.2% in hypertensive patients [2]. Though a majority of pheochromocytomas occur sporadically in the population, 25% can be familial in nature. Genetic mutations associated with the development of these tumors include mutations in VHL, RET, NF1, SDHB or SDHD genes and can be part of von-Hippel-Lindau disease, neurofibromatosis, familial paraganglioma, or the multiple endocrine neoplasia type 2 syndromes. Though mostly located within the adrenal medulla, extra-adrenal pheochromocytomas are well described and referred to as paragangliomas (Fig. 29.1).

The distinction between pheochromocytomas and paragangliomas is important to make as paragangliomas have different implications with regard to risk of malignancy, need for genetic testing, and other associated malignancies. Unlike pheochromocytomas, paragangliomas originate from paraganglia in *chromaffin-negative* glomus cells derived from the embryonic neural crest. While all paragangliomas contain neurosecretory granules, only a small percentage (1–3%) of cases secrete enough hormones (such as catecholamines) to be clinically significant. Most paragangliomas are benign in nature and 85% will develop in the abdomen, 12% in the chest, and 3% in the head and neck region (often as carotid body tumors, glomus

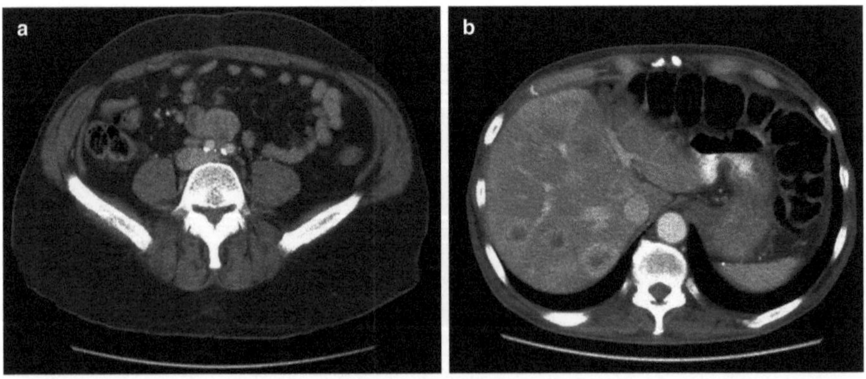

Fig. 29.1 (**a**) CT scan of the abdomen showing a malignant paraganglioma at the aortic bifurcation in a 59 year old male. (**b**) CT scan of liver in the same patient 3 years later showing evidence of metastatic disease

jugulare or globus tympaticum tumors in the middle ear). Given the variable locations of paragangliomas, care must be taken to properly identify and localize these tumors preoperatively.

The 'rule of 10s' has been a popular teaching pearl through the years and holds as a general way to characterize pheochromocytomas. The rule describes that: 10% are bilateral, 10% are extra-adrenal, 10% are familial, and 10% are malignant. With most pheochromocytomas being benign, cure can be achieved by surgical resection; however, malignant pheochromocytmas clearly exist. The diagnosis of malignancy with regard to pheochromocytomas can often be difficult to make. Even when equipped with preoperative imaging, intraoperative findings, and final histopathology, there can be uncertainty. The formal diagnosis of malignant pheochromocytoma requires evidence of metastases to non-chromaffin containing sites at a distant location from the primary tumor. Though local invasion certainly increases the likelihood of malignancy, invasiveness and malignancy are not necessarily associated in this disease. While evidence of metastatic disease is the most commonly accepted definition for a pheochromocytoma being malignant, case numbers are limited. As a result, some authors have included locally invasive tumors in their definition of malignancy.

Metastatic pheochromocytomas may be identified early at the time of initial diagnoses or later, often months to years, during surveillance following initial resection. Given the difficulty with histological confirmation of malignant disease, care must be taken to appropriately provide adequate long-term follow-up. Post-resection occurrences are typically found in the first 5 years but can surface 15 or more years postoperatively as noted by some reports [3]. Unfortunately, there is no effective cure for malignant pheochromocytoma; however, therapeutic interventions play an important role in its management. Treatment can provide the following benefits: decrease of disease burden, minimization of compression on nearby anatomic structures, improvement of symptoms, reduction of catecholamine excess, and potentially improved survival. Therapeutic options should be discussed in a multidisciplinary fashion involving surgeons, endocrinologists, radiologists, nuclear medicine specialists, pathologists, and oncologists. Though there is an array of treatment modalities, therapeutic strategies fall into two basic categories: surgical and non-surgical.

Surgical Therapy

Surgical resection offers the opportunity for remission, decreased biochemical activity, diminished local invasion, and the potential of improved survival. The primary goal of surgical treatment is resection of the primary tumor and, when possible, resection of local and distant metastasis. Data for the surgical management of malignant pheochromocytoma is limited; however, there are studies that can help guide surgeons through the decision-making process.

With regard to biochemical activity, Ellis et al. examined 42 patients following operative intervention for metastatic pheochromocytoma. Patients were stratified in terms of disease extent and degree of operative resection. They found that patients with only intra-abdominal disease (local invasion and metastatic disease confined within the abdominal cavity) were significantly more likely to achieve biochemical response than patients with extra-abdominal disease (74.1% vs 20%, $p = 0.0009$). In addition, patients with only intra-abdominal disease had a substantially more durable response with approximately 40% maintaining a biochemical improvement 5 years postoperatively.

Degree of surgical resection was also found to be an important variable. In patients with a R0/R1 resection, the mean reduction in biochemical value was 70.1% compared to a R2 resection at 12.9%. Additionally, approximately 60% of patients with a R0/R1 resection achieved a biochemical response at 3 years compared to less than 5% of the R2 patient group [4]. Khorram-Manesh et al. provided a series of four patients with metastatic pheochromocytoma who underwent resection. Two patients had locally metastatic disease and both were alive 11 years post-resection—one with disease and one disease-free. The other two patients with distant disease died five and 23 years post-resection [5]. Wan et al. compiled a series of three patients who underwent resection of malignant pheochromocytoma. The first patient had widely metastatic disease to the liver, lung and bone. Due to pain of the liver, a right hepatectomy and adrenalectomy was performed. The patient died of disease progression 1 year later. A second patient had disease invading the retro-hepatic venacava as well as distant metastasis to the lung. Radical resection of the retrocaval disease resulted in a postoperative death 4 days following surgery. A third patient presented with metastatic disease to the pleura and paratracheal nodes in the right chest. A right adrenalectomy and thoracic resection of all visual disease was performed successfully in the form of a R1 resection. Two years postoperatively, the patient had small stable disease in the right lung but was symptom free and required no medical therapy for symptom control [6]. Noda et al. reported a case of a R0 hepatic resection of metastatic pheochromocytoma with good results. The patient was disease free and asymptomatic 3 years postoperatively [7]. Mishra et al. reported a case of locally metastatic bilateral pheochromocytoma. Following a R0 resection, the patient had no biochemical or radiographic evidence of recurrence. Interestingly, the patient had evidence of catecholamine induced cardiomyopathy preoperatively. Following resection and biochemical normalization, the patient's ejection improved from 26% preoperatively to 68% at 3 years postop [8].

Although such data is limited to very small case-series, there remains supportive evidence to offer patients metastatic resection to improve symptoms and potentially survival if a R0 or R1 resection is achieved. Resection may offer biochemical improvement, symptom improvement, prevent local invasion of surrounding structures, and possibly contribute to the efficacy of future non-operative therapies. The goal should be for a R0 or R1 resection if possible, as general debulking is unlikely to provide durable biochemical improvement. Additionally, there is some data to support that improvement in symptoms and survival can be achieved if a R0/R1 resection is performed and the metastatic disease is confined to the abdomen. Surgery for malignant pheochromocytomas can be difficult at times and often requires en-bloc resection resulting in significant morbidity and mortality. As such, advanced operative resources and surgical expertise is necessary and should be provided by centers with experience in taking care of patients with pheochromocytomas. Though not outlined in this chapter, preoperative pharmacologic management should be in place to minimize the risk of complications during surgery such as hypertensive crisis. Most centers use alpha blockade (i.e phenoxybenzamine) titrated to the point of orthostasis, followed by beta-blockade to avoid tachyarrythmias resulting from unopposed alpha blockade.

To our knowledge, no clinical trials exist which specifically evaluate survival in patients with malignant pheochromocytoma. In general, overall 5-year survival is thought to range between 30 and 50%. The course, however, can be highly variable with extra-abdominal metastatic disease carrying a worse prognosis [9–13]. Huang et al. showed a possible survival benefit to resection while following ten patients for a median of 5.5 years. One patient continues to survive 10 years following resection of metastatic disease in the bone and lung [14]. While a laparoscopic approach is typically preferred in patients with a suspected benign pheochromocytoma, this should not be the approach when a malignant pheochromocytoma is known or suspected. Rather, an open approach should be considered to provide the best chance of a R0 or R1 resection along with appropriate regional lympadenectomy. Violation of the capsule likely increases the incidence of recurrence and should be avoided when possible. In contrast to benign disease, malignant pheochromocytomas are often difficult to fully remove and require a skilled and experience surgeon [15–17]. In summary, complete resection of the primary tumor, as well as metastatic disease, should be performed when possible.

Non-operative Therapy

Aside from surgical resection, potential 'non-operative' therapies can be categorized as local therapy or systemic therapy for the treatment of malignant pheochromocytoma. Local therapies include external beam radiation, percutaneous tumor ablation, and directed transarterial chemoembolization. Systemic therapies include cytotoxic chemotherapy, radionucleotide (^{131}I-MIBG), and molecular targeted therapy. Many non-operative treatment modalities are used synchronously to various degrees with other treatment modalities and are difficult to isolate in such a small patient population as being solely beneficial. While often not curative, these therapies can assist with palliation of symptoms. Though non-operative, care should be taken in providing appropriate pre-therapy pharmacologic treatment to avoid complications such as hypertensive crisis and stroke.

One of the more commonly utilized systemic treatment modalities is ^{131}I-MIBG. ^{131}I-MIBG is an analogue of norepinephrine which is found sequestered in chromaffin cells' neurosecretory granules. Thus, ^{131}I-MIBG's efficacy is contingent upon its uptake by malignant pheochromocytoma cells. This uptake can typically be proven on ^{123}I-MIBG scintigraphy. Unfortunately, only approximately 60% of malignant pheochromocytoma tumors display MIBG-uptake [18, 19]. This number falls with previously radiated tumor sites, bone metastasis, or previous treatment with chemotherapy. As such, MIBG is a much less effective therapy in the setting of bone metastases. Gredik et al. found that 47% of patients treated with ^{131}I-MIBG therapy displayed objective radiographic tumor response with survival time between objective responders and non-responders being different, but not statistically significant at 72 months vs 26 months respectively ($p = 0.537$). Eight of 12 patients (67%) that were evaluated for biochemical improvement showed response to therapy. In addition, subjective symptom improvement was seen in 16 of 18 patients (89%) [20]. Safford et al. studied ^{131}I-MIBG therapy in 22 patients and showed an objective radiographic tumor response in 38%; however, response in of itself did not predict survival improvement. Sixty percent of the patients had a significant reduction in catecholamine levels and 86% had symptomatic improvement. Though radiographic tumor response did not correlate with survival benefit, a decrease in catecholamine levels along with a decrease in symptoms was associated with an increase in median survival [21]. Gonias et al. studied 49 patients treated with ^{131}I-MIBG and found an overall radiographic response rate of 63%. Contradictory to Safford et al. Gonias found radiographic response to be an indicator of improved survival and did not find biochemical functionality or patient symptoms to correlate [22]. Though certainly not effective in treating all tumor presentations, those that respond to ^{131}I-MIBG targeted therapy demonstrate a reasonable radiographic decrease in tumor burden, decrease in tumor functionality, and improvement of symptoms. As such, ^{131}I-MIBG therapy remains an important palliative tool in the treatment of malignant pheochromocytoma. Potential safety issues and side effects associated with MIBG include vomiting, nausea, pulmonary toxicity, hypertensive crisis, as well as hematologic and thyroid dysfunction. Patients with a high tumor burden of malignant pheochromocytoma that is unresectable, progressive in

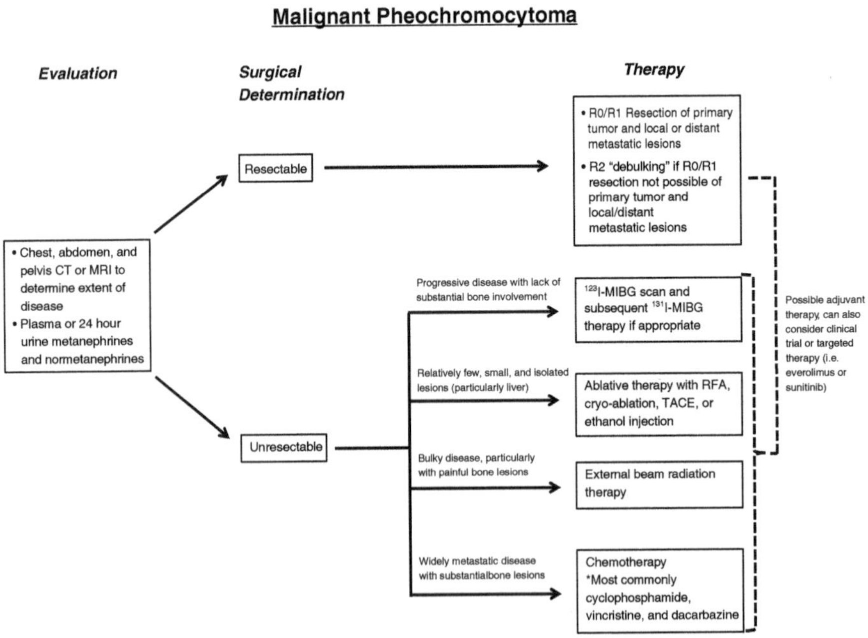

Fig. 29.2 Treatment algorithm for resectable and unresectable malignant pheochromocytoma

nature, lacks substantial bony metastases, and displays MIBG uptake are optimal candidates for ^{131}I-MIBG therapy [23] (Fig. 29.2).

Directed therapies have also been utilized in the treatment of malignant pheochromocytoma. Radiation therapy, ablative therapy, and transarterial chemoembolization are modes of treatment used to assist with both local and distant control. External beam radiation therapy (EBRT) was originally thought to be relatively ineffective for the treatment of malignant pheochromocytoma; however, more recent data suggests that it can have beneficial results giving it resurgence. Fishbein et al. evaluated 17 patients who received a median total dose of 40 Gy in 17 fractions. This study, contrasted with smaller radiation dose studies of the past, employed a higher radiation dose which was felt to contribute to its success. Five of the 17 patients (29%) were also treated with ^{131}I-MIBG therapy. In this subgroup, the areas that were irradiated showed a durable objective response despite experiencing out of field progression of disease. Thus, EBRT can possibly be useful in controlling bulky disease when high doses of radiation are employed (>40 Gy) [24]. The predominant toxicity was due to irradiation of normal tissues adjacent to the field most commonly resulting in nausea and diarrhea. There were no significant episodes of hematologic toxicity in those treated.

Ablative therapy is also being used in the treatment of malignant pheochromocytoma. These techniques, which include radiofrequency ablation (RFA), cryo-ablation, and percutaneous ethanol injection, are best applied to patients with relatively few isolated metastatic lesions. McBride et al. studied ten patients with metastatic pheochromocytoma who received percutaneous ablation. In this group, 47 lesions with an approximate mean tumor size of 2.5 cm were treated within the liver, bone, and retroperitoneum. Liver lesions were treated with RFA or ethanol injection whereas bone and retroperitoneal lesions were treated with either RFA or cryo-ablation. Twenty-seven of the ablated lesions received follow-up imaging that was available for review at a mean interval of 3.7 months. Fifteen of the 27 lesions (56%) in this subgroup were successfully ablated with no evidence of radiographic recurrence [25]. While clearly not a cure, ablative therapy can help control relatively small and discrete local disease. Complications were minimal though one death was recorded as the result of an iatrogenic bowel perforation. For those liver lesions not amendable to local minimally invasive ablation or surgical resection, transarterial chemoembolization (TACE) can be considered and has been shown to be beneficial in several case reports [25–28]. Side effects of this therapy include bleeding, liver injury or infarction, liver failure, systemic absorption of chemotherapy, and vascular injury.

When surgical resection, MIBG, or local treatments are not appropriate options, systemic chemotherapy can be utilized in the treatment of malignant pheochromocytoma. Combination chemotherapy with variations of cyclophosphamide, vincristine, and dacarbazine (CVD) are the most commonly used and well-described regimens. Tanabe et al. evaluated 17 patients with malignant pheochromocytoma receiving chemotherapy. Eight patients (47%) had a partial radiographic response to therapy with five patients (29%) progressing despite treatment. Eight patients (47%) had a complete or partial biochemical response as well. Significant predictors of responsiveness to chemotherapy were found to include younger age and increased time between the diagnosis of pheochromocytoma and the detection of malignant disease. Kaplan-Meier analysis showed that 50% survival was approximately 6 years in patients showing a biochemical and/or radiographic tumor response to treatment, approximately 4 years in patients with no significant change in tumor response, and approximately 3 years in those with continued deterioration of biochemical and tumor responses [29]. Ayala-Ramirez et al. evaluated 52 patients with malignant pheochromocytoma receiving chemotherapy. Thirteen patients (25%) had radiographic response to therapy with eight patients (15%) showing evidence of symptom improvement with normalization of blood pressure [30]. Huang et al. evaluated 18 patients with malignant pheochromocytoma receiving CVD therapy. Ten patients (55%) had a complete or partial objective radiographic response to therapy. All of the patients who responded reported improvement in their symptoms and had objective improvements in blood pressure control. Kaplan-Meier analysis showed that 50% survival was approximately 4 years in responders and approximately 3 years in non-responders [31]. Given the potential for radiographic response, biochemical improvement, and improved survival, chemotherapy should be considered for patients with progressive unresectable disease. It is particularly favorable (when compared to MIBG) in patients with substantial metastatic bone disease. Though chemotherapy can improve patients' biochemistry and symptoms, it can occasionally cause catecholamine excess complication during therapy. It is advised to control symptoms by pharmacologic means prior to initiation of therapy.

Lastly, the newest treatment opportunities have come from the development of targeted therapeutics. In malignant pheochromocytomas, few investigative studies using molecular targeted therapies exist and the ones that have been performed show mixed results. Case series comprising 11 patients treated with everolimus exhibited no significant response to targeted therapy. In one series, five of seven patients did display evidence of disease stabilization; unfortunately, there was no evidence of regression [32, 33]. The largest study examining molecular targeted therapies was performed by Ayala-Ramirez et al. Their group of 14 patients with rapidly progressive malignant pheochromocytoma was treated with sunitinib. Three of the 14 patients (21%) had a partial response and five (36%) had no disease progression. In addition, 43% of the patients had their blood pressure under control and some patients were able to discontinue their antihypertensive medications all together. The median overall survival in the group was 27 months [34]. Additional trials are currently under way to further understand the potential benefits of sunitinib and other molecular targeted therapies.

Recommendations

In summary, malignant pheochromocytoma is a rare condition that carries a poor prognosis. Complete resection of the primary tumor as well as any metastatic lesions should be performed, if possible, to improve symptoms, decrease catecholamine excess, and possibly improve survival. There is a clear difference in outcome between a R0/R1 resection and a R2 resection as 'debulking' operations have not been proven to be effective in isolation of additional therapy. Preoperative decision-making should ideally involve a multidisciplinary team and surgery should be performed by an experience surgeon at a center familiar with managing pheochromocytomas. Such centers should have appropriate OR equipment and anesthesia staff to handle these complex cases. If resection cannot be achieved, additional treatment options include local therapies (external beam radiation, percutaneous ablation, and chemoembolization) as well as systemic therapies (^{131}I-MIBG, chemotherapy, and sunitinib). Systemic therapies can be used as a primary treatment modality in some patients or as adjuvant therapy following surgical resection in others. Regardless of the therapy employed, care should be taken to prepare patients appropriately with pre-treatment pharmacologic therapy to avoid hypertensive crisis or other complications.

References

1. Fränkel F. Ein fall von doppelseitigen vollig latent verlaufen nebennierentumor und gleichseitiger nephritis mit veranderungen am circulation sappart und retinitis. Virchows Arch A. 1886;103:244.
2. Pederson LC, Lee JE. Pheochromocytoma: Current Treat Options. Oncology. 2003;4(4):329–37.
3. Tanka S, Ito T, Tomoda J, Higashi T, Yamada G, Tsuji T. Malignant pheochromocytoma with hepatic metastasis diagnosed 20 years after resection of the primary adrenal lesion. Intern Med. 1993;32:789–94.
4. Ellis RJ, Patel D, Prodanov T, Sadowski S, Nilubol N, Adams K, Steinberg SM, Pacak K, Kebebew E. Response after surgical resection of metastatic pheochromocytoma and paraganglioma: can postoperative biochemical remission be predicted? J Am Coll Surg. 2013;217(3):489–96.
5. Khorram-Manesh A, Ahlman H, Nilsson O, Friberg P, Odén A, Stenström G, Hansson G, Stenquist O, Wängberg B, Tisell LE, Jansson S, Khorram-Manesh A, Ahlman H, Nilsson O, Friberg P, Odén A, Stenström G, Hansson G, Stenquist O, Wängberg B, Tisell LE, Jansson S. Long-term outcome of a large series of patients surgically treated for pheochromocytoma. J Intern Med. 2005;258(1):55–66.
6. Wan WH, Tan KY, Ng C, Tay KH, Mancer K, Tay MH, Chia WK, Soo KC, Ooi LL. Metastatic malignant phaeochromocytoma: a rare entity that underlies a therapeutic quandary. Asian J Surg. 2006;29(4):294–302.
7. Noda T, Nagano H, Miyamoto A, Wada H, Murakami M, Kobayashi S, Marubashi S, Takeda Y, Dono K, Umeshita K, Wakasa K, Monden M. Successful outcome after resection of liver metastasis arising from an extraadrenal retroperitoneal paraganglioma that appeared 9 years after surgical excision of the primary lesion. Int J Clin Oncol. 2009;14(5):473–7.
8. Mishra AK, Agarwal G, Kapoor A, Agarwal A, Bhatia E, Mishra SK. Catecholamine cardiomyopathy in bilateral malignant pheochromocytoma: successful reversal after surgery. Int J Cardiol. 2000;76(1):89–90.
9. Proye C, Vix M, Goropoulos A, Kerlo P, Lecomte-Houcke M. High incidence of malignant pheochromocytoma in a surgical unit. 26 cases out of 100 patients operated from 1971 to 1991. J Endocrinol Investig. 1992;15(9):651–63.
10. Mahoney EM, Harrison JH. Malignant pheochromocytoma: clinical course and treatment. J Urol. 1977;118(2):225–9.
11. Guo JZ, Gong LS, Chen SX, Luo BY, Xu MY. Malignant pheochromocytoma: diagnosis and treatment in fifteen cases. J Hypertens. 1989;7:261–6.
12. Yoshida S, Hatori M, Noshiro T, Kimura N, Kokubun S. Twenty-six-years' survival with multiple bone metastasis of malignant pheochromocytoma. Arch Orthop Trauma Surg. 2001;121:598–600.

13. Pacak K, Eisenhofer G, Ahlman H, et al. Pheochromocytoma: recommendations for clinical practice from the first international symposium. Nat Clin Pract Endocrinol Metab. 2007;3(2):92–102.
14. Huang KH, Chung SD, Chen SC, Chueh SC, Pu YS, Lai MK, Lin WC. Clinical and pathological data of 10 malignant pheochromocytomas: long-term follow up in a single institute. Int J Urol. 2007;14(3):181–5.
15. Joseph L. Malignant pheochromocytoma of the organ of Zuckerkandl with functioning metastases. Br J Urol. 1967;39:221–5.
16. Brauckhoff M, Gimm O, Dralle H. Preoperative and surgical therapy in sporadic and familial pheochromocytoma. Front Horm Res. 2004;31:121–44.
17. Adjallé R, Plouin PF, Pacak K, Lehnert H. Treatment of malignant pheochromocytoma. Horm Metab Res. 2009;41(9):687–96.
18. Pacak K, Ilias I, Adams KT, Eisenhofer G. Biochemical diagnosis, localization and management of pheochromocytoma: focus on multiple endocrine neoplasia type 2 in relation to other hereditary syndromes and sporadic forms of the toumour. J Intern Med. 2005;257:60–8.
19. van der Harst E, de Herder WW, Bruining HA, Bonjer HJ, de Krijger RR, Lamberts SW, van de Meiracker AH, Boomsma F, Stijnen T, Krenning EP, Bosman FT, Kwekkeboom DJ. [(123)I] metaiodobenzylguanidine and [(111)in]octreotide uptake in begnign and malignant pheochromocytomas. J Clin Endocrinol Metab. 2001;86(2):685–93.
20. Gedik GK, Hoefnagel CA, Bais E, Olmos RA. 131I-MIBG therapy in metastatic phaeochromocytoma and paraganglioma. Eur J Nucl Med Mol Imaging. 2008;35(4):725–33.
21. Safford SD, Coleman RE, Gockerman JP, Moore J, Feldman JM, Leight GS Jr, Tyler DS, Olson JA Jr. Iodine -131 metaiodobenzylguanidine is an effective treatment for malignant pheochromocytoma and paraganglioma. Surgery. 2003;134(6):956–62. discussion 962-3.
22. Gonias S, Goldsby R, Matthay KK, Hawkins R, Price D, Huberty J, Damon L, Linker C, Sznewajs A, Shiboski S, Fitzgerald P. Phase II study of high-dose [131I]metaiodobenzylguanidine therapy for patients with metastatic pheochromocytoma and paraganglioma. J Clin Oncol. 2009;27(25):4162–8.
23. Baudin E, Habra MA, Deschamps F, Cote G, Dumont F, Cabanillas M, Arfi-Roufe J, Berdelou A, Moon B, Al Ghuzlan A, Patel S, Leboulleux S, Jimenez C. Therapy of endocrine disease: treatment of malignant pheochromocytoma and paraganglioma. Eur J Endocrinol. 2014;171(3):R111–22.
24. Fishbein L, Bonner L, Torigian DA, Nathanson KL, Cohen DL, Pryma D, Cengel KA. External beam radiation therapy (EBRT) for patients with malignant pheochromocytoma and non-head and -neck paraganglioma: combination with 131I-MIBG. Horm Metab Res. 2012;44(5):405–10.
25. McBride JF, Atwell TD, Charboneau WJ, Young WF Jr, Wass TC, Callstrom MR. Minimally invasive treatment of metastatic pheochromocytoma and paraganglioma: efficacy and safety of radiofrequency ablation and cryoablation therapy. J Vasc Interv Radiol. 2011;22(9):1263–70.
26. Hidaka S, Hiraoka A, Ochi H, Uehara T, Ninomiya T, Miyamoto Y, Hasebe A, Tanihira T, Tanabe A, Ichiryu M, Nakahara H, Tazuya N, Ninomiya I, Michitaka K. Malignant pheochromocytoma with liver metastasis treated by transcatheter arterial chemo-embolization (TACE). Intern Med. 2010;49(7):645–51.
27. Takahashi K, Ashizawa N, Minami T, Suzuki S, Sakamoto I, Hayashi K, Tomiyasu S, Sumikawa K, Kitamura K, Eto T, Yano K. Malignant pheochromocytoma with multiple hepatic metastases treated by chemotherapy and transcatheter arterial embolization. Intern Med. 1999;38(4):349–54.
28. Watanabe D, Tanabe A, Naruse M, Tsuiki M, Torii N, Noshiro T, Takano K. Transcatheter arterial embolization for the treatment of liver metastases in a patient with malignant pheochromocytoma. Endocr J. 2006;53(1):59–66.
29. Tanabe A, Naruse M, Nomura K, Tsuiki M, Tsumagari A, Ichihara A. Combination chemotherapy with cyclophosphamide, vincristine,and dacarbazine in patients with malignant pheochromocytoma and paraganglioma. Horm Cancer. 2013;4(2):103–10.

30. Ayala-Ramirez M, Feng L, Habra MA, Rich T, Dickson PV, Perrier N, Phan A, Waguespack S, Patel S, Jimenez C. Clinical benefits of systemic chemotherapy for patients with metastatic pheochromocytomas or sympathetic extra-adrenal paragangliomas: insights from the largest single-institutional experience. Cancer. 2012;118(11):2804–12.
31. Huang H, Abraham J, Hung E, Averbuch S, Merino M, Steinberg SM, Pacak K, Fojo T. Treatment of malignant pheochromocytoma/paraganglioma with cyclophosphamide, vincristine, and dacarbazine: recommendation from a 22-year follow-up of 18 patients. Cancer. 2008;113(8):2020–8.
32. Druce MR, Kaltsas GA, Fraenkel M, Gross DJ, Grossman AB. Novel and evolving therapies in the treatment of malignant phaeochromocytoma: experience with the mTOR inhibitor everolimus. Horm Metab Res. 2009;41(9):697–702.
33. Oh DY, Kim TW, Park YS, Shin SJ, Shin SH, Song EK, Lee HJ, Lee KW, Bang YJ. Phase 2 study of everolimus monotherapy in patients with nonfunctioning neuroendocrine tumors or pheochromocytomas/paragangliomas. Cancer. 2012;118(24):6162.
34. Ayala-Ramirez M, Chougnet CN, Habra MA, Palmer JL, Leboulleux S, Cabanillas ME, Caramella C, Anderson P, Al Ghuzlan A, Waguespack SG, Deandreis D, Baudin E, Jimenez C. Treatment with sunitinib for patients with progressive metastatic pheochromocytomas and sympathetic paragangliomas. J Clin Endocrinol Metab. 2012;97(11):4040–50.

Alpha Blocker Versus Calcium Channel Blocker for Pheochromocytoma

30

Elizabeth Holt, Jennifer Malinowski,
and Glenda G. Callender

Abstract

The perioperative management of patients undergoing surgical resection of pheochromocytoma is essential to good outcomes. Historically high mortality rates associated with surgery have been mitigated by perioperative management of hemodynamics. Several options exist for the preoperative medical blockade of patients with catecholamine-producing tumors, including non-selective alpha-receptor blockers, selective $alpha_1$-receptor blockers, and calcium channel blockers. In this chapter, we summarize the available data and provide recommendations for the optimal preoperative medical management of patients undergoing surgical resection of pheochromocytoma.

Keywords

Pheochromocytoma · Paraganglioma · Hemodynamic stability · Blood pressure control · Alpha blocker · Beta blocker · Calcium channel blocker

Introduction

Patients undergoing surgical resection of pheochromocytoma require careful preoperative preparation in order to prevent the potentially life-threatening cardiovascular catastrophes that can occur as a result of excess catecholamine secretion during

E. Holt
Department of Internal Medicine, Yale University School of Medicine, New Haven, CT, USA

J. Malinowski · G. G. Callender (✉)
Department of Surgery, Yale University School of Medicine, New Haven, CT, USA
e-mail: glenda.callender@yale.edu

P. Angelos, R. H. Grogan (eds.), *Difficult Decisions in Endocrine Surgery*, Difficult Decisions in Surgery: An Evidence-Based Approach,
https://doi.org/10.1007/978-3-319-92860-9_30

surgery, including hypertensive crisis, cardiac arrhythmia, myocardial infarction, stroke, pulmonary edema, and death. The first successful operations for pheochromocytoma were performed in 1926, by César Roux in Lausanne, Switzerland, and by Charles Mayo in Rochester, Minnesota [1]. By 1951, 125 operations for pheochromocytoma had been performed, with a mortality rate of 26% [2]. In 1956, James Priestley and colleagues at the Mayo Clinic reported a dramatic decrease in intraoperative mortality that accompanied their use of preoperative and intraoperative vasoactive medications for blood pressure control: 61 pheochromocytomas were removed from 51 patients without operative mortality [3]. Today, surgical resection of pheochromocytoma is associated with perioperative mortality of less than 3% and intraoperative mortality of less than 1% [4, 5].

Preoperative medical blockade is one of the fundamental principles of the perioperative management of patients undergoing surgical resection of pheochromocytoma. Patients must undergo some form of preoperative medical blockade to prevent massive catecholamine release on induction of anesthesia or upon manipulation of the tumor, prior to ligation of the adrenal vein. Historically, the non-selective alpha-adrenergic blocker phenoxybenzamine has been used for preoperative preparation of patients with pheochromocytoma. Phenoxybenzamine allows intravascular volume expansion and blocks alpha-adrenergic receptors noncompetitively, which means that catecholamines released by the tumor cannot overcome the blocking effect, at least in theory [6]. However, phenoxybenzamine produces substantial reflex tachycardia and orthostatic hypotension. Dose adjustments must be made slowly, and because the half-life is 24 h, a prolonged hypotensive state can occur following resection of the catecholamine-producing tumor [7]. Selective $alpha_1$-receptor antagonists, such as the oral agents doxazosin, prazosin and terazosin, and the intravenous agent urapidil, have been utilized with greater frequency in recent years in order to circumvent some of the disadvantages of phenoxybenzamine. Although they are competitive blockers of alpha-adrenergic receptors, they do not affect presynaptic $alpha_2$-receptors, and thus they do not enhance norepinephrine release and produce reflex tachycardia. In addition, the half-lives of prazosin, terazosin and urapidil are substantially shorter than that of phenoxybenzamine (2–3, 12 and 2–5 h respectively; the half-life of doxazosin is 22 h), which allows more rapid dose adjustment and decreases the duration of postoperative hypotension [7]. Calcium channel blockers, such as nifedipine and nicardipine, have also been utilized with increasing frequency in the preoperative management of pheochromocytoma. These agents lower blood pressure by inhibiting norepinephrine-mediated release of intracellular calcium and transmembrane calcium influx in vascular smooth muscle, thereby relaxing arteriolar smooth muscle and decreasing peripheral vascular resistance [8]. The half-lives of nifedipine and nicardipine are 0.2–1 and 6–8 h, respectively [9]. The theoretical advantages of calcium channel blockers include less orthostatic hypotension, and prevention of catecholamine-induced coronary vasospasm [7].

Although several options exist for preoperative medical blockade of patients undergoing resection of pheochromocytoma, there are no clear guidelines as to which regimen is optimal. There exists no level one evidence (i.e. data from a randomized, controlled trial) to support the use of any specific agent over another, or even to support the practice of preoperative medical blockade as opposed to no preoperative medical blockade. To date, three sets of clinical practice guidelines for the management of pheochromocytoma have been published: guidelines from the First International Symposium on Pheochromocytoma in 2007, the North American Neuroendocrine Tumor Society (NANETS) in 2010, and the Endocrine Society in 2014 [10–12]. All three sets of guidelines state that preoperative medical blockade is recommended prior to resection of pheochromocytoma and that non-selective alpha-adrenergic blockers, selective $alpha_1$-receptor blockers, and calcium channel blockers are all acceptable options. The purpose of this chapter is to summarize the available data and provide recommendations for the optimal preoperative medical management of patients undergoing surgical resection of pheochromocytoma.

Search Strategy

Current guidelines related to the preoperative management of patients with pheochromocytoma were reviewed. A comprehensive review of the literature was performed in the PubMed database using the following keywords and medical subject headings (MeSH): pheochromocytoma, paraganglioma, hemodynamic stability, blood pressure control, alpha blocker, beta blocker, calcium channel blocker, phenoxybenzamine, dibenzyline, doxazosin, prazosin, cardura, phentolamine, regitine, oraverse, minipress, tolazoline, isoprenaline, isuprel, dexmedetomidine, propanalol, and nifedipine. The initial PubMed search returned 541 articles. The search was then limited to articles in the English language that involved human subjects, were published in the past 30 years, were not case reports, and for which a review of the abstract suggested that they would be applicable to the current question. Of specific interest were articles that directly compared outcomes following different preoperative medical blockade regimens. The quality of each study was determined using the Grades of Recommendation, Assessment, Development, and Evaluation (GRADE) criteria [13]. A total of 73 articles were reviewed critically and 18 articles met inclusion criteria for the analysis performed for this chapter.

No Preoperative Medical Blockade Versus Preoperative Medical Blockade

A total of five articles were identified that addressed the question of whether or not preoperative medical blockade is necessary prior to surgical resection of pheochromocytoma [14–18]. Four are retrospective reviews and one is a prospective case-control study. See Table 30.1.

Stenström et al. [14] reported a retrospective review of a series of 62 patients: 51 patients received phenoxybenzamine (eight of these also received a beta blocker for reflex tachycardia), and 11 patients received no preoperative medical blockade. The different regimens were prescribed based on provider choice. There was a statistically significant reduction in the incidence of intraoperative excessive blood

Table 30.1 Summary of the studies evaluating preoperative medical blockade versus no preoperative medical blockade in patients undergoing surgical resection of pheochromocytoma

Study/Year	Number of patients in each arm		Results favor	Quality of evidence
	Preoperative medical blockade	No preoperative medical blockade		
Stenström et al. (1985) [14]	51	11	Preoperative medical blockade	Low
Boutros et al. (1990) [15]	34	29	No difference	Low
Steinsapir et al. (1997) [16]	27	7	Preoperative medical blockade	Low
Ulchaker et al. (1999) [17]	70% of 113 patients	30% of 113 patients	No difference	Low
Shao et al. (2011) [18]	38	21	No difference (normotensive pheo)	Low

pressure variation in the group treated with phenoxybenzamine, although 69% of the patients treated with phenoxybenzamine still experienced intraoperative systolic blood pressure measurements above 175 mmHg. The authors recommended that all patients with pheochromocytoma be treated preoperatively with an alpha-adrenergic receptor blocker.

Boutros et al. [15] reported a retrospective review of a series of 60 patients who underwent 63 resections of pheochromocytoma: 6 patients received phenoxybenzamine, 28 patients received prazosin (thus, a total of 34 patients received alpha-adrenergic blockade), and 29 patients received no preoperative medical treatment. The different regimens were prescribed based on provider choice. There was no difference between groups in the percent of patients that required intravenous sodium nitroprusside or nitroglycerin intraoperatively to reduce blood pressure, and no patient experienced stroke or myocardial infarction. The authors concluded that patients can safely undergo surgical resection of pheochromocytoma without preoperative alpha blockade.

Steinsapir et al. [16] reported a retrospective review of a series of 34 patients: 6 patients received phenoxybenzamine, 14 patients received phenoxybenzamine and the catecholamine synthesis blocker metyrosine, 6 patients received prazosin and metyrosine, 1 patient received nifedipine and metyrosine, and 7 patients received no preoperative medical blockade. The different regimens were prescribed based on provider choice. Among the patients who received metyrosine as part of their preoperative medical blockade, 95% did not require intraoperative pressors, compared to only 50% in the group that received phenoxybenzamine alone. Among the patients that received metyrosine, 81% did not require intraoperative phentolamine to reduce blood pressure, whereas phentolamine was not required in only 33% and 29% of patients who received phenoxybenzamine alone and no preoperative medical blockade, respectively. Two patients in the group that received no preoperative medical blockade died from hypertensive crisis. The authors concluded that a preoperative treatment regimen including an alpha blocker and metyrosine is necessary in order to reduce surgical morbidity in patients with pheochromocytoma.

Ulchaker et al. [17] reported a retrospective review of a series of 113 patients: 70% of patients received preoperative medical blockade with a combination of alpha blockade (phenoxybenzamine or a selective alpha$_1$-receptor blocker), and/or a calcium channel blocker, and a beta blocker when necessary (exact regimens not specified) and 30% of patients received no preoperative medical blockade (no preoperative blockade was routine if patients were normotensive preoperatively). Different regimens were prescribed based on provider choice and were observed to change over time with respect to method of preoperative fluid expansion and medication choice. There was no statistically significant difference in the intraoperative mean blood pressure between groups. The group of patients that received no preoperative medical blockade required less fluid in the perioperative period. Major cardiovascular complications occurred in 6 patients (pulmonary edema in 3, congestive heart failure in 2, and stroke in 1), all of whom were in the group that received preoperative medical blockade. The authors concluded that preoperative alpha blockade is not necessary prior to surgical resection of pheochromocytoma.

Shao et al. [18] reported a prospective case-control study of 66 patients undergoing resection of adrenal incidentaloma highly suspected to be normotensive pheochromocytoma. Patients were consented and given the option of undergoing preoperative medical blockade with doxazosin versus no preoperative medical blockade. Final pathology revealed pheochromocytoma in 59 patients; of these, 38 received preoperative doxazosin and 21 patients received no preoperative medical blockade. There were no differences found between groups in intraoperative blood pressure and heart rate, and the group that received preoperative doxazosin required more intraoperative nitroglycerin, norepinephrine, phentolamine and colloid fluid. The authors concluded that there is no benefit to preoperative alpha blockade in patients undergoing resection of normotensive pheochromocytoma.

Recommendation

Some evidence exists that preoperative medical blockade may not be necessary prior to resection of pheochromocytoma. These data are strongest for patients who are normotensive preoperatively. However, existing studies have small sample sizes and likely lack sufficient power to detect a difference between preoperative medical blockade and no preoperative medical blockade even if a true difference exists. Therefore, we recommend that all hypertensive patients receive preoperative medical blockade in order to avoid the unpredictable but potentially catastrophic consequences of massive catecholamine release. We recommend that preoperative medical blockade be considered in patients who are normotensive preoperatively, although it may be safe in this patient population to proceed to surgery without preoperative medical blockade.

Preoperative Non-selective Alpha Blockade Versus Preoperative Selective Alpha$_1$ Blockade

A total of 11 articles were identified that compared non-selective alpha-adrenergic blockade to selective alpha$_1$-receptor blockade [19–29]. All are retrospective reviews. See Table 30.2.

Havlik et al. [19] reported a retrospective review of a series of 18 patients who underwent 19 operations: 9 patients received phenoxybenzamine and 6 patients received prazosin (4 patients received no preoperative medical blockade and were excluded from analysis). The different regimens were prescribed based on provider preference. There was no difference between groups in perioperative fluid requirements or intraoperative hemodynamic stability. The authors concluded that either non-selective or selective alpha$_1$-adrenergic blockade is adequate prior to resection of pheochromocytoma.

Russell et al. [20] reported a retrospective review of a series of 14 patients: 12 patients received phenoxybenzamine, and 2 patients received prazosin and labetalol. The different regimens were prescribed based on provider choice. Although the sample size was very small, the authors reported that the intraoperative hemodynamic stability of the patients who received phenoxybenzamine was superior to that of the patients who received prazosin and labetalol.

Kocak et al. [21] reported a retrospective review of a series of 49 patients: 21 patients received phenoxybenzamine, 11 patients received prazosin, and 17 patients received doxazosin. The different regimens were prescribed based on institutional protocol (phenoxybenzamine was routinely used prior to 1994; prazosin between 1994 and 1997; doxazosin after 1997). There was no difference between groups in terms of intraoperative hypertension, postoperative blood pressure, and perioperative fluid requirements. The authors concluded that surgical

Table 30.2 Summary of the studies evaluating preoperative non-selective alpha blockade versus preoperative selective alpha$_1$ blockade in patients undergoing surgical resection of pheochromocytoma

Study/Year	Number of patients in each arm		Results favor	Quality of evidence
	Non-selective alpha blockade	Selective alpha$_1$ blockade		
Havlik et al. (1988) [19]	9	6	No difference	Low
Russell et al. (1998) [20]	12	2	Non-selective	Low
Kocak et al. (2002) [21]	21	28	No difference	Low
Prys-Roberts et al. (2002) [22]	8	27	Selective	Low
Bruynzeel et al. (2010) [23]	31	42	No difference	Low
Weingarten et al. (2010) [24]	50	37	No difference	Low
Zhu et al. (2010) [25]	31	36	No difference	Low
Habbe et al. (2013) [26]	19	11	No difference	Low
Agrawal et al. (2014) [27]	14	13	Non-selective	Low
Kiernan et al. (2014) [28]	71	16	No difference	Low
Li et al. (2014) [29]	70	85	Selective	Low

resection of pheochromocytoma is safe after any of the three regimens used for preoperative medical blockade.

Prys-Roberts et al. [22] reported a retrospective review of a series of 35 patients: 8 patients received phenoxybenzamine and 27 patients received doxazosin. The different regimens were prescribed based on institutional protocol (phenoxybenzamine was routinely used until 1992; doxazosin after 1992). All eight patients treated with phenoxybenzamine experienced orthostatic hypotension during the preoperative period compared with only 2/27 patients treated with doxazosin. There were no differences in intraoperative systolic blood pressure between groups, but in the early postoperative period, the blood pressure was lower in the phenoxybenzamine group than in the doxazosin group. The authors concluded that both regimens provided safe intraoperative blood pressure control, but that doxazosin was associated with fewer adverse side effects and permitted a more rapid postoperative recovery.

Bruynzeel et al. [23] reported a retrospective review of a series of 73 patients: 31 patients received phenoxybenzamine and 42 patients received doxazosin. The different regimens were prescribed based on institutional protocol (phenoxybenzamine was routinely used until 2003; doxazosin after 2003). There were no statistically significant differences between groups in terms of intraoperative blood pressure fluctuations (hypertensive or hypotensive episodes) or fluid administration. However, postoperative mean arterial pressure was statistically significantly higher in the phenoxybenzamine group compared with the doxazosin group. The authors concluded that either non-selective or selective alpha$_1$–adrenergic blockade is adequate prior to resection of pheochromocytoma.

Weingarten et al. [24] reported a retrospective review of a series of 87 patients who underwent surgical resection of pheochromocytoma at two different institutions: 50 patients received the Mayo Clinic protocol with phenoxybenzamine in 98%, a beta blocker in 78%, and a calcium channel blocker in 22% (only one patient received a selective alpha$_1$-receptor blocker); 37 patients received the Cleveland Clinic protocol, with selective alpha$_1$-receptor blockade (doxazosin, prazosin or terazosin) in 65%, beta blockers in 46% and a calcium channel blocker in 30% (only 16% of patients received phenoxybenzamine). Intraoperatively, the maximal and mean blood pressure readings were lower with the Mayo Clinic protocol. Although the lowest intraoperative blood pressure readings did not differ between groups, the Mayo Clinic patients spent relatively more time hypotensive than the Cleveland Clinic patients (as defined by blood pressure episodes ≤30% of baseline); however, the Cleveland Clinic patients received more intraoperative fluids. There was no postoperative myocardial infarction, stroke or death at either institution. The authors concluded that the different regimens for preoperative medical blockade did not result in clinically significant differences in outcome, but did result in differences in intraoperative hemodynamics, with phenoxybenzamine producing better attenuation of intraoperative hypertensive episodes at the cost of longer-lasting hypotension with greater use of vasopressors.

Zhu et al. [25] reported a retrospective review of a series of 67 patients: 31 patients received phenoxybenzamine and 36 patients received doxazosin. The different regimens were prescribed based on institutional protocol (phenoxybenzamine was routinely used until 2005; controlled release doxazosin after 2005). The mean intraoperative systolic arterial blood pressure was higher in the doxazosin group, and the lowest systolic blood pressure after tumor resection was lower in the phenoxybenzamine group. The fluctuation of systolic arterial blood pressure, defined as the change in systolic blood pressure divided by the change in diastolic blood pressure, was greater in the phenoxybenzamine group. There was no difference between groups in volume of intraoperative fluid administered. The authors concluded that both regimens were equally effective, and that phenoxybenzamine provided better arterial pressure control, but doxazosin led to a more stable perioperative hemodynamic course.

Habbe et al. [26] reported a retrospective review of a series of 30 patients: 19 patients received oral phenoxybenzamine for the usual time course and 11 patients received intravenous urapidil for 3 days prior to surgery. The different regimens were prescribed based on institutional protocol (phenoxybenzamine was routinely used until 2007; urapidil after 2007). There were no differences between groups in number of episodes of intraoperative hypertension or hypotension, maximal and minimal intraoperative systolic and diastolic blood pressures, and the use of intraoperative pressors. There was a statistically significant difference in total length of stay (17 days in the phenoxybenzamine group versus 11 days in the urapidil group), which was associated with reduced costs for the urapidil group; however, a critique of these findings is that these lengths of stay from a German study are dramatically longer than the lengths of stay typically seen in patients undergoing resection of pheochromocytoma in the United States. The authors concluded that both regimens prepared patients adequately for surgical resection of pheochromocytoma.

Agrawal et al. [27] reported a retrospective review of a series of 27 patients: 14 patients received phenoxybenzamine and 13 patients received prazosin. The different regimens were prescribed based on provider preference. Patients in the prazosin group had a statistically significantly higher median intraoperative systolic blood pressure as well as more episodes of systolic blood pressure $\geq$ 160 mmHg, $\geq$180 mmHg, and $\geq$ 220 mmHg. The median lowest intraoperative systolic blood pressure was also lowest in the prazosin group. There were no significant differences between groups in heart rate, postoperative blood pressure alterations, or arrhythmias. The authors concluded that phenoxybenzamine was superior to prazosin because it better controlled intraoperative hemodynamic fluctuations.

Kiernan et al. [28] reported a retrospective review of a series of 91 patients: 71 patients received phenoxybenzamine and 16 patients received selective alpha$_1$ blockade with prazosin, doxazosin, or terazosin (4 patients who underwent no preoperative medical blockade were not included in the analysis). The different regimens were prescribed based on provider preference. The use of selective alpha$_1$ blockade was associated with increased incidence of episodes of systolic blood pressure > 200, but there were no other differences between groups in other measures of hemodynamic instability. The authors concluded that selective alpha$_1$ blockade was associated with significantly more episodes of intraoperative hypertension, but no perioperative adverse outcomes.

Li et al. [29] reported a retrospective review of a series of 155 patients: 70 patients received phenoxybenzamine and 85 patients received doxazosin. Although it is not clearly stated in the manuscript, the different regimens appear to have been prescribed based on provider preference, as both medications were utilized in the authors' institution during the study time period. The patients in the phenoxybenzamine group experienced a statistically significantly greater incidence of blood pressure fluctuations (14% versus 2%; defined as systolic blood pressure $\geq$ 200 mmHg or $\leq$ 110 mmHg), but there was no difference between groups in postoperative hemodynamic stability or postoperative adverse outcomes. The authors concluded that doxazosin was preferred to phenoxybenzamine for preoperative alpha blockade.

Recommendation

The majority of the studies reviewed concluded that non-selective alpha blockade and selective $alpha_1$ blockade are equivalent in terms of preparing patients for surgical resection of pheochromocytoma. General recurring themes included better control of maximal intraoperative blood pressures but lower postoperative blood pressure with phenoxybenzamine compared to the selective agents. Both types of preoperative medical blockade are associated with rare adverse postoperative outcomes. Studies are again generally plagued with the limitation of small sample size, and because serious perioperative complications are rare in the modern era, it is certainly possible that a difference between groups was not detected even if a true difference exists. Overall, we recommend that either a non-selective alpha blocker or a selective $alpha_1$ blocker can be used to provide safe preoperative medical blockade prior to surgical resection of pheochromocytoma.

Preoperative Alpha Blockade Versus Preoperative Calcium Channel Blockade

Two retrospective reviews that included 10 patients and 105 patients who received only a calcium channel blocker and no form of alpha blocker have reported that surgical resection of pheochromocytoma is safe after preoperative medical blockade with calcium channel blocker only [30, 31]. However, only three articles were identified that compared preoperative medical blockade with an alpha-adrenergic blocker versus a calcium channel blocker [17, 32, 33]. All are retrospective reviews. See Table 30.3.

Ulchaker et al. [17] reported a retrospective review of a series of 113 patients, described in the previous section that addressed the need for preoperative medical blockade versus no preoperative medical blockade, but included in this section as well because both alpha blockers and calcium channel blockers were included in this study. To summarize the findings specifically as they pertain to the question of alpha blockers versus calcium channel blockers, exact regimens are not specified in

Table 30.3 Summary of the studies evaluating preoperative alpha blockade versus preoperative calcium channel blockade in patients undergoing surgical resection of pheochromocytoma

	Number of patients in each arm			
Study/Year	Alpha blockade	Calcium channel blockade	Results favor	Quality of evidence
Ulchaker et al. (1999) [17]	40% of 113 patients	26% of 113 patients	No difference	Low
Siddiqi et al. (2012) [32]	57	7	No difference	Low
Brunaud et al. (2014) [33]	41	110	No difference	Low

the manuscript, but 70% of patients received preoperative medical blockade with a combination of alpha blockade (phenoxybenzamine or a selective alpha$_1$ blocker), and/or a calcium channel blocker, and a beta blocker when necessary. Institutional protocol was to utilize a calcium channel blocker as the treatment of choice, with the addition of a selective alpha blocker (or rarely phenoxybenzamine) if hypertension was not adequately controlled with the calcium channel blocker alone. Beta blockers were utilized only when a cardiac dysrhythmia was noted. Overall, in the 24 h prior to surgery, 26% of patients received calcium channel blockers, 30% received selective alpha$_1$ blockers, 10% received phenoxybenzamine, and 20% received a beta blocker (some patients received multiple medications). In addition, 30% of patients received no preoperative medical blockade, as this was routine protocol if patients were normotensive preoperatively. There was no statistically significant difference in the intraoperative mean blood pressure between groups. The group of patients that received no preoperative medical blockade required less fluid in the perioperative period. Major cardiovascular complications occurred in six patients (pulmonary edema in three, congestive heart failure in two, and stroke in one), all of whom were in the group that received preoperative medical blockade; the authors do not specify which of these patients were receiving calcium channel blockers versus alpha blockers. The authors concluded that preoperative alpha blockade is not necessary prior to surgical resection of pheochromocytoma. The authors also concluded that calcium channel blockers are equally effective but safer than alpha blockers when used as the primary mode of antihypertensive therapy, although they published no data that specifically support this conclusion.

Siddiqi et al. [32] reported a retrospective review of a series of 64 patients: 57 patients received phenoxybenzamine and 7 patients received oral nicardipine. The different regimens were prescribed based on provider preference. There were no differences between groups in intraoperative hemodynamic stability, defined as the fraction of patients with, or number of episodes of, sustained or transient hypertension or hypotension, or sustained tachycardia. The percent of patients in each group requiring intraoperative medications for blood pressure control was not different between groups. Postoperative outcomes were similar between groups: there were no differences in rates of hemodynamic instability, length of hospital stay, stroke, myocardial infarction, pulmonary edema, or death. In spite of the recognized limitation of the very small sample size in the nicardipine group, the authors concluded that nicardipine is an equivalent alternative to phenoxybenzamine for preoperative medical blockade in patients undergoing surgical resection of pheochromocytoma.

Brunaud et al. [33] reported a retrospective review of a series of 155 patients across three institutions: 41 patients from a center in the United States received phenoxybenzamine, 110 patients from two different centers in France received oral nicardipine, and 4 patients received no preoperative medical blockade. This article was not included in the previous section that addressed the need for preoperative medical blockade versus no preoperative medical blockade, as the number of patients who received no preoperative medical blockade was so small. The different regimens were prescribed based on provider preference. Overall, there was no difference between groups in terms of the percent of patients that experienced intraoperative hemodynamic instability, defined as the occurrence of both hypertensive and hypotensive episodes during the same procedure. However, the phenoxybenzamine group experienced statistically significantly higher mean maximal systolic blood pressures, greater number and duration of episodes of systolic blood pressure > 200 mmHg, more frequent and longer episodes of severe hypotension (mean arterial pressure < 60 mmHg), more use of intraoperative vasoactive agents, and greater mean volumes of intraoperative fluid. The authors concluded that there was no difference between groups on intraoperative hemodynamic instability and postoperative morbidity, and that calcium channel blockers are a safe alternative to phenoxybenzamine for the preoperative preparation of patients undergoing surgical resection of pheochromocytoma.

Recommendation

The very few studies that have examined this question concluded that alpha blockade and calcium channel blockade are equivalent in terms of preparing patients for surgical resection of pheochromocytoma. Again, because of the small sample sizes, and because serious perioperative complications are rare in the modern era, it is certainly possible that a difference between groups was not detected even if a true difference exists. Overall, we recommend that either an alpha blocker or a calcium channel blocker can be used to provide safe preoperative medical blockade prior to surgical resection of pheochromocytoma.

Summary of Recommendations

No Preoperative Medical Blockade Versus Preoperative Medical Blockade

Preoperative medical blockade is recommended over no preoperative medical blockade for hypertensive patients undergoing surgical resection of pheochromocytoma (evidence quality low; strong recommendation). Consideration of preoperative medical blockade is recommended in patients with pheochromocytoma who are normotensive preoperatively, although it may not be necessary in this patient population (evidence quality low; weak recommendation).

Preoperative Non-selective Alpha Blockade Versus Preoperative Selective Alpha$_1$ Blockade

Non-selective alpha blockade and selective alpha$_1$ blockade are recommended equally for the preoperative medical preparation of patients undergoing surgical resection of pheochromocytoma (evidence quality low; weak recommendation).

Preoperative Alpha Blockade Versus Preoperative Calcium Channel Blockade

Alpha blockade and calcium channel blockade are recommended equally for the preoperative medical preparation of patients undergoing surgical resection of pheochromocytoma (evidence quality low; weak recommendation).

Conclusion

The perioperative management of patients undergoing surgical resection of pheochromocytoma is essential to good outcomes. Several options exist for the preoperative medical blockade of patients with catecholamine-producing tumors, including non-selective alpha-receptor blockers, selective alpha$_1$-receptor blockers, and calcium channel blockers. In this chapter, we have summarized the available data and have provided recommendations for the optimal preoperative medical management of patients undergoing surgical resection of pheochromocytoma. In brief, it appears that preoperative medical blockade of some type offers an advantage over no preoperative blockade, at least for hypertensive patients; however, there is insufficient data to recommend one specific agent over another. No data exist from randomized controlled trials. The studies that have been reported in the literature are virtually all retrospective case series, with small sample sizes and frequent serious design flaws predisposing to bias. The authors of the majority of the studies report that either no clinically significant difference or no statistically significant difference exists between groups, and therefore conclude that indeed no true difference exists, yet not a single study reports a power calculation, and therefore, no certainty exists that a Type II error is not being made. We know that patients with pheochromocytoma undergo medical and surgical procedures prior to their diagnosis on a regular basis, even biopsy of the tumor itself, and often experience no consequence; however, the rare instances of catastrophic cardiovascular collapse are so undesirable that it makes intuitive sense to employ preoperative medical blockade in order to avoid these, even though the data are limited. The agent for which the greatest body of literature exists is phenoxybenzamine, but there are no clear, consistent data that phenoxybenzamine is superior to selective alpha$_1$-receptor blockers or calcium channel blockers. No agent appears to eliminate hemodynamic instability completely. The possibility exists that the intravenous agents used to treat intraoperative and postoperative hypertension and hypotension on a minute-by-minute basis are so effective that the type of preoperative medical blockade is of no consequence, but a larger, better-designed study than what currently exists in the literature would be needed in order to draw such a conclusion, ideally a randomized, controlled trial. In summary, when dealing with an entity such as pheochromocytoma, for which complications are rare but devastating, the most conservative approach is likely the optimal approach in the absence of better data.

References

1. Welbourn RB. Early surgical history of phaeochromocytoma. Br J Surg. 1987;74(7):594–6.
2. Graham JB. Pheochromocytoma and hypertension; an analysis of 207 cases. Int Abstr Surg. 1951;92(2):105–21.
3. Kvale WF, Manger WM, Priestley JT, Roth GM. Pheochromocytoma. Circulation. 1956;14(4 Part 1):622–30.
4. Kinney MA, Warner ME, vanHeerden JA, et al. Perianesthetic risks and outcomes of pheochromocytoma and paraganglioma resection. Anesth Analg. 2000;91(5):1118–23.
5. Plouin PF, Duclos JM, Soppelsa F, Boublil G, Chatellier G. Factors associated with perioperative morbidity and mortality in patients with pheochromocytoma: analysis of 165 operations at a single center. J Clin Endocrinol Metab. 2001;86(4):1480–6.
6. Hamilton CA, Reid JL, Sumner DJ. Acute effects of phenoxybenzamine on alpha-adrenoceptor responses in vivo and in vitro: relation of in vivo pressor responses to the number of specific adrenoceptor binding sites. J Cardiovasc Pharmacol. 1983;5:868–73.
7. Bravo EL. Pheochromocytoma: an approach to antihypertensive management. Ann N Y Acad Sci. 2002;970:1–10.
8. Lehmann HU, Hochrein H, Witt E, Mies HW. Hemodynamic effects of calcium antagonists. Hypertension. 1983;5:1166–73.
9. Elliott WJ, Ram CV. Calcium channel blockers. J Clin Hypertens. 2011;13:687–9.
10. Pacak K, Eisenhofer G, Ahlman H, et al. Pheochromocytoma: recommendations for clinical practice from the first international symposium. Nat Clin Pract Endocrinol Metab. 2007;3:92–102.
11. Chen H, Sippel RS, Pacak K. The NANETS consensus guideline for the diagnosis and management of neuroendocrine tumors: pheochromocytoma,paraganglioma & medullary thyroid cancer. Pancreas. 2010;39:775–83.
12. Lenders JWM, Duh Q-Y, Eisenhofer G, et al. Pheochromocytoma and paraganglioma: an endocrine society clinical practice guideline. J Clin Endocrinol Metab. 2014;99:1915–42.
13. Jaeschke R, Guyatt GH, Dellinger P, Schunemann H, Levy MM, Kunz R, Norris S, Bion J., GRADE working group. Use of GRADE grid to reach decisions on clinical practice guidelines when consensus is elusive. BMJ. 2008;337:a744.
14. Stenström G, Haljamäe H, Tisell LE. Influence of pre-operative treatment with phenoxybenzamine on the incidence of adverse cardiovascular reactions during anaesthesia and surgery for pheochromocytoma. Acta Anaesthesiol Scand. 1985;29:797–803.
15. Boutros AR, Bravo EL, Zanettin G, Straffon RA. Perioperative management of 63 patients with pheochromocytoma. Cleve Clin J Med. 1990;57(7):613.
16. Steinsapir J, Carr AA, Prisant M, Bransome ED Jr. Metyrosine and pheochromocytoma. Arch Intern Med. 1997;157:901–6.

17. Ulchaker JC, Goldfarb DA, Bravo EL, Novick AC. Successful outcomes in pheochromocytoma surgery in the modern era. J Urol. 1999;161:764–7.
18. Shao Y, Chen R, Shen Z, et al. Preoperative alpha blockade for normotensive pheochromocytoma: is it necessary? J Hypertens. 2011;29:2429–32.
19. Havlik RJ, Cahow E, Kinder BK. Advances in the diagnosis and treatment of pheochromocytoma. Arch Surg. 1988;123:626–30.
20. Russell WJ, Metcalfe IR, Tonkin AL, Frewin DB. The preoperative management of phaeochromocytoma. Anaesth Intensive Care. 1998;26:196–200.
21. Kocak S, Aydintug S, Canakci N. α blockade in preoperative preparation of patients with pheochromocytomas. Int Surg. 2002;87:191–4.
22. Prys-Roberts C, Farndon JR. Efficacy and safety of doxazosin for perioperative management of patients with pheochromocytoma. World J Surg. 2002;26:1037–42.
23. Bruynzeel H, Reelders RA, Groenland THN, et al. Risk factors for hemodynamic instability during surgery for pheochromocytoma. J Clin Endocrinol Metab. 2010;95:678–85.
24. Weingarden TN, Cata JP, O'Hara JF, et al. Comparison of two preoperative medical management strategies for laparoscopic resection of pheochromocytoma. Urology. 2010;76:508e6–11.
25. Zhu Y, He H, Su T, et al. Selective α_1-adrenoceptor antagonist (controlled release tablets) in preoperative management of pheochromocytoma. Endocrine. 2010;38:254–9.
26. Habbe N, Ruger F, Bojunga J, et al. Urapidil in the preoperative treatment of pheochromocytomas: a safe and cost-effective method. World J Surg. 2013;37:1141–6.
27. Agrawal R, Mishra SK, Bhatia E, et al. Prospective study to compare peri-operative hemodynamic alterations following preparation for pheochromocytoma surgery by phenoxybenzamine or prazosin. World J Surg. 2014;38:716–23.
28. Kiernan CM, Du L, Chen X, et al. Predictors of hemodynamic instability during surgery for pheochromocytoma. Ann Surg Oncol. 2014;21:3865–71.
29. Li J, Yang C-H. Improvement of preoperative management in patients with adrenal pheochromocytoma. Int J Clin Exp Med. 2014;7:5541–6.
30. Proye C, Thevenin D, Cecat P, et al. Exclusive use of calcium channel blockers in preoperative and intraoperative control of pheochromocytomas: hemodynamics and free catecholamine assays in ten consecutive patients. Surgery. 1989;106:1149–54.
31. Lebuffe G, Dosseh ED, Tek G, et al. The effect of calcium channel blockers on outcome following the surgical treatment of phaeochromocytomas and paragangliomas. Anaesthesia. 2005;60:439–44.
32. Siddiqi HD, Yang H, Laird AM, et al. Utility of oral nicardipine and magnesium sulfate infusion during preparation and resection of pheochromocytomas. Surgery. 2012;152:1027–36.
33. Brunaud L, Boutami M, Nguyen-Thi P-L, et al. Both preoperative alpha and calcium channel blockade impact intraoperative hemodynamic stability similarly in the management of pheochromocytoma. Surgery. 2014;156:1410–8.

Surgery Versus Nonsurgical Therapy for Recurrent Adrenocortical Carcinoma

31

Zahraa Al-Hilli and Melanie L. Lyden

Abstract

Adrenocortical carcinoma is a rare endocrine neoplasm associated with poor prognosis. Complete surgical resection is the only potential cure for the disease. Unfortunately, a significant number of patients develop disease relapse and present with local or systemic recurrence. Close follow-up with regular clinical examination aided by radiological imaging and blood investigations is crucial for the early detection of recurrent disease. The best treatment options for recurrent disease remain unclear and these include surgery, chemotherapy, and radiotherapy, in addition to new and upcoming treatments. This chapter will focus on the treatment of recurrent ACC including a discussion of surgical and non-surgical therapy options.

Keywords

Adrenocortical carcinoma · Recurrence · Surgery · Mitotane · Chemotherapy · Radiotherapy · Radiofrequency ablation · Treatment

Introduction

Adrenocortical carcinoma (ACC) is a rare and aggressive endocrine malignancy. Approximately 0.7–2.0 per million individuals are diagnosed with ACC each year [1, 2]. The prognosis of patients with ACC is poor, with an overall 5-year

Z. Al-Hilli (✉)
Department of General Surgery, Cleveland Clinic, Cleveland, OH, USA
e-mail: ALHILLZ@ccf.org

M. L. Lyden
Department of Surgery, Mayo Clinic Hospital, Rochester, MN, USA
e-mail: Lyden.Melanie@mayo.edu

P. Angelos, R. H. Grogan (eds.), *Difficult Decisions in Endocrine Surgery*, Difficult Decisions in Surgery: An Evidence-Based Approach,
https://doi.org/10.1007/978-3-319-92860-9_31

survival of less than 35% [3–5]. Patients with stage IV ACC have a 5-year survival rate of less than 15% [6, 7]. A bimodal age distribution is described, with a peak frequency at ages younger than 5 years and a second peak most commonly in the fourth and fifth decades [1, 3]. Females are slightly more frequently affected than males [1].

This chapter will focus on the treatment of recurrent ACC including a discussion of surgical and non-surgical therapy options (Table 31.1).

Adrenocortical carcinomas present as a functional tumor related to excess adrenal hormone production, as a result of mass effect most often in cases of a non-functional tumor, or found incidentally on radiological imaging. Up to 60% of patients present with the hormonal symptoms of the functional tumor (most commonly Cushing's syndrome) [8]. Unfortunately, when these tumors are non-functional, they may not be detected until they develop into a large mass that may invade into adjacent structures with possible metastases.

The etiology of ACC is unclear, but smoking and the use of oral contraceptives have been described as risk factors [9]. The majority of ACCs are sporadic. Familial association has been shown in patients with Li-Fraumeni syndrome [10]. Progress is being made in recent years in the understanding of the molecular mechanisms of ACC tumor development and genetic profiling [11].

Historically, the McFarlane classification as modified by Sullivan was used for staging in ACC (Table 31.2) [12, 13]. Subsequent modifications restricted stage IV disease to include patients with metastatic disease. Current classifications include the World Health Organization and the Union for International Cancer Control classification which is based on the McFarlane/Sullivan system and the European Network for the Study of Adrenal Tumor (ENSAT) classification (Tables 31.3 and 31.4) [14, 15].

The management of patients with ACC requires a multi-disciplinary approach. Surgical resection of disease is the main treatment modality in patients with limited disease. Adjuvant therapy includes chemotherapy and/or radiation. Although complete surgical resection offers the best chance of cure in patients who present with localized disease, recurrence following surgery is common. Unfortunately, up to 75–85% of patients with ACC develop local and/or distant metastases, despite initial pathological evidence of a complete R0 resection [16, 17]. Disease recurrence is most common within the first 2 years following surgery, with 40% of patients recurring within this time period [18]. Unfortunately, tumor recurrence is likely to be followed by further relapses, with a shortened disease-free interval (DFI) between these episodes. Literature on the treatment of recurrent ACC is scarce, and level I evidence is lacking. Treatment can be broadly divided into surgical or non-surgical options. Non-surgical treatment encompasses chemotherapy, radiation therapy, radiofrequency ablation and cryosurgery. This chapter will focus on the treatment options for the treatment of recurrent ACC. The available evidence for these treatment modalities will be discussed (Table 31.5).

Table 31.1 PICO table

*P*opulation	Patients with recurrent adrenocortical carcinoma
*I*ntervention	Surgical resection
*C*omparator	Chemotherapy, radiotherapy, tumor ablation, targeted therapies
*O*utcomes	Surgical resection is recommended for patients with recurrent adrenocortical carcinoma who are suitable for further intervention and who develop a recurrence after 6–12 months of initial treatment. Treatment with chemotherapy and/or radiotherapy may be of benefit following surgery

Table 31.2 The MacFarlane classification modified by Sullivan for staging adrenocortical carcinoma

Stage	Size	Lymph nodes	Local invasion	Metastases	TNM
I	<5 cm	–	–	–	T1, N0, M0
II	>5 cm	–	–	–	T2, N0, M0
III	Any size	+	+	–	T1–2, N1, M0
IV	Any size	+	+	+	T1–2, N1, M1

Table 31.3 Union for International Cancer Control (UICC)/World Health Organization (WHO) 2004 staging system for adrenocortical carcinoma, derived from the MacFarlane classification as modified by Sullivan

Stage	UICC/WHO
I	T1, N0, M0
II	T2, N0, M0
III	T1–2, N1, M0 or T3, N0, M1
IV	T4, N0, M0 or T3, N1,M0 or T1–4, N0–1, M1

T1 tumor ≤5 cm, *T2* tumor >5 cm, *T3* tumor infiltration locally reaching neighboring organs, *T4* tumor invasion of neighboring organs, *N0* no positive lymph nodes, *N1* positive lymph nodes, *M0* no distant metastases, *M1* distant metastasis

Table 31.4 European Network for the Study of Adrenal Tumors (ENSAT) 2008 staging system for adrenocortical carcinoma

Stage	ENSAT
I	T1, N0, M0
II	T2, N0, M0
III	T1–2, N1, M0 or T3–4, N0–1, M0
IV	T1–4, N0–1, M1

T1 tumor ≤5 cm, *T2* tumor >5 cm, *T3* tumor infiltration into surrounding tissue, *T4* tumor invasion into adjacent organs or venous tumor thrombus in vena cava or adrenal vein, *N0* no positive lymph nodes, *N1* positive lymph nodes, *M0* no distant metastases, *M1* distant metastasis

Table 31.5 Studies reporting treatment of recurrent adrenocortical carcinoma

First author	Year	Type	Number of patients included with recurrent disease	Treatment modality	Outcome
Linos [19]	1986	Retrospective case series	1	Surgical resection	– Alive at 16 months follow-up
Decker [20]	1991	Retrospective case series	Includes patients treated for primary disease, recurrence both local and distant	Surgical resection and/or mitotane	– Resection for local recurrence may prolong survival
Jensen [21]	1991	Retrospective case series	15 patients treated with surgical resection plus chemotherapy and 18 patients treated with chemotherapy alone	Surgical resection plus chemotherapy	– Improved survival in the surgical group compared with chemotherapy alone – 5 patients (33%) were alive at 5-year follow-up
Icard [6]	1992	Retrospective case series	Includes patients treated for primary disease, recurrence both local and distant	Surgery and/or medical therapy	– 5-year survival 27% with reoperation – Mitotane improved the survival rate only in patients with metastases who received it after operation (vs non-mitotane-treated patients)
Pommier [16]	1992	Retrospective case series	45 treated for recurrent disease (19 treated medically and 26 surgically)	Surgical resection or chemotherapy	– 5-year survival 47% with complete resection – Mean survival of 56 months for patients who underwent reoperation compared with 19 months for patients treated medically – Mitotane had a 24% partial response rate. Other chemotherapeutic agents were ineffective – Surgery superior to medical treatment
Van Aalderen [22]	1992	Case report	1	Mitotane	Long term survival noted
Ahlman [23]	1993	Retrospective case series	2	Surgical resection	

Haak [24]	1994	Retrospective case series	Includes patients treated for primary disease and recurrence 38 with recurrence	26 patients treated with mitotane at recurrence	Tumor response was only observed in patients with high maintenance mitotane levels. Five of these patients had a complete remission lasting 2–120 months at the time of reporting
Sakamoto [25]	1995	Case report	1	Surgical resection	Alive at 18 years follow-up
Crucitti [18]	1996	Retrospective case series	Includes patients treated for primary disease, recurrence both local and distant	Surgery and/or medical therapy	– Re-operated patients experienced better survival (mean, 41.5 months) than non-re-operated cases (mean, 15.6 months)
Bellantone [26]	1997	Retrospective case series	52 patients with recurrence (20 treated with surgical resection)	Surgery or no surgery for recurrence	– Mean survival in 20 patients who underwent reoperation was significantly higher (15.85 ± 14.9 months) than in non-reoperated cases (3.2 ± 2.9 months) – 5-year actuarial survival in re-operated patients is significantly better than in nonreoperated patients (49.7% versus 8.3%, respectively)
Khorram-Manesh [27]	1998	Retrospective case series	5	Surgery	Positive correlation between DFI and survival after repeat surgery
Schulick [28]	1999	Retrospective case series	47	Surgery	– Median survival of 47 months with complete second resection and 16 months with incomplete second resection – 5-year survival 57% with complete resection and 0% for incomplete resection
Seki [29]	1999	Case report	1	Mitotane at recurrence	Recurrence 2 years after mitotane for first recurrence and death 4 months later
Langer [30]	2000	Retrospective case series	1	Surgical resection	Surgery is recommended for recurrent disease if resectable
Ilias [31]	2001	Retrospective case series	One treated with surgery followed by mitotane and second treated with mitotane	One patient who had surgery followed by mitotane and a second treated with mitotane	First patients alive at 16 years and second patient alive at 14 year
Fujii [32]	2003	Case report	1	Radiotherapy, chemotherapy then surgery	Alive at 5-year follow-up

(continued)

Table 31.5 (continued)

First author	Year	Type	Number of patients included with recurrent disease	Treatment modality	Outcome
Tauchmanova [33]	2004	Retrospective case series	2	Surgical resection and chemotherapy	Overall survival was 96 months for one patients and 39 months for the second
Matsumoto [34]	2005	Case report	1	Surgery then chemotherapy	Alive at 3-year follow-up
Palazzo [35]	2006	Retrospective case series	1	Surgery	Outcome following surgery not reported
Schlamp [36]	2007	Case report	1	Surgery followed by radiotherapy and chemotherapy	Alive at 21 month
Tan [37]	2009	Retrospective case series	2	Surgery followed by chemotherapy and radiotherapy	– Outcome for first patient not reported – Second patient overall survival of 35 months
Sabolch [38]	2011	Retrospective case series	27 (out of a total of 58 patients studied)	Surgery alone (n = 8), surgery with radiotherapy (n = 7), radiotherapy alone (n = 12)	– Overall results reported (primary and recurrent) – Local failure occurred in 16 of the 48 instances of treatment with surgery alone, in 2 of the 10 instances of surgery plus adjuvant radiotherapy, and in one of the instances of definitive radiotherapy – Lack of radiotherapy use was associated with 4.7 times the risk of local failure compared with treatment regimens that involved radiotherapy – In patients receiving radiation to the tumor bed, tumors of a maximum dimension greater than 10 cm were 4.3 times more likely to fail locally than those with smaller tumors

Datrice [39]	2012	Retrospective case series	19 treated for local recurrence and 38 had distant metastases	Surgery (and/or radiofrequency ablation in 3 patients)	– Overall results reported for treatment of local and distant disease – The median overall survival for patients with a DFI less than 12 months was 1.7 years (range: 2.8 months to >12 years), compared to 6.6 years (range: 3.6 months to >12 years) for a DFI greater than 12 months The median DFS of patients rendered with no evidence of disease (NED) after first metastectomy was 6 months. The median PFS of the population not rendered NED was 2.4 months
Dy [40]	2013	Retrospective case series	67 treated with surgical resection and 26 had non-operative therapy or no intervention (Includes local and distant recurrence)	Surgery or no surgery (medical therapy or no intervention)	– A comparison of survival for these three groups (surgery, non-surgical therapy and no intervention) at 1,2 and 5 years of patients was 82%, 67%, and 30% in the surgery group, 26%, 13%, and 0% in the non-surgical therapy group, and 30%, 10% and 0% in those patients treated with supportive care alone
Erdogen [41]	2013	Retrospective case series	101 had surgical resection of recurrence and 53 treated medically	Surgery followed by chemotherapy or chemotherapy only	– Patients who underwent either incomplete (R2-resection or tumor debulking) or no surgery had a similar progression-free survival, whereas overall survival was worst in patients who were not operated at all

DFI disease free interval, *DFS* disease free survival, *NED* no evidence of disease, *PFS* progression free survival

Search Strategy

A focused review of available literature was conducted. Original articles were identified using a PubMed search strategy. The following search terms were used in combinations: recurrent adrenocortical carcinoma, surgery, chemotherapy, radiation, radiofrequency ablation, mitotane and treatment.

Surgical Management

The management of patients with ACC requires a multi-disciplinary approach. The main goal of treatment in patients with limited disease is complete surgical resection with negative margins (R0). Surgery should involve an *en bloc* resection of the tumor with involved adjacent structures. It is crucial to take caution in preserving the integrity of the tumor capsule to prevent tumor spillage, which may lead to future tumor recurrence [4, 5]. Studies have shown a correlation between the ability to achieve clear margins and prognosis [18, 28, 40]. In addition to careful pathological assessment, evaluation of hormone levels post-operatively can be used to assess the completeness of surgical resection. In patients who present with metastatic disease or advanced tumors, then tumor debulking may be of benefit, specifically when control of excess hormone secretion is required. However, data on this is scare and a survival data is controversial [3, 40].

Despite having an adequate resection, up to 85% of patients with ACC will develop a local or distant recurrence (Fig. 31.1) [16, 17, 42]. Traditionally, surgical resection was thought to be contraindicated in patients with recurrent and metastatic disease. More recently, our understanding of the biology of ACC has improved and criteria such as DFI and resectability of the tumor recurrence has evolved as predictors of a possible improved outcome with re-operation.

An earlier study by Jensen et al., compared treatment with chemotherapy and surgical resection followed by chemotherapy in recurrent ACC [21]. Survival following

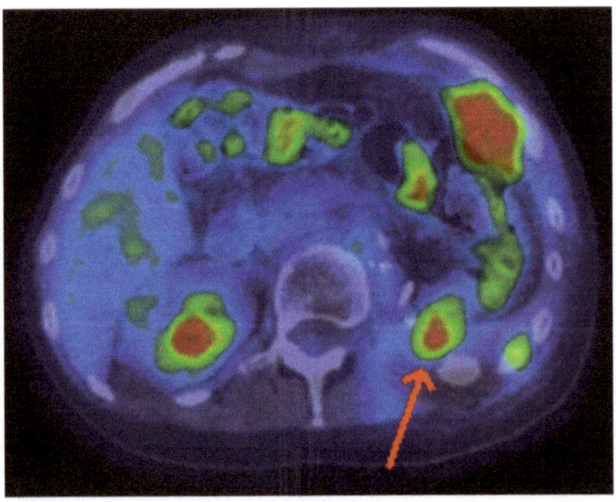

Fig. 31.1 PET-CT image showing a retroperitoneal ACC recurrence

first recurrence was significantly longer in patients treated with chemotherapy plus aggressive surgical resection of recurrent disease than in patients treated with chemotherapy alone (27 vs 11 months, $p < 0.05$). Five patients in the study (33%) survived greater than 5 years from the time of first recurrence. In addition, the authors noted that an initial time to recurrence of greater than 12 months was associated with a significantly improved overall survival. More recently, Erdogen et al., published a larger series showing similar findings [41]. The study represented the collective experience from the German Adrenocortical Carcinoma Registry and found that a time to first recurrence greater than 12 months as well as a complete R0 resection of the recurrent tumor was associated with improved patient survival and outcome. In addition, a recurrence that occurred early within the first 6 months indicated a poor prognosis with a progression-free survival (PFS) of 3 months and an overall survival of 13 months, compared with patients who developed a recurrence after more than 24 months where the PFS was 17 months and overall survival was 115 months.

When performed, surgical resection for ACC recurrence has been shown to be associated with low post-operative mortality. Schulick et al. published a retrospective series from Memorial Sloan Kettering Cancer Center which included 47 patients who underwent a second resection for locally recurrent of metastatic disease [28]. Of a total of 83 repeat resections in this cohort, the authors reported a 30-day mortality of 3.6%. In this study, stratification of patients by completeness of the repeat resection revealed a higher median survival of 74 months in patients undergoing a complete resection compared with 16 months when the resection was incomplete. Thus, emphasizing the prognostic value of achieving a complete resection in patients with recurrent ACC as described by other authors. Similar results were seen in a study by Cricitti et al., where a complete resection was associated with a longer-disease free survival and overall survival than in those patients who have recurrent disease that is not amenable to surgical resection (DFS 41.5 months versus 15 months and OS at 5 years of 50% versus 8% respectively) [18].

Our experience at Mayo Clinic was recently published and included 67 patients who underwent reoperation for recurrence and 26 patients who had non-operative therapy or no intervention [40]. A comparison of survival for these three groups (surgery, non-surgical therapy and no intervention) at 1, 2 and 5 years of patients was 82%, 67%, and 30% in the surgery group, 26%, 13%, and 0% in the non-surgical therapy group, and 30%, 10% and 0% in those patients treated with supportive care alone ($p < 0.0001$). In addition, the study showed that patients who did not achieve an R0 resection for recurrent disease had a reduced overall survival compared with those achieving a complete resection. Furthermore, debulking surgery was found to be associated with an improved medial survival of 3.5 years compared with patients who did not undergo surgery ($p = 0.002$). In contrast to the studies discussed earlier showing an improved survival in patients who had an initial DFI of more than 12 months, a time period of greater than 6 months was identified in this study to be independently associated with improved survival among patients proceeding with surgical resection of recurrent tumor [40]. Hence, these results in addition to other reports, support a role for surgical intervention in recurrent ACC.

The use of laparoscopic surgery for ACC is a subject of ongoing controversy. Open adrenalectomy is generally the preferred procedure for patients with proven ACC or where there is a high suspicion for this diagnosis. It also is the procedure of choice in cases where the tumor is larger than 10–12 cm, there is evidence of invasion of adjacent structures, and lymphadenopathy [43, 44]. Studies to date have shown an increased local recurrence rate and intra-peritoneal dissemination of disease in cases of ACC resected by a laparoscopic approach [45]. Therefore, data extrapolated from these experiences do not support a laparoscopic approach in the recurrent setting.

Recommendation

A number of case reports and retrospective case series have been published showing a benefit for re-operation for recurrent ACC. In these studies, a complete resection was associated with an improved overall survival compared with an incomplete resection. A complete surgical resection, therefore, is recommended for patients who develop a recurrence of ACC more than 6–12 months following their initial therapeutic resection (evidence quality low, weak recommendation).

Non-surgical Management

Chemotherapy

To date, mitotane (ortho,para'-DDD or 1,1-dichloro-2-[*o*-chlorophenyl]-2-[*p*-chlorophenyl] ethane) has been shown to be the only adrenal specific agent for the treatment of ACC. Mitotane acts through several different mechanisms which include decreasing cortico-steroid biosynthesis and by inducing structural damage to the mitochondria in the zona reticularis and zona fasciculata, thereby leading to necrosis of both normal and tumor tissue [46, 47]. The actions of mitotane appear to be dose dependent. A correlation between plasma serum levels and survival have been shown with serum levels of more than 14 μg/mL [24]. As a result of improved understanding of the variability of response in patients with ACC, as well as the increasing half-life with prolonged administration of mitotane, various dosing regimens have been proposed [48, 49]. Side effects of mitotane are also dose dependent and are reversed by stopping therapy. The most common of these include gastrointestinal symptoms such as nausea, vomiting, diarrhea and anorexia [4, 42, 46]. Others include neuropsychiatric symptoms, hepatotoxicity, hematologic abnormalities, renal abnormalities and skin rashes [4, 46]. In addition, glucocorticoid replacement is warranted in patients treated with mitotane due to the suppressive effects on health adrenal tissue. The reported efficacy of mitotane in the treatment of patients with ACC is variable and unclear. It has been shown to be effective in inducing tumor response in 33% of patients treated [50]. Terzolo et al., reviewed the outcomes of patients with ACC who had undergone radical surgery and treated with mitotane compared with patients who were not treated with mitotane [42]. The study revealed that PFS was significantly prolonged in the mitotane group compared with the two control groups (42 months vs 10 and 25 months respectively). Multivariate analysis indicated that mitotane treatment had a significant advantage for PFS.

In addition to mitotane, chemotherapeutic agents have been shown to be of benefit in patients with ACC, especially those patients that do not responds to mitotane, experience severe side effects or patients advanced disease. Various combinations have been used and reported in retrospective series. These include cisplatin-based therapy in combination with etoposide, 5-fluorouracil and doxorubicin or streptozocin. The First International Randomized Trial in Locally Advanced and Metastatic Adrenocortical Carcinoma Treatment (FIRM-ACT) study is the only phase III randomized controlled trial in the treatment of ACC to be reported to date. This study compared two of the most successful regimen in the treatment of patients with advanced ACC (etoposide, doxorubicin and cisplatin (EDP) with mitotane and streptozocin with mitotane) and aimed to establish a treatment standard for advanced disease [51–53]. An objective tumor response was noted in 23.2% of patients in the EDP-mitotane group compared with 9.2% of patients in the streptozocin-mitotane group. The median DFI was 5.0 months in the EDP-mitotane group compared with 2.1 months in the streptozocin group [53]. The 12-month survival and median overall survival between the EDP-mitotane group and streptozocin-mitotane group was 26.1% and 14.8 months vs 7.2% and 12.0 months respectively. The study concluded that EDP-mitotane as first-line treatment reduced the risk of death by 21% as compared with streptozocin-mitotane [53]. Despite this small benefit, this trial is important in setting a standard for current practice (EDP-mitotane as first line combination treatment of advanced ACC) as well as providing a platform for further research in this area. The European Society of Medical Oncology (ESMO) guidelines recommend combination chemotherapy and mitotane for patients with inoperable ACC with high tumor volume and rapid disease, whilst mitotane alone can be used initially for patients with low tumor volume, slow progression or those patients who are unfit for surgery [54].

In the setting of tumor recurrence, the role of mitotane or chemotherapy-mitotane combinations, as well as consensus on the best treatment is yet to be fully elucidated. Reports of chemotherapy in recurrent ACC have not been consistent and have shown no increase in survival rates, long term disease control, as well as disease remission [4, 24, 31, 46, 55]. In addition, studies comparing medical treatment and surgery have consistently shown a survival benefit in patients treated with surgery (with or without further medical therapy) compared with no surgery [16, 21, 34]. Therefore, it is accepted that an evaluation of patients at the time of recurrence is important to establish the resectability of recurrent disease and patient fitness for surgery. Factors discussed in the previous section including DFS and tumor biology should be considered. Following surgical resection, patients may receive mitotane with or without chemotherapy and/or radiation.

In patients with excess hormone secretion, additional pharmacologic agents are available for use and have a role in controlling the production of steroids. This is particularly important in patients who may be unsuitable for further surgery or who have disease that in no amenable to a complete R0 resection. Such agents include metyrapone and ketoconazole. Metyrapone inhibits cortisol production, while ketoconazole is an imidazole antifungal agent that has a role in suppressing corticosteroid and androgen production and has an important role in benign adrenal disease. These agents, unfortunately, do not inhibit tumor growth. Other agents include etomidate and mifepristone.

Recommendation

The use of chemotherapy and other medical therapy in recurrent ACC is unclear and evidence to support its use is limited to retrospective case series and reports. These therapies should be considered in the following reoperation for recurrent ACC and for the treatment of patients who have disease that is not amenable to surgical resection (evidence quality low, weak recommendation).

Radiotherapy

The role of radiation treatment in ACC is yet to be fully elucidated. Radiotherapy has been traditionally reserved for the palliative treatment of patients with ACC. The main challenges in its utilization include the lack of clear treatment benefit as well as radiation effects on adjacent organs such as the kidney, liver and small bowel. A recommendation from a review of data from the German ACC Registry includes consideration of radiotherapy within 3 months of surgery to the tumor bed in patients at high risk of local resection, such as those with an incomplete resection (microscopically involved or indeterminate resection margins), stage III disease, tumors greater than 8 cm, or a Ki 67% of greater than 10%. A total dose of >40 Gy with single fractions of 1.8–2 Gy are suggested (including a boost volume to reach from 50 to 60 Gy) [56]. In addition radiotherapy is recommended for use for symptomatic metastases to bone, brain or vena cava obstruction [56].

A search of the literature regarding the use of radiotherapy in recurrent adrenocortical carcinoma is limited to retrospective case series. A retrospective series of patients with primary and recurrent ACC compared treatment with surgery alone, surgery plus adjuvant radiotherapy and definitive radiotherapy for unresectable disease [38]. This study showed that the lack of radiotherapy use was associated with 4.7 times the risk of local failure compared with treatment regimens that involved radiotherapy (95% CI, 1.2–19.0; $p = 0.030$). In patients receiving radiation to the tumor bed, tumors of a maximum dimension greater than 10 cm were 4.3 times more likely to fail locally than those with smaller tumors (95% CI, 1.5–13.0; $p = 0.004$). The heterogenous nature (primary vs recurrent, various treatment modalities) of the patients included is a limitation of this study.

Recommendation

The use of radiotherapy in recurrent ACC is unclear and evidence to support its use is limited to retrospective case series and reports. Radiotherapy should be considered in the following reoperation for recurrent ACC and for the treatment of patients who have disease that is not amenable to surgical resection (evidence quality low, weak recommendation).

Tumor Ablation

Radiofrequency ablation (RFA) delivers minimally invasive local treatment utilizing high frequency alternating current. It works by transforming radiofrequency energy into heat, which is deposited into the tumor. It has been shown to be safe and effective treatment for a variety of tumors. In patients with ACC, it may constitute part of the treatment of patients of patients who are deemed as poor candidates for surgical resection and also as part of multimodality treatment. In the primary setting, evidence to date has shown that RFA is well tolerated with 53% of patients demonstrating a reduction in the size of their tumor (more notable response in tumors <5 cm, 67% complete response) or loss of enhancement on imaging [57]. Side effects reported include bleeding, infection, and injury to adjacent organs [58, 59]. Datrice et al. reported on the use of RFA in a cohort of patients with recurrent and metastatic ACC [39]. The authors reported on the safety and feasibility of this procedure when performed at a specialized institution and when combined with surgery to treat lesions that might otherwise be considered unresectable. It is unclear however from this report as to how many patients had RFA specifically for recurrence rather than treatment of metastasis.

Cryoablation is another form of ablative treatment (Fig. 31.2). This causes tumor necrosis as a result of rapid cell freezing. To our knowledge there is no data available of the use of cryoablation in the treatment of recurrent ACC. Its use, however, has been demonstrated in the treatment of adrenal metastasis from other tumors [60]. Xiao et al. reported on the use of cryoablation for benign adrenal tumors and adrenal metastasis [61]. This study revealed a complete response of 92.3% and a partial response of 7.7% with its use for primary adrenal lesions. In the setting of metastasis a complete response was seen in 30% and a partial response in 70%. A third method of ablation that can be used for adrenal gland disease is chemical ablation. This is performed using image-guided instillation of a chemical agent, most commonly ethanol or acetic acid. Li et al. reported a case of a patient with recurrent and metastatic ACC in which survival of 58 months was achieved with aggressive multiple trans-arterial embolization [62]. Addressing the role of these treatments in patients with ACC recurrence is challenging and further studies and reports are needed.

Recommendation

Evidence on the use of RFA in recurrent ACC is very limited. Further investigation is needed to address the long-term efficacy of this technique and its role in improving disease free and overall survival. As such, radiofrequency ablation may be considered alone or in combination with surgery in patients with recurrent ACC (evidence quality low, weak recommendation). There is no evidence to suggest that this treatment is superior to surgery alone or other treatment modalities.

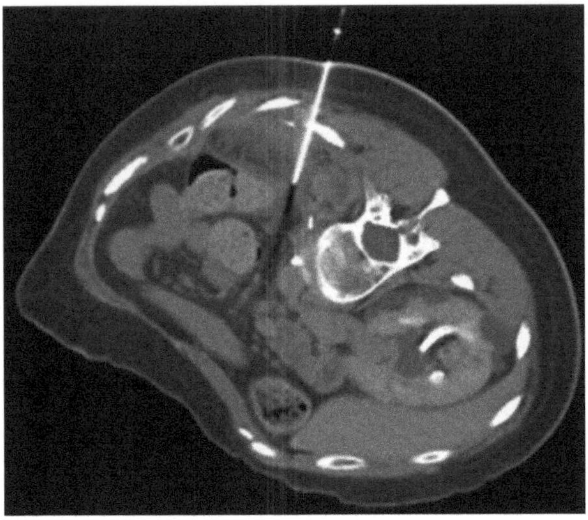

Fig. 31.2 CT-guided cryoprobe for ablation

Novel Therapies

A number of novel therapies are currently being investigated for the treatment of advanced ACC. These include the use of inhibitors of vascular endothelial growth factor (VEGF), epidermal growth factor receptor (EGFR), insulin-like growth factor receptor 1 (IGFR1) and mammalian target of rapamycin (mTOR). Other targets of interest include micro RNA therapies, targeting the Wnt/B-catenin pathway, interleukin-13 receptor alpha 2, and dimethylating agents. There is no evidence as yet to support their use in recurrent adrenocortical carcinoma and further research is needed.

Recommendation

There is no evidence for the use of novel targeted therapies in the treatment of recurrent ACC.

Conclusions

The management of patients with recurrent ACC poses a great challenge for the treating physician. Despite achieving a complete resection of the primary tumor and receiving adjuvant therapy, up to 85% of patients with ACC experience disease relapse. Appropriate patient referral to a specialized unit and a multidisciplinary approach to patient treatment are crucial. Surgical resection is recommended for patients with recurrent ACC who are suitable for further intervention and who develop a recurrence after 6–12 months of initial treatment (Fig. 31.3).

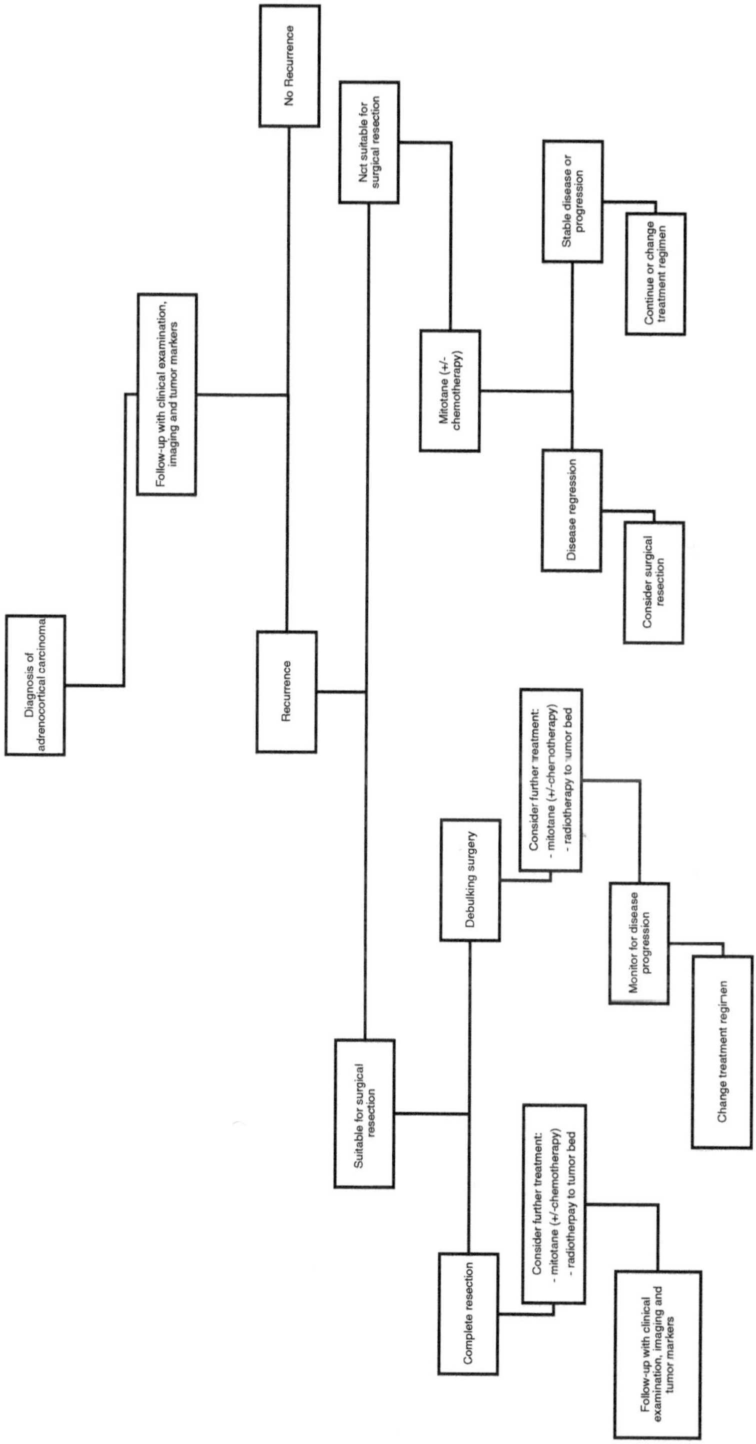

Fig. 31.3 Suggested algorithm for the treatment of patients with ACC

Recommendations Summary

Surgery

A number of case reports and retrospective case series have been published showing a benefit for re-operation for recurrent ACC. In these studies a complete resection was associated with an improved overall survival compared with an incomplete resection. A complete surgical resection, therefore, is recommended for patients who develop a recurrence of ACC more than 6–12 months following their initial therapeutic resection (evidence quality low, weak recommendation).

Chemotherapy

The use of chemotherapy and other medical therapy in recurrent ACC is unclear and evidence to support its use is limited to retrospective case series and reports. These therapies should be considered in the following reoperation for recurrent ACC and for the treatment of patients who have disease that is not amenable to surgical resection (evidence quality low, weak recommendation).

Radiotherapy

The use of radiotherapy in recurrent ACC is unclear and evidence to support its use is limited to retrospective case series and reports. Radiotherapy should be considered in the following reoperation for recurrent ACC and for the treatment of patients who have disease that is not amenable to surgical resection (evidence quality low, weak recommendation).

Tumor Ablation

Evidence on the use of RFA in recurrent ACC is very limited. Further investigation is needed to address the long-term efficacy of this technique and its role in improving disease free and overall survival. As such, radiofrequency ablation may be considered alone or in combination with surgery in patients with recurrent ACC (evidence quality low, weak recommendation). There is no evidence to suggest that this treatment is superior to surgery alone or other treatment modalities.

Targeted Therapies

There is no evidence for the use of novel targeted therapies in the treatment of recurrent ACC.

References

1. Kebebew E, Reiff E, Duh QY, Clark OH, McMillan A. Extent of disease at presentation and outcome for adrenocortical carcinoma: have we made progress? World J Surg. 2006;30:872–8.
2. Golden SH, Robinson KA, Saldanha I, Anton B, Ladenson PW. Clinical review: prevalence and incidence of endocrine and metabolic disorders in the United States: a comprehensive review. J Clin Endocrinol Metab. 2009;94:1853–78.
3. Wajchenberg BL, Albergaria Pereira MA, Medonca BB, Latronico AC, Campos Carneiro P, Alves VA, et al. Adrenocortical carcinoma: clinical and laboratory observations. Cancer. 2000;88:711–36.
4. Allolio BFM. Clinical review: adrenocortical carcinoma: clinical update. J Clin Endocrinol Metab. 2006;91(6):2027–37.
5. Dackiw APB, Lee JE, Gagel RF, Evans DB. Adrenal cortical carcinoma. World J Surg. 2001;25:914–26.
6. Icard P, Goudet P, Charpenay C, Andreassian B, Carnaille B, Chapuis Y, et al. Adrenocortical carcinomas: surgical trends and results of a 253-patient series from the French Association of Endocrine Surgeons study group. World J Surg. 2001;25:891–7.
7. Lughezzani G, Sun M, Perrotte P, Jeldres C, Alasker A, Isbarn H, et al. The European Network for the Study of Adrenal Tumors staging system is prognostically superior to the international union against cancer-staging system: a North American validation. Eur J Cancer. 2010;46:713–9.
8. Koschker A-C, Fassnacht M, Hahner S, Weismann D, Allolio B. Adrenocortical carcinoma – improving patient care by establishing new structures. Exp Clin Endocrinol Diabetes. 2006;114:45–51.
9. Hsing AW, Nam JM, Co Chien HT, McLaughlin JK, Fraumeni JF. Risk factors for adrenal cancer: an exploratory study. Int J Cancer. 1996;65:432–6.
10. Hisada M, Garber JE, Fung CY, Fraumeni JF, Li FP. Multiple primary cancers in families with Li-Fraumeni syndrome. J Natl Cancer Inst. 1998;90:606–11.
11. Fassnacht M, Libé R, Kroiss M, Allolio B. Adrenocortical carcinoma: a clinician's update. Nat Rev Endocrinol. 2011;7:323–35.
12. McFarlane D. Cancer of the adrenal cortex; the natural history, pronosis and treatment in a study of fifty-five cases. Ann R Coll Surg Engl. 1958;23:155–86.
13. Sullivan M, Boileau MHC. Adrenal cortical carcinoma. J Urol. 1978;120:660–5.
14. DeLellis RA, Lloyd RV, Heitz PU, Eng C. World Health Organization classification of tumours. Pathology and genetics of tumours of endocrine organs. Lyon: IARC; 2004.
15. Fassnacht M, Johanssen S, Quinkler M, Bucsky P, Willenberg HS, Beuschlein F, et al. Limited prognostic value of the 2004 international union against cancer staging classification for adrenocortical carcinoma. Cancer. 2009;115:243–50.
16. Pommier RF, Brennan MF. An eleven-year experience with adrenocortical carcinoma. Surgery. 1992;112:963–70. Discussion 970–1.
17. Stojadinovic A, Ghossein RA, Hoos A, Nissan A, Marshall D, Dudas M, et al. Adrenocortical carcinoma: clinical, morphologic, and molecular characterization. J Clin Oncol. 2002;20:941–50.
18. Crucitti F, Bellantone R, Ferrante A, Boscherini M, Crucitti P, Carbone G, et al. The italian registry for adrenal cortical carcinoma: analysis of a multiinstitutional series of 129 patients. Surgery. 1996;119:161–70.
19. Linos D, Vassilopoulos P, Papadimitriou J, Tountas K. The surgical management of adrenal cortical carcinoma. Int Surg. 1986;71(2):104–6.
20. Decker R, Kuehner M. Adrenocortical carcinoma. Am Surg. 1991;57(8):502–13.
21. Jensen C. Recurrent or metastatic disease in select patients with adrenocortical carcinoma adrenocortical. Arch Surg. 1991;126:457–61.

22. Van Aalderen W, Van Seters AP, Backer ET, Chang PC, Van Krieken JHJM, Moolenaar AJ. A case of recurrent adrenocortical carcinoma, with observations on long-term o,p'-DDD therapy and complications. Neth J Med. 1992;41:161–70.
23. Ahlman H, Jansson S, Wangberg B, Tisell L, Schersten T, Hansson G, et al. Adrenocortical carcinoma – diagnostic and therapeutical implications. Eur J Surg. 1993;159(3):149–58.
24. Haak HR, Hermans J, van de Velde CJ, Lentjes EG, Goslings BM, Fleuren GJ, et al. Optimal treatment of adrenocortical carcinoma with mitotane: results in a consecutive series of 96 patients. Br J Cancer. 1994;69:947–51.
25. Sakamoto K, Ariyoshi A, Okazaki M. Metastatic adrenocortical carcinoma treated by repeated resection: a case report of long-term survival over 18 years. Int J Urol. 1995;2:50–2.
26. Bellantone R, Ferrante A, Boscherini M, Lombardi CP, Crucitti P, Crucitti F, et al. Role of reoperation in recurrence of adrenal cortical carcinoma: results from 188 cases collected in the Italian National Registry for Adrenal Cortical Carcinoma. Surgery. 1997;122:1212–8.
27. Khorram-Manesh A, Ahlman H, Jansson S, Wängberg B, Nilsson O, Jakobsson CE, et al. Adrenocortical carcimona: surgery and mitotane for treatment and steroid profiles for follow-up. World J Surg. 1998;22:605–12.
28. Schulick RD, Brennan MF. Long-term survival after complete resection and repeat resection in patients with adrenocortical carcinoma. Ann Surg Oncol. 1999;6:719–26.
29. Seki M, Nomura K, Hirohara D, Kanazawa M, Sawada T, Takasaki K, et al. Changes in neoplastic cell features and sensitivity to mitotane during mitotane-induced remission in a patient with recurrent, metastatic adrenocortical carcinoma. Endocr Relat Cancer. 1999;6(4):529–33.
30. Langer P, Bartsch D, Moebius E, Rothmund M, Nies C. Adrenocortical carcinoma – our experience with 11 cases. Langenbeck's Arch Surg. 2000;385:393–7.
31. Ilias I, Alevizaki M, Philippou G, Anastasiou E, Souvatzoglou A. Sustained remission of metastatic adrenal carcinoma during long-term administration of low-dose mitotane. J Endocrinol Investig. 2001;24:532–5.
32. Fujii Y, Kageyama Y, Kawakami S, Masuda H, Arisawa C, Akamatsu H, et al. Successful long-term disease-free survival following multimodal treatments in a patient with a repeatedly recurrent refractory adrenal cortical carcinoma. Int J Urol. 2003;10(8):445.
33. Tauchmanovà L, Colao A, Marzano LA, Sparano L, Camera L, Rossi A, et al. Andrenocortical carcinomas: twelve-year prospective experience. World J Surg. 2004;28:896–903.
34. Matsumoto K, Egawa S, Satoh T, Okuno N, Kaseda S, Baba S. Thoracoscopic transdiaphragmatic adrenalectomy for isolated locally recurrent adrenal carcinoma. Int J Urol. 2005;12:1055–7.
35. Palazzo FF, Sebag F, Sierra M, Ippolito G, Souteyrand P, Henry JF. Long-term outcome following laparoscopic adrenalectomy for large solid adrenal cortex tumors. World J Surg. 2006;30:893–8.
36. Schlamp A, Hallfeldt K, Mueller-Lisse U, Pfluger T, Reincke M. Recurrent adrenocortical carcinoma after laparoscopic resection. Nat Clin Pract Endocrinol Metab. 2007;3:191–5.
37. Tan CT, Meyer-Rochow GY, Sywak MS, Delbridge LW, Sidhu SB. Reoperative adrenal surgery: lessons learnt. ANZ J Surg. 2009;79:371–7.
38. Sabolch A, Feng M, Griffith K, Hammer G, Doherty G, Ben-Josef E. Adjuvant and definitive radiotherapy for adrenocortical carcinoma. Int J Radiat Oncol Biol Phys. 2011;80:1477–84.
39. Datrice NM, Langan RC, Ripley RT, Kemp CD, Steinberg SM, Wood BJ, et al. Operative management for recurrent and metastatic adrenocortical carcinoma. J Surg Oncol. 2012;105:709–13.
40. Dy BM, Wise KB, Richards ML, Young WF, Grant CS, Bible KC, et al. Operative intervention for recurrent adrenocortical cancer. Surgery. 2013;154:1292–9.
41. Erdogan I, Deutschbein T, Jurowich C, Kroiss M, Ronchi C, Quinkler M, et al. The role of surgery in the management of recurrent adrenocortical carcinoma. J Clin Endocrinol Metab. 2013;98:181–91.
42. Terzolo M, Angeli A, Fassnacht M, Daffara F, Tauchmanova L, Conton PA, et al. Adjuvant mitotane treatment for adrenocortical carcinoma. N Engl J Med. 2007;356:2372–80.
43. Saunders BD, Doherty GM. Laparoscopic adrenalectomy for malignant disease. Lancet Oncol. 2004;5:718–26.

44. Shen WT, Lim RC, Siperstein AE, Clark OH, Schecter WP, Hunt TK, et al. Laparoscopic vs open adrenalectomy for the treatment of primary hyperaldosteronism. Arch Surg. 1999;134:628–31.
45. Cobb WS, Kercher KW, Sing RF, Heniford BT. Laparoscopic adrenalectomy for malignancy. Am J Surg. 2005;189(4):405–11.
46. Hahner S, Fassnacht M. Mitotane for adrenocortical carcinoma treatment. Curr Opin Investig Drugs. 2005;6:386–94.
47. Kopf D, Goretzki PE, Lehnert H. Clinical management of malignant adrenal tumors. J Cancer Res Clin Oncol. 2001;127:143–55.
48. Terzolo M, Pia A, Berruti A, Osella G, Alì A, Carbone V, et al. Low-dose monitored mitotane treatment achieves the therapeutic range with manageable side effects in patients with adrenocortical cancer. J Clin Endocrinol Metab. 2000;85:2234–8.
49. Faggiano A, Leboulleux S, Young J, Schlumberger M, Baudin E. Rapidly progressing high o,p'DDD doses shorten the time required to reach the therapeutic threshold with an acceptable tolerance: preliminary results. Clin Endocrinol. 2006;64:110–3.
50. Schteingart DE. Conventional and novel strategies in the treatment of adrenocortical cancer. Braz J Med Biol Res. 2000;33:1197–200.
51. Berruti A, Terzolo M, Sperone P, Pia A, Della Casa S, Gross DJ, et al. Etoposide, doxorubicin and cisplatin plus mitotane in the treatment of advanced adrenocortical carcinoma: a large prospective phase II trial. Endocr Relat Cancer. 2005;12:657–66.
52. Khan TS, Imam H, Juhlin C, Skogseid B, Gröndal S, Tibblin S, et al. Streptozocin and o,p'DDD in the treatment of adrenocortical cancer patients: long-term survival in its adjuvant use. Ann Oncol. 2000;11:1281–7.
53. Fassnacht M, Terzolo M, Allolio B, Baudin E, Haak H, Berruti A, et al. Combination chemotherapy in advanced adrenocortical carcinoma. N Engl J Med. 2012;366:2189–97.
54. Berruti A, Baudin E, Gelderblom H, Haak HR, Porpiglia F, Fassnacht M, et al. Adrenal cancer: ESMO clinical practice guidelines for diagnosis, treatment and follow-up. Ann Oncol. 2012;23(suppl 7):vii131–8.
55. Kornely E, Schlaghecke R. Complete remission of metastasized adrenocortical carcinoma under o,p'-DDD. Exp Clin Endocrinol. 1994;102:50–3.
56. Polat B, Fassnacht M, Pfreundner L, Guckenberger M, Bratengeier K, Johanssen S, et al. Radiotherapy in adrenocortical carcinoma. Cancer. 2009;115:2816–23.
57. Wood BJ, Abraham J, Hvizda JL, Alexander HR, Fojo T. Radiofrequency ablation of adrenal tumors and adrenocortical carcinoma metastases. Cancer. 2003;97:554–60.
58. Venkatesan AM, Locklin J, Dupuy DE, Wood BJ. Percutaneous ablation of adrenal Tumors. Tech Vasc Interv Radiol. 2010;13:89–99.
59. Beland MD, Mayo-Smith WW. Ablation of adrenal neoplasms. Abdom Imaging. 2009;34:588–92.
60. Atwell TD, Wass CT, Charboneau JW, Callstrom MR, Farrell MA, Sengupta S. Malignant hypertension during cryoablation of an adrenal gland tumor. J Vasc Interv Radiol. 2006;17:573–5.
61. Xiao YY, Tian JL, Li JK, Yang L, Zhang JS. CT-guided percutaneous chemical ablation of adrenal neoplasms. Am J Roentgenol. 2008;190:105–10.
62. Li SH, Huang CH, Ko SF, Chou FF, Huang SC. Extended survival in a patient with recurrent and metastatic adrenal cortical carcinoma by aggressive transarterial embolization – a case report. J Surg Oncol. 2005;90:101–5.

Resection Versus Observation for Adrenal Gland Metastasis

32

Frédéric Mercier, Liane S. Feldman, and Elliot J. Mitmaker

Abstract

The adrenal glands are frequently the site of metastasis from several different types of cancers, including lung, breast, melanoma, renal cell, and colon. Traditionally, the finding of adrenal metastasis was believed to portend end-stage disease and consequently surgery was rarely performed. Since the introduction of laparoscopic adrenalectomy in 1992, resection for isolated adrenal metastases is being reported with increasing frequency, and several authors have even reported improved outcomes and survival in selected patients. Presently the evidence for this recommendation is based solely on published anecdotal reports and retrospective series. Hence prospective studies are desperately needed so that formal guidelines can be established in the decision-making process for patients with adrenal metastases.

Keywords

Adrenal metastases · Oligometastases · Stereotactic ablative body radiotherapy · Adrenalectomy · Laparoscopic adrenalectomy · Radiofrequency ablation

F. Mercier
Department of Surgical Oncology, Centre Hospitalier de l'université de Montréal, Montreal, QC, Canada

L. S. Feldman
Department of Surgery, McGill University Health Center, Montreal, QC, Canada

Steinberg-Bernstein Centre for Minimally Invasive Surgery and Innovation, McGill University, Montreal, QC, Canada

E. J. Mitmaker (✉)
Department of Surgery, Royal Victoria Hospital – Glen Site, McGill University Health Center, Montreal, QC, Canada
e-mail: elliot.mitmaker@mcgill.ca

P. Angelos, R. H. Grogan (eds.), *Difficult Decisions in Endocrine Surgery*, Difficult Decisions in Surgery: An Evidence-Based Approach,
https://doi.org/10.1007/978-3-319-92860-9_32

Introduction

In the past, most if not all of the evidence reporting metastasis to the adrenal glands have come from autopsy series. A review of the literature in the first half of the twentieth century has documented the presence of metastatic lesions to the adrenal glands from almost all malignant epithelial tumors. All of these studies showed the metastatic potential of these invasive cancers and how they were able to establish a tumor "niche" in this small retroperitoneal endocrine gland [1, 2].

However, all of this did not provide any pathophysiologic dynamic that would help relate this phenomenon to the natural history of metastases to the adrenal glands [3]. The incidence of metastases to the adrenal gland is only second to the presence of non-functioning adrenal adenomas found at autopsy. Unraveling this problem had to await the imaging revolution in the last quarter of the twentieth century. The key was to be found in modern technology—the CT scan, the MRI and the PET scan [4].

With the recent emphasis on cancer surveillance, modern imaging methods have revealed the surprising fact that there is an increasing incidence of both synchronous and metachronous lesions in the adrenal gland of cancer patients. Modern radiological modalities (CT, MRI, PET scans) allow for early detection of isolated metastatic lesions to the adrenal glands. In view of the above, the surgeon is now confronted with a new clinical conundrum, what to do with the incidental adrenal nodule in a patient with a history of prior malignancy [4]?

The decision to operate on patients with disseminated metastatic disease is not an easy one. If one limits the discussion to adrenal metastasis only, whether the incidental nodule be a synchronous or metachronous lesion, it is becoming apparent that certain options are available for these patients. For patients with disseminated metastatic disease, surgery is generally not a viable option. In a subset of patients that have only a single metastatic lesion to the adrenal gland, then surgery is a viable option. Modern imaging has identified a new entity, whereby the primary cancer is in a state between locoregional extension and disseminated disease. This phase of the cancer is referred to as the stage of oligometastasis, corresponding to 1–5 macroscopic lesions. The surgical oncology literature has reported long disease-free survival following resection of isolated metastatic lesions to the adrenals [5]. Although there is no evidence that resection of isolated metastatic lesions offers any survival benefit compared to observation alone, the National Comprehensive Cancer Network (NCCN) already recommends resection of oligometastases. What data support these recommendations [6]? (Table 32.1).

Table 32.1 PICO table

*P*opulation	Patients with metastasis to the adrenal gland
*I*ntervention	Surgical resection
*C*omparator	Ablative techniques and medical management
*O*utcomes	Survival

Methods

Search Strategy

A systematic literature search was performed for all articles published relating to the management of adrenal gland metastases. We searched bibliographic databases (MEDLINE, EMBASE, Cochrane Collaboration, PubMed) as well as conference proceedings, using electronic search terms and keywords: adrenal gland metastases, adrenal neoplasms, catheter ablation, laparoscopy, adrenalectomy (resection, surgery, surgical). Total retrieval within each database was 78 articles in MEDLINE, 112 articles in EMBASE and 1 in the Cochrane Library. The search was limited to papers published in English, involving adult subjects (18+ years of age) and relevant articles from a 10-year period up to and including January 2015. Studies were initially screened for relevance based on title and abstract. All studies deemed relevant that met the study inclusion criteria were retained, totaling 53 articles.

Characterization of Adrenal Gland Metastasis

Incidence

The incidence of adrenal metastases is difficult to determine because most adrenal metastases are discovered at autopsy. In a retrospective series that followed patients for 30 years, 94% of adrenal metastases were discovered at autopsy (435/464), while only 4.3% (20/464) were symptomatic from their disease. Amongst those patients presenting with metastatic disease to the adrenal gland, 49% had bilateral metastases. In addition, approximately two-thirds of patients presented with synchronous disease, while one-third presented as metachronous disease, with a median time to presentation of 7 months [7].

Prevalence

The prevalence of adrenal gland metastases is quite variable. The largest study to date is from 1950, deriving data from 1000 autopsies performed on patients diagnosed with an epithelial carcinoma. The likelihood of finding adrenal metastases was 27% in that study. However, the prevalence of adrenal metastases is difficult to define as it depends on the population of patients that are studied [1].

Etiology

Historically, autopsy series found that adrenal metastases arise most commonly from the lung, breast, kidney, gastro-intestinal tract and skin (melanoma), with lung cancer representing up to 39% of cases and breast cancer up to 35% of cases [1, 2, 7]. One thousand autopsies were performed on patients who died from a variety of epithelial malignancies. In those 1000 patients, 270 presented with metastases to the adrenal gland (27%), while other autopsy series report lower rates of adrenal gland metastases (8.6%) [2]. Out of the 270 patients, 90 were from breast cancer, 57 were from lung cancer, 25 from gastric cancer and 17 from colon cancer. It is of interest to note that adrenal metastases occurred in 57% (90/167) of breast cancer patients, 33% of lung cancer patients (57/160), 21% of gastric cancer patients (25/119) and 15% of colon cancer patients (17/117) in this autopsy series from the 1950s. The etiology of adrenal gland metastases is reflective of the era of cancer therapeutics as the rate of adrenal gland metastases from breast cancer is now rare (<3%) [8]. Potential bias may exist in studies like these, as autopsies were performed on the first consecutive 1000 patients from a cancer center, suggesting that the sample may not be representative from a general population diagnosed with cancer. Given that all of these patients died from diffuse metastatic disease, one can ask if these metastatic findings are clinically relevant. In addition, the pathological techniques for detecting metastases (like immunohistochemistry) were not as developed in the 1950s. Finally melanoma, known to be a common primary that metastasizes to the adrenal gland, was not included in this study [1]. Furthermore, a review of 2833 autopsies reported by Bullock et al., showed different results in which the overall rate of adrenal metastases was 8.6% (244/2833) compared to 27% in the Abrams study. The most noticeable differences in prevalence of metastases were related to breast and gastric cancers. Abrams reported 53% and 21%, whereas Bullock showed a prevalence of 12.8% and 4.7%, respectively. Bullock was the first to report on metastatic adrenal lesions in melanoma in 10 of 32 cases. The results of these two historical studies are quite different therefore making it difficult to establish a precise prevalence of adrenal metastases. Still, these reports set the general rule for the average probability of metastases to the adrenal glands [2]. Finally, the anatomic site of the primary cancer that leads to adrenal metastases differs depending on geographic location. In comparison to the above-mentioned North American series, a study from Hong Kong revealed that the majority of adrenal metastasis came from the lung (149/421, 35%), followed by the stomach (60/421, 14.3%), oesophagus (51/421 12.1%), liver/bile duct cancer (45/421, 10.7%) pancreas, colon, kidney and breast. Hence, the pattern of adrenal metastatic disease seems to be influenced by geographic location [7].

There are three distinct patient presentations. The first presentation is when patients with a prior history of cancer are discovered to have a metachronous lesion in the adrenal gland during the postoperative surveillance period. Lenert et al. studied this population and found that 42 of 81 patients (52%) presented with adrenal metastases related to their primary cancer [9]. The prevalence rate appears to be high, and the authors do suggest that this may represent an overestimate of the real prevalence of adrenal gland metastases due to the fact that they excluded those patients discovered to have benign lesions from the analysis. In addition, this study was conducted over a 30-year period dating back to the 1970s. This represents another confounding variable, as considerable improvements with radiological imaging have been able to distinguish a benign from a likely malignant adrenal mass. As such, benign lesions would be underrepresented, leading to an overestimation of malignant lesions in this patient population. Therefore, the overall risk of an adrenal metastasis in a patient with a proven cancer is likely below 50%.

The second presentation is when the patient with a highly suspected cancer (or a proven cancer) is found with a synchronous adrenal lesion during cancer staging. The management of these patients will depend on the extent of the metastatic burden. Resection could be proposed if the adrenal gland is the only site of metastasis [10].

Finally the third presentation can be defined as a patient with an incidentally discovered adrenal lesion in the context of an unknown primary cancer. In this population, is it useful to perform a fine needle aspiration of the adrenal mass in order to diagnose the unknown primary malignancy? Lee et al. have studied this question by analyzing 1715 cases with unknown primary cancers and found only four patients (0.2%) whereby the adrenal incidentaloma uncovered the nature of the primary cancer. However, these four cases were clinically symptomatic due to the size of the adrenal lesion (>6 cm). This suggests that for asymptomatic incidentalomas, screening for an unknown primary extra-adrenal malignancy is not necessary [11].

Defining the Extent of the Disease in the Context of Adrenal Metastasis

Solitary Metastases

A solitary metastasis represents a rare occurrence of a single and isolated metastatic lesion to the adrenal gland from an occult or known primary malignancy.

Oligometastases

Hellman and Weichselbaum defined the term oligometastases in reference to an intermediary state between locoregional and disseminated metastatic disease, defined as the existence of one to five isolated macroscopic metastases [12].

Diffuse Metastatic Disease

This situation is most commonly seen when the patient presents with metastases in multiple organs, including the adrenal gland.

Adrenal Metastases and the "Seed and Soil" Theory

Paget's "seed and soil" hypothesis states that the interaction between the primary cancer (seed) and its organ microenvironment (soil) influences the pattern of metastases. The microenvironment of the adrenal gland appears to have the necessary components to favor metastatic growth. The adrenal gland has an extensive blood supply, exposing this endocrine organ to a significant tumor emboli transit. In addition, the adrenal gland has a vast lymphatic network throughout the cortex and medulla. Given these anatomical features, several studies have shown a predilection for metastatic deposits as they correlate with the number of capillary and lymphatic networks (3). Currently, there has been an investigation into the use of molecular markers to help predict the likelihood that a given cancer would metastasize to the adrenal gland [13].

Radiological Imaging Characterization

CT Scan

This imaging modality is most commonly used for the identification of adrenal masses. Specifically, adrenal metastases and primary adrenal cancer contain no fat as compared to benign adrenal lesions. Studies have identified cutoff values for density being 10 Hounsfield units (HU). A value below 10 HU allows for the diagnosis of an adrenal adenoma with 95% sensitivity and 80% specificity. Another useful imaging characteristic is the contrast washout behavior. Malignant lesions have an abnormal vasculature pattern, described by a high microvascular density and a high endothelial permeability resulting in slow blood flow with accumulation of contrast material within the lesion as compared to benign adrenal nodules [14]. A 50% washout value at 10 min has a sensitivity and specificity of 100% for differentiating between benign adenomas and malignant lesions [15].

MRI

MRI imaging readily identifies the lipid rich adenoma in comparison to lipid poor lesions such as primary and metastatic adrenal lesions. MRI scans achieve 89% sensitivity and 100% specificity in differentiating between benign and malignant adrenal nodules [16].

PET-CT Scan

This method is capable of detecting neoplastic lesions of the adrenal gland. When adding a low resolution CT scan with the PET scan, sensitivity and specificity are in the range of 95% [14]. This test is only useful in tumors that are FDG avid and is useful for patients with a history of prior malignancy [17].

Biopsy of an Adrenal Mass

Biopsy of the adrenal gland is generally not recommended [11, 18]. However, those patients with indeterminate adrenal lesions on imaging that prove to be non-functional, biopsy can be useful in the right setting. When an indeterminate adrenal lesion is discovered in the context of a known extra-adrenal malignancy, adrenal biopsy does have a high sensitivity and specificity (~90–95%) [4]. Therefore adrenal biopsy can be resorted to in specific clinical situations (i.e. needing a diagnosis in the setting of diffuse metastases). However, given the current advances in adrenal imaging, biopsy is rarely indicated.

Synchronous vs. Metachronous Metastases

Synchronous metastases are defined as lesions appearing within 6 months of diagnosis of the primary malignancy. Metachronous metastases are lesions appearing more than 6 months following the initial diagnosis of the malignancy. There are some reports indicating that the outcomes are significantly better for patients with non-small cell lung cancer who present with resectable metachronous metastases as compared to synchronous metastatic lesions within the first 3 years. Consequently, there is some clinical relevance in determining the status of the patient with adrenal metastasis as far as non-small cell lung cancer is concerned. This is in concordance with other types of tumors such as colorectal cancer with liver metastasis, renal cell cancer with brain metastasis or non-small cell lung cancer with brain metastases. Even though some reports suggest that survival following resection of metachronous lesions is better in the short term (up to 3 years from initial diagnosis), a systematic review revealed that long-term results were similar with a 25% survival rate at 5 years for both synchronous and metachronous lesions [19, 20]. For patients presenting with bilateral adrenal metastases that undergo bilateral adrenalectomy, there is a survival benefit in a select group of patients [20]. Therefore, bilateral adrenal metastases are not an absolute contraindication to surgical resection.

Surgical and Ablative Therapies in the Treatment of Adrenal Gland Metastases

Surgical Resection

Who Are the Candidates?

First and foremost, patients must be fit for surgery in order to undergo a major abdominal organ resection under general anesthesia. Contraindications to surgery include cardiac and pulmonary comorbidities, local invasion of other organs by the tumor and disseminated metastases. Optimal control of the primary malignancy is also a prerequisite for enrolling patients for an adrenal resection [4, 10].

Solitary vs. Oligometastases vs. Diffuse Metastatic Disease

As defined earlier, a solitary adrenal metastasis corresponds to the adrenal gland being the only site of metastasis. Oligometastases is an intermediate state between loco-regional and disseminated metastatic disease, usually defined as the existence of 1–5 isolated macroscopic metastases. Diffuse metastases are when the adrenal gland is part of multiple metastatic sites. There is no report that differentiates between all these subgroups primarily because the diffuse state is always seen as a contraindication to surgery except for symptomatic palliation.

The goal of surgery depends on the differences with respect to the biology of the primary lesions as discussed in the review by Sancho et al. An illustration of resecting oligometastases can be found in non-small cell lung cancer where there is anecdotal evidence of a short-term survival benefit from adrenalectomy following resection of brain metastases [21]. On the other hand, no benefit was seen for performing adrenalectomy in the setting of metastatic melanoma if complete surgical control of the primary tumor was not possible [22]. Yet, others suggest that resection of oligometastases seem to benefit from adrenalectomy if all other metastatic sites are potentially resectable [23].

Synchronous vs. Metachronous Adrenal Metastases

The 6-month cut-off that distinguishes synchronous from metachronous metastatic lesions is important for establishing prognosis as some studies report the metachronous group fares better when compared to the synchronous group. Earlier series from MSKCC found that a disease-free interval of greater than 6 months was a predictor for improved survival [24]. However, when the MSKCC group analyzed a larger cohort of patients with metastatic adrenal lesions, the disease-free interval was no longer considered a significant predictor of survival [25]. The authors explained this discrepancy due to a short follow-up period in their initial publication. Despite this finding, many other studies found a significant difference between the synchronous and metachronous groups [19, 26]. Although there is controversy surrounding the prognostic significance of the disease-free interval, subgroup analysis of the individual primary malignancies may reveal a more accurate prognosis when accounting for tumor biology [26]. Yet a greater disease-free interval may still be viewed as a surrogate marker for a primary tumor that is less aggressive [5].

Outcomes: Morbidity of Surgery, Local Control, Overall Survival

Morbidity is inconsistently reported in the different surgical retrospective studies. An exhaustive meta-analysis reviewed 30 surgical cohorts of patients. Only 60% (18/30) reported complications in their series. From the 18 studies totaling 491 patients, there were six reported deaths. The total reported complication rate was 17% and the major complication rate was 7.5% [5].

To add to the difficulties in interpreting these studies, the local control rate was reported even less frequently. The local control rate ranged from 82.6% to 100% for a 2-year period, this being reported in only 11 studies out of the 30 cohorts included in the Gunjur meta-analysis [5].

Survival rates (overall survival) varied widely between studies and the one-year survival rate was reported to range from 55% to 100%. Not surprisingly, the one-year survival rate is the lowest for non-small cell lung cancer patients and highest in the renal cell cancer patients. The rate at 5 years had similar variability, ranging from 10 to 45% [5]. Although some series report up to a 60% rate of survival at 5 years, these studies included patients who had different primary malignancies at variable stages of disease progression [10]. Therefore, it is difficult to obtain a realistic estimate of survival at 5 years. Still, it is important to note that there is the possibility of long-term survivorship. The major issue lies in patient selection. (Table 32.2).

Table 32.2 Summary data from surgical and ablative studies in the treatment of adrenal metastasis

Study	Patients	Methods	Histology	Follow-up (months)	OS
Branum et al. [29]	8	Surgery (OP)	Melanoma	NR	50% crude median 59 months
Lo et al. [30]	52	Surgery (OP)	RCC, NSCLC, CRC, melanoma	NR	73% 1 year 40% 2 years
Wade et al. [31]	47	Surgery (OP)	NSLC, RCC, melanoma, CRC, esophagus, liver	NR	10% 5 years
Haigh et al. [22]	27	Surgery (OP)	Melanoma	NR	59% 1 year
Heniford et al. [32]	10	Surgery (LSC)	RCC, NSCLC, colon, melanoma	8.3	100% crude
Harrison et al. [33]	8	Surgery (OP)	NSCLC, RCC, CRC	Median 42	NR
Bretcha-Boix et al. [34]	5	Surgery (OP)	NSCLC	NR (8–52)	NR
Porte et al. [35]	43	Surgery (OP)	NSCLC	23.8 (2–94)	29% 2 years 11% 4 years
Momoi et al. [36]	13	Surgery (OP)	HCC	NR	68% 1 year 34% 5 years
Pfannschmidt et al. [37]	11	Surgery (OP)	NSCLC	21 (2–72)	55% 1 year
Lucchi et al. [38]	11	Surgery (LSC)	NSCLC	NR	55% 2 years
Mercier et al. [19]	23	Surgery (OP)	NSCLC	26 (0.3–110)	37% 2 years 23% 5 years
Sebag et al. [39]	16	Surgery (LSC)	NSCLC, melanoma, RCC	21 (1–68)	33% 5 years
Kita et al. [40]	8	Surgery (OP)	Lung, RCC, melanoma	NR	33% 2 years
Mittendorf et al. [23]	22	Surgery (OP and LSC)	Melanoma	12.6	61% crude
Park et al. [41]	5	Surgery	HCC	NR	Median 21.4 months
Strong et al. [25]	92	Surgery (OP and LSC)	NSCLC, RCC, CRC, melanoma	51.3	80% 1 year
Adler et al. [42]	17	Surgery (OP and LSC)	RCC, NSCLC, melanoma, breast, CRC	12.5	47% 2 years
Collinson et al. [43]	23	Surgery (OP and LSC)	Melanoma	NR	61% 1 year 39% 2 years

(continued)

Table 32.2 (continued)

Study	Patients	Methods	Histology	Follow-up (months)	OS
Bonnet et al. [44]	11	Surgery (OP and LSC)	RCC	34 (15–60)	100% 1 year
Mourra et al. [45]	8	Surgery	CRC	NR	NR
Marangos et al. [46]	31	Surgery (LSC)	CRC, RCC, lung, melanoma HCC	25 (3–70)	22% 3 years
De Haas et al. [47]	10	Surgery (OP and LSC)	CRC	NR	Median 23 months
Muth et al. [48]	30	Surgery (OP and LSC)	RCC, melanoma, NSCLC, CRC	19.5 (2–120)	23% 5 years
Pascual Piedrola et al. [49]	10	Surgery (LSC)	Lung, RCC, CRC	23 (2–38)	NR
Wu et al. [50]	12	Surgery (LSC)	RCC, NSCLC, melanoma, CRC	17.2 (2–56)	NR
Raz et al. [51]	20	Surgery (OP and LSC)	NSCLC	NR	34% 5 years
Crenn et al. [52]	14	Surgery (LSC)	RCC, NSCLC, melanoma, breast, eye	NR	Median 14 months
Zerwek et al. [53]	65	Surgery (OP and LSC)	RCC, NSCLC, melanoma, sarcoma, CRC pancreas	NR	68% 1 year 17% 5 years
Katoh et al. [54]	8	SABR	NSCLC, SCLC, HCC, RCC	16 (3–21)	78% 1 year
Chawla et al. [55]	30	SABR	Lung, HCC, breast, pancreas melanoma	9.8 (0,8–35)	44% 1 year 25% 2 years
Torok et al. [56]	7	SABR	NSCLC, SCLC, HCC	14	63% 1 year
Oshiro et al. [57]	11	SABR	NSCLC, SCLC	10.1 (0.7–87.8)	55% 1 year 33% 2 years 22% 5 years
Holy et al. [58]	18	SABR	NCSLC	12 (–61)	Median 21 months
Casamassima et al. [59]	48	SABR	Lung, CRC, melanoma, breast, kidney	16.2 (3–63)	40% 1 year 14% 2 years
Guiou et al. [60]	9	SABR	NSCLC, SCLC	7.3 (0–26)	52% 1 year 13% 2 years
Ahmed et al. [61]	13	SABR	NSCLC, SCLC, skin, RCC	12.3 (3.1–18)	63% 1 year
Scorsetti et al. [62]	34	SABR	NSCLC, SCLC, melanoma	41 (12–75)	Median 22.8 months

(continued)

Table 32.2 (continued)

Study	Patients	Methods	Histology	Follow-up (months)	OS
Mayo-Smith et al. [63]	10	RFA	NSCLC, RCC, melanoma	11.2 (1–46)	Median 8 months
Carafiello et al. [64]	6	RFA	RCC, breast, ovarian, NSCLC	24 (6–36)	NR
Wang et al. [65]	5	RFA	HCC, RCC	19 (8–31)	NR
Mouracade et al. [66]	5	RFA	RCC	NR	NR
Yamakado et al. [67]	6	RFA	HCC	37.7 (4–70.9)	NR
Wolf et al. [68]	19	RFA	RCC, lung, melanoma, HCC	NR	NR

OS overall survival, *SABR* stereotactic ablative body radiotherapy, *RFA* radiofrequency ablation, *OP* open, *LSC* laparoscopic, *RCC* renal cell carcinoma, *NSCLC* Non small cell lung cancer, *SCLC* small cell lung cancer, *CRC* colorectal cancer, *NR* no results
Table adapted from Gunjur et al. [5]; with permission

Non Invasive Options: Curative vs Palliative

Stereotactic Ablative Body Radiotherapy and Percutaneous Catheter Ablation

The non-surgical options for treating adrenal gland metastases include ablative techniques in the form of stereotactic ablative body radiotherapy and percutaneous catheter ablation. In general, ablative techniques in metastatic disease are feasible and can be offered to a carefully select group of patients, usually after consultation with a local interdisciplinary tumor board.

The principle of stereotactic ablative body radiotherapy (SABR) is to deliver a form of external beam radiotherapy with accuracy and precision using a high dose of radiation to a given target in one or few treatment fractions [27]. This technique uses a multiple number of beams that each deliver a small dose of irradiation, but when combined will result in a much larger dose at a given focal area of treatment [5].

The percutaneous ablation techniques include radiofrequency ablation (RFA) and microwave ablation (MWA). Through image guidance, these thermal ablative techniques to the adrenal gland, can deliver thermal energy of greater than 50 °C thereby exerting cytotoxic effects by denaturing intra- and extracellular proteins leading to cell dessication and coagulative necrosis.

Nine trials were evaluated in the Gunjur meta-analysis, which totaled 178 patients. The majority of patients had lung cancer primaries (68%) [5]. Fractioned doses of radiotherapy were quite different ranging from 10 to 60 Gy with body equivalent dosing of 28 to 110 Gy. The local control rate ranged from 55% to 100% at 1 year. Overall survival was quite low, with a reported rate of 55% at 1 year to 14% at 2 years. In these studies no serious adverse events were reported. Only grade one and two toxicities were reported at a rate of 6%. It has been suggested that a total body equivalent dosage greater or equal to 100 Gy is necessary to get local control of non-small cell lung cancer [28]. Due to the lower dose of radiation used in these studies, this can explain the low complication rate as well as the low overall survival rate. The lower dose of radiation given in the majority of these studies reflects a palliative dose, thus providing an explanation for the poor local control and overall survival rates.

Outcomes: Local Control Versus Overall Survival from Surgical and Ablative Treatments

There is a paucity of data concerning the newer ablative techniques regarding local control and overall survival. The majority of outcome data were derived from surgical series that examined disease control. In a recent review of 30 retrospective studies, a total of 818 patients were evaluated [5]. The three most common malignancies were lung (non-small cell), renal cell carcinoma and melanoma. 75% of these patients presented with isolated adrenal metastases. A third of the patients underwent laparoscopic surgery despite the debate between open and minimally invasive techniques. Local control was rarely reported in these studies. The compilation of the local control data, representing a total of 93 patients (11% of the total patients), gave a local control rate of 84% at 2 years. The overall survival rate, which is the more frequently reported value, was 46% at 2 years. Of note, the follow up period for the majority of these studies was less than 2 years [5].

The data for stereotactic ablative body radiotherapy (SABR) was not as robust when compared to surgery as a treatment for adrenal metastases. A total of 178 patients from nine different studies were examined. The majority of adrenal metastases treated by SABR were from a lung cancer primary (68%) while 4% were of renal origin. Local control was reported in eight out of nine studies, with a local control rate of 63% at 2 years. The overall survival at 2 years was 19%. Although the overall survival was much lower in the SABR series, the surgery treatment group could not really be compared to the SABR group, as the clinical characteristics of these populations were not equivalent [5].

Percutaneous radiofrequency ablation or microwave ablation are other methods of local control. Only six studies with a total of 51 patients were identified. Adrenal metastasis from renal cell carcinoma was the most common primary malignancy treated (45%), while lung cancer was the second most common metastatic lesion treated (27%). Local control was only reported in one of six studies, examining only five patients. Of this small cohort, a local control rate of 80% was achieved. The overall survival rate was not reported in any of these studies [5].

Even if the populations are difficult to compare, the local control and overall survival rates seem to be highest in the surgical cohort which could be partially explained by the better overall health and performance of the surgically-treated patients (Table 32.2).

Outcomes: Morbidity from Surgery Compared with SABR and Percutaneous Ablation

Complications from each of the different modalities are inconsistently reported in the literature. The systematic review by Gunjur et al. looked at a total of 30 studies but the complications were not systematically reported. Of the studies reporting complications in the surgery cohort, a wide range of major and minor complications were recorded. Major complications included: 4 bowel perforations (0.84%) (1 gastric, 1 duodenal and 2 small bowel), 1 vena cava laceration (0.2%), 1 bronchopleural fistula (0.2%), 1 evisceration (0.2%) and 1 diaphragmatic tear (0.2%). Minor complications included 1 surgical site infection but the majority of the studies did not specify minor complications [5].

For the SABR group, complications were categorized as either acute or late toxicity. These complications were reported for all nine studies. Five studies reported no acute complications. Combining the remaining four studies, GI toxicity (grade 2) was reported in 4.5% of patients. For complications regarding late toxicity, there were 1.7% of patients with GI toxicity (grade 2), 0.5% reported fatigue (grade 2) and another 0.5% reported adrenal insufficiency (grade 2).

Overall complications were minimal when patients underwent percutaneous radiofrequency ablation. Amongst the reported complications, there were 8% hypertensive crises, 8% back pain, 4% retroperitoneal hematomas, 2% abscesses, 2% pleural effusions and 2% myocardial infarctions.

As expected, the complication rate was higher in the surgery group. The only deaths reported were in the surgical cohort representing a 1.25% mortality rate. There were more major complications in the surgical group as compared to the SABR and percutaneous ablation groups. When comparing non-surgical local control techniques, the complication rate was higher in the percutaneous ablation group as compared to the SABR group [5] (Table 32.2).

Summary Recommendations

The choice between an invasive or non-invasive approach in the treatment algorithm for adrenal gland metastases remains a challenge. This is due primarily to the lack of strong evidence in support of either surgical resection, focused ablative techniques or systemic therapies. With the majority of evidence composed of retrospective reviews and meta-analyses, it appears that surgical resection offers the best chance of improved survival when compared to other therapeutic modalities. Selection criteria for any type of adrenal-directed therapy for metastasis must ensure that the patient is fit to undergo a particular treatment. The literature suggests that surgical resection should be considered when faced with the single metachronous lesion or isolated adrenal metastasis, and for patients with resectable oligometastases. If the metastases are synchronous, unresectable or diffuse, palliative treatments should be considered, including ablative or systemic therapies, based on the origin of the primary malignancy. The best therapeutic strategy for the treatment of adrenal gland metastases is yet to be determined. Hopefully this will be based on information forthcoming from prospective trials thereby providing evidence-based guidelines for the treatment of this problem.

References

1. Abrams HL, Spiro R, Goldstein N. Metastases in carcinoma; analysis of 1000 autopsied cases. Cancer. 1950;3(1):74–85.
2. Bullock WK, Hirst AE. Metastatic carcinoma of the adrenal. Am J Med Sci. 1953;226(5):521–4.
3. Onuigbo WI. Lymphangiogenesis may explain adrenal selectivity in lung cancer metastases. Med Hypotheses. 2010;75(2):185–6.
4. McLean K, Lilienfeld H, Caracciolo JT, Hoffe S, Tourtelot JB, Carter WB. Management of isolated adrenal lesions in cancer patients. Cancer Control. 2011;18(2):113–26.
5. Gunjur A, Duong C, Ball D, Siva S. Surgical and ablative therapies for the management of adrenal 'oligometastases' - a systematic review. Cancer Treat Rev. 2014;40(7):838–46.
6. Kulke MH, Shah MH, Benson AB, Bergsland E, Berlin JD, Blaszkowsky LS, et al. Neuroendocrine tumors, version 1.2015. J Natl Compr Cancer Netw. 2015;13(1):78–108.
7. Lam KY, Lo CY. Metastatic tumours of the adrenal glands: a 30-year experience in a teaching hospital. Clin Endocrinol. 2002;56(1):95–101.
8. Liu XJ, Shen P, Wang XF, Sun K, Sun FF. Solitary adrenal metastasis from invasive ductal breast cancer: an uncommon finding. World J Surg Oncol. 2010;8:7.
9. Lenert JT, Barnett CC, Kudelka AP, Sellin RV, Gagel RF, Prieto VG, et al. Evaluation and surgical resection of adrenal masses in patients with a history of extra-adrenal malignancy. Surgery. 2001;130(6):1060–7.
10. Sancho JJ, Triponez F, Montet X, Sitges-Serra A. Surgical management of adrenal metastases. Langenbeck's Arch Surg. 2012;397(2):179–94.
11. Lee JE, Evans DB, Hickey RC, Sherman SI, Gagel RF, Abbruzzese MC, Abbruzzese JL. Unknown primary cancer presenting as an adrenal mass: frequency and implications for diagnostic evaluation of adrenal incidentalomas. Surgery. 1998;124(6):1115–22.
12. Hellman S, Weichselbaum RR. Oligometastases. J Clin Oncol. 1995;13(1):8–10.
13. Raynaud CM, Mercier O, Dartevelle P, Commo F, Olaussen KA, de Montpreville V, et al. Expression of chemokine receptor CCR6 as a molecular determinant of adrenal metastatic relapse in patients with primary lung cancer. Clin Lung Cancer. 2010;11(3):187–91.
14. Blake MA, Holalkere NS, Boland GW. Imaging techniques for adrenal lesion characterization. Radiol Clin N Am. 2008;46(1):65–78. vi.
15. Caoili EM, Korobkin M, Francis IR, Cohan RH, Platt JF, Dunnick NR, Raghupathi KI. Adrenal masses: characterization with combined unenhanced and delayed enhanced CT. Radiology. 2002;222(3):629–33.
16. Haider MA, Ghai S, Jhaveri K, Lockwood G. Chemical shift MR imaging of hyperattenuating (>10 HU) adrenal masses: does it still have a role? Radiology. 2004;231(3):711–6.
17. Metser U, Miller E, Lerman H, Lievshitz G, Avital S, Even-Sapir E. 18F-FDG PET/CT in the evaluation of adrenal masses. J Nucl Med. 2006;47(1):32–7.
18. Lee JE, Evans DB, Sherman SI, Gagel RF. Evaluation of the incidental adrenal mass. Am J Med. 1997;103(3):249–50.
19. Mercier O, Fadel E, de Perrot M, Mussot S, Stella F, Chapelier A, Dartevelle P. Surgical treatment of solitary adrenal metastasis from non-small cell lung cancer. J Thorac Cardiovasc Surg. 2005;130(1):136–40.
20. Tanvetyanon T, Robinson LA, Schell MJ, Strong VE, Kapoor R, Coit DG, Bepler G. Outcomes of adrenalectomy for isolated synchronous versus metachronous adrenal metastases in non-small-cell lung cancer: a systematic review and pooled analysis. J Clin Oncol. 2008;26(7):1142–7.
21. Sugimura H, Nichols FC, Yang P, Allen MS, Cassivi SD, Deschamps C, et al. Survival after recurrent nonsmall-cell lung cancer after complete pulmonary resection. Ann Thorac Surg. 2007;83(2):409–17. discussion 417-8.
22. Haigh PI, Essner R, Wardlaw JC, Stern SL, Morton DL. Long-term survival after complete resection of melanoma metastatic to the adrenal gland. Ann Surg Oncol. 1999;6(7):633–9.

23. Mittendorf EA, Lim SJ, Schacherer CW, Lucci A, Cormier JN, Mansfield PF, et al. Melanoma adrenal metastasis: natural history and surgical management. Am J Surg. 2008;195(3):363–8. discussion 368-9.
24. Sarela AI, Murphy I, Coit DG, Conlon KC. Metastasis to the adrenal gland: the emerging role of laparoscopic surgery. Ann Surg Oncol. 2003;10(10):1191–6.
25. Strong VE, D'Angelica M, Tang L, Prete F, Gönen M, Coit D, et al. Laparoscopic adrenalectomy for isolated adrenal metastasis. Ann Surg Oncol. 2007;14(12):3392–400.
26. Moreno P, de la Quintana BA, Musholt TJ, Paunovic I, Puccini M, Vidal O, et al. Adrenalectomy for solid tumor metastases: results of a multicenter european study. Surgery. 2013;154(6):1215–22. discussion 1222-3.
27. Guckenberger M, Andratschke N, Alheit H, Holy R, Moustakis C, Nestle U, et al. Definition of stereotactic body radiotherapy: principles and practice for the treatment of stage I non-small cell lung cancer. Strahlenther Onkol. 2014;190(1):26–33.
28. Onishi H, Araki T, Shirato H, Nagata Y, Hiraoka M, Gomi K, et al. Stereotactic hypofractionated high-dose irradiation for stage I nonsmall cell lung carcinoma: clinical outcomes in 245 subjects in a japanese multiinstitutional study. Cancer. 2004;101(7):1623–31.
29. Branum GD, Epstein RE, Leight GS, Seigler HF. The role of resection in the management of melanoma metastatic to the adrenal gland. Surgery. 1991;109(2):127–31.
30. Lo CY, van Heerden JA, Soreide JA, Grant CS, Thompson GB, Lloyd RV, Harmsen WS. Adrenalectomy for metastatic disease to the adrenal glands. Br J Surg. 1996;83(4):528–31.
31. Wade TP, Longo WE, Virgo KS, Johnson FE. A comparison of adrenalectomy with other resections for metastatic cancers. Am J Surg. 1998;175(3):183–6.
32. Heniford BT, Arca MJ, Walsh RM, Gill IS. Laparoscopic adrenalectomy for cancer. Semin Surg Oncol. 1999;16(4):293–306.
33. Harrison J, Ali A, Bonomi P, Prinz R. The role of positron emission tomography in selecting patients with metastatic cancer for adrenalectomy. Am Surg. 2000;66(5):432–6. discussion 436-7.
34. Bretcha-Boix P, Rami-Porta R, Mateu-Navarro M, Hoyuela-Alonso C, Marco-Molina C. Surgical treatment of lung cancer with adrenal metastasis. Lung Cancer. 2000;27(2):101–5.
35. Porte H, Siat J, Guibert B, Lepimpec-Barthes F, Jancovici R, Bernard A, et al. Resection of adrenal metastases from non-small cell lung cancer: a multicenter study. Ann Thorac Surg. 2001;71(3):981–5.
36. Momoi H, Shimahara Y, Terajima H, Iimuro Y, Yamamoto N, Yamamoto Y, et al. Management of adrenal metastasis from hepatocellular carcinoma. Surg Today. 2002;32(12):1035–41.
37. Pfannschmidt J, Schlolaut B, Muley T, Hoffmann H, Dienemann H. Adrenalectomy for solitary adrenal metastases from non-small cell lung cancer. Lung Cancer. 2005;49(2):203–7.
38. Lucchi M, Dini P, Ambrogi MC, Berti P, Materazzi G, Miccoli P, Mussi A. Metachronous adrenal masses in resected non-small cell lung cancer patients: therapeutic implications of laparoscopic adrenalectomy. Eur J Cardiothorac Surg. 2005;27(5):753–6.
39. Sebag F, Calzolari F, Harding J, Sierra M, Palazzo FF, Henry JF. Isolated adrenal metastasis: the role of laparoscopic surgery. World J Surg. 2006;30(5):888–92.
40. Kita M, Tamaki G, Okuyama M, Saga Y, Kakizaki H. Adrenalectomy for metastatic adrenal tumors. Hinyokika Kiyo. 2007;53(11):761–6.
41. Park JS, Yoon DS, Kim KS, Choi JS, Lee WJ, Chi HS, Kim BR. What is the best treatment modality for adrenal metastasis from hepatocellular carcinoma? J Surg Oncol. 2007;96(1):32–6.
42. Adler JT, Mack E, Chen H. Equal oncologic results for laparoscopic and open resection of adrenal metastases. J Surg Res. 2007;140(2):159–64.
43. Collinson FJ, Lam TK, Bruijn WM, de Wilt JH, Lamont M, Thompson JF, Kefford RF. Long-term survival and occasional regression of distant melanoma metastases after adrenal metastasectomy. Ann Surg Oncol. 2008;15(6):1741–9.
44. Bonnet S, Gaujoux S, Leconte M, Thillois JM, Tissier F, Dousset B. Laparoscopic adrenalectomy for metachronous metastasis from renal cell carcinoma. World J Surg. 2008;32(8):1809–14.

45. Mourra N, Hoeffel C, Duvillard P, Guettier C, Flejou JF, Tiret E. Adrenalectomy for clinically isolated metastasis from colorectal carcinoma: report of eight cases. Dis Colon Rectum. 2008;51(12):1846–9.
46. Marangos IP, Kazaryan AM, Rosseland AR, Røsok BI, Carlsen HS, Kromann-Andersen B, et al. Should we use laparoscopic adrenalectomy for metastases? Scandinavian multicenter study. J Surg Oncol. 2009;100(1):43–7.
47. de Haas RJ, Rahy Martin AC, Wicherts DA, Azoulay D, Castaing D, Adam R. Long-term outcome in patients with adrenal metastases following resection of colorectal liver metastases. Br J Surg. 2009;96(8):935–40.
48. Muth A, Persson F, Jansson S, Johanson V, Ahlman H, Wängberg B. Prognostic factors for survival after surgery for adrenal metastasis. Eur J Surg Oncol. 2010;36(7):699–704.
49. Pascual Piédrola JI, Rincón Mayans A, Tolosa Eizaguirre E, Barba Abad J, Romero Vargas L, Rosell Costa D. Laparoscopic adrenalectomy for metachronous metastasis. Experience in 12 cases. Actas Urol Esp. 2010;34(2):201–5.
50. Wu HY, Yu Y, Xu LW, Li XD, Yu DM, Zhang ZG, Li GH. Transperitoneal laparoscopic adrenalectomy for adrenal metastasis. Surg Laparosc Endosc Percutan Tech. 2011;21(4):271–4.
51. Raz DJ, Lanuti M, Gaissert HC, Wright CD, Mathisen DJ, Wain JC. Outcomes of patients with isolated adrenal metastasis from non-small cell lung carcinoma. Ann Thorac Surg. 2011;92(5):1788–92. discussion 1793.
52. Crenn G, Delaunay B, Salloum A, Vezzosi D, Bellec L, Thoulouzan M, et al. Carcinological results of laparoscopic adrenalectomy for adrenal metastasis. Prog Urol. 2011;21(9):607–14.
53. Zerrweck C, Caiazzo R, Clerquin B, Donatini G, Lamblin A, El Khatib Z, et al. Renal origin and size are independent predictors of survival after surgery for adrenal metastasis. Ann Surg Oncol. 2012;19(11):3621–6.
54. Katoh N, Onimaru R, Sakuhara Y, Abo D, Shimizu S, Taguchi H, et al. Real-time tumor-tracking radiotherapy for adrenal tumors. Radiother Oncol. 2008;87(3):418–24.
55. Chawla S, Chen Y, Katz AW, Muhs AG, Philip A, Okunieff P, Milano MT. Stereotactic body radiotherapy for treatment of adrenal metastases. Int J Radiat Oncol Biol Phys. 2009;75(1):71–5.
56. Torok J, Wegner RE, Burton SA, Heron DE. Stereotactic body radiation therapy for adrenal metastases: a retrospective review of a noninvasive therapeutic strategy. Future Oncol. 2011;7(1):145–51.
57. Oshiro Y, Takeda Y, Hirano S, Ito H, Aruga T. Role of radiotherapy for local control of asymptomatic adrenal metastasis from lung cancer. Am J Clin Oncol. 2011;34(3):249–53.
58. Holy R, Piroth M, Pinkawa M, Eble MJ. Stereotactic body radiation therapy (SBRT) for treatment of adrenal gland metastases from non-small cell lung cancer. Strahlenther Onkol. 2011;187(4):245–51.
59. Casamassima F, Livi L, Masciullo S, Menichelli C, Masi L, Meattini I, et al. Stereotactic radiotherapy for adrenal gland metastases: university of Florence experience. Int J Radiat Oncol Biol Phys. 2012;82(2):919–23.
60. Guiou M, Mayr NA, Kim EY, Williams T, Lo SS. Stereotactic body radiotherapy for adrenal metastases from lung cancer. J Radiat Oncol. 2012;1(2):155–63.
61. Ahmed KA, Barney BM, Macdonald OK, Miller RC, Garces YI, Laack NN, et al. Stereotactic body radiotherapy in the treatment of adrenal metastases. Am J Clin Oncol. 2013;36(5):509–13.
62. Scorsetti M, Alongi F, Filippi AR, Pentimalli S, Navarria P, Clerici E, et al. Long-term local control achieved after hypofractionated stereotactic body radiotherapy for adrenal gland metastases: a retrospective analysis of 34 patients. Acta Oncol. 2012;51(5):618–23.
63. Mayo-Smith WW, Dupuy DE. Adrenal neoplasms: CT-guided radiofrequency ablationpreliminary results. Radiology. 2004;231(1):225–30.
64. Carrafiello G, Laganà D, Recaldini C, Giorgianni A, Ianniello A, Lumia D, et al. Imaging-guided percutaneous radiofrequency ablation of adrenal metastases: preliminary results at a single institution with a single device. Cardiovasc Intervent Radiol. 2008;31(4):762–7.
65. Wang Y, Liang P, Yu X, Cheng Z, Yu J, Dong J. Ultrasound-guided percutaneous microwave ablation of adrenal metastasis: preliminary results. Int J Hyperth. 2009;25(6):455–61.

66. Mouracade P, Dettloff H, Schneider M, Debras B, Jung JL. Radio-frequency ablation of solitary adrenal gland metastasis from renal cell carcinoma. Urology. 2009;74(6):1341–3.
67. Yamakado K, Anai H, Takaki H, Sakaguchi H, Tanaka T, Kichikawa K, Takeda K. Adrenal metastasis from hepatocellular carcinoma: radiofrequency ablation combined with adrenal arterial chemoembolization in six patients. AJR Am J Roentgenol. 2009;192(6):W300–5.
68. Wolf FJ, Dupuy DE, Machan JT, Mayo-Smith WW. Adrenal neoplasms: effectiveness and safety of ct-guided ablation of 23 tumors in 22 patients. Eur J Radiol. 2012;81(8):1717–23.

Routine Versus Selective Adrenal Vein Sampling for Primary Aldosteronism

33

Sarah C. Oltmann, Alan Dackiw, and Fiemu E. Nwariaku

Abstract

Primary aldosteronism (PA) represents a spectrum of conditions characterized by autonomous adrenal aldosterone secretion, and hypertension. Adrenalectomy is associated with excellent outcomes in patients with unilateral autonomous primary aldosteronism, whereas bilateral adrenal aldosteronism does not respond to unilateral adrenalectomy and such patients are better managed using medical therapy. Given the importance of lateralization on therapeutic decision-making and outcomes, the accuracy of lateralization tests is crucial.

Cross-sectional imaging techniques such as CT and MRI suffer from poor accuracy, particularly because of the prevalence of non-functional adrenal nodules in many patients. As such, much interest exists regarding adrenal vein sampling (AVS) for lateralization. Routine AVS is associated with excellent surgical outcomes, however AVS is invasive, technically demanding and requires expertise. In addition, AVS is not widely available.

In an attempt to better define which population of patients require AVS, we reviewed the literature to provide evidence of the use of routine versus selective AVS. We find that patients with young patients with very high serum aldosterone levels in the context of suppressed plasma renin activity, who have a defined unilateral adrenal nodule and a normal contralateral adrenal gland, can undergo adrenalectomy without AVS. We recommend AVS for lateralization for all other patients with PA.

Keywords

Primary aldosteronism · Conn's syndrome · Aldosteronoma · Adrenal vein sampling · Adrenal incidentaloma · Adrenalectomy

S. C. Oltmann · A. Dackiw · F. E. Nwariaku (✉)
Department of Surgery, University of Texas Southwestern Medical Center, Dallas, TX, USA
e-mail: fiemu.nwariaku@utsouthwestern.edu

P. Angelos, R. H. Grogan (eds.), *Difficult Decisions in Endocrine Surgery*,
Difficult Decisions in Surgery: An Evidence-Based Approach,
https://doi.org/10.1007/978-3-319-92860-9_33

Introduction

Primary aldosteronism, PA (Conn's syndrome) represents a spectrum of disease entities characterized by autonomous adrenal aldosterone production, concomitant hypertension, and hypokalemia [1, 2]. While the exact prevalence of PA varies worldwide, most reports support a prevalence rate of 5–20% among hypertensive patients, with higher rates within clinical practices that specialize in treating hypertensive patients. High prevalence populations also include subjects with resistant hypertension, older age, known adrenal tumor, family-history of PA, or young-onset hypertension. Furthermore, the prevalence of PA varies depending on the cutoff thresholds used for PA screening.

The spectrum of PA includes two conditions; SRA (surgically remediable aldosteronism) and IHA (bilateral idiopathic aldosteronism). While these two clinical scenarios may not always be distinguishable, it is important to determine if autonomous adrenal aldosterone production is predominantly unilateral or bilateral. The therapeutic implications are important because unilateral adrenal aldosterone production is surgically-curable with minimal morbidity, whereas bilateral adrenal aldosterone production is better managed with mineralocorticoid receptor antagonists [3].

The appropriate management of patients with PA requires biochemical confirmation of autonomous adrenal aldosterone production, as well as lateralization studies to confirm unilateral PA. Patients with biochemical confirmation and lateralization benefit from surgical adrenalectomy, whereas those in whom lateralization is equivocal or impossible can be treated with a mineralocorticoid receptor (MR) antagonist.

Lateralization is commonly performed by a combination of cross-sectional imaging (CT or MRI) and/or adrenal vein sampling (AVS). Imaging is the traditional mainstay of lateralization; however the presence of incidental and non-functioning adrenal lesions, frequently confounds clinical decision-making. Recently, the accuracy of image-guided lateralization has been questioned, and the use of routine adrenal vein sampling (AVS) has increased significantly. However, AVS is technically demanding, procedure methods and threshold values for confirming lateralization are variable, and failure to lateralize aldosterone production and complications are significant. Therefore, it would seem prudent to identify patients in whom AVS is not necessary, and perform AVS selectively only in patients who are likely to benefit from AVS.

In this chapter, we review the current literature to determine the role of AVS in lateralization of aldosterone production in PA, provide evidence to support selective AVS and review the potential pitfalls in procedure performance and interpretation of results (Table 33.1). There are no randomized controlled to address the question of routine, versus selective AVS. Therefore our conclusions are based on retrospective studies and cohort studies.

Table 33.1 PICO table

*P*opulation	Patients with primary aldosteronism
*I*ntervention	Routine adrenal vein sampling
*C*omparator	Selective adrenal vein sampling
*O*utcome	Recurrence, cure

Search Strategy

We performed a focused review of the current literature regarding primary aldosteronism utilizing the PubMed database, using the following keywords; adrenal vein sampling, primary aldosteronism, primary hyperaldosteronism, adrenal incidentaloma, computed tomography, adrenal adenoma and adrenalectomy. We critically reviewed 38 articles as well as the guidelines on the management of adrenal incidentalomas and primary aldosteronism published by the American Association of Clinical Endocrinologists, American Association of Endocrine Surgeons, and the Endocrine Society [2, 4].

Diagnosing Primary Aldosteronism

The clinical presentation of PA is usually associated with the presence of hypertension, and/or hypokalemia. PA screening is associated with high yields among high-prevalence populations, therefore we recommend screening in this group. These include young (<40 years old) onset hypertensive patients, those with known adrenal tumors, family history of PA or resistant hypertension or hypokalemia. Screening is generally successful with minimal or no preparation. A generally accepted screening algorithm is to calculate the aldosterone-to-renin ratio (ARR). While the 'accepted' ARR ratio to suspect PA is variable, the *most sensitive threshold* to maximize case detection and minimize false negatives is the presence of suppressed renin activity (<0.3 ng/ml/h) associated with a simultaneous serum aldosterone level of at least 6 ng/dl, resulting in an ARR that is greater than 20 [5]. Higher ARR (>30) and associated renin suppression is the most acceptable criteria for a positive screen [1, 4, 6–8]. It is important to note that, lower ARR thresholds (~20) may increase the false positive rate of screening tests [2, 4]. Furthermore, there needs to be a high aldosterone concentration in the ARR calculation. Many endocrinologists and endocrine surgeons require PAC concentration to be in the range of greater than 10–15 ng/dl in the context of a suppressed PRA [2, 6].

A major benefit of screening in the ambulatory setting is the high accuracy of screening despite ongoing use of antihypertensive medication. Specifically, there is no need to discontinue MR. However, an important caveat is the need for correction of hypokalemia prior to screening, because hypokalemia impairs aldosterone biosynthesis. In addition, dietary sodium intake can influence PA screening results particularly in patients with milder disease. Dietary sodium restriction (which is common among patients with hypertension), can result in false-negative screening [9].

A common question is whether antihypertensive medications need to be discontinued prior to PA screening. In general, patients with PA have a positive ARR screen regardless of antihypertensive medication. The most common cause of a false-negative screen is the use of a medication that raises renin. These include MR, sodium channel inhibitors, ACEIs and ARBs. However, *if the PRA is suppressed, then the ARR is interpretable and the screen is valid.* If the renin is low but not suppressed, and the PAC and ARR are high, then PA cannot be excluded, and then antihypertensive medications can be discontinued for 4–6 weeks. For patients with difficult to control hypertension, close monitoring must be provided to ensure this withdraw from medication does not provoke a hypertensive crisis. When ongoing antihypertensive therapy is necessary, calcium channel blockers (Verapamil, etc.), alpha blockers (Prazosin, Doxazosin, etc.) and vasodilators (Hydralazine) can be used with minimal effect on serum aldosterone levels.

A positive ARR screen needs to be followed up by confirmatory testing, except in situations with excessively high PAC (>20 ng/dl), concomitant renin suppression with an ARR > 20 and hypokalemia [2].

Confirmatory Testing

Confirmation, of PA is usually performed by dynamic testing to confirm autonomous aldosterone excess. This can be accomplished by oral or intravenous salt loading, fludrocortisone suppression or captopril challenge [5]. Of these tests, salt loading is the most common test in clinical practice. Oral salt loading is preferred because it can be accomplished in the ambulatory setting and does not require admission to a health facility.

Patients undergoing the saline infusion test should suppress their PAC to <5–10 ng/dl, unless they have primary aldosteronism which prevents suppression [8]. Dietary salt loading for 3–5 days, followed by a 24-h urinary collection for measurement of aldosterone levels is the preferred method of oral salt loading [1, 4]. Failure to suppress 24 h urine aldosterone levels to less than 12 mcg after 24 h of salt loading, confirms the diagnosis, of primary aldosteronism.

Lateralization

Following confirmation of PA, identifying which adrenal gland is the source of autonomous aldosterone secretion is crucial to determine appropriate treatment. Cross-sectional imaging (particularly CT and MRI), has been the mainstay of lateralization for many years. However, recent reports have questioned the accuracy of CT and MRI for localization. Ironically, the improved spatial resolution has increased identification of nonfunctional adrenal adenomas that confound surgical decision-making.

Cross-Sectional Imaging

After confirming the diagnosis of primary aldosteronism, the first step in subtype classification involves a thin cut (2–3 mm slice) adrenal CT to evaluate the adrenal glands for underlying masses [1, 2, 10]. The underlying dilemma with cross-sectional imaging for primary aldosteronism is that an underlying APA is often less than 1 cm in size [11]. Even with the thin slice, dedicated adrenal protocols for both CT and MRI, APAs 4–8 mm in size may be over looked, or confused with nodularity of the gland [8].

Several studies have found CT and MRI imaging to be less sensitive and specific than AVS for the prediction of SRA [5, 11, 12] (Table 33.2). One retrospective study found CT alone to be misleading, and AVS altered decision making in more than one-third of 34 patients [13]. Similarly, others have observed a false positive lateralization rate of 25–28% among large cohorts of patients with PA [14, 15]. See Fig. 33.1a for an example of appropriate lateralization of a right APA despite a contralateral abnormality. This patient underwent successful right adrenalectomy with surgical cure of PA.

Although most guidelines recommend the use of AVS in addition to CT or MRI to optimize localization of PA, this recommendation has been recently challenged by the first large randomized controlled trial to assess the utility of AVS for predicting SRA [16]. In brief, this study (The SPARTACUS trial) showed that patients who had PA treatment decisions made using CT alone, versus CT with AVS together, had nearly the same clinical outcome 1 year later [16]. Patients treated with CT had an 80% rate of biochemical cure when compared to 89% with AVS, and after 1 year of follow up, there were no differences in the number of antihypertensive medications used or in blood pressure control. Clinical outcomes beyond 1 year were not available to assess the long-term durability of the results.

Unfortunately, this trial suffered from a few shortcomings namely (1), Only 50% of patients met criteria for the CT-guided arm (>7 mm mass in one adrenal gland and a normal contralateral gland), and only 80% of those patients were cured with surgery, (2) CT and AVS were discordant in 50% of patients with conclusive data from both procedures. Given the fact that 50% of patients in the study met criteria for CT-guided therapy, it is unknown how many patients in that arm were inappropriately denied potentially curative surgery.

Table 33.2 Criteria to consider screening for primary aldosteronism as recommended by the 2016 Endocrine Society Clinical Practice Guideline [5]

• Severe hypertension (>150/100 mmHg)
• Hypertension resistant to three or more anti-hypertensive medications or hypertension requiring four or more medications to achieve control
• Hypertension with spontaneous or diuretic-induced hypokalemia
• Hypertension with an incidentally discovered adrenal mass
• Hypertension with sleep apnea
• Hypertension with a family history of early onset hypertension or cerebrovascular disease
• Family history of PA

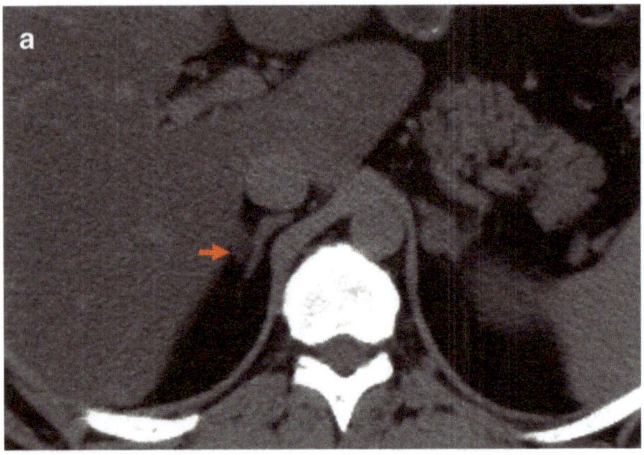

b

Laboratory Evaluation of Adrenal Gland Lateralization

Patient's Name	Medical Record Number	Physician/Mail Code	Date of Surgery
[redacted]	[redacted]	[redacted]	13 Apr 01

Specimen Source	Post-ACTH [Aldosterone], ηg/dL	Post-ACTH [Cortisol], μg/dL	A/C (x 10^{-3})	C_{RAV} and $C_{LAV} \geq 3C_{IVC}$	Adrenal Vein A/C Ratio: Dominant	D/IVC	Nondominant	ND/IVC	$\frac{(A/C)_{Dominant}}{(A/C)_{Nondominant}}$
RAV	4555.0	707.9	6.4	Yes	6.4	4.5	1.2	0.8	5.3
LAV	836.0	691.5	1.2	Yes					
IVC	36.5	25.5	1.4	Yes	☜ Overall AVS successful?				
PV	33.3	26.5	1.3	Yes	☜ $C_{PV} \geq 20$ ug/dL?				

Interpretive Notes:

AVS is considered successful if $C_{RAV} \geq 3C_{IVC}$ and $C_{LAV} \geq 3C_{IVC}$.

If $(A/C)_{Dominant}/(A/C)_{Nondominant} \geq 4$ and $(A/C)_{Nondominant} \leq (A/C)_{IVC}$ and dominant (A/C) value is from *RAV*, then laterality is *right* adrenal gland.

If $(A/C)_{Dominant}/(A/C)_{Nondominant} \geq 4$ and $(A/C)_{Nondominant} \leq (A/C)_{IVC}$ and dominant (A/C) value is from *LAV*, then laterality is *left* adrenal gland.

Diagnosis	Criteria	Criteria Met
APA or PAH	$(A/C)_{Dominant}/(A/C)_{Nondominant} \geq 4$ AND $(A/C)_{Nondominant} \leq (A/C)_{IVC}$	Yes
	Laterality [Right or Left Adrenal Gland (AG)]	*Right AG*
BAH	$(A/C)_{RAV} > (A/C)_{IVC}$ AND $(A/C)_{LAV} > (A/C)_{IVC}$	No

Abbreviations: A, aldosterone; C, Cortisol; LAV, left adrenal vein; RAV, right adrenal vein; D, dominant; ND, nondominant; LAPA, left aldosterone-producing adenoma; RAPA, right aldosterone-producing adenoma; PAH, primary adrenal hyperplasia; BAH, bilateral adrenal hyperplasia; n.d., not done.

Fig. 33.1 (**a**) Appropriate lateralization of a right APA despite a contralateral abnormality. This patient underwent successful right adrenalectomy with surgical cure of PA. Red arrow points to side with highest aldosterone levels. (**b**) Lateralization of the right APA

The SPARTACUS study highlights the complexity of the decision making process in regards to PA localization. For clinicians' at specialized medical centers with expertise with AVS, the use of AVS is common prior to adrenalectomy, since a failure rate of 20–30% is generally viewed as unacceptable. Furthermore, most of these centers have observed that the sensitivity of AVS exceeds that of CT and that the rate of biochemical cure following AVS directed adrenalectomy is >95%.

In summary current guidelines recommend AVS for the most accurate selection of patients with SRA [5]. Despite this, cross sectional imaging still plays an important role in the assessment of the patient with PA because it provides anatomic information about the gland location which may alter operative approach, and can also assess adrenal masses concerning for adrenal cortical carcinoma [8, 10, 17]. Also a well-defined adrenal adenoma on CT imaging, in a young patient (<40 years old), with extremely high aldosterone levels, suppressed renin levels and hypokalemia, may be all the localization necessary for appropriate treatment.

Technique of Adrenal Vein Sampling

Another confounding factor in AVS is the institutional variability in sampling protocols. One study of AVS techniques showed that approximately one-third of centers performed bilateral AVS sequentially following Cosyntropin stimulation, one-third performed bilateral AVS simultaneously without Cosyntropin stimulation, and about one-third performed bilateral AVS simultaneously following Cosyntropin stimulation [3]. The value of Cosyntropin is an increase in adrenal blood flow and constant aldosterone and cortisol production resulting in less variability during sequential catheterization of the right and left adrenal veins.

The AVS criteria that best predict SRA continue to evolve. Serum aldosterone concentrations from each adrenal vein and from the peripheral vein are divided by the respective cortisol concentrations to calculate the cortisol-corrected aldosterone concentration (A/C). The ratio of dominant A/C to non-dominant A/C is referred to as the lateralization index (LI). See Fig. 33.1b for example of lateralization of the right APA. Under Cosyntropin stimulation, a LI < 2 demonstrates bilateral disease, while a LI > 4 is usually predictive of a good response to adrenalectomy [5]. An additional finding of a suppressed non-dominant A/C (below the IVC A/C ratio), provides greater confidence of lateralization, and better prediction of surgical response [18, 19]. Most patients with SRA meet both criteria. Because aldosterone and cortisol values are generally much lower, LI criteria without Cosyntropin are generally lower, as low as two for lateralization [3]. Figure 33.2(a–d) show concordant CT and AVS lateralization of a left APA.

Patients with an LI of 2–4 are considered to have indeterminate lateralization. However, evaluation of all clinical and biochemical factors can facilitate better prediction of surgical response. For instance, if the LI is 3–4 and significant contralateral suppression is observed, adrenalectomy is likely to yield significant clinical benefits. Similarly, several factors are known to predict the clinical response to adrenalectomy, including age, duration of hypertension, number of antihypertensive medications, and hypokalemia.

Finally, measurement of additional biomarkers in the AVS samples such as 18-hydroxycorticosterone can provide additional evidence of lateralization [20].

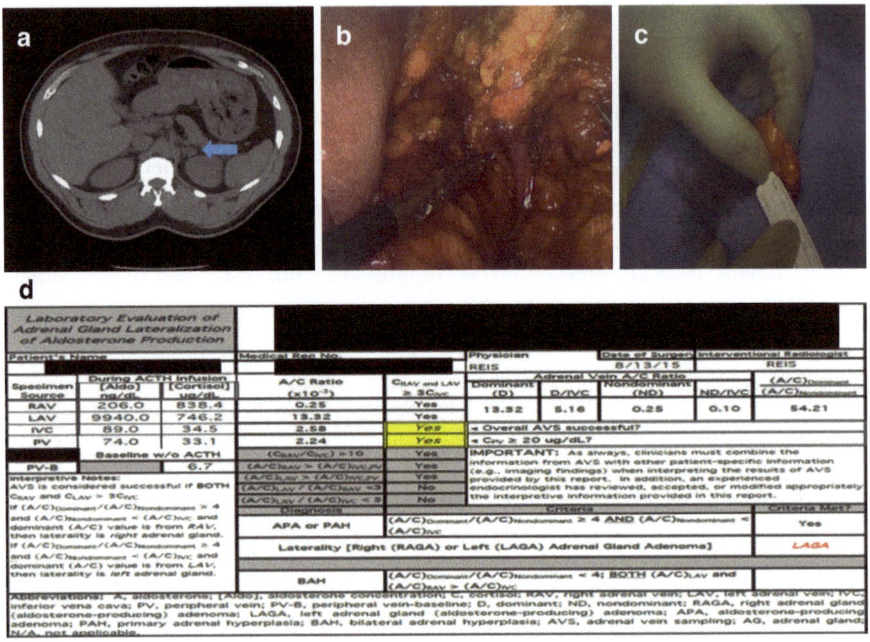

Laboratory Evaluation of Adrenal Gland Lateralization of Aldosterone Production [redacted]

Patient's Name: [redacted] | Medical Rec No. [redacted] | Physician: REIS | Date of Surgery: 8/13/15 | Interventional Radiologist: REIS

Specimen Source	During ACTH Infusion [Aldo] ng/dL	During ACTH Infusion [Cortisol] ug/dL	A/C Ratio (x10⁻³)	C_{RAV} and LAV ≥ $3C_{IVC}$
RAV	206.0	838.4	0.25	Yes
LAV	9940.0	746.2	13.32	Yes
IVC	89.0	34.5	2.58	Yes ◂ Overall AVS successful?
PV	74.0	33.1	2.24	Yes ◂ C_{PV} ≥ 20 ug/dL?
[redacted]	Baseline w/o ACTH		$(C_{RAV}/C_{IVC}) > 10$	Yes
PV-B		6.7	$(A/C)_{RAV} > (A/C)_{IVC,PV}$	Yes
			$(A/C)_{LAV} > (A/C)_{IVC,PV}$	Yes
			$(A/C)_{LAV} / (A/C)_{RAV} < 3$	No
			$(A/C)_{LAV} / (A/C)_{IVC} < 3$	No

Adrenal Vein A/C Ratio: Dominant (D)	D/IVC	Nondominant (ND)	ND/IVC	$(A/C)_{Dominant}/(A/C)_{Nondominant}$
13.32	5.16	0.25	0.10	54.21

IMPORTANT: As always, clinicians must combine the information from AVS with other patient-specific information (e.g., imaging findings) when interpreting the results of AVS provided by this report. In addition, an experienced endocrinologist has reviewed, accepted, or modified appropriately the interpretive information provided in this report.

Interpretive Notes:
AVS is considered successful if BOTH C_{RAV} and C_{LAV} > $3C_{IVC}$
If $(A/C)_{Dominant}/(A/C)_{Nondominant}$ ≥ 4 and $(A/C)_{Nondominant}$ < $(A/C)_{IVC}$ and dominant (A/C) value is from *RAV*, then laterality is *right* adrenal gland.
If $(A/C)_{Dominant}/(A/C)_{Nondominant}$ ≥ 4 and $(A/C)_{Nondominant}$ < $(A/C)_{IVC}$ and dominant (A/C) value is from *LAV*, then laterality is *left* adrenal gland.

Diagnosis	Criteria	Criteria Met?
APA or PAH	$(A/C)_{Dominant}/(A/C)_{Nondominant}$ ≥ 4 AND $(A/C)_{Nondominant}$ < $(A/C)_{IVC}$	Yes
Laterality [Right (RAGA) or Left (LAGA) Adrenal Gland Adenoma]		LAGA
BAH	$(A/C)_{Dominant}/(A/C)_{Nondominant}$ < 4; BOTH $(A/C)_{LAV}$ and $(A/C)_{RAV}$ > $(A/C)_{IVC}$	

Abbreviations: A, aldosterone; [Aldo], aldosterone concentration; C, cortisol; RAV, right adrenal vein; LAV, left adrenal vein; IVC, inferior vena cava; PV, peripheral vein; PV-B, peripheral vein-baseline; D, dominant; ND, nondominant; RAGA, right adrenal gland (aldosterone-producing) adenoma; LAGA, left adrenal gland (aldosterone-producing) adenoma; APA, aldosterone-producing adenoma; PAH, primary adrenal hyperplasia; BAH, bilateral adrenal hyperplasia; AVS, adrenal vein sampling; AG, adrenal gland; N/A, not applicable.

Fig. 33.2 (**a–d**) Concordant CT and AVS lateralization of a left APA. Arrow demonstrates left adrenal aldosteronoma

Safety of AVS

When performed by experienced interventional radiologists, adrenal vein sampling can be successfully performed with minimal morbidity. Potential complications include adrenal infarction (venous thrombosis), or hemorrhage from adrenal vein rupture. However, a large study from 20 international, high-volume centers which performed over 2600 procedures over a 6 year period, noted a rate of adrenal vein rupture of only 0.61%, [3]. No deaths were observed in this trial. The author(s) also note that patients who undergo AVS may demonstrate peri-venous adhesions during surgery. Therefore we recommend an appropriate interval of 2–4 weeks between AVS and adrenalectomy, when possible.

Conclusion

Primary aldosteronism is a significant contributor to hypertension in 5–20% of hypertensive patients. Given the potential for surgical cure in this group of patients, the imperative of accurate diagnosis of PA and lateralization cannot be overemphasized. For patients with unilateral excessive aldosterone secretion, unilateral adrenalectomy is safe, cost-effective and curative.

As the spatial resolution of cross-sectional imaging has improved, the potential for poor, image-guided lateralization (due to incidental, non-functioning, structural adrenal abnormalities) has increased significantly. This has placed a

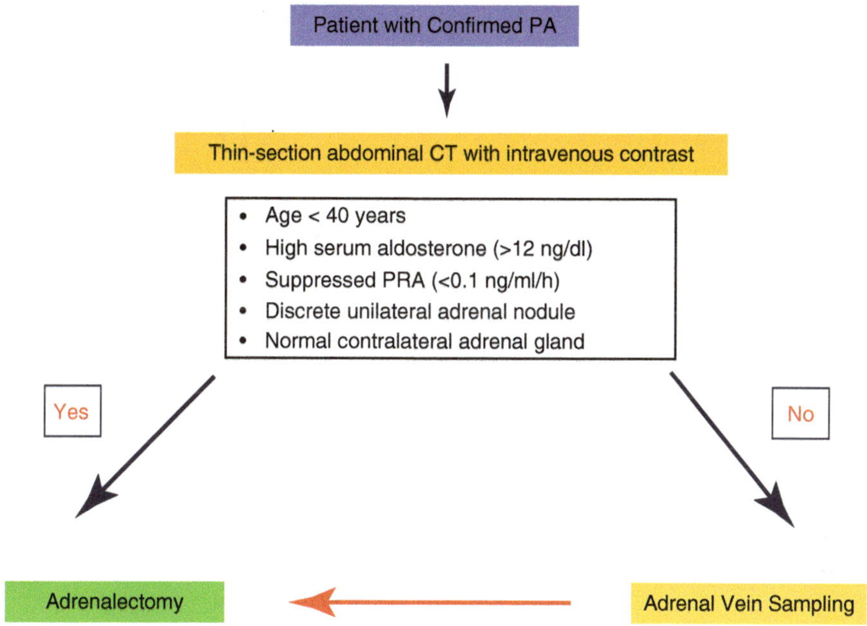

Fig. 33.3 Diagnostic algorithm for PA

greater burden on adrenal vein sampling to appropriately identify autonomous unilateral adrenal secretion.

For young patients with high serum aldosterone levers associated with an elevated ARR, clear unilateral adrenal nodules and normal contralateral adrenal glands on appropriate cross-sectional imaging, and demonstrable hypokalemia, we believe that adrenalectomy without AVS is associated with a good response. However, we recommend AVS for all other patients with PA because of the importance on accurate lateralization. Figure 33.3 outlines our diagnostic algorithm for PA.

When performed in specialized centers by experienced providers, AVS is a safe, effective and powerful tool to lateralize aldosterone production in PA. Controversy persists regarding most appropriate protocols (Cosyntropin administration), lateralization thresholds and management of patients with an indeterminate lateralization index.

References

1. Rossi GP, Bernini G, Caliumi C, Desideri G, Fabris B, Ferri C, et al. A prospective study of the prevalence of primary aldosteronism in 1,125 hypertensive patients. J Am Coll Cardiol. 2006;48(11):2293–300.
2. Funder JW, Carey RM, Fardella C, Gomez-Sanchez CE, Mantero F, Stowasser M, et al. Case detection, diagnosis, and treatment of patients with primary aldosteronism: an endocrine society clinical practice guideline. J Clin Endocrinol Metab. 2008;93(9):3266–81.

3. Rossi GP, Barisa M, Allolio B, Auchus RJ, Amar L, Cohen D, et al. The adrenal vein sampling international study (AVIS) for identifying the major subtypes of primary aldosteronism. J Clin Endocrinol Metab. 2012;97(5):1606–14.
4. Zeiger MA, Thompson GB, Duh QY, Hamrahian AH, Angelos P, Elaraj D, et al. The American Association of Clinical Endocrinologists and American Association of endocrine surgeons medical guidelines for the management of adrenal incidentalomas. EndocrPract. 2009;15(Suppl 1):1–20.
5. Funder JW, Carey RM, Mantero F, Murad MH, Reincke M, Shibata H, et al. The management of primary aldosteronism: case detection, diagnosis, and treatment: an endocrine society clinical practice guideline. J Clin Endocrinol Metab. 2016;101(5):1889–916.
6. Lee JI, Oltmann SC, Woodruff SL, Nwariaku FE, Holt SA, Rabaglia JL. Contralateral adrenal abnormalities in Conn's syndrome. J Surg Res. 2015;200(1):183–8.
7. White ML, Gauger PG, Doherty GM, Cho KJ, Thompson NW, Hammer GD, et al. The role of radiologic studies in the evaluation and management of primary hyperaldosteronism. Surgery. 2008;144(6):926–33. discussion 33.
8. Mulatero P, Bertello C, Rossato D, Mengozzi G, Milan A, Garrone C, et al. Roles of clinical criteria, computed tomography scan, and adrenal vein sampling in differential diagnosis of primary aldosteronism subtypes. J Clin Endocrinol Metab. 2008;93(4):1366–71.
9. Baudrand R, Guarda FJ, Torrey J, Williams G, Vaidya A. Dietary sodium restriction increases the risk of misinterpreting mild cases of primary aldosteronism. J Clin Endocrinol Metab. 2016;101(11):3989–96.
10. Magill SB, Raff H, Shaker JL, Brickner RC, Knechtges TE, Kehoe ME, et al. Comparison of adrenal vein sampling and computed tomography in the differentiation of primary aldosteronism. J Clin Endocrinol Metab. 2001;86(3):1066–71.
11. Rossi GP, Sacchetto A, Chiesura-Corona M, De Toni R, Gallina M, Feltrin GP, et al. Identification of the etiology of primary aldosteronism with adrenal vein sampling in patients with equivocal computed tomography and magnetic resonance findings: results in 104 consecutive cases. J Clin Endocrinol Metab. 2001;86(3):1083–90.
12. Phillips JL, Walther MM, Pezzullo JC, Rayford W, Choyke PL, Berman AA, et al. Predictive value of preoperative tests in discriminating bilateral adrenal hyperplasia from an aldosterone-producing adrenal adenoma. J Clin Endocrinol Metab. 2000;85(12):4526–33.
13. Harper R, Ferrett CG, McKnight JA, McIlrath EM, Russell CF, Sheridan B, et al. Accuracy of CT scanning and adrenal vein sampling in the pre-operative localization of aldosterone-secreting adrenal adenomas. QJM. 1999;92(11):643–50.
14. Harvey A, Pasieka JL, Kline G, So B. Modification of the protocol for selective adrenal venous sampling results in both a significant increase in the accuracy and necessity of the procedure in the management of patients with primary hyperaldosteronism. Surgery. 2012;152(4):643–9. discussion 9-51.
15. Kempers MJ, Lenders JW, van Outheusden L, van der Wilt GJ, Schultze Kool LJ, Hermus AR, et al. Systematic review: diagnostic procedures to differentiate unilateral from bilateral adrenal abnormality in primary aldosteronism. Ann Intern Med. 2009;151(5):329–37.
16. Dekkers T, Prejbisz A, Kool LJ, Groenewoud HJ, Velema M, Spiering W, et al. Adrenal vein sampling versus CT scan to determine treatment in primary aldosteronism: an outcome-based randomised diagnostic trial. Lancet Diabetes Endocrinol. 2016;4(9):739–46.
17. Agcaoglu O, Sahin DA, Siperstein A, Berber E. Selection algorithm for posterior versus lateral approach in laparoscopic adrenalectomy. Surgery. 2012;151(5):731–5.
18. El Ghorayeb N, Mazzuco TL, Bourdeau I, Mailhot JP, Zhu PS, Therasse E, et al. Basal and post-ACTH aldosterone and its ratios are useful during adrenal vein sampling in primary aldosteronism. J Clin Endocrinol Metab. 2016;101(4):1826–35.
19. Wolley MJ, Ahmed AH, Gordon RD, Stowasser M. Does ACTH improve the diagnostic performance of adrenal vein sampling for subtyping primary aldosteronism? Clin Endocrinol. 2016;85(5):703–9.
20. Vaidya A, Malchoff CD, Auchus RJ, Committee AAS. An individualized approach to the evaluation and management of primary aldosteronism. Endocr Pract. 2017;23(6):680–9.

Surgery Versus Observation for Asymptomatic Nonfunctioning Pancreatic Neuroendocrine Tumors

34

Carlos R. Cordón-Fernández and Miguel F. Herrera

Abstract

Non-functioning pancreatic neuroendocrine tumors account for 2% of all pancreatic malignancies, most of them are benign and sporadic. The most common image studies for their characterization are CT, MRI, endoscopic ultrasound, and PET. Serum Chromogranine A is the most common tumor marker for PNETs and it is used for the diagnosis as well as for surveillance. Surgical resection, either open or laparoscopic is the treatment of choice for all symptomatic sporadic tumors as well as for malignant tumors in the absence of extra pancreatic extension, lymph node or hepatic metastases.

Keywords

Non-functioning PNET · CT · MRI · Endoscopic ultrasound · PET · Chromogranine A

Introduction

Non-functioning pancreatic neuroendocrine tumors account for 2% of all pancreatic malignancies, most of them are benign and sporadic. The most common image studies for their characterization are CT, MRI, endoscopic ultrasound, and PET. Serum Chromogranine A is the most common tumor marker for PNETs and it is used for the

C. R. Cordón-Fernández
Department of Surgical Oncology, Instituto Guatemalteco de Seguridad Social, Guatemala City, Guatemala

M. F. Herrera (✉)
UNAM at the Instituto Nacional de Ciencias Médicas y Nutrición Salvador Zubirán, Mexico City, Mexico

P. Angelos, R. H. Grogan (eds.), *Difficult Decisions in Endocrine Surgery*, Difficult Decisions in Surgery: An Evidence-Based Approach,
https://doi.org/10.1007/978-3-319-92860-9_34

diagnosis as well as for surveillance. Surgical resection, either open or laparoscopic is the treatment of choice for all symptomatic sporadic tumors as well as for malignant tumors in the absence of extra pancreatic extension, lymph node or hepatic metastases. With the idea that most asymptomatic, small NF-PNETs may be benign, there has been an increasing interest in avoiding unnecessary surgery in selected patients. Some studies have found that surgical resections are significantly associated to a longer survival whereas others have shown that tumors smaller than 2 cm have excellent long term survival despite non-operative treatment. Based on the existing literature, we believe that it seems reasonable to propose non surgical treatment for NF-PNETs tumors less than 2 cm in size, provided that patients are asymptomatic, that tumors do not have radiologic features suggestive of malignancy and that either the Ki-67 index or the mitotic count on FNA are <2%. Patients selected for surveillance need a close follow-up both, clinical and radiological, perhaps every 6 months for at least 2 years.

Neuroendocrine tumors have been described to originate in many tissues including the bronchial epithelium, the thyroid, the parathyroid glands, the thymus, both the adrenal cortex and the medulla, and the sympathetic nervous system [1]. However, the majority of these tumors develop in the gastrointestinal tract, being the stomach and the pancreas the two most frequent locations [1, 2].

Pancreatic neuroendocrine tumors (PNETs) arise from the endocrine tissues of the pancreas. They may secrete a variety of hormones such as Insulin, Gastrin, Glucagon or the Vasoactive intestinal peptide resulting in a myriad of clinical syndromes. Some pancreatic neuroendocrine tumors lack of symptoms of hormone overproduction and are named Non-functioning pancreatic neuroendocrine tumors (NF-PNETs). Despite the absence of symptoms, NF-PNETs may produce a variety of non-specific peptides such as Chromogranin A (CgA), Pancreatic polypeptide and Calcitonin. The purpose of the present chapter is to review general characteristics of PNETs with emphasis to the surgical versus observational management of NF-PNETs (Table 34.1).

NF-PNET account for 2% of all pancreatic malignancies [3], the annual incidence increased from 1.4 to 3.0 per million in the last three decades probably due to the more extensive use of advanced imaging studies [3–5]. The malignancy rate of NF-PNETs is 40% [6, 7], and half of the patients present with distant metastasis at the time of the diagnosis [7]. Despite considerable research, knowledge of tumor behavior, treatment efficacy and prognosis are still limited.

Although there is not a uniform terminology for grading or staging PNETs, some features such as the mitotic count, the Ki-67 proliferative index and the extent of local spread are shared by most classification systems. NF-PNETs can range from well to poorly differentiated and according to the World Health Organization (WHO) criteria they have been divided into three groups as shown in table 1 [8].

Table 34.1 PICO table

*P*opulation	Patients with non-functioning PNET
*I*ntervention	Surgery
*C*omparator	Medical management
*O*utcomes	Survival, complications, QOL

Clinical Presentation

Most NF-PNETs are sporadic and tend to affect individuals of advanced age. There is a slight increased incidence in men compared to women (55% vs. 45%) [9, 10]. Since NF-PNETs do not produce hormones or do not produce the necessary amount of hormones to produce clinical signs, they are usually silent and their symptoms are mainly related to the local mass effect or the presence of metastatic disease (Table 34.2). Tumor related symptoms are dependent of tumor location. When tumors arise from the head of the pancreas, patients present back pain or jaundice, tumors in the pancreatic tail can be asymptomatic until they grow enough to become palpable at the physical exam to produce pain or hemorrhage due to erosion to adjacent vessels [10]. However, with the widespread use of abdominal imaging, the number of tumors incidentally identified in asymptomatic patients is on the rise. Distribution of NF-PNETs throughout the pancreas is shown in Table 34.3.

Most NF-PNETs are sporadic, but close to 10% can be associated to familial syndromes including the Multiple Endocrine Neoplasia type 1 (MEN1), the von Hippel-Lindau type 1 (VHL), the Von Recklinghausen disease or neurofibromatosis type 1 (NF-1) and the tuberous sclerosis complex [11]. These patients are usually diagnosed at younger age and the lesions are multiple throughout the pancreas. NF-PNETs are more common in MEN1 than in VHL, and they are uncommon in NF-1 and the tuberous sclerosis complex [14].

Table 34.2 Classification of PNETs according to the ENETs and WHO 2010

ENETS/WHO2010	Differentiation grade	Mitotic count	Ki-67 (%)
Neuroendocrine tumor grade 1	Low grade (G1)	<2 per 10 HPF	<2
Neuroendocrine tumor grade 2	Intermediate grade (G2)	2–20 per 10 HPF	2–20
Neuroendocrine carcinoma grade 3 (small cell)	High grade (G3)	>20 per 10 HPF	>20
Neuroendocrine carcinoma grade 3 (large cell)	High grade (G3)	>20 per 10 HPF	>20

HPF High Power Field, *WHO* World Health Organization, *ENETS* European Neuronedocrine tumour society
References [8, 11]

Table 34.3 Main symptoms of NF-PNET at diagnosis

First author (Reference)	*n*	Study period	Abdominal mass on physical examination (%)	Abdominal pain (%)	Jaundice	Anorexia and weight loss (%)	No symptoms (%)
Yang et al. [10]	55	2000–2013	30.3	56.4	14.5	–	–
Gullo et al. [12]	184	1987–2001	–	50.5	7.1	7.6	34.8
Phan et al. [13]	58	1949–1996	–	56	35	46	–

Diagnosis

The disease spectrum of PNETs extends from poorly differentiated carcinomas, which are rapidly progressive and seldom resectable, to small, apparently innocent nodules that could remain unchanged for years. Non-functional islet cell malignant tumors tend to be larger than ordinary pancreatic adenocarcinomas at the time of diagnosis. CT scan is the study of choice for the initial study of NF-PNET. Modern equipment like the multidetector CT, (MDCT) minimizes the breathing effect artifact because of the short scanning time [15]. Because of the hipervascular nature, PNETs exhibits robust contrast enhancement in the late arterial phase, showing a well circumscribed, and hypervascular lesion [16]. Larger NF-PNETs are usually not as well vascularized and may comprise areas of necrosis, they frequently present calcifications that are best depicted in the non-contrast enhanced examination. The differential diagnosis includes: serous cystic adenoma, solid pseudo papillary neoplasm and intrapancreatic accessory spleens among others [17].

The sensitivity and specificity of CT to localize a PNET vary between 63–82% and 83–100% respectively for tumors larger than 3 cm and decreases for lesions smaller than 2 cm, whereas the detection rate of PNETs ranges between 39 and 94% [15] (Table 34.4).

MRI has a sensitivity and specificity of PNETs localization between 85–100% and 75–100% respectively with a detection rate for PNETs between 50 and 94% [15, 16]. NET presents a low signal lesion in T1 and a high signal lesion in T2 weighted images. The MRI characteristics are very similar to CT, but MRI has greater sensitivity for the detection of liver metastasis than CT and Scintigraphy [14, 15].

Endoscopic ultrasound (EUS) is able to detect lesions between 2 and 3 mm and has the advantage to provide guidance for Fine needle aspiration or trucut biopsies. EUS is the most sensitive method for diagnosing PNETs with a 90% rate of detection [17]. Unfortunately, it is highly operator dependent [15–18].

PNETs express Somatostatin receptors in 50–90% of the tumors. Functional imaging can be obtained using radiolabeled SSA. The most frequently used is Ocreotide. Both PET and SPECT have better spatial resolution and faster image acquisition than scintigraphy. The radiotracers most commonly used are: ^{68}Ga-DOTATOC, ^{68}Ga-DOTANOC and 68Ga-DOTATATE. The sensitivities for PNET detection range from 75 to 100% [16, 19].

PET and SPECT have the additional benefit of detecting metastatic disease outside the abdomen. On the other hand, they do not provide information on tumor size, relationship with the pancreatic duct and resectabillity. Therefore the best image studies to assess surgical resection are CT and MRI.

Table 34.4 Location of NF-PNET

First author (Reference)	*n*	Head (%)	Body (%)	Tail (%)	Multiple (%)
Gullo et al. [12]	184	33.2	14.1	10.9	0.5
Yan et al. [10]	55	51.5	27.3	21.2	–
Bilimoria et al. [7]	8344	34.6	7.9	21.4	36
Franko et al. [3]	2158	42	11	27	20

Serum CgA is the most common tumor marker for PNETs and it is used for the diagnosis as well as for surveillance. In general, high levels of CgA are associated with poor prognosis. However, significant decrease of CgA after surgery value is associated with favorable outcomes [20]. Elevation of the Pancreatic Polypeptide is found in 50–100% of the patients with PNETs. However, it is not a specific marker [2].

Treatment

Surgical resection either open or laparoscopic is the treatment of choice for all symptomatic sporadic tumors as well as for malignant tumors in the absence of extra pancreatic extension, lymph node or hepatic metastases. If a solid PNET is not functional, the optimal treatment depends on its size. Considering the limited aggressiveness of malignant NF-PNETs, surgical treatment is also indicated in some patients with metastatic or extra pancreatic disease [21].

The choice of the surgical procedures depends on the size, the type of tumor and its anatomical location. Surgical procedures include, tumor enucleation pancreatoduodenectomy (Whipple procedure), distal pancreatectomy, subtotal pancreatectomy and central pancreatectomy.

Solorzano et al. in a retrospective study found that tumor size was not a predictor of survival. By contrast Bettini [22], Gullo et al. [12] and Bilimoria et al. [7] found that tumors less than 3 cm are associated with a longer survival. Franco and colleagues [3] in a study on 2158 patients with NF-PNETs demonstrated that patients with non-metastatic malignant tumors had a longer survival after resection (11.3 years) when compared with patients with distant metastases (1.6 years). In both groups, patients without distant metastasis and with metastasis who had surgical resection had a longer median survival.

Little is known about the natural history of small lesions in asymptomatic patients. With the idea that most asymptomatic, small NF-PNETs may be benign and that pancreatic resections may lead to complications in up to 64% of the patients [23], there has been an increasing interest in avoiding unnecessary surgery in selected patients. A European study that collected patients from 2000 to 2011 showed that in a median follow up of 34 months, patients NF-PNETs smaller than 2 cm selected for non-operative treatment had excellent longterm survival despite the presence of nodal metastasis in 10% of the patients [24]. Lee et al. [25] conducted a study in 133 patients with NF-PNETs <2 cm. Patients were divided into two groups. The first group consisted of 56 patients who underwent tumor resection. The second group was conformed by 77 patients elected for close observation without treatment. Almost half of the patients in the surgical group experienced morbidity. In a mean follow-up of 45 months, there was no recurrence or metastatic disease in the treated group and tumor size remained stable without any evidence of local invasion or metastases in the untreated group. By contrast, Sharpe and colleagues performed a study on 380 patients with PNETs ≤2 cm who were treated either by observation (19%) or resection (81%). Neither the functional status nor the radiologic characteristics were analyzed. Overall 5-year survival for the patients who underwent surgery was 82.2% and it was 34.3% for those observed [26]. In a similar study on 251 patients where 195 were treated surgically and 56 observed, Zhang et al. found that surgical resection was significantly associated to a longer survival only in the group of patients with tumors ≥1 cm [27].

Based on the low frequency of malignancy in small tumors, the accuracy of radiologic characteristics to identify invasion and the high sensitivity of the differentiation grade, the Ki-67 index and the mitotic count to distinguish benign from malignant lesions, it seems reasonable to propose non surgical treatment for NF-PNETs tumors less than 2 cm in size, provided that patients are asymptomatic, that tumors do not have radiologic features suggestive of malignancy and either the Ki-67 index or the mitotic count on FNA are <2%. Patients selected for surveillance need close follow-up both, clinical and radiological, perhaps every 6 months for at least 2 years [4].

Surgery for Hepatic Metastasis

In the absence of extra hepatic disease, the resection of the primary tumor and the hepatic metastasis can be considered [28] since the 5-year survival of patients with hepatic resection ranges from 47 to 76% compared with the 30–40% in untreated patients. To attempt a hepatic resection 90% of the tumor must be removed and sufficient hepatic reserve has to be maintained [28]. Kim et al. [29] in a series of 125 patients with NF-PNET found that repeated operations for recurrence led patients to a prolonged survival.

When surgery is not possible, other therapeutic approaches may also impact favorably survival duration [30]. Among the available palliative procedures, hepatic artery embolization has a response rate of 50% [14, 31] and can be performed also using cytotoxic drugs or radioactive isotopes. For deep intraparenchimal metastases radiofrequency ablation is a good option.

Chemotherapy

There is limited response to conventional therapeutic agents for neuroendocrine tumors. In the last two decades, the combination of Doxorubicin and Streptozocine has shown good results in long-term survival [32, 33].

Targeted therapy is still under investigation but seems to have also a promising effect on survival in patients with metastasic disease especially with the use of Everolimus and Sunitinib. Two other drugs, Bevacizumab and Sorafenib alone or in combination have also shown benefits on progression and free of disease survival.

References

1. Massironi S, Sciola V, Peracchi M, Ciafardini C, Spampatti MP, Conte D. Neuroendocrine tumors of the gastro-entero-pancreatic system. World J Gastroenterol. 2008;14(35):5377–84.
2. Kulke MH, Anthony LB, Bushnell DL, de Herder WW, Godsmith SJ, Klimstra DS, et al. NANETS treatment guidelines: well-differenciated neuroendocrine tumors of the stomach and pancreas. Pancreas. 2010;39(6):735–52.

3. Franko J, Weantao F, Genovese E, Moser J. Non functional neuroendocrine carcinoma of the pâncreas: incidence, tumor biology and outcomes in 2158 patients. J Gastrointest Surg. 2009;14(3):541–8.
4. Herrera MF, Akerstrom G, Angelos P, Grant CS, Hoff AO, Pantoja JP, et al. AACE/ACE disease state clinical review: pancreatic neuronedocrine incidentalomas. Endocr Pract. 2015;21:546–53.
5. Yao JC, Hassan M, Phan A, et al. One hundred years after "carcinoid": epidemiology of and prognostic factors for neuroendocrine tumors in 35,825 cases in the United States. J Clin Oncol. 2008;26(18):3063.
6. Kent RB, Van Heerden JA, Weiland LH. Nonfuctionning islet cell tumors. Ann Surg. 1981;193:185–90.
7. Bilimoria KY, Tomlinson JS, Merkow RP. Clinocopathologic features and treatment trends of pancreatic neuroendocrine tumors: analysis of 9821 patients. J Gastrointest Surg. 2007;11:1460–7.
8. Falconi M, Barstsch DF, Eriksson B, et al. ENETS concensus guidelines for the management of patients with digestive neuroendocrine neoplasm of the digestive system: well differenciated pancreatic non-functionning tumors. Neuroendocrinology. 2012;95:120–34.
9. Halfdanarson TR, Rabe KG, Rubin J, et al. Pancreatic neuroendocrine tumors (PNETs): incidence, prognosis and recent trend toward improved survival. Ann Oncol. 2008;19(10):1727–33.
10. Yan M, Zeng L, Zhang Y, et al. Surgical treatment and clinical outcomes of nonfunctional pancreatic neuroendocrine tumors. A 14 year experience from a single center. Medicine. 2014;93(22):1–7.
11. Klimstra DS, Modlin IR, Coppola D, et al. The pathologic classification of neuroendocrine tumors: a review of nomenclature, grading, and staging systems. Pancreas. 2010;39:707–12.
12. Gullo L, Migliori M, Falconi M, et al. Nonfunctioning pancreatic tumors: a multicenter clínical study. Am J Gastroent. 2003;98(11):2435–9.
13. Phan GQ, Yeo CJ, Hruban RH, et al. Surgical experience with pancreatic and peripancreatic neuroendocrine tumors: review of 125 patients. J Gastrointest Surg. 1998;2(5):473–82.
14. Kuo J, Lee J, Chabot J. Nonfunctional pancreatic neuroendocrine tumors. Surg Clin North Am. 2014;94(3):689–708.
15. Kartalis N, Pozzi RM, Sundin A. Recent developments in imaging of pancreatic neuroendocrine tumors. Ann Gastroenterol. 2015;28(2):193–202.
16. Hochwald S, Conlon K, Brennan M. Nonfunctional pancreatic islet cell tumors. In: Doherty G, Skogseid B, editors. Surgical endocrinology. Philadelphia: Lippincot Williams &Wilkins; 2001. p. 362–73.
17. Sundin A, Vullierme MP, Kaltsas G, et al. ENETS consensus guidelines for the standards of care in neuroendocrine tumors: radiological examinations. Neuroendocrinology. 2009;90(2):167–83.
18. Chatzipantelis P, Salla C, Konstantinou P, et al. Endoscopic ultrasound-guided fine-needle aspiration cytology of pancreatic neuroendocrine tumors: a study of 48 cases. Cancer. 2008;114(4):255–62.
19. Miderer M, Weber MM, Fottner C. Molecular imaging of gastroenteropancreatic neuroendocrine tumors. Gastroenterol Clin N Am. 2010;39:923–35.
20. Ter-Minassian M, Chan J, Hooshmand S, et al. Clinial presentation, survival and recurrence in patients with neuroendocrine tumors: results from a prospective institutional database. Endocr Relat Cancer. 2013;20:187–96.
21. Bettini R, Boninsegna L, Mantovani W, et al. Prognostic factors at diagnosis and value of WHO classification in a mono-institutional series of 180 non functioning pancreatic endocrine tumors. Ann Oncol. 2008;19:903–8.
22. Touzios JG, Kiely JM, Pitt SC, et al. Neuroendocrine hepatic metastases: does aggressive management improve survival? Ann Surg. 2005;241:776–85.
23. Lee LC, Grant CS, Salomao DR, et al. Small, nonfunctioning, asymptomatic pancreatic neuroendocrine tumors (PNETs): role of non-operative management. Surgery. 2012;152:965–74.
24. Sallinen V, Haglund C, Sepannen H. Outcomes of resected nonfunctional pancreatic neuroendocrine tumors: do size and symptoms matter? Surgery. 2015;158(6):1556–63.

25. Gaujoux S, Partelli S, Maire F, et al. Observational study of natural history of small sporadic nonfuntioning pancreatic neuroendocrine tumors. J Clin Endocrinol Metab. 2013;98(12):4784–9.
26. Zhang IY, Fernandez-del Castillo C, Zhao J, et al. Operative vs. non-operative management of nonfunctioning pancreatic neuroendocrine tumors. In: 49th annual meeting of the pancreas club syllabus. 2015. p. S001.
27. Falconi M, Plockinger U, Kwekkemboom D, et al. Well differenciated pancreatic nonfunctioning tumors/carcinoma, ENETS guidelines. Neuroendocrinology. 2006;84:196–211.
28. Kim MJ, Choi DW, Heo JS, et al. Surgical strategies for nonfunctioning pancreatic neuroendocrine tumors. Br J Surg. 2012;99:1562–8.
29. Sharpe SM, In H, Winchester DJ, Talamonti MS, et al. Surgical resection provides an overall survival benefit for patients with small pancreatic neuroendocrine tumors. J Gastrointest Surg. 2015;19:117–23.
30. Solorzano CC, Lee JE, Pisters PWT, et al. Nonfunctioning islet cell carcinoma of the páncreas: survival results in a contemporary series of 163 patiens. Surgery. 2011;130:1078–85.
31. Toumpanakis C, Meyer T, Caplin ME. Citotoxic treatment including embolization/chemoembolization for neuroendocrine tumors. Best Pract Res Clin Endocrinol Metab. 2007;21:131.
32. Moertel CG, Lefkopoulo M, Lipsitz S, et al. Streptozocina-doxorubicina, streptozocina-fluoracil or chlorozotocina in the treatment of advanced islet cell carcinoma. N Engl J Med. 1992;326:519–23.
33. Moertel CG, Kvols LK, Oconnell MJ, et al. Treatment of neuroendocrine carcinoma with combined etoposide and cisplatin. Cancer. 1991;68:227.

Routine Lymph Node Dissection Versus Duodenal Inspection Alone for the Treatment of Multiple Endocrine Neoplasia Type 1 Patients with Hypergastrinemia

35

Paxton V. Dickson

Abstract

Gastrinomas represent the most common funtional pancreaticoduodenal neuroendocrine tumor in MEN1 patients, however, there is lack of consensus regarding appropriate timing and extent of operation for these patients. An optimal strategy has been difficult to define due to the uncommon nature of the disease, inconsistency of operative approaches, absence of controlled studies, limited follow-up, and incomplete understanding of the natural history of the disease. It has been demonstrated that the majority of MEN1-associated gastrinomas are located in the duodenum and often occur concomitantly with non-gastrin producing pancreatic neoplasms. Therefore, evaluation of the duodenum for removal of these tumors is critical to the operative strategy, regardless of the extent of pancreatectomy planned. This chapter reviews outcomes of studies focused on MEN1 patients with hypergastrinemia with particular attention to the incidence of gastrinoma-associated nodal metastases and the rationale for performance of a regional lymphadenectomy at the time of operative exploration. Although there are relatively few studies examining this issue, available data demonstrate a high occurrence of gastrinoma lymph node metastases in MEN1 patients. Furthermore, these are often micrometastases and commonly used preoperative imaging modalities have a low sensitivity for detecting this disease. Collectively, the available evidence suggest that in addition to removal of the primary tumor(s), a formal anatomically based regional lymphadenectomy may result in more durable reduction of gastrin hypersecretion and offer potential long-term oncologic benefit (GRADE B).

P. V. Dickson
Division of Surgical Oncology, University of Tennessee Health Science Center, Memphis, TN, USA
e-mail: pdickso1@uthsc.edu

P. Angelos, R. H. Grogan (eds.), *Difficult Decisions in Endocrine Surgery*, Difficult Decisions in Surgery: An Evidence-Based Approach,
https://doi.org/10.1007/978-3-319-92860-9_35

Keywords
Multiple endocrine neoplasia type 1 · Gastrinoma · Hypergastrinemia · Lymph node metastases

Background

In 1955, Drs. Zollinger and Ellison described two patients, likely with multiple endocrine neoplasia type I (MEN1), found to have atypical peptic ulceration, gastric acid hypersecretion, and neuroendocrine tumors of the pancreas [1]. Since this initial description, substantial advances have been made in understanding the biology of gastrinomas and gastric physiology, as well as improvements in treating gastric acid hypersecretion with potent anti-secretory medications and operative therapy [2]. In addition, considerable progress has occurred in the comprehensive management of MEN1 patients. Pancreaticoduodenal neuroendocrine tumors (PDNETs) occur in 30–75% of patients with MEN1 and metastases from these neoplasms represent the leading cause of disease-specific mortality [3]. Gastrinomas represent the most common functional PDNETs in this population, causing symptoms and complications related to gastric acid hypersecretion. While the use of anti-secretory agents in patients with gastrinomas has made complications from ulcer disease a rare cause of death, morbidity related to hormone excess does occur [4].

The management of MEN1 patients with hypergastrinemia remains controversial, with ongoing debate regarding the role, timing, and extent of operative therapy [5]. An optimal strategy for these patients has been difficult to define due to the uncommon nature of the disease, inconsistency of operative approaches, absence of controlled studies, limited follow-up, and incomplete understanding of the natural history of the disease [6]. Recommendations for management of MEN1 patients with hypergastrinemia have varied widely and included: withholding exploration until neoplasms reach ≥2–3 cm in size [7]; routine early exploration with performance of a distal pancreatectomy, enucleation of neoplasms in the pancreatic head or uncinate combined with duodenotomy and excision of any duodenal neoplasms, and peri-pancreatic LN dissection [8]; routine performance of pancreaticoduodenectomy [9, 10], and non-operative management with proton-pump inhibitors. This chapter reviews evidence related to the role and rationale for routine performance of regional lymphadenectomy in patients with MEN1 and hypergastrinemia who undergo operative intervention (Table 35.1).

Table 35.1 PICO table

*P*opulation	Multiple endocrine neoplasia type I patients with hypergastrinemia undergoing surgery
*I*ntervention	Routine lymph node dissection
*C*omparator	Duodenal inspection and selective lymph node resection
*O*utcome	Survival, recurrence, complications

Surgical Series Evaluating Outcomes for MEN-1 Patients with Hypergastrinemia

Although several institutional series have studied operative outcomes of MEN1-associated PDNETs, few have specifically examined outcomes for patients with MEN1-related gastrinomas (Table 35.2). These reports have primarily examined surgical strategies and rates of achieving eugastrinemia or "biochemical cure" following surgery. A close look at these series, however, demonstrates these neoplasms have a propensity for malignant transformation, with 40–80% of patients harboring lymph node (LN) metastases [8–13]. Moreover, in their respective manuscripts, the authors of these studies address the importance of removing these nodes at the time of exploration for MEN1 patients with hypergastrinemia.

Thompson endorsed routine early exploration for MEN1 patients with hypergastrinemia [8]. His recommended operative approach for these patients included performance of a distal pancreatectomy, enucleation of neoplasms in the pancreatic head or uncinate combined with duodenotomy with excision of any duodenal neoplasms, and peripancreatic LN dissection. In his seminal series, 40% of patients with duodenal gastrinomas were found to have LN metastases. In performing his described operation in 34 patients with MEN1 and ZES over a 20-year period, he reported that 68% were eugastrinemic and 33% had negative secretin stimulation tests at follow up (longest follow up 19 years).

In 1999, Norton et al. reported on 28 patients with MEN1 and ZES treated at the NIH [11]. In this study, patients were operated if a tumor of 3 cm or larger was detected by imaging. Operations included enucleation or resection of pancreatic neoplasms and evaluation of the duodenum. In this series prior to 1987 duodenal evaluation involved kocherizing and externally palpating the duodenum while subsequent procedures included endoscopic transillumination and/or duodenotomy with intraluminal digital inspection. In this study, 61% of patients had LN metastases and 7% had tumor bearing lymph nodes with no identifiable primary gastrinoma. Furthermore, in the discussion of the manuscript, the authors emphasized the importance of removing lymph nodes in the region of the head of the pancreas and duodenum even if they appear normal because of the propensity for microscopic nodal metastases. Patients underwent rigorous post-operative biochemical evaluation with serum gastrin and secretin stimulation tests performed 3–6 months after operation and then yearly. They found that all but one patient demonstrated biochemical recurrence by 3 years and that every patient had recurred by 10 years.

Bartsch et al. detailed their results in using an aggressive surgical approach over a 23-year period (1981–2004) for 26 MEN1 patients with duodenopancreatic neoplasms [10]. Eleven patients in this series underwent surgery for ZES. Patients treated prior to 1997 had an operative approach similar to that described by Thompson [8] while pylorus-preserving pancreaticoduodenectomy with regional lymphadenectomy was performed in subsequent years. LN metastases were identified in 7/11 (64%) of patients with gastrinomas, including 3/4 patients whose primary tumor size was <1 cm. Only one patient with ZES was found to have distant metastatic disease in this series. At a median follow up of 123 months, 7/11 patients remained without

Table 35.2 Surgical series evaluating outcomes for patients with MEN1 and hypergastrinemia

Series	No MEN1 patients with HG	RLND described	Incidence of gastrinoma lymph node metastases (%)	Incidence of gastrinoma liver metastases (%)	Reported outcomes
Thompson [8]	34	Yes	40	3	68% were EG and 33% had negative secretin stimulation tests (longest fu 19 years). 5-year and 10-year disease specific survival 100%
Norton et al. [11]	28	Yes	68[a]	14	27/28 relapsed HG by 3 years, all relapsed HG by 10 years. 5-year and 10-year disease specific survival 100% and 86%, respectively
Bartsch et al. [10]	11	Yes	64	9	At a median follow up of 123 months, 7/11 patients remained "biochemically cured"
Tonelli et al. [9]	13	Yes	54[b]	0	Reported 10/13 patients with normal basal and stimulated gastrin levels at last follow up. No reported disease-specific deaths
Imamura et al. [12]	16	Yes	63	6	Follow up ranging from 2 months—18 years, 14/16 patients reported as EG. 10-year overall survival 90%
Dickson et al. [13]	20	Yes	80[b]	NR	12/20 patients rendered EG, at median fu of 44 months, 10/12 remained EG. RLND and duodenal inspection were significantly associated with achieving EG

One patient had tumor found in LN, but no duodenal or pancreatic primary
[a]Two patients had tumor found in LN, but no duodenal or pancreatic primary
[b]One patient had tumor found in LN, but no duodenal or pancreatic primary

biochemical evidence of recurrence. There were no peri-operative mortalities and they reported a 58% surgical complication rate, primarily related to pancreatectomy.

Tonelli et al. reported their operative experience from 13 MEN1 patients with hypergastrinemia over an 11-year period (1992–2003) [9]. They performed standard or pylorus preserving pancreaticoduodenectomy in the majority of patients and lymphadenectomy of the peripancreatic region, hepatoduodenal ligament, and hepatic and celiac arteries in all patients. Fifty-four percent (7/13) were found to have gastrinoma nodal metastases. At the time of publication, 10/13 patients had normal basal and stimulated gastrin levels. In two patients with recurrent hypergastrinemia, CT demonstrated regional nodal recurrence at 18 months post-operatively. In their series, 38/41 identified gastrinomas were duodenal, 2 were documented "ectopic" (1 in the gallbladder and 1 in the extrahepatic biliary tree), and 1 was considered a nodal primary gastrinoma. Two patients were found to have hepatic metastases that did not stain for gastrin and were believed to arise from nonfunctional pancreatic neoplasms. No pancreatic gastrinomas were identified in this series. There were no post-operative mortalities and the reported operative morbidity was 37% (all related to pancreatectomy). The authors advocated an aggressive surgical approach, recommending pancreaticoduodenectomy with regional lymphadenectomy when hypergastrinemia is detected in these patients.

Imamura et al. reported their 18-year experience (1991–2009) of 16 patients with MEN1 and ZES who underwent operative intervention [12]. Over the reported time period, their operative approach evolved from performance of pancreaticoduodenectomy (three patients) to local tumor resection with transduodenal excision or partial duodenectomy (six patients) to pancreas-preserving total duodenectomy [14] (seven patients) with regional lymphadenectomy performed in all patients. Gastrinoma nodal metastases were identified in 10/16 (63%). With a follow up range from 2 months to 18 years, 14 of 16 patients were reported as eugastrinemic. One patient developed suspected gastrinoma-related liver metastases and in a second patient distant lymph node metastases developed. Based on their results, the authors recommended early and aggressive surgical intervention with MEN1 patients with hypergastrinemia.

In a review from MD Anderson Cancer Center 20 patients with MEN1 and hypergastrinemia underwent surgical exploration between 1980 and 2010 [13]. This study specifically evaluated the impact of duodenal evaluation and formal regional lymphadenectomy on achieving eugastrinemia. The limits of an anatomically based regional lymph node dissection (RLND) described in this study are shown in Fig. 35.1. The authors recommended a generous Kocher maneuver and dissection to ensure removal of periduodenal and peripancreatic LNs posterior to the duodenum and head, uncinate, and neck of the pancreas and anterior to the vena cava and aorta; portal nodes from the right lateral border and posterior aspect of the portal vein; hepatic arterial nodes immediately caudal to the proper hepatic artery and cephalad to the pancreas; and resection of the cephalad 4–5 cm of the right gonadal vein and its associated soft tissue to ensure clearance of lateral peri-duodenal and para-caval nodes. In this study the median number of lymph nodes identified for patients undergoing a formal RLND was 16 (range 4–41) versus 1 (range 0–19) for those

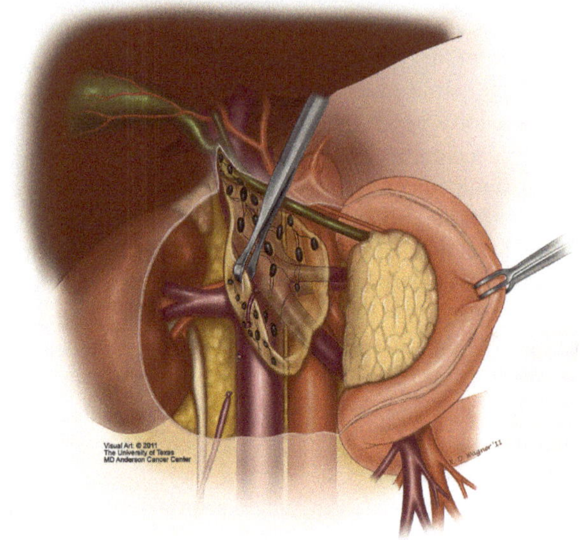

Fig. 35.1 Anatomic boundaries of recommended formal regional lymphadenectomy for patients with MEN1-associated hypergastrinemia who undergo operative intervention [13, with permission]

who did not. Eighty percent of patients were found to have LN metastases and the median number of LN involved was 3 (range 1–15). Eugastrinemia was achieved in 12 patients (60%), while 8 (40%) had persistent hypergastrinemia. Compared to patients with persistent hypergastrinemia, patients rendered eugastrinemic more often underwent intra-operative duodenal evaluation (11/12; 92% versus 2/8; 25%, $p = 0.01$) and RLND (11/12; 92% versus 3/8; 38%, $p = 0.03$). There was no relationship between pancreatic resection and achievement of eugastrinemia (9/12; 75% versus 8/8; 100%, $p = 0.32$). After a median follow up of 44 months, 10/12 (80%) patients rendered eugastrinemic remained eugastrinemic; including 3 patients (25%) with follow up of ≥5 years (5, 6, and 24 years).

This study also evaluated the utility of pre-operative EUS, CT, and octreoscan in these patients. Although EUS (90%) and CT (71%) were reasonably sensitive in detecting pancreatic neoplasms, no imaging technique was highly sensitive for detecting duodenal tumors (EUS 12.5%, CT 30%, Octreoscan 14%) or regional nodal metastases (EUS 40%, CT 46%, Octreoscan 33%). Given these findings as well as the high incidence of gastrinoma nodal metastases, and the impact of duodenal evaluation and regional lymphadenectomy in achieving eugastrinemia, the authors note the necessity of both formal duodenal evaluation as well as anatomic RLND at the time of operative exploration for MEN1 patients with hypergastrinemia.

Rationale for Duodenal Inspection and Routine Lymphadenectomy in MEN1 Patients with Hypergastrinemia

Although the above-mentioned series have inherent limitations of any smaller, single institution, retrospective (with the exception of the study by Norton et al.) analyses, several conclusions can be the drawn from the collective experience.

The majority of MEN1-associated gastrinomas arise within the duodenum rather than the pancreas. They likely arise from proliferation of gastrin cells within the normal duodenal mucosa [15]. These neoplasms are generally small (<1 cm) and commonly multifocal. In this patient population, duodenal gastrinomas often occur concomitantly with non-gastrin producing pancreatic neuroendocrine tumors. Furthermore, standard pre-operative imaging modalities have a low sensitivity for detecting these small duodenal lesions. Therefore, if the decision is made to explore MEN1 patients with hypergastrinemia, thorough evaluation and removal of any duodenal gastrinomas is necessary, regardless of the distribution of additional pancreatic neoplasms and extent of pancreatectomy planned.

MEN1-associated gastrinomas have a propensity for nodal metastases (40–80% in the above mentioned series). In some circumstances, bulky nodal disease may be easily detected on pre-operative imaging or at the time of exploration. However, LN micrometastases are often present and failure to extirpate these nodes likely results in less durable reduction of gastrin hypersecretion and potentially adverse oncologic outcomes. Most authors would advocate that adequate clearance of this disease requires a formal, anatomically based, regional lymphadenectomy. This should occur, regardless of the primary pancreaticoduodenal resection being performed. The "gastrinoma triangle", originally described by Passaro et al. is bound superiorly by the junction of the cystic and common duct, inferiorly by the junction of the second and third portions of the duodenum, and medially by the anatomic neck of the pancreas [16]. A lymphadenectomy that considers these boundaries would involve thorough clearance of nodes within the hepatoduodenal ligament, along the common hepatic artery towards the celiac axis, retroduodenal and retropancreatic nodes lying along the pancreaticoduodenal arteries, and clearance of aortocaval nodes behind the neck of the pancreas (Fig. 35.1).

In addition to considering the potential for clinically meaningful reduction of gastrin hypersecretion, extirpation of regional lymph nodes in MEN 1 patients with gastrinoma may offer an oncologic benefit. The most important predictor of survival in patients with MEN1 and pancreaticoduodenal neuroendocrine tumors is liver metastases. Jensen et al. recently reported on 326 patients with PDNETs from the NIH and Stanford University Hospital, the majority of which had gastrinomas [17]. They specifically examined the impact of LN metastases on overall and disease-related survival and development of metachronous hepatic metastases. When evaluating the entire cohort, there was no difference in survival between patients with or without LN metastases. However, patients with LN metastases were found to have a shorter interval to the development of metachronous liver metastases. In the subset of patients from the NIH who had longer follow-up (mean 11 years), disease-specific survival was significantly decreased among patients with LN metastases versus those without. Furthermore, they found that disease-related survival decreased as a function of the number of metastatic nodes. In patients with duodenal or pancreatic gastrinomas, the incidence of lymph node metastases was 71% and 76%, respectively. Those with pancreatic gastrinomas did have a significantly higher incidence of liver metastases and disease-related death. Although only some of these were MEN1 patients, the data does suggest that standard performance of a regional lymphadenectomy in these patients offers both prognostic and therapeutic value.

None of the above-mentioned studies specifically examined morbidity associated with performance of removing regional lymph nodes. However, it is unlikely that including a regional lymphadenectomy as part of the operation for MEN1 patients with hypergastrinemia adds much, if any, morbidity over that related to the primary resection being performed.

Conclusion

Although controversy exists regarding appropriate timing and extent of operation in MEN1 patients with hypergastrinemia, review of the current literature clearly demonstrates a propensity for gastrinoma-associated regional LN metastases. Standard preoperative imaging modalities (CT, EUS, Octreoscan) are not particularly sensitive in detecting these nodal metastases. Failure to remove regional lymph nodes at the time of exploration may result in persistent hypergastrinemia and potentially adverse long-term oncologic outcomes. If a decision is made to explore MEN1 patients with hypergastrinemia, in addition to resection of the primary tumor(s), performance of an anatomically based regional lymphadenectomy is recommended (GRADE B).

References

1. Zollinger RM, Ellison EH. Primary peptic ulcerations of the jejunum associated with islet cell tumors of the pancreas. Ann Surg. 1955;142(4):709–28.
2. Yeung MJ, Pasieka JL. Gastrinomas: a historical perspective. J Surg Oncol. 2009;100(5):425–33.
3. Brandi ML, Gagel RF, Anteli A, Bilezikian JP, Beck-Peccoz P, Bordi C, et al. Guidelines for diagnosis and therapy of MEN type 1 and type 2. J Clin Endocrinol Metab. 2001;86(12):5658–71.
4. Carty SE, Helm AK, Amico JA, Clarke MR, Foley TP, Watson CG, Mulvihill JJ. The variable penetrance and spectrum of manifestations of multiple endocrine neoplasia type 1. Surgery. 1998;124(6):1106–14.
5. Norton JA, Jensen RT. Resolved and unresolved controversies in the surgical management of pateints with Zollinger-Ellison syndrome. Ann Surg. 2004;240(5):757–73.
6. Ellison EC, Sparks J, Verducci JS, Johnson JA, Muscarella P, Bloomston M, Melvin WS. 50-year appraisal of gastrinoma: recommendations for staging and treatment. J Am Coll Surg. 2006;202(6):897–905.
7. Norton JA, Alexander HR, Fraker DL, Venzon DJ, Gibril F, Jensen RT. Does the use of routine duodentotomy (DUODZ) affect rate of cure, development of liver metastases, or survival in patients with Zollinger-Ellison syndrome? Ann Surg. 2004;239(5):617–26.
8. Thompson NW. Current concepts in the surgical management of multiple endocrine neoplasia type 1 pancreatic-duodenal disease. Results in the treatment of 40 patients with Zollinger-Ellison syndrome, hypoglycaemia or both. J Intern Med. 1998;243(6):495–500.
9. Tonelli F, Fratini G, Nesi G, Tommasi MS, Batignani G, Falchetti A, Brandi ML. Pancreatectomy in multiple endocrine neoplasia type 1-related gastrinomas and pancreatic endocrine neoplasias. Ann Surg. 2006;244(1):61–70.
10. Bartsch DK, Fendrich V, Langer P, Celik I, Kann PH, Rothmund M. Outcome of duodenopancreatic resections in patients with multiple endocrine neoplasia type 1. Ann Surg. 2005;242(6):757–66.
11. Norton JA, Franker DL, Alexander HR, Venzon DJ, Doppman JL, Serrano J, et al. Surgery to cure the Zollinger-Ellison syndrome. N Engl J Med. 1999;341(9):635–44.

12. Imamura M, Komoto I, Ota S, Hiratsuka T, Kosugi S, Doi R, et al. Biochemically curative surgery for gastrinoma in multiple endocrine neoplasia type 1 patients. World J Gastroenterol. 2011;17(10):1343–53.
13. Dickson PV, Rich TA, Xing Y, Cote GJ, Wang H, Perrier ND, et al. Achieving eugastrinemia in MEN1 patients: both duodenal inspection and formal lymph node dissection are important. Surgery. 2011;150(6):1143–52.
14. Imamura M, Komoto I, Doi R, Onodera H, Kobayashi H, Kawai Y. New pancreas-preserving total duodenectomy technique. World J Surg. 2005;29(2):203–7.
15. Anlauf M, Perren A, Meyer CL, Schmid S, Saramaslani P, Kruse ML, et al. Precursor lesions in patients with multiple endocrine neoplasia type 1-associated duodenal gastrinomas. Gastroenterology. 2005;128(5):1187–98.
16. Stabile BE, Morrow DJ, Passaro E Jr. The gastrinoma triangle: operative implications. Am J Surg. 1984;147(1):25–31.
17. Krampitz GW, Norton JA, Poultsides GA, Visser BC, Sun L, Jensen RT. Lymph nodes and survival in pancreatic neuroendocrine tumors. Arch Surg. 2012;147(9):820–7.

Resection Versus Chemotherapy for Metastatic Neuroendocrine Tumors of the Pancreas

36

Kathleen K. Christians, George Younan, Ben George, Susan Tsai, and Douglas B. Evans

Abstract

Pancreatic neuroendocrine tumors (PNET) represent a broad spectrum of disease with behavior ranging from benign to highly malignant. Treatment strategies are quite variable and frequently lack consensus. This chapter focuses on the debate between surgery and chemotherapy for metastatic PNET. We summarize the evidence for both strategies including which treatment is appropriate in each clinical setting.

Keywords

Pancreatic neuroendocrine tumor · Neuroendocrine carcinoma · Ki67 · mTOR inhibitors · MGMT

Introduction

Pancreatic neuroendocrine tumors (PNET) account for only 1–4% of all clinically apparent pancreatic tumors [1–3]. The majority are sporadic in inheritance, although 10% may be part of inherited disorders such as neurofibromatosis, tuberous sclerosis, multiple endocrine neoplasia (MEN) type 1 or von Hippel-Lindau (VHL) syndrome. PNETs arise from islet cells of the pancreas and may or may not secrete functionally active hormones (classified as functional versus nonfunctional

K. K. Christians (✉) · G. Younan · B. George · S. Tsai · D. B. Evans
Pancreatic Cancer Program, Medical College of Wisconsin; Department of Surgery (Division of Surgical Oncology), Milwaukee, WI, USA
e-mail: kchristi@mcw.edu

P. Angelos, R. H. Grogan (eds.), *Difficult Decisions in Endocrine Surgery*, Difficult Decisions in Surgery: An Evidence-Based Approach,
https://doi.org/10.1007/978-3-319-92860-9_36

Table 36.1 PICO table

*P*opulation	Patients with metastatic PNET
*I*ntervention	Surgical resection
*C*omparator	Medical management
*O*utcomes	Survival, recurrence, complications, QOL

[majority]). In 2010, the World Health Organization developed another clinically relevant classification based on tumor grade (G) and Ki-67 index. A G1 tumor was defined as having a mitotic count <2/10 high powered fields (hpf) and a Ki-67 index <3%. G2 tumors were defined as having a mitotic count of 2–20/10 hpf and a Ki-67 of 3–20%. G3 tumors were defined as having a mitotic count of >20/10 hpf and/or a Ki-67 index >20%. In general, well differentiated PNETs are either low or intermediate grade (G1 or G2), whereas poorly differentiated PNETS are high grade (G3) and considered carcinomas [4]. The older literature references to high-grade neuroendocrine carcinoma, small cell carcinoma, undifferentiated carcinoma, anaplastic carcinoma and large cell neuroendocrine carcinoma are all included in the current nomenclature of poorly differentiated PNET [5]. This terminology can be confusing since all well differentiated PNETs have malignant potential (defined as the ability to metastasize to regional lymph nodes and/or distant organs). The exception is small, nonmetastatic insulinomas which in general, carry no risk for metachronous distant organ recurrence. Tumor grade has significant prognostic value and is particularly important for treatment decisions because well differentiated PNETs are managed very differently relative to poorly differentiated tumors [5–10]. All patients with a PNET who have advanced disease should undergo a biopsy of their tumor and have proper histologic assessment (Ki-67/mitotic index) in order to classify the tumor as a guide for further therapy.

Surgical resection of PNETs remains the only curative therapy for this disease and represents the current standard of care [11–16]. A complete resection of all visible disease controls tumor growth, reduces excess hormone production in patients with liver metastases and provides a 5-year overall survival exceeding 60% [17–19]. This chapter summarizes the current literature in the debate of surgery versus systemic therapy for the treatment of metastatic PNET (Table 36.1).

Search Strategy

We conducted a focused review of current guidelines related to the surgical and medical management of metastatic PNET. The PubMed database was searched for the past 20 years for the following key words: pancreatic neuroendocrine tumor, pancreatic neuroendocrine carcinoma, chemotherapy, pancreatectomy, resection, enucleation, transplantation, mTOR inhibitors, somatostatin analogues, and tyrosine kinase inhibitors. Emphasis was placed on national and international guidelines and recommendations.

Surgical Resection of PNET

Patients with well-differentiated PNETs or those "tumors" that are G1 or G2 with Ki67 < 20% should be treated differently from patients with poorly differentiated "neuroendocrine carcinomas" that are grade G3 and have Ki67 indices >20% [5, 8, 20, 21]. Poorly differentiated PNETs have a high rate of metastatic spread even in patients that appear to have localized disease and therefore surgical resection is rarely curative [5, 22]. Surgical resection is, however, generally recommended if all or >90% of the imageable disease can be removed [11, 13, 16, 19, 23]. In general, surgery is not recommended where resection cannot be complete or results in removal of >90% of the metastatic tumor as this does not improve survival [11, 13, 16]. Less than a complete resection (debulking) is considered in patients with functional tumors where hormone secretion is causing significant symptoms; we rarely consider surgery for nonfunctional PNETs if a complete gross resection of all disease cannot be accomplished.

Minimal Resection for Early Disease

Benign biologic behavior is exhibited in 10–40% of PNETs and is uniformly seen in nonmetastatic insulinomas [24]. Solitary PNETs located >2–3 mm from the pancreatic duct are frequently enucleated, as opposed to resected with a margin of normal pancreas [11, 25]. For tumors in the pancreatic neck or proximal body of the pancreas, parenchymal preservation in the form of middle segment pancreatectomy is an option when enucleation is not feasible due to ductal proximity [26]. The disadvantage of any operation which requires transection of the pancreatic duct is the risk of a pancreatic fistula [27]. Pancreatic endocrine and exocrine function is preserved with any operation that is able to preserve pancreatic parenchyma, which is very important in young patients [27]. Minimally invasive approaches are ideal for tumors that are small, benign and located in the pancreatic body or tail [28, 29]. More recently, robotic-assisted minimally invasive pancreatic resections have been advocated as superior to laparoscopic approaches due to decreased rates of conversion to open laparotomy (0% vs 16%) without adding increased morbidity [30].

Lymph Node Resection

With the exception of sporadic nonmetastatic insulinoma, positive regional lymph nodes are found in up to 23% of patients with low risk PNETs and result in a significantly shorter disease-free survival than in patients who are node negative (4.5 vs 14.6 years; $P < 0.0001$) [31]. Node positivity occurs more frequently in tumors with the following characteristics: >15 mm in size, located in the pancreatic head, G3 and exhibiting lymphatic invasion [31, 32]. Although Partelli and colleagues attempted to develop predictive models of risk for lymph node involvement, preoperative variables did not reliably predict the probability of nodal involvement to the extent that surgeons could omit regional lymphadenectomy at the time of pancreatic resection for PNET [33, 34]. Clearly, there is a huge selection bias in this literature as lymph nodes cannot be assessed for the presence of metastases unless they are both surgically excised and pathologically assessed. It is perhaps best to conclude that all PNETs, except for small insulinomas, are associated with a significant risk of regional lymph node metastases and these nodes should be removed at the time of surgery whenever possible. This surgical practice prevents a metachronous recurrence in regional nodes which could have been removed at the first operation.

High Risk/Malignant Disease

In the setting of neuroendocrine carcinoma, surgery is superior to conservative therapies in extending survival and controlling local and metastatic disease [34]. A retrospective study utilizing the Surveillance, Epidemiology and End Results (SEER) database demonstrated a survival benefit of 79 months for resected patients compared to those who were recommended to undergo surgery but were not resected (114 months vs 35 months; $P < 0.0001$) [35]. This survival advantage held true for the subgroup of patients with distant metastases (60 vs 31 months; $P = 0.01$) [35]. In addition, surgical resection reduced the risk of metachronous liver metastases in patients with gastrinoma (5% vs 29%) [36]. In patients with more advanced/larger local disease, aggressive resection when possible, in carefully selected patients, offers optimal disease control [37]. Interestingly, in some reports, a margin-positive resection in patients with large, regionally advanced PNETs had a similar overall survival benefit compared to a margin negative resection [38]. This finding clearly reflects the more indolent biology of this disease compared to pancreatic adenocarcinoma.

Liver Metastases

Liver metastases are present in up to 60% of patients with PNET at the time of initial diagnosis and such synchronous liver metastases are not a contraindication to surgical treatment [19, 39, 40]. However, it remains controversial as to whether the primary tumor should be removed in the setting of unresectable metastatic disease. Some reports conclude that removal of the primary tumor in the setting of unresectable distant disease does not improve survival compared to the use of nonsurgical therapies [41, 42]. In contrast, if the liver metastases are able to be completely resected, a much higher 5 year survival (72 vs 25%) and longer median survival (96 vs 20 months) is observed compared to patients treated nonoperatively [43]. Extended liver resections for metastatic disease can be performed safely with acceptable morbidity (21%) and mortality (5% or less) [44–48]. In sharp contrast to most other solid tumors, 5-year survival is both possible and probable after resection of PNET liver metastases; one series reported a 5-year survival of 66% [44]. The European Neuroendocrine Tumor Society (ENETs) guidelines take the role for surgery even further and extend it to patients with liver metastases who may not be eligible for complete resection and can undergo surgical debulking of >90% of liver metastases [13, 49, 50]. The authors of this review are not comfortable with this recommendation in most situations and largely limit elective liver resections to those patients who can receive a complete gross resection of all image positive disease. Surgical resection may be complemented by ablation or transarterial chemoembolization (TACE) [12, 43].

Extended Resections of the Primary

Major vascular involvement (portal/superior mesenteric vein, superior mesenteric artery, inferior vena cava) does not preclude resection and may result in 30% of patients with PNETs being disease-free at 5 years [37, 51, 52]. This is particularly important for PNETs involving the splenic vein (SV) or portal vein/superior mesenteric vein (PV/SMV) resulting in extrahepatic portal hypertension with resultant gastroesophageal varices and gastrointestinal bleeding, as the bleeding resolves with resection of the PNET and the spleen [37, 53, 54]. Current evidence stems from retrospective nonrandomized studies as ethical and feasibility considerations preclude realization of a prospectively controlled randomized trial. PNETs with a Ki-67 index >5%, positive lymph nodes, and a size >4 cm have a significantly higher risk of metachronous disease recurrence [55, 56].

Liver Transplantation

Liver transplantation is an option, but evidence is limited, oncologic outcome is uncertain and its use is controversial [12, 57–59]. A recent study of 17 patients who underwent liver transplantation for metastatic PNET reported a 1-, 5-, and 10-year survival of 89%, 80% and 50% respectively which may not be much better than other forms of therapy. However, these patients may have had very large tumor burdens and the highly selected nature of these results makes further interpretation very difficult [13, 49, 60, 61]. Risk factors for a poor prognosis after transplantation include: extrahepatic disease at the time of transplant; abdominal exenteration or multivisceral transplant at the time of the liver transplant; metastatic PNET (as opposed to gastrointestinal carcinoid); age > 50; >50% of the liver involved; Ki 67 > 10%; and, aberrant E-cadherin staining [12, 14, 58, 59, 62]. ENETs 2012 consensus guidelines therefore, recommend liver transplantation only for patients with life-threatening hormonal disturbances refractory to other treatments, or for patients with nonfunctional PNET with diffuse liver metastases refractory to all other treatments [12]. PNET liver metastases are not considered a standard exception that would yield more points by Eurotransplant or UNOS criteria.

High Grade Pancreatic Neuroendocrine Carcinomas

Patients with a high Ki-67 index have increased risk of recurrence and metastatic disease with resultant poor survival. In patients with poorly differentiated carcinomas with a high Ki-67, surgery should only be undertaken if an R0 resection is possible; there is no role for cytoreductive (<R0) surgery in these patients [13, 55]. Conventional systemic chemotherapy and less frequently, targeted systemic therapies such as multityrosine kinase inhibitors and mTOR inhibitors are the standard in these settings [34].

Summary of Recommendations

The biology of PNETs is different based on tumor grade and Ki 67 index and therefore tumor biopsy at the time of diagnosis is critically important. Surgical resection is the only curative treatment modality and is the current standard of care for patients who appear eligible for a complete gross resection of all local and distant disease. Resection of PNETs with low malignant potential should be done with the goal of parenchymal preservation (enucleation or limited resection) and with minimally invasive surgery if possible (robotically or laparoscopically). Lymph node metastases are present in up to one fourth of PNETs and regional lymphadenectomy is recommended for all diagnoses other than sporadic insulinoma. In the setting of well to moderately differentiated (G1 or G2) PNETs, surgery when feasible, is superior to nonoperative therapies in extending survival and controlling local and metastatic disease. In addition, surgery is often the optimal treatment for large G1 or G2 PNETs with local extension requiring vascular resection and reconstruction; in such situations, the role of pre-operative/adjunctive systemic therapies should be explored in a multidisciplinary setting. Liver transplantation is reserved for those patients with life-threatening hormonal imbalances or nonfunctional PNETs refractory to all other treatments. High grade, poorly differentiated tumors should not be treated with surgical resection unless an R0 status can be achieved.

Medical Management of Metastatic PNET

Chemotherapy for PNETs

Cytotoxic chemotherapy continues to play an important role in patients with advanced metastatic PNET. The regimens utilized differ based on several factors, most notably, the degree of differentiation of the neuroendocrine carcinoma [5, 12, 14, 63–65]. Chemotherapy is usually reserved for palliative intent treatment of patients with inoperable disease. Currently, there is no defined role for systemic therapy in the adjuvant setting (post resection of PNETs) outside of clinical trials, however, it is increasingly used in a neoadjuvant fashion to (1) assess tumor biology in patients that present with synchronous metastatic disease prior to offering them a resection and (2) to induce response in patients with a large tumor burden if they require a complex operation for removal of the primary tumor with or without concomitant liver resection [12, 14, 64–66]. Because of significant treatment-related toxicities, cytotoxic chemotherapy is recommended for PNETs in the following situations: (1) metastatic poorly differentiated PNETS (G3, Ki 67 index > 20%), (2) unresectable G1 or G2 PNETS (Ki 67 < 20%) after failure of biotherapy and/or targeted systemic therapy, (3) neoadjuvant therapy for G1 or G2 PNETS that present with synchronous metastatic disease or bulky primary tumors mandating complex surgery/vascular reconstruction to assess tumor biology and/or to induce a response prior to offering resection [12, 14, 67–69].

In G1–G2 (Ki67 < 3 or 3–20%) well differentiated metastatic PNETs, the combination of streptozotocin and 5-fluorouracil (FU) with/without doxorubicin has an objective response rate of 20–45%. Responses can be relatively short lived (6–20 months), and patients may experience side effects including but not limited to nausea and emesis (70–100%) and renal toxicity (15–40%) [12, 14, 65, 70]. A relatively new combination of temozolomide and capecitabine has shown efficacy with improved response rates and less toxicity based on early non-randomized data. A retrospective study of 30 patients with metastatic well differentiated PNETs treated with capecitabine and temazolomide demonstrated a partial response rate of 70% with a median PFS of 18 months, a 2 year survival of 92%, and only 13% developed grade three or four adverse events [71–74]. The ongoing randomized, phase II, Eastern Cooperative Oncology Group (ECOG) 2211 trial evaluates the efficacy of temozolimide with or without capecitabine in patients with G1 or G2 metastatic PNETs, with progression free survival (PFS) being the primary endpoint.

Kulke et al. showed that low levels of the DNA repair enzyme 06-methylguanine DNA methyltransferase (MGMT) in the tumor were associated with response to alkylating agents such as temozolomide [74]. This correlation between low tumoral expression of MGMT by immunohistochemistry and response to temozolomide has been noted in glioblastoma as well, but MGMT has thus far not been prospectively validated as a predictive biomarker for temozolomide therapy.

Both ENETS 2012 and the North American Neuroendocrine Tumor Society (NANETS) 2010 guidelines recommend chemotherapy in selected patients with advanced, metastatic, inoperable, well-differentiated (G1 or G2) PNETs—especially if rapidly growing, symptomatic, or if a large volume of disease is present [12, 16].

Biotherapy for Advanced/Metastatic PNETs

Somatostatin Analogues

Somatostatin analogues (SSAs) help control the hormone-excess state in functional PNETs and also have anti-tumor growth effects [12, 14, 16, 75–78]. PNETS overexpress one or more of the five subtypes of somatostatin receptors (SSTR 1–5) in 70–100% of patients [14, 75–78]. The PROMID study, which included patients (*N* = 85, 74% octreoscan positive, 39% with carcinoid syndrome) with well differentiated metastatic midgut NETs tumors (but did not include patients with PNETs), demonstrated that octreotide LAR extended time to tumor progression (14.3 vs 6 months, $p < 0.000072$) resulting in 67% of treated patients having stable disease at 6 months compared to 37% of controls ($p = 0.0079$) [79]. Tumor response was significant only in patients with low hepatic tumor burden (<10%) and was more favorable in the setting of a resected primary tumor. Objective decrease in tumor size was uncommon (<10%) but tumor stabilization was frequent (40–80%) [12, 14, 16, 75, 77, 78]. Another SSA (lanreotide) was investigated in the phase III, CLARINET trial that compared lanreotide versus placebo in patients with advanced, well to moderately differentiated (Ki-67 < 10%), non-functioning, gastroenteropancreatic NETs [80]. Notably, the majority of the patients (96%) had no tumor progression in 3–6 months prior to randomization and a third of the patients had hepatic tumor burden >25%. Lanreotide when compared to placebo, was associated with a significantly prolonged median PFS (median not reached vs. 18.0 months, hazard ratio (HR) 0.47, 95% confidence interval (CI) 0.30–0.73, $p < 0.01$). The estimated rate of PFS at 2 years in the lanreotide arm was 65% (95% CI, 54.0–74.1%) compared to 33% (95% CI, 23.0–43.3%) in the placebo group. While there were some key differences between the patient populations evaluated in the PROMID and CLARINET trials that were reflected in the outcomes noted in the placebo and interventional arms, these two trials unequivocally established a therapeutic role for SSAs in treatment of patients with well to moderately differentiated gastroenteropancreatic NETs.

National Comprehensive Cancer Network (NCCN) guidelines state that somatostatin analogues should be considered (level 2A evidence) for local-regional, unresectable, and/or metastatic well-moderately differentiated PNETs [81, 82]. ENETS 2012 guidelines support somatostatin if tumors are G1 and NANETS 2010 uses somatostatin analogues for antiproliferative effects and their low side effect profile [12, 81, 82]. Both octreotide and lanreotide have high affinity for somatostatin receptor subtypes two and five, however PNETS frequently possess other subtypes [14, 76, 83]. Pasireotide has high affinity for somatostatin receptors one, two, three and five and is being evaluated for enhanced anti-growth effects on neuroendocrine tumors and for its antisecretory effects [84–86]. However, Pasireotide is currently not recommended for treatment of well-moderately differentiated PNETs outside of a clinical trial.

Targeted Therapy

mTOR Inhibitors (Everolimus)

Everolimus is an oral mTOR inhibitor with efficacy demonstrated in several recent trials evaluating patients with metastatic PNETs, including the pivotal phase III RADIANT-3 trial [86–89]. In this report, 410 patients with low to intermediate grade metastatic PNETs were assigned to everolimus (10 mg, orally, once daily) or placebo, both in conjunction with best supportive care. Patients treated with everolimus, compared to placebo, showed a significant improvement in PFS (11 vs 4.6 months, HR 0.35, 95% CI, 0.27–0.45, $p < 0.0001$) and PFS rate at 18 months

(34%, 95% CI 26–43% vs 9%, 95% CI, 4–16%). The significant improvement in PFS and low rate of grade 3 or 4 adverse events (stomatitis 7%, anemia 6% and hyperglycemia 5%) led to everolimus being approved in Europe and the United States for use in patients with low to intermediate grade metastatic PNETs. This strategy is endorsed by both ENETS and NCCN.

Tyrosine Kinase Inhibitors (Sunitinib)

Tyrosine kinase receptors are a family of receptors (20 members) which include epidermal growth factor, platelet derived growth factor, hepatocyte growth factor (c-MET), stem cell factor (c-KIT) and VEGFRs among others. These receptors function as tyrosine kinases when activated and downstream effects include mediation of growth-related cascades, angiogenesis, apoptosis and cellular differentiation [90, 91]. PNETs frequently possess a number of tyrosine kinase receptors [91–95]. Sunitinib is an oral inhibitor of tyrosine kinase activity of PDGFRs, VEGFR-1, VEGFR-2, c-KIT and FLT3 [91]. An international, double-blind, multicenter Phase III study randomly assigned 171 patients with metastatic well differentiated PNETs to Sunitinib (37.5 mg/day, orally) or placebo in conjunction with SSA (at the investigator's discretion, in both arms). The primary end point (median PFS) was significantly improved in the Sunitinib arm compared to the placebo arm (11.4 vs. 5.5 months, HR 0.42, 95% CI, 0.26–0.66, $p < 0.001$). This study was discontinued early, after an independent data and safety monitoring committee observed more serious adverse events in the placebo group and a favorable PFS in the Sunitinib group. The demonstrated efficacy and relative paucity of grade 3 or 4 adverse events (neutropenia 12%, hypertension 10%, and palmar-plantar erythro-dysesthesia 6%) resulted in approval for the use of Sutent in both Europe and the United States, in patients with metastatic well-differentiated PNETS. This was subsequently endorsed by both ENETS and NCCN. In addition to sunitinib, numerous tyrosine kinase inhibitors have demonstrated activity in NETS (imatinib, sorafenib, vatalanib, pazopanib) [90, 91, 95–97] but none of these agents are recommended for use outside of clinical trials.

Summary of Targeted Therapy

For patients with metastatic low to intermediate grade PNETs, the authors recommend initiation of therapy with either a SSA or combination of SSA and everolimus/sunitinib based on disease burden and symptomatology. Patients with bulky disease and/or symptoms from their low-intermediate grade metastatic PNETs may benefit from combining SSA with either a targeted agent or cytotoxic chemotherapy, at presentation, based on the rapidity of response desired.

While the addition of these targeted therapies have led to significant improvements in the overall survival of patients with low-intermediate grade PNETs, there is a crucial need for newer therapeutic strategies to further the oncologic outcome in these patients. Disease progression while on these agents occurs either due to development of resistance to therapy and/or intolerance to the side effects. Strategies that attempt to overcome acquired/intrinsic resistance to available therapies and explore new therapeutic opportunities based on our evolving understanding of the development and progression of PNETs are being evaluated in clinical trials. These efforts include both individual and combined strategies aimed at targeting candidate genes/proteins involved in alternate tumor survival pathways.

Peptide Receptor Radionuclide Therapy with Radiolabeled Somatostatin (PRRT)

This treatment is based on the over/ectopic expression of somatostatin receptors by 60–100% of PNETs which in turn, allows for targeting of the tumor by cytotoxic, radiolabeled somatostatin analogues [14, 83, 98, 99]. Two different radiolabels are commonly used in combination with SSAs (1) ^{90}Y which strongly emit beta particles or (2) ^{177}Lu which emit B particles and gamma rays. A number of different somatostatin analogues and attached chelators (to allow binding of the radioisotope) have been used in various studies (DTPA, DOTA and peptide-chelator combinations DOTATATE, DOTATOC). Although a number of reports support the role of PRRT in the treatment of metastatic low-intermediate grade PNETs (European Studies), it is still considered investigational in the United States [99–101].

Treatment of Metastatic Poorly Differentiated PNETs

Poorly differentiated PNETs account for <1% of all malignant PNETS and 2–3% of all PNETS [5]. They have histologic and radiologic/clinical features of aggressive growth (G3, Ki 67 > 20% but usually 50–90%, necrosis, nuclear atypia), and carry a poor prognosis [5, 7, 20, 102]. Poorly differentiated PNETs have low densities of (or absent) somatostatin receptors and thus somatostatin scintigraphy is rarely useful and somatostatin analogues are not clinically effective. Most patients have regional or distant metastases at the time of presentation and surgery is rarely curative [5, 7]. Systemic chemotherapy is the treatment of choice and commonly used drugs include various combinations of platinum agents (Cisplatin, Carboplatin), Etoposide, topoisomerase inhibitors (Irinotecan, Topotecan) and Paclitaxel. Such treatments induce response in 14–80% of patients with a mean duration of response of <12 months [5, 20, 21, 64, 103]. Major toxicity can occur including myelosuppression and nausea/emesis [21, 11, 104].

Summary of Recommendations for Medical Management

Somatostatin analogues are commonly used at the time of initial diagnosis for patients with unresectable and/or metastatic PNETs to control the hormone excess state and for their antiproliferative effects. Octreotide and lanreotide have the most data in support of their use however, newer agents with higher affinity for other somatostatin receptors are currently being evaluated. NCCN guidelines recommend targeted therapy with mTOR inhibitors (Everolimus) or tyrosine kinase inhibitors (Sunitinib), either as first-line treatment for unresectable and/or metastatic well-moderately differentiated PNETs in combination with SSAs or sequentially following progression on SSAs.

Cytotoxic chemotherapy is recommended for use in patients with well-moderately differentiated metastatic/unresectable PNETs due to (1) failure of SSAs and/or targeted therapy and (2) presentation with initial bulky or symptomatic disease mandating disease response to facilitate cytoreduction or symptom control. The use of Streptozotocin, 5FU, and doxorubicin (FAS) as well as the combination of capecitabine and temozolomide are supported by non-randomized data. Peptide receptor radionuclide therapy while promising, remains in the experimental realm to date. Metastatic high grade/poorly differentiated PNETs are treated with cytotoxic chemotherapy alone.

Personal View of the Data/How We Do It

Initial Evaluation

Patients with functional PNETs usually present with symptoms caused by hormone hypersecretion. Patients with nonfunctional PNETs may present with vague abdominal complaints or have no symptoms whatsoever, having their tumors incidentally discovered on cross-sectional imaging obtained for unrelated conditions. If there is no evidence of metastatic disease, workup includes endoscopic ultrasound (EUS) with fine needle aspiration (FNA) for tissue diagnosis and assessment of Ki-67/mitotic index. If the patient has metastatic disease, a metastatic lesion may be targeted for biopsy, if readily accessible. Multiphasic cross-sectional imaging (computed tomography or magnetic resonance imaging) with emphasis on an early arterial phase is critical to assess the lesion(s) and to rule out metastatic disease. Laboratory evaluation should include serum levels of chromogranin A, neuron specific enolase, gastrin, human pancreatic polypeptide, serotonin, calcium and possibly others, if a particular symptom complex related to hormonal hypersecretion is present (i.e. insulinoma, gastrinoma, VIPoma among others). The Chromogranin A suppression test is also frequently performed, especially if metastatic disease is discovered, as a guide to the use of octreotide or lanreotide [105]. Finally, an octreotide scan is completed to assess otreotide avidity of the primary and assess metastatic disease burden. This is particularly helpful for surveillance after resection.

Single Small Pancreatic PNET

In the setting of a single tumor confined to the pancreas, we prefer a minimally invasive, parenchymal-sparing approach to resection. Our preferred technique is laparoscopic or robotic resection either by enucleation (if eccentric, away from the pancreatic duct) or a limited parenchyma-sparing resection (margin negative, spleen-preserving). The advantages of 3-D, high magnification vision, wristed motion and precision in limited space makes the robotic platform quite attractive in this patient population and certainly in those patients with small volume disease. As the patients are frequently younger and the disease course is often measured in many years, parenchyma preservation is very important to minimize the risk of insulin dependence.

Larger Volume Tumors with Vascular Involvement and/or Metastatic Disease

As most of these patients will survive for years (not months), even in the absence of surgery, it is critically important that the treatment not worsen survival and/or cause undue morbidity; the treatment should not be worse than the disease itself. For patients with large tumors and/or metastatic PNETs at diagnosis, the disease has either been indolent for years and progressed slowly until mass effect has occurred, or is highly aggressive and has spread rapidly. This reality underscores the need for biopsy with assessment of tumor differentiation and Ki-67/mitotic index. Patients with a resectable primary and somewhat limited metastatic disease, with moderate or well differentiated tumors (GI/G2, Ki-67 $< 20\%$) are frequently taken to the operating room for a combined liver/pancreas resection. If both the liver and the pancreas require an extensive operation (for example, a formal lobectomy or more in the liver, or a Whipple procedure with vascular resection/reconstruction in the pancreas) we may two-stage the operation based on the surgical risk and technical complexity of the procedure. If a biliary-enteric anastomosis is required/anticipated for resection of the primary pancreatic tumor, we may treat the liver first (with liver directed therapies, if mandated by multidisciplinary evaluation/discussion) to avoid the risk of liver abscess from biliary contamination.

In contrast, patients with moderate to poorly differentiated (Ki-67 $> 20\%$) will be assessed for cytotoxic therapy with capecitabine/temozolomide (based on MGMT status), or other agents if MGMT is not deficient. In situations where the liver is diffusely involved and the patient is unlikely to ever be taken for surgical resection, transarterial chemoembolization (TACE) or yttrium90 is attractive early in the treatment course to control hepatic disease progression, especially in those patients with hormone secretion as their major symptom.

References

1. Yao JC, Hassan M, Phan A, Dagohoy C, Leary C, Mares JE, Abdalla EK, Fleming JB, Vauthey JN, Rashid A, Evans DB. One hundred years after "carcinoid": epidemiology of and prognostic factors for neuroendocrine tumors in 35,825 cases in the United States. J Clin Oncol. 2008;26:3063–72.
2. Halfdanarson TR, Rabe KG, Rubin J, Petersen GM. Pancreatic neuroendocrine tumors (PNETs): incidence, prognosis and recent trend toward improved survival. Ann Oncol. 2008; 19:1727–33.

3. Milan SA, Yeo CJ. Neuroendocrine tumors of the pancreas. Curr Opin Oncol. 2012;24:46–55.
4. Klimstra DS, Modlin IR, Coppola D, Lloyd RV, Suster S. The pathologic classification of neuroendocrine tumors: a review of nomenclature, grading, and staging systems. Pancreas. 2010;39:707–12.
5. Nilsson O, Van Cutsem E, Delle Fave G, et al. Poorly differentiated carcinomas of the foregut (gastric, duodenal and pancreatic). Neuroendocrinology. 2006;84:212–5.
6. Ekeblad S, Skogseid B, Dunder K, et al. Prognostic factors and survival in 324 patients with pancreatic endocrine tumor treated at a single institution. Clin Cancer Res. 2008;14:7798–803.
7. Hentic O, Couvelard A, Rebours V, et al. Ki-67 index, tumor differentiation, and extent of liver involvement are independent prognostic factors in patients with liver metastases of digestive endocrine carcinomas. Endocr Relat Cancer. 2011;18:51–9.
8. Oberg K. Pancreatic endocrine tumors. Semin Oncol. 2010;37:594–618.
9. Bettini R, Boninsegna L, Mantovani W, et al. Prognostic factors at diagnosis and value of WHO classification in a mono-institutional series of 180 non-functioning pancreatic endocrine tumours. Ann Oncol. 2008;19:903–8.
10. Panzuto F, Boninsegna L, Fazio N, et al. Metastatic and locally advanced pancreatic endocrine carcinomas: analysis of factors associated with disease progression. J Clin Oncol. 2011;29:2372–7.
11. Jensen RT, Cadiot G, Brandi ML, et al. ENETS Consensus Guidelines for the management of patients with digestive neuroendocrine neoplasms: functional pancreatic endocrine tumor syndromes. Neuroendocrinology. 2012;95:98–119.
12. Pavel M, Baudin E, Couvelard A, et al. ENETS Consensus Guidelines for the management of patients with liver and other distant metastases from neuroendocrine neoplasms of foregut, midgut, hindgut, and unknown primary. Neuroendocrinology. 2012;95:157–76.
13. Falconi M, Bartsch DK, Eriksson B, et al. ENETS Consensus Guidelines for the management of patients with digestive neuroendocrine neoplasms of the digestive system: well-differentiated pancreatic non-functioning tumors. Neuroendocrinology. 2012;95:120–34.
14. Metz DC, Jensen RT. Gastrointestinal neuroendocrine tumors: pancreatic endocrine tumors. Gastroenterology. 2008;135:1469–92.
15. Sundin A, Vullierme MP, Kaltsas G, Plockinger U. ENETS guidelines for the standards of care in patients with neuroendocrine tumours: radiological examinations in patients with neuroendocrine tumours. Neuroendocrinology. 2009;90:167–83.
16. Kulke MH, Anthony LB, Bushnell DL, et al. NANETs treatment guidelines: well-differentated neuroendocrine tumors of the stomach and pancreas. Pancreas. 2010;39:735–52.
17. Frilling A, Li J, Malamutmann E, et al. Treatment of liver metastases from neuroendocrine tumours in relation to the extent of hepatic disease. Br J Surg. 2009;96:175–84.
18. Schurr PG, Strate T, Rese K, et al. Aggressive surgery improves long-term survival in neuroendocrine pancreatic tumors: an institutional experience. Ann Surg. 2007;245:273–81.
19. Sarmiento JM, Heywood G, Rubin J, et al. Surgical treatment of neuroendocrine metastases: a plea for resection to increase survival. J Am Coll Surg. 2003;197:29–37.
20. Strosberg JR, Coppola D, Klimstra DS, et al. The NANETS consensus guidelines for the diagnosis and management of poorly differentiated (high-grade) extrapulmonary neuroendocrine carcinomas. Pancreas. 2010;39:799–800.
21. Iwasa S, Morizane C, Okusaka T, et al. Cisplatin and etoposide as a first-line chemotherapy for poorly differentiated neuroendocrine carcinoma of the hepatobiliary tract and pancreas. Jpn J Clin Oncol. 2010;40:313–8.
22. Kvols LK, Turaga KK, Strosberg J, Choi J. Role of interventional radiology in the treatment of patients with neuroendocrine metastases in the liver. J Natl Compr Canc Netw. 2009;7:765–72.
23. Norton JA, Warren RS, Kelly MG, et al. Aggressive surgery for metastatic liver neuroendocrine tumors. Surgery. 2003;134:1057–65.
24. Ito T, Igarashi H, Jensen RT. Therapy of metastatic pancreatic neuroendocrine tumors (pNETs): recent insights and advances. J Gastroenterol. 2012;47:941–60.

25. Cauley CE, Pitt HA, Ziegler KM, Nakeeb A, Schmidt CM, Zyromski NJ, House MG, Lillemoe KD. Pancreatic enucleation: improved outcomes compared to resection. J Gastrointest Surg. 2012;16:1347–53.
26. Müller MW, Friess H, Kleeff J, Hinz U, Wente MN, Paramythiotis D, Berberat PO, Ceyhan GO, Büchler MW. Middle segmental pancreatic resection: an option to treat benign pancreatic body lesions. Ann Surg. 2006;244:909–18. discussion 918–920.
27. Cherif R, Gaujoux S, Couvelard A, Dokmak S, Vuillerme MP, Ruszniewski P, Belghiti J, Sauvanet A. Parenchymasparing resections for pancreatic neuroendocrine tumors. J Gastrointest Surg. 2012;16:2045–55.
28. Isla A, Arbuckle JD, Kekis PB, Lim A, Jackson JE, Todd JF, Lynn J. Laparoscopic management of insulinomas. Br J Surg. 2009;96:185–90.
29. España-Gómez MN, Velázquez-Fernández D, Bezaury P, Sierra M, Pantoja JP, Herrera MF. Pancreatic insulinoma: a surgical experience. World J Surg. 2009;33:1966–70.
30. Daouadi M, Zureikat AH, Zenati MS, Choudry H, Tsung A, Bartlett DL, Hughes SJ, Lee KK, Moser AJ, Zeh HJ. Robot-assisted minimally invasive distal pancreatectomy is superior to the laparoscopic technique. Ann Surg. 2013;257:128–32.
31. Hashim YM, Trinkaus KM, Linehan DC, Strasberg SS, Fields RC, Cao D, Hawkins WG. Regional lymphadenectomy is indicated in the surgical treatment of pancreatic neuroendocrine tumors (PNETs). Ann Surg. 2014;259:197–203.
32. Tsutsumi K, Ohtsuka T, Mori Y, Fujino M, Yasui T, Aishima S, Takahata S, Nakamura M, Ito T, Tanaka M. Analysis of lymph node metastasis in pancreatic neuroendocrine tumors (PNETs) based on the tumor size and hormonal production. J Gastroenterol. 2012;47:678–85.
33. Partelli S, Gaujoux S, Boninsegna L, Cherif R, Crippa S, Couvelard A, Scarpa A, Ruszniewski P, Sauvanet A, Falconi M. Pattern and clinical predictors of lymph node involvement in nonfunctioning pancreatic neuroendocrine tumors (NFPanNETs). JAMA Surg. 2013;148:932–9.
34. D'Haese JG, Tosolini C, Ceyhan GO, et al. Update on surgical treatment of pancreatic neuroendocrine neoplasms. World J Gastroenterol. 2014;20(38):13893–8.
35. Hill JS, McPhee JT, McDade TP, Zhou Z, Sullivan ME, Whalen GF, Tseng JF. Pancreatic neuroendocrine tumors: the impact of surgical resection on survival. Cancer. 2009;115:741–51.
36. Norton JA, Fraker DL, Alexander HR, Gibril F, Liewehr DJ, Venzon DJ, Jensen RT. Surgery increases survival in patients with gastrinoma. Ann Surg. 2006;244:410–9.
37. Norton JA, Harris EJ, Chen Y, Visser BC, Poultsides GA, Kunz PC, Fisher GA, Jensen RT. Pancreatic endocrine tumors with major vascular abutment, involvement, or encasement and indication for resection. Arch Surg. 2011;146:724–32.
38. Pomianowska E, Gladhaug IP, Grzyb K, Røsok BI, Edwin B, Bergestuen DS, Mathisen O. Survival following resection of pancreatic endocrine tumors: importance of R-status and the WHO and TNM classification systems. Scand J Gastroenterol. 2010;45:971–9.
39. Panzuto F, Nasoni S, Falconi M, et al. Prognostic factors and survival in endocrine tumor patients: comparison between gastrointestinal and pancreatic localization. Endocr Relat Cancer. 2005;12:1083–92.
40. Fendrich V, Langer P, Celik I, Bartsch DK, Zielke A, Ramaswamy A, Rothmund M. An aggressive surgical approach leads to long-term survival in patients with pancreatic endocrine tumors. Ann Surg. 2006;244:845–51. discussion 852–853.
41. Capurso G, Bettini R, Rinzivillo M, Boninsegna L, Delle Fave G, Falconi M. Role of resection of the primary pancreatic neuroendocrine tumour only in patients with unresectable metastatic liver disease: a systematic review. Neuroendocrinology. 2011;93:223–9.
42. Bettini R, Mantovani W, Boninsegna L, et al. Primary tumour resection in metastatic nonfunctioning pancreatic endocrine carcinomas. Dig Liver Dis. 2009;41:49–55.
43. Touzios JG, Kiely JM, Pitt SC, Rilling WS, Quebbeman EJ, Wilson SD, Pitt HA. Neuroendocrine hepatic metastases: does aggressive management improve survival? Ann Surg. 2005;241:776–83. discussion 783–785.
44. Birnbaum DJ, Turrini O, Vigano L, et al. Surgical management of advanced pancreatic neuroendocrine tumors: short-term and long-term results from an international multi-institutional study. Ann Surg Oncol. 2015;22:1000–7.

45. Ahmed A, Turner G, King B, et al. Midgut neuroendocrine tumours with liver metastases: results of the UKINETS study. Endocr Relat Cancer. 2009;16:885–94.
46. Norton JA, Kivlen M, Li M, et al. Morbidity and mortality of aggressive resection in patients with advanced neuroendocrine tumors. Arch Surg. 2003;138:859–66.
47. Nguyen SQ, Angel LP, Divino CM, et al. Surgery in malignant pancreatic neuroendocrine tumors. J Surg Oncol. 2007;96:397–403.
48. Fischer L, Kleeff J, Esposito I, et al. Clinical outcome and long-term survival in 118 consecutive patients with neuroendocrine tumours of the pancreas. Br J Surg. 2008;95:627–35.
49. Mayo SC, de Jong MC, Pulitano C, et al. Surgical management of hepatic neuroendocrine tumor metastasis: results from an international multiinstitutional analysis. Ann Surg Oncol. 2010;17:3129–36.
50. Cusati D, Zhang L, Harmsen WS, Hu A, Farnell MB, Nagorney DM, Donohue JH, Que FG, Reid-Lombardo KM, Kendrick ML. Metastatic nonfunctioning pancreatic neuroendocrine carcinoma to liver: surgical treatment and outcomes. J Am Coll Surg. 2012;215:117–24. discussion 124–125.
51. Tsuchikawa T, Kondo S, Hirano S, et al. Distal pancreatectomy and portal vein resection without vascular reconstruction for endocrine tumors with massive intraportal growth: report of a case. Hepatogastroenterology. 2011;58:1029–31.
52. Ochiai T, Masuda T, Nishizawa M, et al. Curative resection of a huge malignant pancreatic endocrine tumor by pancreaticoduodenectomy with portal and superior mesenteric vein resection and reconstruction using the right ovarian vein: report of a case. Surg Today. 2011;41:1260–5.
53. Okuno M, Sakaguchi S, Nagayama M, et al. Nonfunctioning islet cell carcinoma presenting bleeding gastric varices and splenomegaly. Jpn J Surg. 1984;14:244–7.
54. Yamaguchi T, Takahashi H, Kagawa R, et al. Nonfunctioning pancreatic endocrine tumor presenting with hemorrhage from isolated gastric varices. Am Surg. 2005;71:1027–30.
55. Hamilton NA, Liu TC, Cavatiao A, Mawad K, Chen L, Strasberg SS, Linehan DC, Cao D, Hawkins WG. Ki-67 predicts disease recurrence and poor prognosis in pancreatic neuroendocrine neoplasms. Surgery. 2012;152:107–13.
56. Boninsegna L, Panzuto F, Partelli S, Capelli P, Delle Fave G, Bettini R, Pederzoli P, Scarpa A, Falconi M. Malignant pancreatic neuroendocrine tumour: lymph node ratio and Ki67are predictors of recurrence after curative resections. Eur J Cancer. 2012;48:1608–15.
57. Pascher A, Klupp J, Neuhaus P. Endocrine tumours of the gastrointestinal tract. Transplantation in the management of metastatic endocrine tumours. Best Pract Res Clin Gastroenterol. 2005;19:637–48.
58. Harring TR, Nguyen NT, goss JA. Treatment of liver metastases in patients with neuroendocrine tumors: a comprehensive review. Int J Hepatol. 2011,2011:154541.
59. Gregoire E, Le Treut YP. Liver transplantation for primary or secondary endocrine tumors. Transpl Int. 2010;23:704–11.
60. Rosenau J, Bahr MJ, von Wasielewski R, Mengel M, Schmidt HH, Nashan B, Lang H, Klempnauer J, Manns MP, Boeker KH. Ki67, E-cadherin, and p53 as prognostic indicators of long-term outcome after liver transplantation for metastatic neuroendocrine tumors. Transplantation. 2002;73:386–94.
61. Mazzaferro V, Pulvirenti A, coppa J. Neuroendocrine tumors metastatic to the liver: how to select patients for liver transplantation? J Hepatol. 2007;47:460–6.
62. Steinmuller T, Kianmanesh R, Falconi M, et al. Consensus guidelines for the management of patients with liver metastases from digestive (neuro) endocrine tumors: foregut, midgut, hindgut, and unknown primary. Neuroendocrinology. 2008;87:47–62.
63. Riccardi F, Rizzo M, Festino L, et al. Therapy innovation for the treatment of pancreatic neuroendocrine tumors. Expert Opin Ther Targets. 2012;16(Suppl 2):S91–102.
64. Eriksson B, Annibale B, Bajetta E, et al. ENETs consensus guidelines for the standards of care in neuroendocrine tumors: chemotherapy in patients with neuroendocrine tumors. Neuroendocrinology. 2009;90:214–9.

65. Toumpanakis C, Meyer T, Caplin ME. Cytotoxic treatment including embolization/chemoembolization for neuroendocrine tumours. Best Pract Res Clin Endocrinol Metab. 2007;21:131–44.
66. Maire F, Hammel P, Kianmanesh R, et al. Is adjuvant therapy with streptozotocin and 5-fluorouracil useful after reseection of liver metastases from digestive endocrine tumors? Surgery. 2009;145:69–75.
67. Kos-Kudla B, O'Tool D, Falconi M, et al. ENETS consensus guidelines for the management of bone and lung metastases from neuroendocrine tumors. Neuroendocrinology. 2010;91:341–50.
68. Yu F, Venzon DJ, Serrano J, et al. Prospective study of the clinical course, prognostic factors and survival in patients with longstanding Zollinger-Ellison syndrome. J Clin Oncol. 1999;17:615–30.
69. Sutliff VE, Doppman JL, Gibril F, et al. Growth of newly diagnosed, untreated metastatic gastrinomas and predictors of growth patterns. J Clin Oncol. 1997;15:2420–31.
70. Kouvaraki MA, Ajani JA, Joff P, et al. Fluorouracil, doxorubicin and streptozocin in the treatem of patients with locally advanced and metastatic pancreatic endocrine carcinomas. J Clin Oncol. 2004;22:4762–71.
71. Strosberg JR, Fine RL, Choi J, et al. First-line chemotherapy with capecitabine and temozolomide in patients with metastatic pancreatic endocrine carcinomas. Cancer. 2011;117:268–75.
72. Maire F, Hammel P, Faivre S, et al. Temozolomide: a safe and effective treatment for malignant digestive endocrine tumors. Neuroendocrinology. 2009;90:67–72.
73. Ekeblad S, sundin A, Janson ET, et al. Temozolomide as monotherapy is effective in treatment of advanced malignant neuroendocrine tumors. Clin Cancer Res. 2007;13:2986–91.
74. Kulke MH, Hornick JL, Frauenhoffer C, et al. 06-methylguanin DNA methyltransferase deficiency and response to temozolomide-based therapy in patients with neuroendocrine tumors. Clin Cancer Res. 2009;15:338–45.
75. Sideris L, Dube P, Rinke A. Antitumor effects of somatostatin analogs in neuroendocrine tumors. Oncologist. 2012;17:747–55.
76. Appetecchia M, Baldelli R. Somatostatin analogues in the treatment of gastroenteropancreatic neuroendocrine tumours, current aspects and new perspectives. J Exp Clin Cancer Res. 2010;29:19–31.
77. Strosberg J, Kvols L. Antiproliferative effect of somatostatin analogs in gastroenteropancreatic neuroendocrine tumors. World J Gastroenterol. 2010;16:2963–70.
78. Panzuto F, Di Francesco V, Iannicelli E, et al. Long-term clinical outcome of somatostatin analogues for treatment of progressive, metastatic, well-differentiated entero-pancreatic endocrine carcinoma. Ann Oncol. 2006;17:461–6.
79. Rinke A, Muller HH, Schade-Brittinger C, et al. Placebo-controlled, double-blind prospective randomized study on the effect of octreotide LAR in the control of tumor growth in patients with metastatic neuroendocrine midgut tumors: a report from the PROMID Study Group. J Clin Oncol. 2009;27:4656–63.
80. Caplin ME, Pavel M, Cwikla JB, et al. Lanreotide in metastatic enteropancreatic neuroendocrine tumors. NEJM. 2014;371(3):224–33.
81. The NCCN clinical practice guidelines in oncology for neuroendocrine tumors version 1.1.2012.Version1.2012.2012.online. go to www.nccn.org.
82. Miljkovic MD, Girotra M, Abraham RR, Erlich RB. Novel medical therapies of recurrent and metastatic gastroenteropancreatic neuroendocrine tumors. Dig Dis Sci. 2012;57:9–18.
83. Oberg K. Somatostatin analog octreotide LAR in gastro-enteropancreatic tumors. Expert Rev Anticancer Ther. 2009;9:557–66.
84. Pavel M. Translation of molecular pathways into clinical trials of neuroendocrine tumors. Neuroendocrinology. 2013;97(1):99–112.
85. Eriksson B. New drugs in neuroendocrine tumors: rising of new therapeutic philosophies. Curr Opin Oncol. 2010;22:381–6.
86. Yao JC. Molecular targeted therapy for carcinoid and islet-cell carcinoma. Best Pract Res Clin Endocrinol Metab. 2007;21:163–72.

87. Vargas M, Gornals J, Ponseti JM, et al. Pancreatic endocrine tumors or apudomas. Rev Esp Enferm Dig. 2011;103:184–90.
88. Yao JC, Phan AT, Chang DZ, et al. Efficacy of RAD001(everolimus) and octreotide LAR in advanced low- to intermediate grade neuroendocrine tumors: results of a phase II study. J Clin Oncol. 2008;26:4311–8.
89. Yao JC, Shah MH, Ito T, et al. Everolimus for advanced pancreatic endocrine tumors. N Engl J Med. 2011;364:514–23.
90. Capurso G, Fazio N, Festa S, et al. Molecular target therapy for gastroenteropancreatic endocrine tumors: biological rationale and clinical perspectives. Crit Rev Oncol Hematol. 2009;72:110–24.
91. Raymond E, Hobday T, Castellano D, et al. Therapy innovations: tyrosine kinase inhibitors for te treatment of pancreatic neuroendocrine tumors. Cancer Metastasis Rev. 2011;30(Suppl 1):19–26.
92. Faivre S, Sablin MP, Dreyer C, Raymond E. Novel anticancer agents in clinical trials for well-differentiated neuroendocrine tumors. Endocrinol Metab Clin N Am. 2010;39:811–26.
93. Pavel ME, Wiedenmann B. Novel therapeutic agents for the treatment of gastroenteropancreatic neuroendocrine tumors. Horm Metab Res. 2011;43:844–53.
94. Fjallskog ML, Lejonklou MH, Oberg KE, et al. Expression of molecular targets for tyrosine kinase receptor antagonists in malignant endocrine pancreatic tumors. Clin Cancer Res. 2003;9:1469–73.
95. Raymond E, Dahan L, Raoul JL, et al. Sunitinib malate for the treatment of pancreatic neuroendocrine tumors. N Engl J Med. 2011;364:501–13.
96. Chan JA, Kulke MH. New treatment options for patients with advanced neuroendocrine tumors. Curr Treat Options Oncol. 2011;12:136–48.
97. Raut CP, Kulke MH. Targeted therapy in advanced well-differentiated neuroendocrine tumors. Oncologist. 2011;16:286–95.
98. Van Vliet EI, Teunissen JJ, Kam BL, et al. Treatment of gastroenteropancreatic neuroendocrine tumors with peptide receptor radionuclide therapy. Neuroendocrinology. 2013; 97(1):74–85.
99. Van Essen M, Krenning EP, Kam BL, et al. Peptide-receptor radionuclide therapy for endocrine tumors. Nat Rev Endocrinol. 2009;5:382–93.
100. Kwekkeboom DJ, de Herder WW, Krenning EP. Somatostatin-receptor targeted radionuclide therapy in patients with gastroenteropancreatic neuroendocrine tumors. Endocrinol Metab Clin North Am. 2011;40:173–85.
101. Oberg KE, Reubi JC, Kwekkeboom DJ, Krenning EP. Rol of somatostatins in gastroenteropancreatic neuroendocrine tumor development and therapy. Gastroenterology. 2010;139:742–53.
102. Basuroy R, Srirajaskanthan R, Ramage JK. A multimodal approach to the management of neuroendocrine tumour liver metastases. Int J Hepatol. 2012,2012:819193.
103. Hainsworth JD, Spigel DR, Litchy S, Greco FA. Phase II trial of paclitaxel, carboplatin and etoposide in advanced poorly differentiated neuroendocrine carcinoma: a Minnie Pearl Cancer Research Network Study. J Clin Oncol. 2006;24:3548–54.
104. Olsen IH, Langer SW, Jepsen I, et al. First line treatment of patients with disseminated poorly differentiated neuroendocrine carcinomas with carboplatin, etoposide and vincristine: a single institution experience. Acta Oncol. 2012;51:97–100.
105. Massironi S, Conte D, Sciola V, et al. Plasma Chromogranin A response to octreotide test: prognostic value for clinical outcome in endocrine digestive tumors. Am J Gastroenterol. 2010;105:2072–8.

Observation Versus Surgery for Nonlocalized Insulinoma

37

Anthony J. Chambers and Janice L. Pasieka

Abstract

Insulinoma are rare neuroendocrine tumors that almost always occur in the pancreas. They produce symptoms of episodic hypoglycemia secondary to the uncontrolled release of insulin. Using contemporary non-invasive and invasive investigations, insulinoma can be localized in as many as 97% of cases preoperatively. Insulinoma that cannot be localized preoperatively can be identified at the time of surgery with the aid of intraoperative ultrasound in more than 90% of cases and successfully removed. Surgery for insulinoma is associated with significant rates of morbidity (up to 68%), but a low mortality (0–5%). When surgery is not performed, long-term symptom control of hypoglycemia is achieved in only 55–78% of cases using medical management alone. Surgery is therefore recommended for the small percentage of insulinoma that are non-localized, and should be considered preferable to observation. The strength of this recommendation by GRADE criteria is assessed as weak. Given the paucity of evidence in the literature, the overall quality of the evidence supporting this recommendation is assessed as low by GRADE criteria. The investigation and management of patients with insulinoma should be performed at specialized institutions by experienced clinicians.

Keywords

Hyperinsulinism · Insulinoma · Neuroendocrine tumors

A. J. Chambers (✉)
Department of Surgical Oncology, St Vincent's Hospital and University of New South Wales, Sydney, NSW, Australia
e-mail: anthony.chambers@svha.org.au

J. L. Pasieka
Faculty of Medicine, University of Calgary and Tom Baker Cancer Centre, Calgary, AB, Canada

P. Angelos, R. H. Grogan (eds.), *Difficult Decisions in Endocrine Surgery*, Difficult Decisions in Surgery: An Evidence-Based Approach,
https://doi.org/10.1007/978-3-319-92860-9_37

Table 37.1 PICO table

*P*opulation	Patients with non-localized (occult) insulinoma
*I*ntervention	Intraoperative pancreatic exploration with intraoperative ultrasound
*C*omparator	No surgery unless positive preoperative localization studies
*O*utcomes	Complications of persistent hypoglycemia and the control of hypoglycemia with medical management versus the complications of surgery and likelihood of successful operation

Introduction

Insulinoma are rare neuroendocrine tumors, occurring with an approximate incidence of four cases per million population annually [1]. They are the most common type of functional neuroendocrine tumor of the pancreas. Insulinoma may be associated with the multiple endocrine neoplasia type 1 (MEN1) syndrome in 3–11% of cases [2, 3]. Insulinoma typically present with symptoms of episodic hypoglycemia secondary to the uncontrolled release of insulin from these tumors.

For patients with benign insulinoma, surgery to excise the tumor offers the only cure for this condition, and is successful in more than 98% of cases [3–6]. Successful surgical excision is facilitated by the localization of the primary tumor either by preoperative investigations, or at the time of surgical exploration. This chapter deals with the question of whether patients with biochemical confirmation of endogenous hyperinsulinism (insulinoma) where the tumor is not localized on preoperative investigations (occult insulinoma) should be managed by surgical exploration or should be managed conservatively with observation and best medical management. The evidence in the literature in support of these alternative strategies is reviewed in order to arrive at an evidence-based recommendation (Table 37.1).

Pathophysiology of Insulinoma

Insulinoma are located in the pancreas in 99% of cases, with 1% occurring in ectopic locations [7]. Most insulinoma are benign, with only 3–14% of tumors demonstrating malignant behavior [5, 8]. In such cases, metastases to regional lymph nodes or the liver may occur. Insulinoma are relatively small in size, with a median size of 15 mm and 90% of tumors being less than 20 mm [5, 7]. They occur within the regions of the head, neck, body and tail of the pancreas in roughly equal frequencies [3, 7]. Insulinoma may be multiple in as many as 12% of cases, particularly in the setting of MEN1 [2].

Clinical Features of Insulinoma

Insulinoma manifest clinically with episodic symptoms of hypoglycemia secondary to the uncontrolled release of insulin by these tumors. Symptoms of neuroglycopenia such as fatigue, dizziness, clouded sensorium, confusion, visual changes, behavioral change and tremor commonly occur [4]. Symptoms related to the sympathetic response to hypoglycemia such as palpitations, chest pain, pallor, anxiety, sweating and hunger may also be seen. These symptoms are typically episodic in nature and associated with fasting and exercise. In severe cases seizures, reduction in the level of consciousness, loss of consciousness or death may result.

The diagnosis of insulinoma is confirmed by the measurement of blood glucose, insulin, C-peptide and proinsulin concentrations during a supervised period of fasting. Fasting blood glucose level of less than 45 mg/dl associated with an elevated insulin concentration of greater than 3 μIU/ml, C-peptide level of greater than 200 pmol/l and proinsulin level greater than 5 pmol/l is considered diagnostic for insulinoma [9]. Anti-insulin antibodies should also be measured to rule out this rare cause of hypoglycemia. It is critical that the diagnosis of insulinoma is confirmed with certainty on biochemical grounds to rule out other causes of hypoglycemia prior to undertaking further extensive investigations to localize an insulinoma or considering surgery for this condition.

Localization of Insulinomas

Insulinoma can be localized within the pancreas by non-invasive and invasive imaging studies (Table 37.2). Cross-sectional imaging with either triple-phase helical computed tomography (CT) or magnetic resonance (MR) are the investigations of choice in the first instance for the detection of the primary tumor and to evaluate for any metastatic disease within the liver or regional lymph nodes. Primary tumors and their metastases are best visualized after the administration of intravenous contrast in the arterial phase due to their hypervascular nature (Fig. 37.1). CT and MR each have sensitivities of 60–80% for the localization of insulinoma, and are primarily limited by the small size of these lesions [9, 10]. MR appears to be more sensitive for the detection of smaller lesions when compared to CT, yet may not be as widely available [11].

Somatostatin receptor scintigraphy has been used to localize insulinoma however somatostatin-2 receptors are present in as few as 50% of these tumors and at low levels of density, limiting the efficacy of this test [12, 13]. Newer compounds such as

Table 37.2 Localization investigations for insulinoma

Investigation	Sensitivity	References
Non-invasive tests		
Computed tomography	60–80%	[9, 10, 17, 18]
Magnetic resonance	60–80%	[9–11, 18]
Somatostatin receptor scintigraphy	24–60%	[12, 31]
Invasive tests		
Endoscopic ultrasound	83–95%	[15, 16]
Transhepatic portal venous sampling	55–100%	[3, 18]
Selective arterial calcium stimulation with hepatic venous sampling	89–100%	[18, 19]
Intraoperative		
Intraoperative ultrasound	92–100%	[2, 3, 5, 6, 26]

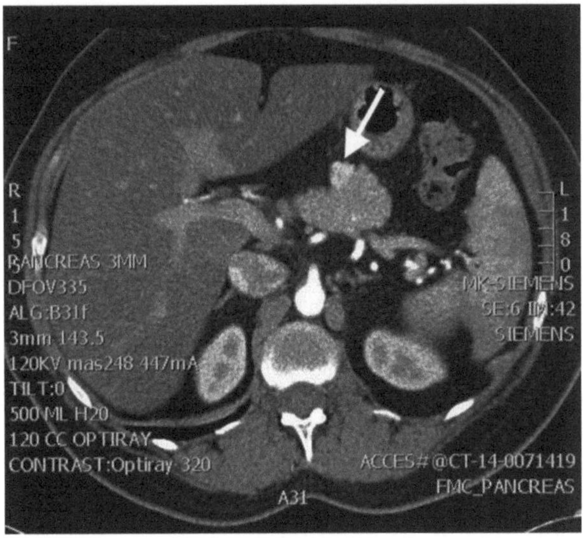

Fig. 37.1 Arterial phase contrast-enhanced computed tomography scan showing insulinoma in the body of the pancreas (*arrow*) with typical hypervascular appearance

Gallium-DOTATATE have recently demonstrated promise as a non-invasive means of localizing insulinomas, but these compounds are not yet widely utilized [14].

Invasive studies are indicated in those patients where CT and MR fail to localize the primary tumor. Endoscopic ultrasound (EUS) is the most commonly employed technique and can successfully localize 83–94% of insulinoma [15, 16]. EUS is particularly useful in localizing lesions within the head of the pancreas. Tumors in the distal body and tail of the pancreas are more difficult to image using this technique. Combined preoperative imaging using both CT and EUS was able to localize 100% of insulinoma in a series reported by Gouya and coworkers [17].

In patients where CT, MR and EUS are unable to localize the primary tumor, interventional radiology techniques can be used to 'regionalize' the insulinoma to within the head, body or tail of the pancreas. Although some centers reserve these techniques following a failed exploration, others believe the regionalization of the lesion preoperatively allows for a more focused exploration and a greater likelihood of success [3, 4, 9, 18].

The technique of transhepatic portal venous sampling involves the measurement of levels of insulin, proinsulin and C-peptide within tributaries of the portal, superior mesenteric and splenic veins draining the different regions of the pancreas. This technique can successfully identify the region of the pancreas involved with insulinoma in 55–100% of cases [3, 18].

Selective arterial calcium stimulation with hepatic venous sampling has largely replaced this technique to become the interventional procedure of choice for localizing insulinoma at specialized centers [18]. This procedure avoids the morbidity associated with transhepatic access to the portal venous system, is easier to perform and is associated with higher rates of successful localization. It involves the selective catheterization of branches of the hepatic, gastroduodenal, superior mesenteric and splenic arteries supplying regions of the pancreas. Calcium, a potent stimulator of insulin secretion, is injected into each of these branches sequentially, and insulin levels are measured from the hepatic veins via a second catheter. A step-up in the level of insulin in the hepatic veins will occur after calcium infusion into the region where the insulinoma is located. This technique can successfully 'regionalize' insulinoma in 89–100% of cases, and is the invasive investigation of choice where CT, MR and EUS fail to localize the lesion [9, 19, 20]. A number of large series from specialized Centers of Excellence have demonstrated that almost all insulinoma can be localized preoperatively when CT, MR, EUS and selective arterial calcium stimulation are all utilized [3, 5, 21].

Intraoperative Localization of Insulinoma

Surgical exploration for insulinoma requires mobilization of the entire pancreas to allow the careful palpation of all regions of the gland. Surgeons experienced in these procedures can identify the primary tumor by palpation alone in as many as 61% of cases [21]. The use of intraoperative ultrasound (IOUS) facilitates the detection of small impalpable tumors as well as those located within regions of the pancreas where palpation is difficult, namely the head, neck and uncinate process. With the aid of IOUS, insulinoma can be successfully located intraoperatively in 92–100% of cases [3, 5, 21, 22]. IOUS is also useful in delineating the relationship of the tumor to critical structures including the pancreatic duct, common bile duct, and portal vein tributaries prior to enucleation of the lesion in order to prevent injury to any of these structures [23].

It has been suggested in some studies that extensive preoperative investigations to localize insulinoma are not necessary or cost effective given the high rates of successful identification of these tumors at the time of operation with the aid of IOUS [24, 25]. Although the evidence for the use of invasive localization techniques in all cases prior to surgery is confined to observational case series, recent larger studies from specialized centers have recommended preoperative localization as an important contributor to the high rates of successful surgery for these tumors [3, 5, 26]. In these studies it is argued that the preoperative localization of the tumor allows the intraoperative search for the lesion to be focused, and facilitates a strategy for resection of the involved region of the gland if a lesion cannot be found at the time of surgical exploration. Preoperative localization also allows for surgical planning, assisting in the decision of which operative technique, open versus laparoscopic, would be the best approach.

Surgery for Insulinoma

Surgical exploration and excision for benign insulinoma is associated with successful and long-term cure in between 95% and 100% of cases (Table 37.3). Insulinoma can be removed using a number of surgical approaches after they have been localized. Most insulinoma are suitable for enucleation, and this is the preferred approach for lesions in the head and neck of the gland as it spares the morbidity associated with formal resection of this region [27]. For larger lesions in the head or neck of the pancreas or those associated with nodal metastases, formal resection of this region by panceatico-duodenectomy is indicated. Lesions located in the tail and distal body of the pancreas may be managed by distal pancreatectomy rather than enucleation.

Surgery for insulinoma is associated with significant rates of morbidity (11–68%) (Table 37.3). This is due mostly to the formation of pancreatic fistula and the resulting associated complications, occurring in 11–42% of cases. The complication rates are not significantly different for cases where laparoscopic techniques are utilized. Despite these high levels of complications, mortality in contemporary series is rare, occurring in 0–5% of cases performed at specialist centers (Table 37.3).

Observation and Conservative Management of Insulinoma

Modern series from Centers of Excellence have demonstrated that surgical intervention is successful in curing more than 95% of patients with benign insulinoma [3, 6, 21]. For this reason, the literature describing the conservative and medical management of patients with these tumors is confined to a few small observational case series only [28–30]. These consist of patients who had undergone failed surgery for insulinoma, were considered unfit for surgery or who had refused operation. Many series that describe the conservative and medical management of insulinoma include patients with benign tumors being managed for short durations prior to definitive surgery, and therefore provide little evidence regarding the efficacy of long-term control of symptoms [28]. Many of these series also contain patients with malignant insulinoma with unresectable metastatic disease, limiting their relevance to the management of benign lesions.

The mainstay of medical management of insulinoma is with diazoxide, a benzothiadizine derivative that reduces the release of insulin from these tumors [30]. Diazoxide can control symptoms of hypoglycemia in 55–78% of patients with insulinoma [28–30]. Acceptable control of symptoms can be maintained in the long-term in the majority of patients [28]. Side effects are seen in up to 56% of patients, particularly hirsuitism, fluid retention and weight gain, however they are generally tolerable and rarely require cessation of this agent [28, 29].

Treatment with somatostatin analogs can also be used to control symptoms from insulinoma by acting on somatostatin receptors to inhibit the release of insulin from these tumors [31]. Short-acting agents such as octreotide can achieve symptom control initially in 80% of cases, however tachyphylaxis commonly occurs requiring increasing dosage, leading to long-term rates of symptom control in only 57% of cases [31]. Longer-acting somatostatin analogs such as octreotide LAR have also been used successfully for the long-term control of hypoglycemia in patients with benign insulinoma [32, 33]. In 10% of patients paradoxical hypoglycemia may occur as a result of the inhibition of glucagon and growth hormone as well as insulin by these longer-acting agents. For this reason, a test dose of short-acting octreotide should always be given prior to the administration of a long-acting formula.

Table 37.3 Case series of surgery for insulinoma with more than 20 cases published in English language literature 2000–2014

Author	Year	No. of cases	% Cases localized preoperatively	% Cases localized intraoperatively	% Cases successful	Morbidity	Mortality	References
Crippa	2012	198	97%	100%	100%	52%	0%	[5]
Zhang	2012	147	–	–	100%	–	–	[39]
Richards	2011	215	–	–	98%	–	0%	[21]
Varma	2011	40	–	100%	100%	43%	–	[40]
Zhao	2011	328	–	–	–	54%	1%	[41]
Espana-Gomez	2009	34	97%	97%	97%	68%	3%	[42]
Nikfarjam	2008	61	98%	92%	98%	–	0%	[3]
Liu	2007	52	–	–	100%	32%	0%	[43]
Ravi	2007	20	75%	97%	95%	45%	5%	[37]
Chung	2006	20	–	100%	100%	10%	0%	[44]
Chen	2002	74	–	–	97%	–	–	[45]
Hirshberg	2002	99	–	98%	100%	–	–	[6]
Hiramoto	2001	37	77–37%	95%	100%	11%	0%	[26]
Hellman	2000	65	–	98%	100%	–	0%	[2]

– not stated in article

More recently, the utilization of mammalian target of rapamycin (mTOR) inhibitors such as everolimus have been shown to provide glycemic control in unresectable insulinomas [34]. mTOR inhibition appears to be a promising drug in situations where resecting the insulin-secreting tissue and controlling hypoglycaemia by classic pharmacologic agents is not possible [35]. However this chemotherapeutic drug is associated with adverse reactions such as somatitis, rash, diarrhea and edema in more than 30% of patients.

Management of Non-localized Insulinoma

It should be recognized that with contemporary imaging techniques and the use of invasive localization procedures, only a small proportion of patients with insulinoma will be non-localized. Several large series have shown that as few as 2–3% of insulinoma cannot be localized or 'regionalized' at specialized centers where advanced localization techniques are employed [3, 5].

There are few studies in the literature that have examined the outcomes of surgery for patients with non-localized insulinoma. In a series of 198 patients with insulinoma undergoing surgery at the University of Verona, Crippa and co-workers reported only six patients (3%) where the tumor could not be localized prior to surgery [5]. In all of these cases the tumor was subsequently identified at surgery with the aid of IOUS and successfully removed. In smaller series, Lo and co-workers reported that 30% of cases were non-localized and all of these were subsequently successfully identified at operation using IOUS and removed [36]. Similarly, Ravi et al. reported that 25% of cases were non-localized, and in all but one of these cases surgery was successful [37]. In addition, several series from Centers of Excellence have reported a high level of success in their cohort of patients referred to them following a failed operation [3, 6].

In summary, although the evidence in the literature is confined to a small number of observational case series such as these, it would be reasonable to conclude that for patients with non-localized insulinoma, surgical exploration with the aid of IOUS at specialist centers can be performed with a very high rate of success (greater than 90%) (Fig. 37.2).

Recommendations

Although the evidence-base is limited to observational case series, surgery is to be recommended for the management of non-localized insulinoma and should be considered preferable to observation in those patients fit for surgery. Intraoperative exploration using IOUS can successfully identify more than 90% of insulinoma, even where the tumor cannot be localized before surgery. Surgery for both localized and non-localized insulinoma is associated with successful cure in more than 95% of cases. Although there are significant risks of complications from surgery, mostly from pancreatic fistula, these are generally transient and mortality is rare. This

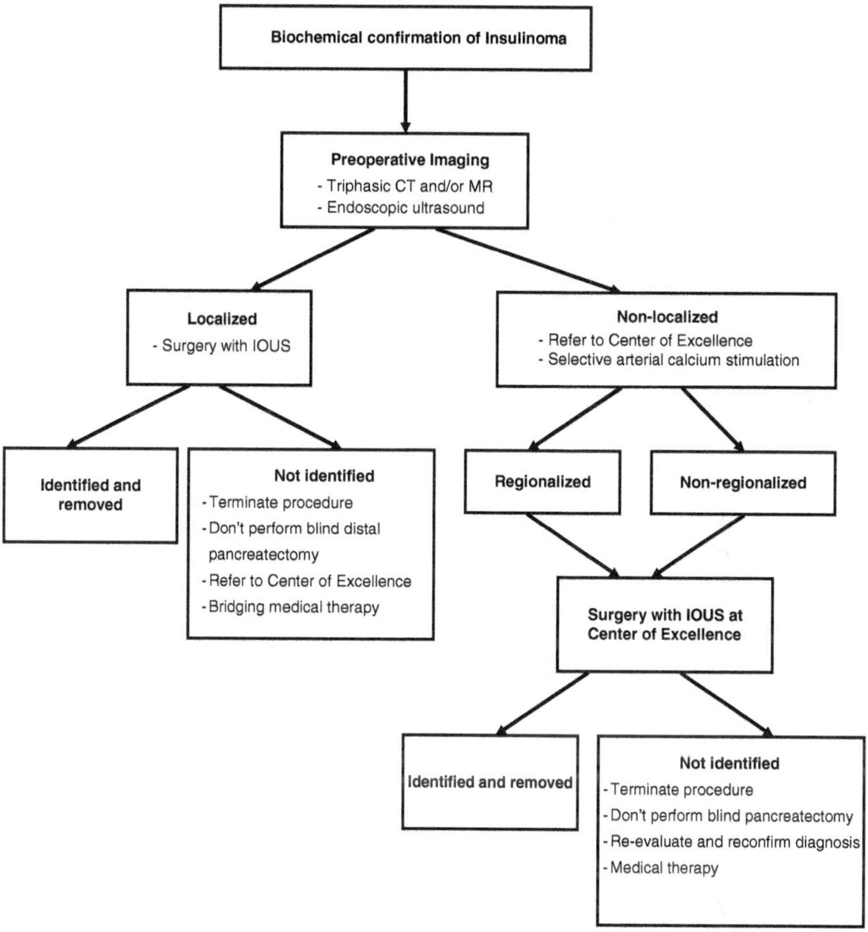

Fig. 37.2 Algorithm showing the recommended management of patients with biochemically proven insulinoma

compares favorably with the medical management of this condition, where long-term symptom control can be maintained in only 55–78% of cases. Furthermore, the symptoms of hypoglycemia associated with insulinoma are debilitating and may even be life-threatening.

In qualifying this recommendation, the supporting evidence in the literature is confined to observational case series, many being retrospective in nature, and therefore subject to multiple sources of bias. These series are also almost entirely from specialized institutions experienced in the management of these rare tumors, and therefore the findings should be applied with caution to other clinical settings. For this reason, the investigation and management of patients with insulinoma should be performed only at specialized Centers of Excellence by experienced clinicians.

In summary, the overall quality of the evidence supporting the recommendation for surgery for non-localized insulinoma is assessed as low using the Grading of Recommendations Assessment, Development and Evaluation (GRADE) system [38]. Given the limited evidence supporting this recommendation and the fact that the recommendation is qualified, the strength of the recommendation using GRADE criteria is assessed as weak.

Summary

- Insulinoma are rare neuroendocrine tumors, almost always occurring in the pancreas. They produce episodic symptoms of hypoglycemia secondary to the uncontrolled release of insulin.
- Using a combination of contemporary non-invasive and invasive investigations, insulinoma can be localized in as many as 97% of cases preoperatively.
- Insulinoma that cannot be localized preoperatively can be identified at the time of surgery with the aid of intraoperative ultrasound in more than 90% of cases and successfully removed.
- Surgery for insulinoma is associated with significant rates of morbidity (11–68%), but low mortality (0–5%).
- Long-term control of symptoms is achieved in only 55–78% of cases of insulinoma using medical agents.
- Surgery in specialized centers is recommended for non-localized insulinoma, and should be considered preferable to observation. The strength of this recommendation by GRADE criteria is assessed as weak.
- The overall quality of the evidence supporting this recommendation is assessed as low by GRADE criteria.
- The investigation and management of patients with insulinoma should be performed at specialized Centers of Excellence by experienced clinicians.

References

1. Service FJ, McMahon MM, O'Brien PC, Ballard DJ. Functioning insulinoma – incidence recurrence, and long-term survival of patients: a 60-year study. Mayo Clin Proc. 1991;66:711–9.
2. Hellman P, Goretski P, Dietmar S, Dotzenrath C, Roher HD. Therapeutic experience of 65 cases with organic hyperinsulinism. Langenbecks Arch Surg. 2000;385:329–36.
3. Nikfarjam M, Warshaw AL, Axelrod L, Deshpande V, Thayer SP, Ferrone CR, et al. Improved contemporary surgical management of insulinomas: a 25-year experience at the Massachusetts General Hospital. Ann Surg. 2008;247:165–72.
4. Tucker ON, Crotty PL, Conlon KC. The management of insulinoma. Br J Surg. 2006;93:264–75.
5. Crippa S, Zerbi A, Boninsegna L, Capitanio V, Partelli S, Balzano G, et al. Surgical management of insulinoma: short and long-term outcomes after enucleations and pancreatic resections. Arch Surg. 2012;147:261–6.
6. Hirshberg B, Libutti SK, Alexander HR, Bartlett DL, Cochran C, Livi A, Chang R, Shawker T, et al. Blind distal pancreatectomy for occult insulinoma, an inadvisable procedure. J Am Coll Surg. 2002;194:761–4.

7. Rothmund M, Angelini L, Brunt LM, Farndon JR, Geelhoed G, Grama D, et al. Surgery for benign insulinoma: an international review. World J Surg. 1990;14:393–9.
8. Bottger TC, Weber W, Beyer J, Junginger T. Value of tumor localization in patients with insulinoma. World J Surg. 1990;14:107–14.
9. Rostambiegi N, Thompson GB. What should be done in an operating room when an insulinoma cannot be found? Clin Endocrinol. 2009;70:512–5.
10. Noone TC, Hosey J, Firat Z, Semelka RC. Imaging and localization of islet-cell tumours of the pancreas on CT and MRI. Best Pract Res Clin Endocrinol Metab. 2005;19:195–211.
11. Hamoud AK, Khan MF, Aboalmaali N, Usadel KH, Wullstein C, Vogl TJ. Mangan-enhanced MR imaging for the detection and localisation of small pancreatic insulinoma. Eur Radiol. 2004;14:923–5.
12. Krenning EP, Kwekkeboom DJ, Bakker WE, Breeman WA, Kooij PP, Oei HY, van Hagen M, et al. Somatostatin receptor scintigraphy with [111In-DTPA-D-Phe1]-and [123I-Tyr3]-octreotide: the Rotterdam experience with more than 1000 patients. Eur J Nucl Med. 1993;20:716–31.
13. van der Lely AJ, de Herder WW, Krenning EP, Kwekkeboom DJ. Octreoscan radioreceptor imaging. Endocrine. 2003;20:307–11.
14. Sadowski SM, Neychev V, Cottle-Delisle C, Merkel R, Yang LA, Quezado MM, Chang R, Kebebew E. Detection of insulinoma using 68Gallium-DOTATATE PET/CT: a case report. Gland Surg. 2014;3:E1.
15. McLean AM, Fairclough PD. Endoscopic ultrasound in the localisation of pancreatic islet cell tumours. Best Pract Res Clin Endocrinol Metab. 2005;19:177–93.
16. Sotoudehmanesh R, Hedayat A, Shirazian N, Shahraeeni S, Ainechi S, Zeinali F, Kolahdoozan S. Endoscopic ultrasonography (EUS) in the localization of insulinoma. Endocrine. 2007;31:238–41.
17. Gouya H, Vignaux O, Augui J, Dousset B, Palazzo L, Louvel A, Chaussade S, Legmann P. CT, endoscopic sonography, and a combined protocol for preoperative evaluation of pancreatic insulinomas. Am J Roentgenol. 2003;181:987–92.
18. Abboud B, Boujaoude J. Occult sporadic insulinoma: localization and surgical strategy. World J Gastroenterol. 2008;14:657–65.
19. Lo CY, Chan FL, Tam SC, Cheng PW, Fan ST, Lam KS. Value of intra-arterial calcium stimulated venous sampling for regionalization of pancreatic insulinomas. Surgery. 2000;128:903–9.
20. Brändle M, Pfammatter T, Spinas GA, Lehmann R, Schmid C. Assessment of selective arterial calcium stimulation and hepatic venous sampling to localize insulin secreting tumours. Clin Endocrinol. 2001;55:357–62.
21. Richards ML, Thompson GB, Farley DR, Kendrick ML, Service JF, Vella A, Grant CS. Setting the bar for laparoscopic resection of sporadic insulinoma. World J Surg. 2011;35:785–9.
22. Norton JA, Shawker TH, Doppman JL, Miller DL, Fraker DL, Cromack DT, Gorden P, Jensen RT. Localization and surgical treatment of occult insulinomas. Ann Surg. 1990;212:615–20.
23. Boukhman MP, Karam JM, Shaver J, Siperstein AE, DeLorimier AA, Clark OH. Localization of insulinomas. Arch Surg. 1999;134:818–23.
24. Hashimoto LA, Walsh RM. Preoperative localization of insulinomas is not necessary. J Am Coll Surg. 1999;189:368–73.
25. van Heerden JA, Grant CS, Czako PF, Charboneau JW. Occult functioning insulinomas: which localizing studies are indicated? Surgery. 1992;112:1010–4.
26. Hiramoto JS, Feldstein VA, LaBerge JM, Norton JA. Intraoperative ultrasound and preoperative localization detects all occult insulinomas. Arch Surg. 2001;136:1020–6.
27. Pasieka JL, McLeod MK, Thompson NW, Burney RE. Surgical approach to insulinomas: assessing the need for preoperative localization. Arch Surg. 1992;127:442–7.
28. Goode PN, Farndon JR, Anderson J, Johnston ID, Morte JA. Diazoxide in the management of patients with insulinoma. World J Surg. 1986;10:586–92.
29. Gill GV, Rauf O, MacFarlane IA. Diazoxide treatment for insulinoma: a national UK survey. Postgrad Med J. 1997;73:640–1.
30. Stefanini P, Carboni M, Patrassi N, Bernardinis GD, Negro P. Problems of the management of insulinomas: review of 132 cases treated with medical measures. Acta Diabetol Lat. 1974;11:71–7.

31. Vezzosi D, Bennet A, Rochaix P, Courbon F, Selves J, Pradere B, Buscail L, et al. Octreotide in insulinoma patients: efficacy on hypoglycemia, relationships with Octreoscan scintigraphy and immunostaining with anti-sst2A and anti-sst5 antibodies. Eur J Endocrinol. 2005;152:757–67.
32. Usukura M, Yoneda T, Yamamoto N, Takata H, Hasatani K, Takeda Y. Medical treatment of benign insulinoma using octreotide LAR: a case report. Endocr J. 2007;54:95–101.
33. Kishikawa H, Okada Y, Hirose A, Tanikawa T, Kanda K, Tanaka Y. Successful treatment of insulinoma by a single daily dose of octreotide in two elderly female patients. Endocr J. 2006;53:79–85.
34. Kulke MH, Bergsland EK, Yao JC. Glycemic control in patients with insulinoma treated with everolimus. N Engl J Med. 2009;360:195–7.
35. de Herder WW, van Schaik E, Kwekkeboom D, Feelders RA. New therapeutic options for metastatic malignant insulinomas. Clin Endocrinol. 2011;75:277–84.
36. Lo CY, Lam KY, Kung AW, Lam KS, Tung PH, Fan ST. Pancreatic insulinomas: a 15-year experience. Arch Surg. 1997;132:926–30.
37. Ravi K, Britton BJ. Surgical approach to insulinomas: are pre-operative localization tests necessary? Ann R Coll Surg Engl. 2007;89:212–7.
38. Guyatt G, Oxman AD, Akl EA, Kunz R, Vist G, Brozek J, Norris S, et al. GRADE guidelines: 1. Introduction – GRADE evidence profiles and summary of findings tables. J Clin Epidemiol. 2011;64:383–94.
39. Zhang T, Mu Y, Qu L, Wang X, Lv Z, Du J, Guo Q, Ba J, et al. Accurate combined preoperative localization of insulinomas aid the choice for enucleation: a single institution experience over 25 years. Hepatogastroenterol. 2012;59:1282–5.
40. Varma V, Tariciotti L, Coldham C, Taniere P, Buckels JA, Bramhall SR. Preoperative localisation and surgical management of insulinoma: single centre experience. Dig Surg. 2010;28:63–73.
41. Zhao YP, Zhang HX, Cong L, Dai MH, Liao Q, Cai LX. Surgical management of patients with insulinomas: results of 292 cases in a single institution. J Surg Oncol. 2011;103:169–74.
42. Espana-Gomez MN, Velazquez-Fernandez D, Bezaury P, Sierra M, Pantoja JP, Herrera MF. Pancreatic insulinoma: a surgical experience. World J Surg. 2009;33:1966–70.
43. Liu H, Peng C, Zhang S, Wu Y, Fang H, Sheng H, Peng S. Strategy for the surgical management of insulinomas: analysis of 52 cases. Dig Surg. 2007;24:463–70.
44. Chung JC, Choi SH, Jo SH, Heo JS, Choi DW, Kim YI. Localization and surgical treatment of the pancreatic insulinomas. ANZ J Surg. 2006;76:1051–5.
45. Chen X, Cai WY, Yang WP, Li HW. Pancreatic insulinomas: diagnosis and surgical treatment of 74 patients. Hepatobiliary Pancreat Dis Int. 2002;1:458–61.

Index

P. Angelos, R. H. Grogan (eds.), *Difficult Decisions in Endocrine Surgery*, Difficult Decisions in Surgery: An Evidence-Based Approach,
https://doi.org/10.1007/978-3-319-92860-9

Q

R

FSC
www.fsc.org
MIX
Papier | Fördert
gute Waldnutzung
FSC® C083411

Kolibri 360 GmbH
Ferdinand-Jühlke-Straße 7
99095 Erfurt, Deutschland
produktsicherheit@kolibri360.de